Fracture Management
for Primary Care

THIRD EDITION

Fracture Management *for* Primary Care

M. Patrice Eiff, MD
Professor
Department of Family Medicine
Oregon Health and Science University
Portland, Oregon

Robert Hatch, MD, MPH
Professor
Department of Community Health and Family Medicine
University of Florida
Gainesville, Florida

Mariam K. Higgins
Medical Illustrator
Portland, Oregon

ELSEVIER
SAUNDERS

1600 John F. Kennedy Blvd.
Ste 1800
Philadelphia, PA 19103-2899

Notices

Knowledge and best practice in this field are constantly changing. As new research and experience broaden our understanding, changes in research methods, professional practices, or medical treatment may become necessary.

Practitioners and researchers must always rely on their own experience and knowledge in evaluating and using any information, methods, compounds, or experiments described herein. In using such information or methods they should be mindful of their own safety and the safety of others, including parties for whom they have a professional responsibility.

With respect to any drug or pharmaceutical products identified, readers are advised to check the most current information provided (i) on procedures featured or (ii) by the manufacturer of each product to be administered, to verify the recommended dose or formula, the method and duration of administration, and contraindications. It is the responsibility of practitioners, relying on their own experience and knowledge of their patients, to make diagnoses, to determine dosages and the best treatment for each individual patient, and to take all appropriate safety precautions.

To the fullest extent of the law, neither the Publisher nor the authors, contributors, or editors, assume any liability for any injury and/or damage to persons or property as a matter of products liability, negligence or otherwise, or from any use or operation of any methods, products, instructions, or ideas contained in the material herein.

Library of Congress Cataloging-in-Publication Data

Eiff, M. Patrice.
   Fracture management for primary care / M. Patrice Eiff, Robert Hatch.—3rd ed.
      p. ; cm.
   Includes bibliographical references and index.
   ISBN 978-1-4377-0428-0 (pbk.)
   1. Fractures.   2. Primary care (Medicine)   I. Hatch, Robert, 1957- II. Title.
   [DNLM: 1. Fractures, Bone—diagnosis. 2. Fractures, Bone—therapy. 3. Primary Health Care—methods. WE 180]
   RD101.E34 2012
   617.1'5—dc23

                                              2011017590

Senior Acquisitions Editor: Kate Dimock
Senior Developmental Editor: Janice Gaillard
Publishing Services Manager: Patricia Tannian
Team Manager: Hemamalini Rajendrababu
Senior Project Manager: Sharon Corell
Project Manager: Deepthi Unni
Design Direction: Ellen Zanolle

Printed in the United States of America

Last digit is the print number: 9 8 7 6 5

contributors

M. Patrice Eiff, MD
Professor
Department of Family Medicine
Oregon Health and Science University
Portland, Oregon

Robert L. Hatch, MD, MPH
Professor
Department of Community Health and Family
  Medicine
University of Florida
Gainesville, Florida

John Malaty, MD
Assistant Professor
Department of Community Health and Family
  Medicine
Shands Hospital at University of Florida
Gainesville, Florida

Ryan C. Petering, MD
Clinical Instructor
Department of Family Medicine
Oregon Health and Science University
Portland, Oregon

Michael J. Petrizzi, MD
Clinical Professor
Department of Family Medicine
Virginia Commonwealth University School
  of Medicine
Richmond, Virginia

Adam Prawer, MD
Family Medicine Resident
Department of Family Medicine
Bayfront Medical Center
St. Petersburg, Florida

Michael Seth Smith, MD, PharmD
University of Florida
Department of Community Health and
  Family Medicine
Gainesville, Florida

Charles W. Webb, DO, FAAFP
Associate Professor
Director, Sports Medicine
Department of Family Medicine
Associate Professor
Department of Family Medicine and Orthopedics
Oregon Health and Science University
Portland, Oregon

preface

From the earliest conception of this book through the publication of this third edition, it has always been our intent to produce a practical user-friendly book that helps clinicians manage their patients who have fractures. We have accomplished this through a systematic approach to each fracture that enables you to find the information you need quickly, including what to look for, what to do in the acute setting, how to manage the fracture long term, and when to refer. The many high-quality radiographs and illustrations help clinicians properly identify those fractures that can be managed by primary care providers and those that need to be referred. The basic systematic format of the text has been retained, but information from the second edition has been significantly revised to include current evidence and references. We have expanded the discussion in the imaging sections for each fracture to include evidence regarding preferred modalities for identifying fractures. Aspects of the emergency care of fractures, including guidelines for emergent referral and greater detail regarding methods for closed reductions for fractures and dislocations, are featured in this edition. New radiographs and illustrations have been added to give you optimal examples of the fractures you will encounter.

This edition builds on the success of the second edition and gives you an even better reference for your practice. One of the most notable changes is the addition of an entire section devoted to step-by-step instructions on applying a variety of splints and casts. Another update in this edition is the inclusion of patient education handouts that can be downloaded from the online version of the book. These handouts will give your patients information about the healing process and the kinds of rehabilitation exercises they can do to return to full activity after an injury. The online book also includes videos covering techniques for splinting and reducing dislocations.

We would like to thank the many individuals who helped us in the preparation of this edition. We thank our contributing authors for their assistance with individual chapters and the appendix: Ryan Petering, MD (Finger Fractures and Carpal Fractures), Charles Webb, MD (Metacarpal Fractures), John Malaty, MD (Facial and Skull Fractures), Adam Prawer, MD (Radius and Ulna Fractures), Michael Seth Smith, MD (Metatarsal Fractures), and Michael Petrizzi, MD, and Timothy Sanford, MD (Appendix). We thank Walter Calmbach, MD, for his contribution to the first two editions of the book. We also thank Janice Gaillard, senior developmental editor, at Elsevier for her guidance and advice. And finally, we are grateful to the many practicing clinicians who have encouraged us to take this next step in pursuit of our vision to give you the most accurate and practical working guide to fracture management.

M. Patrice Eiff
Robert L. Hatch

introduction

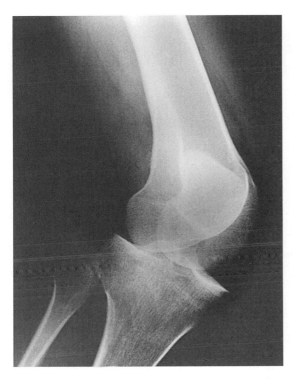

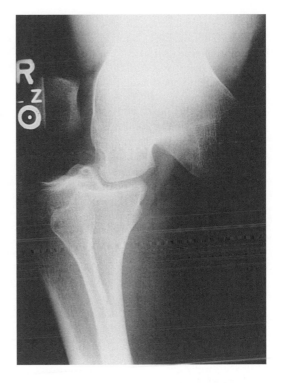

FRACTURE MANAGEMENT: A PERSONAL VIEW

I've always enjoyed teaching sports medicine and fracture management, but I never aspired to become an orthopedic teaching case. That was all to change on the Mambo Run in January 1988.

While I was lying in the snow awaiting transport, my mind quickly began running through a differential diagnosis. My first thought was a femur or tibia fracture. A few torn ligaments were certainly a possibility. After the Ski Patrol member said, "Something doesn't feel quite right," I revised my differential to put patellar dislocation at the top of the list. Of course, that must be it. I wanted that to be it.

In the emergency department of the local hospital, I got the first glimpse of my knee. Admittedly it didn't look right, but I was unwilling to broaden my differential. The physician on duty pulled the sheet back and said something like, "Oooh! Give her some morphine and call the orthopedic surgeon." My concern was mounting. As I was wheeled back from the X-ray department, I overheard my surgeon and skiing companion

remark to the ED physician, "I don't look at bone films too often, but even I can tell that these don't look quite right."

My X rays that "don't look quite right" provide an excellent tool to reinforce the orthopedic principle that one should always obtain two views taken at 90-degree angles from each other when evaluating skeletal injuries. At first glance the X rays tend to create confusion and some head scratching. Confusion turns to a somewhat queasy feeling when viewers realize that they are looking at the femur and tibia at 90-degree angles from each other on the same view.

One's own joint injury or fracture can certainly generate interest in orthopedics. In my case, my knee dislocation fueled a passion to write this book and help others manage patients with orthopedic injuries. There have been many advances in the management of fractures and imaging techniques since the first edition of this book was published in 1998, but plain films can still tell a story. Even if my X-ray picture isn't worth a thousand words, it might be worth a teaching point or two.

M. Patrice Eiff, MD

contents

video contents

Videos courtesy of *Procedures Consult*, Elsevier Inc.

FRACTURE MANAGEMENT BY PRIMARY CARE PROVIDERS

The evaluation and management of patients with acute musculoskeletal injuries is a routine part of most primary care practices. Distinguishing a fracture from a soft tissue injury is an essential part of clinical decision making for these injuries. To provide physicians, nurse practitioners (NPs), and physician assistants (PAs) with adequate training and continuing education in fracture care, we need to know more about the scope, content, and outcome of this aspect of their practices.

PRIMARY CARE PHYSICIANS

Determining the extent of fracture management performed by primary care providers starts with a query of large databases that catalogue the most common diagnoses encountered in primary care. The National Ambulatory Medical Care Survey (NAMCS) is the most comprehensive database available to characterize visits to office-based physicians in many specialties.[1,2] Based on the author's (MPE) analysis of 2005 data, in a representative national sample of more than 25,000 patient visits, fractures and dislocations made up 1.2% of all visits and ranked 18th of the top 20 diagnoses. As expected, orthopedic surgeons saw most of the patients with fractures (68%). Family physicians handled the majority of the remaining visits (10% of the total fracture visits). Visits to family physicians, general internists, and general pediatricians accounted for approximately 18% of the total visits for fracture treatment. Fracture diagnoses rank thirteenth among children younger than 17 years of age. Orthopedic surgeons provided 65%, family physicians provided 6%, and pediatricians provided 17% of the visits for pediatric fractures.

In a 1979 study using national, regional, and individual practice data, orthopedic problems constituted approximately 10% of all visits to family physicians, and fractures accounted for 6% to 14% of the orthopedic problems encountered.[3] In studies done in the early 1980s, fracture care varied in rank from 19th to 28th in relation to other diagnoses made by family physicians.[4,5] A 1995 survey of West Virginian family physicians revealed that 42% provided fracture care.[6] The majority of the respondents of the survey practiced in rural areas.

The distribution of various types of fractures managed by family physicians has been reported in a few studies.[7-9] Two of these studies were done in military family practice residency programs, and the other was performed in a rural residency practice in Virginia. The distribution of fractures is presented in Table 1-1. The most common injuries encountered were fractures of the fingers, radius, metacarpals, toes, and fibula. A report of the epidemiology of nearly 6000 fractures seen in an orthopedic trauma unit in Scotland during the year 2000 found the top five fracture locations to be the distal radius, metacarpal, proximal femur, finger, and ankle.[10]

Family physicians vary in which fractures they manage and which they refer. This is often based on the accessibility of orthopedic specialists, practical experience with fractures, and amount of fracture management taught during family medicine residency training. In settings in which family physicians have considerable experience in fracture management, the overall rate of fracture referral to orthopedists varies from 16% to 25% (excluding fractures of the hip and face).[6,8,11] Most fractures are referred because of the presence of at least one complicated feature, such as angulation or displacement requiring reduction, multiple fractures, intraarticular fractures, tendon or nerve disruption, or epiphyseal plate injury.

Although we have an understanding of the common types of fractures seen by family physicians, less is known about the outcomes of fractures managed by family physicians. In a study of 624 fractures treated by family physicians, healing times for nearly all fractures were consistent with standard healing times reported in a primary care orthopedic textbook (Table 1-2).[8] In a retrospective study, Hatch and Rosenbaum[9] collected information about the outcomes of 170 fractures managed by family physicians. Only four patients

Table 1-1	*Percentage Distribution of Fractures Seen by Family Physicians*		
FRACTURE	EIFF AND SAULTZ[8] (N = 624)*	HATCH AND ROSENBAUM[9] (N = 268)*	ALCOFF AND IBEN[7] (N = 411)[†]
Finger	17	18	12
Metacarpal	16	7	5
Radius	14	10	16
Toe	9	9	1
Fibula	7	7	7
Metatarsal	6	5	4
Clavicle	5	6	7
Radius and ulna	4	6	4
Carpal	2	1	5
Ulna	2	2	3
Humerus	2	4	3
Tibia	2	4	4
Tarsal	1	1	2

*Number of fractures.
[†]Number of fracture visits.

had a significant decrease in range of motion, and only 10 patients had marked symptoms at the end of the follow-up period. Fractures requiring reduction, intraarticular fractures, and scaphoid fractures had the worst outcomes. Complications noted in the total group were minor and with rare exception resolved fully during treatment. The authors concluded that the vast majority of fractures treated by family physicians heal well and that most adverse outcomes can be avoided if family physicians carefully select which fractures they manage.

NURSE PRACTITIONERS AND PHYSICIAN ASSISTANTS

As more and more NPs and PAs join primary care teams, especially in rural communities, they will need skills in managing fractures. PAs and NP's

have been found to provide care similar to one another and physicians in regards to diagnostic, therapeutic, and preventive services in a primary care setting.[12]

A few studies have documented how often NPs encounter acute orthopedic problems in practice. A study of a nurse-managed health center in rural Tennessee found that minor trauma and acute musculoskeletal problems represented 8.5% of all acute conditions treated.[13] The incidence of fractures encountered was not specifically stated. Respondents to a survey study of family nurse practitioners throughout the United States reported "neurologic/ musculoskeletal" problems as the second most common category of cases seen in their practices.[14] Accidental injuries were encountered at least one to three times a month. In another national survey study, fractures ranked 13th out of the top 15 diagnoses in patients seen by 356 family nurse

Table 1-2	*Healing Time of Acute Nonoperative Fractures*	
FRACTURE	ACTUAL HEALING TIME* (WEEKS)	RECOMMENDED LENGTH OF IMMOBILIZATION[†] (WEEKS)
Proximal phalanx	4.1	4
Middle phalanx	3.7	4
Distal phalanx	4.4	3
Metacarpal (excluding fifth)	4.9	4
Fifth metacarpal (boxers)	5.1	4
Scaphoid	7.7	6-12
Distal radius	5.6	6
Distal radius and ulna	6.7	6
Clavicle	3.9	4-6
Fibula	5.9	7-8
Metatarsal	5.9	4-6
Toes	3.6	3-4

*Median values for time from injury to clinical healing (see Alcoff and Iben[7]).
[†]Eiff MP, Saultz JW. Fracture care by family physicians. *J Am Board Fam Pract.*, 1993;6(2):179-181.

practitioners.[15] Data from the NAMCS found that symptoms referable to the musculoskeletal system were the most common category of emergency department (ED) visits for patients who saw nurse practitioners, and "orthopedic care" procedures were performed in 27.6% of the visits related to musculoskeletal symptoms.[16] Results from another national survey found that orthopedic procedures such as reduction of a nursemaid's elbow; splinting an extremity; and reduction of finger, shoulder, and patellar dislocations are performed commonly by nurse practitioners in EDs.[17] According to the American Academy of Physician Assistants 2009 Census survey, 36% practice in a primary care setting and 10% in an ED setting.[18] Today the PA's role is determined by his or her supervising physician within the bounds of the PA's training and experience and in accordance with state laws. Certainly in the primary care or ED setting, NPs and PAs care for patients with a variety of musculoskeletal conditions, including fractures.

Generalizing the results of the studies mentioned is difficult, and the percentages given should be used as only rough estimates of the amount of fracture care provided by primary care providers. Even so, the data support the fact that primary care providers encounter patients with fractures as a routine part of their practices. Even though primary care providers have a large role in managing musculoskeletal problems, some reports have demonstrated a mismatch between the level of skill required in practice and the adequacy of training and self-assessed musculoskeletal knowledge.[19-21] Skills in recognizing and managing fractures should be an essential part of formal education in musculoskeletal medicine in residency to adequately train our primary care workforce.[22,23] The Society of Teachers of Family Medicine Group on Hospital Medicine and Procedural Training considers the initial management of simple fractures, applying splints and casts, and performing closed reductions to be core skills that all family medicine residents should be able to perform independently by graduation.[24]

The content of individual chapters in this book reflects the known distribution of fractures in a primary care setting, and the most commonly encountered fractures are discussed in the most detail. Chapter 2, "General Principles of Fracture Care," covers the features of uncomplicated and complicated fractures to assist primary care providers in the selective management of fractures. The discussion of individual fractures emphasizes aspects of the initial and follow-up care that contribute to proper healing and return to full function while minimizing adverse outcomes. Pediatric fractures are discussed in each chapter after the description of adult fractures.

REFERENCES

1. Rosenblatt RA, Hart LG, Gamliel S, et al. Identifying primary care disciplines by analyzing the diagnostic content of ambulatory care. *J Am Board Fam Pract.* 1995; 8(1):34-45.
2. Binns HJ, Lanier D, Pace WD, et al. Describing primary care encounters: the Primary Care Network Survey and the National Ambulatory Medical Care Survey. *Ann Fam Med.* 2007;5:39-47.
3. Geyman JP, Gordon MJ. Orthopedic problems in family practice: incidence, distribution, and curricular implications. *J Fam Pract.* 1979;8(4):759-765.
4. Geyman JP, Rosenblatt RA. The content of family practice: current status and future trends. *J Fam Pract.* 1982;15(4):677-737.
5. Kirkwood CR, Clure HR, Brodsky R, et al. The diagnostic content of family practice: 50 most common diagnoses recorded in the WAMI community practices. *J Fam Pract.* 1982;15(3):485-492.
6. Swain R, Ashley J. Primary care orthopedics and sports medicine in West Virginia. *West Virginia Med J.* 1995;99: 98-100.
7. Alcoff J, Iben G. A family practice orthopedic trauma clinic. *J Fam Pract.* 1982;14(1):93-96.
8. Eiff MP, Saultz JW. Fracture care by family physicians. *J Am Board Fam Pract.* 1993;6(2):179-181.
9. Hatch RL, Rosenbaum CI. Fracture care by family physicians. *J Fam Pract.* 1994;38(3):238-244.
10. Court-Brown CM, Caesar B. Epidemiology of adult fractures: a review. *Injury.* 2006;37:691-697.
11. Manusov EG, Pearman D, Ross S, et al. Orthopedic trauma: a family practice perspective. *Mil Med.* 1990; 155(7):314-316.
12. Hooker RS, McCaig LF. Use of physician assistants and nurse practitioners in primary care, 1995-1999. *Health Affairs.* 2001;20(4):231-238.
13. Ramsey P, Edwards J, Lenz C, et al. Types of health problems and satisfaction with services in a rural nurse managed clinic. *J Community Health Nurs.* 1993;10(3):161-170.
14. Ward MJ. Family nurse practitioners: perceived competencies and recommendations. *Nurs Res.* 1979;28(6):343-347.
15. Draye MA, Pesznecker BL. Diagnostic scope and certainty: an analysis of FNP practice. *Nurse Pract.* 1979;4(15): 42-43.
16. Mills AC, McSweeney M. Primary reasons for ED visits and procedures performed for patients who saw nurse practitioners. *J Emerg Nurse.* 2005;31:145-149.
17. Wood, C, Wettlaufer J, Shaha SH, Lillis K. Nurse practitioner roles in pediatric emergency departments: a national survey. *Pediatr Emerg Care.* 2010;26:406-407.
18. American Academy of Physician Assistants. National Physician Assistant Census Report. Accessed August 8, 2010, at http://www.aapa.org/images/stories/Data_2009/National_Final_with_Graphics.pdf.
19. Lynch JR, Schmale GA, Schaad DC, Leopold SS. Important demographic variables impact the musculoskeletal knowledge and confidence of academic primary care physicians. *J Bone Joint Surg Am.* 2006;88(7): 1589-1595.
20. Lynch JR, Gardner GC, Parsons RR. Musculoskeletal workload versus musculoskeletal clinical confidence among primary care physicians in rural practice. *Am J Orthop.* 2005;34(10):487-491.
21. Matheny JM, Brinker MR, Elliott MN, et al. Confidence of graduating family practice residents in their management of musculoskeletal conditions. *Am J Orthop.* 2000;29(12):945-952.

22. Haywood BL, Porter SL, Grana WA. Assessment of musculoskeletal knowledge in primary care residents. *Am J Orthop.* 2006;35(6):273-275.

23. Manning RL, DePiero AD, Sadow KB. Recognition and management of pediatric fractures by pediatric residents. *Pediatrics.* 2004;114:1530-1533.

24. Nothnagle M, Sicilia JM, Forman S, et al. Required procedural training in family medicine residency: a consensus statement. *Fam Med.* 2008;40(4):248-252.

GENERAL PRINCIPLES OF FRACTURE CARE

Although each fracture requires individual evaluation and management, general principles of fracture assessment and fracture healing can be applied to aid providers in the proper care of patients with fractures. Accurate fracture identification is the first step in deciding whether to treat the fracture or refer the patient to a specialist. After carefully selecting which fractures to manage, the primary care provider can follow general guidelines for initial and definitive treatment, immobilization, and follow-up evaluation. Keeping in mind the different healing mechanisms and healing rates of various types of fractures also helps guide decisions about immobilization, duration of treatment, and radiographic follow-up.

BONE COMPOSITION

Bone consists of cells imbedded within an abundant extracellular matrix of mineral and organic elements. Mineral in the matrix lends strength and stiffness in compression and bending. The organic component, primarily type I collagen, gives bone great strength in tension. The outer covering of bone, the periosteum, consists of two layers—an outer fibrous layer and an inner more vascular and cellular layer. The inner periosteal layer in infants and children is thicker and more vascular and therefore is more active in healing. This difference partially explains why the periosteal reaction and callus formation after many pediatric fractures are more pronounced than those in adults.

FRACTURE HEALING

Bone has the remarkable and unique ability to heal by complete regeneration rather than by scar tissue formation. Fractures in bones initiate a continuous sequence of healing that includes inflammation, repair, and remodeling.[1] The inflammation phase is relatively short, constituting only about 10% of the total healing time. Bone repair continues for several weeks after the injury. Remodeling of bone begins before repair is complete and may continue for several months to years after a fracture.

Inflammation

Inflammation is the shortest phase of healing and begins immediately after injury. Release of chemical mediators, migration of inflammatory cells to the injury site, vasodilatation, and plasma exudation occur during this phase. Signs and symptoms include swelling, erythema, bruising, pain, and impaired function. After impact to the bone, a hematoma forms between the fracture ends and beneath the elevated periosteum. In a closed fracture, increased interstitial pressure within the hematoma compresses the blood vessels, limiting the size of the hematoma. Nevertheless, the bleeding associated with a closed fracture can still be substantial. For example, a closed fracture of the femoral shaft can result in up to 3 L of blood loss. Generally, open fractures result in much greater blood loss because the tamponade effect of the surrounding soft tissue is absent.

Repair

The bone reparative process is stimulated by chemotactic factors released during inflammation. Electrical stimuli may also play a role. As the inflammatory response subsides, necrotic tissue at the bone ends is resorbed. This resorption of 1 to 2 mm of the fracture ends makes fracture lines more distinct radiographically 5 to 10 days after injury. Fibroblasts appear and start building a new reparative matrix. The fracture hematoma provides a fibrin scaffold for the formation of the fracture callus. The new tissue that arises, the soft callus, is primarily cartilage and acts to stabilize and bridge the fracture gap. As new blood vessels develop that supply nutrients to the cartilage, immobilization of the fracture site is desirable during this phase to allow for revascularization. Bone begins to replace the cartilage approximately 2 to 3 weeks after injury, forming a hard callus.

This process continues until continuity is reestablished between the cortical bone ends.

Mineralization of the fracture callus by chondrocytes and osteoblasts mimics similar events in the normal growth plate. As mineralization proceeds, stability of the fracture fragments progressively increases, and eventually clinical union occurs. Clinical union is demonstrated by lack of movement or pain at the fracture site and radiographs showing bone crossing the fracture site. At this stage, fracture healing is not yet complete. The fracture callus is weaker than normal bone and regains full strength only during the remodeling process.

Remodeling

The final phase of fracture healing begins approximately 6 weeks after the injury. During the repair phase, woven bone is deposited rapidly and has an irregular pattern of matrix collagen. Remodeling reshapes the repair tissue by replacing irregular, immature woven bone with lamellar or mature bone and by resorbing excessive callus. Osteoclasts resorb unnecessary or poorly placed trabeculae and form new bony struts oriented along the lines of stress. Although most remodeling that is apparent on plain radiographs ceases within months of injury, removal and reorganization of repair tissue may continue for several years. Bone scans will continue to show increased uptake at the fracture site during this lengthy period of remodeling.

Factors That Influence Fracture Healing

Fracture healing is a complex process and can be influenced by a number of injury, patient, and treatment factors. Severe injuries with significant soft tissue and bone damage, open fractures, segmental fractures, inadequate blood supply, and soft tissue interposition adversely affect healing. Fracture healing ranges from rapid and complete to delayed or incomplete. When fracture healing progresses more slowly than usual, it is referred to as *delayed union*. When the healing process is arrested, a nonunion occurs, and a pseudarthrosis or fibrous tissue that does not progress to complete healing forms at the fracture site. Intraarticular fracture healing may be delayed because of excessive motion of fracture fragments or synovial fluid collagenases that weaken the fracture callus. Because of this, intraarticular fractures must be in excellent alignment and sufficiently stabilized to reduce the possibility of poor healing.

Age is one of the most important factors that influence bone healing. Whereas children's fractures heal rapidly, fractures heal much more slowly in older persons. Hormonal factors also affect healing. Growth hormone, thyroid hormone, insulin, calcitonin, cortisol, anabolic steroids, and gonadal steroids all play roles.[2] Fractures in patients with a hormonal imbalance generally heal, although union may be delayed. Nutritional factors are also important in the healing process. An adequate balanced diet and sufficient amounts of vitamin D and vitamin C are essential for normal fracture healing. Conditions that compromise fracture healing include diabetes, hypothyroidism, excessive chronic alcohol use, and smoking. Corticosteroids compromise fracture healing, and patients who use steroids on a long-term basis are at increased risk of fractures because of the increased risk of osteoporosis.[3] A causal relationship between nonsteroidal antiinflammatory drugs (NSAIDs) and an increased risk of nonunion has not been established despite some reports of an effect on fracture healing.[4]

The treatment factors that promote bone healing include adequate fragment apposition, weight bearing or fracture loading, and proper fracture stabilization. For most fractures, inappropriate or ineffective stabilization slows healing and may lead to nonunion. Some fractures heal well even though the fracture remains mobile until callus forms. This is true of clavicle, some metacarpal, and many humeral shaft fractures.

POTENTIAL FRACTURE SITES

Identifying the specific location of the fracture within a bone is the first step in the proper evaluation of fractures. In a skeletally mature adult, fractures may occur in the diaphysis (e.g., shaft of long bones) or in the metaphysis (e.g., neck of long bones or short, flat bones) or may extend into the joint (intraarticular). Fractures in children may also involve the growth plate (physis) or the epiphysis. Fig. 2-1 shows the potential fracture locations in adult and growing bone.

Bone tissue is of two types: cortical or compact bone and cancellous or trabecular bone. The diaphysis is made up mostly of solid, hard, cortical bone. Metaphyseal bone consists of a thin shell of cortical bone surrounding primarily spongy, cancellous bone. Differences in the distribution of cortical and cancellous bone in various locations result in differences in healing mechanisms and rates.

In a diaphyseal fracture with minimal separation in cortical bone, healing occurs by formation of callus that progressively stabilizes the fracture fragments. In shaft fractures that require surgery and rigid internal fixation, healing can occur without callus formation. In this type of healing (called *primary bone healing*), the bone surfaces are in direct contact, and lamellar bone forms directly across the fracture line. In cancellous bone, which consists of a labyrinth of trabeculae lined by

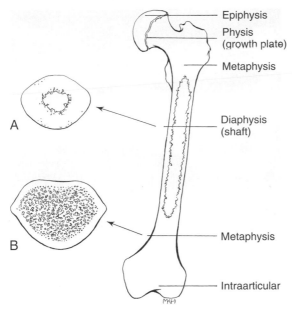

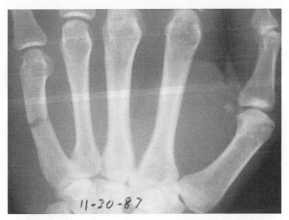

FIGURE 2-2 A transverse fracture of the fifth metacarpal shaft.

FIGURE 2-1 Potential fracture sites. **A,** Section through the diaphysis revealing mostly cortical bone. **B,** Section through the metaphysis showing mostly cancellous bone.

osteoblastic cells, new bone is created in all areas after a fracture. Healing in cancellous bone is usually much more rapid and complete than cortical bone healing, but it is more difficult to evaluate radiographically because it does not produce an external callus.

FRACTURE DESCRIPTION

The management of fractures begins with proper identification and description, including fracture location, fracture type, and the amount of displacement. Learning to describe fractures accurately and precisely is essential for primary care providers. Effective communication with consultants who provide advice over the telephone or receive the patient in referral is difficult without this skill.

Fracture Type

Many terms are used to describe fractures. Using precise language and avoiding vague terminology help ensure proper treatment, especially when the primary care practitioner is relying on telephone advice. Fracture type includes description of the direction of the fracture line, the number of fragments, and the injury force applied to the bone. A transverse fracture has a fracture line oriented perpendicular to the long axis of the bone. Fracture lines can be transverse, oblique, or spiral. A true spiral fracture involves a fracture line that traverses in two different oblique directions. A long oblique fracture line is often mistakenly called a spiral fracture. Both of these fracture types are

relatively unstable and can result from a rotational force applied to the bone. An intraarticular fracture extends into the joint space and is typically described in relation to the percentage of the joint space that is disrupted. A comminuted fracture has multiple fragments, and a segmental fracture is a type of comminuted fracture in which large well-defined fragments occur. Radiographic examples of these fracture types are shown in Figs. 2-2 to 2-6.

Other terms used to describe fracture types relate to the deforming forces applied to the

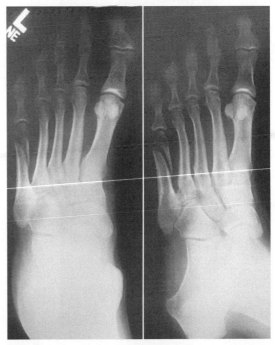

FIGURE 2-3 An oblique fracture of the fifth metatarsal shaft.

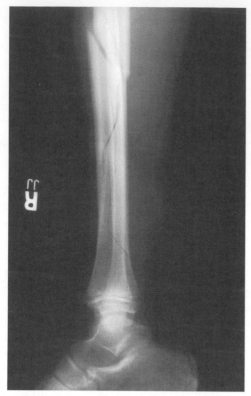

FIGURE 2-4 A spiral fracture of the tibial shaft.

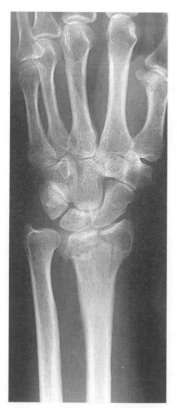

FIGURE 2-5 A comminuted intraarticular fracture of the distal radius.

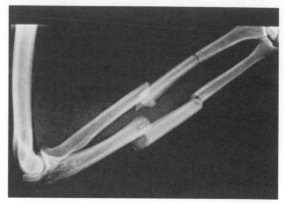

FIGURE 2-6 A segmental fracture of the radius and ulna. (From Browner BD, Jupiter JB, Levine AM, Trafton PG [eds]. Skeletal Trauma: Fractures, Dislocations, Ligamentous Injuries. Philadelphia, WB Saunders, 1992.)

fracture fragments (Fig. 2-7). In an impacted fracture, a direct force applied down the length of the bone results in a telescoping of one fragment on the other. An avulsion fracture occurs after a forceful contraction of the muscle that tears its bony attachment loose. Compression fractures are common in cancellous flat bones because they are spongy. A pathologic fracture occurs at the site of bone weakened by tumor or osteoporosis. A stress fracture results from chronic or repetitive overloading of the bone (Fig. 2-8).

The fracture types unique to growing bone are torus (buckle), greenstick, and plastic deformation. These are discussed in the Pediatric Fracture section at the end of this chapter.

Fracture Displacement

Fracture displacement occurs when one fragment shifts in relation to the other through translation, angulation, shortening, or rotation. In general, displacement is described by referring to the movement of the distal fragment relative to the proximal fragment. Translation can occur in either the anteroposterior (AP) plane or the medial-lateral plane. In the description of displacement of hand and wrist fractures, the terms volar and dorsal are commonly used instead of anterior and posterior, and ulnar and radial are used instead of medial and lateral. In addition to a description of the direction of translation, the amount of translation should be reported. This can be measured on the radiograph in millimeters, or the percentage of apposition can be estimated (Fig. 2-9). Generally speaking, 3 mm or less of translation is considered "minimally displaced."

Angulation at the fracture site may be in the frontal or sagittal plane or both. True AP and lateral radiographs, at 90 degrees from each other,

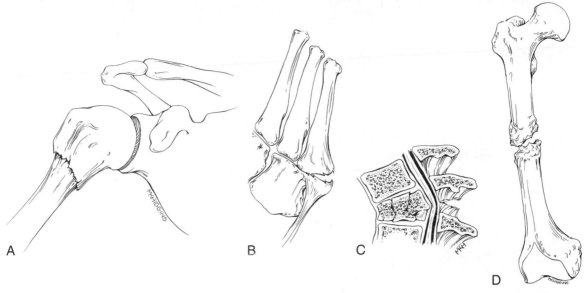

FIGURE 2-7 Fracture types. **A,** Impacted. **B,** Avulsion. **C,** Compression. **D,** Pathologic.

are necessary to accurately estimate angulation of a fracture. Angulation cannot be assessed from an oblique film. In the description of angulation, the direction in which the apex of the angle (i.e., the point of the "V" formed by the angulated

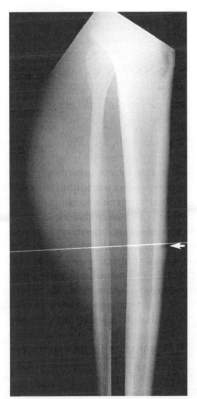

FIGURE 2-8 A stress fracture of the anterior midshaft of the tibia (*arrow*).

fragments) is pointing should be stated. Fig. 2-10 is an example of apex medial angulation. Fig. 2-11 demonstrates apex dorsal angulation. The amount of angulation is measured in degrees with the aid of a goniometer (Fig. 2-12).

Shortening of the bone is another type of displacement. A change in bone length occurs in an impacted fracture or in bayonet-type apposition. Fractures vary as to how much shortening is acceptable for proper healing. The deforming forces of trauma, gravity, or muscle pull can cause rotational displacement of fracture fragments. Rotation is difficult to visualize radiographically and is more often detected clinically (Fig. 2-13).

Radiographic Interpretation

Using proper terminology as already described leads to accurate and clear descriptions of radiographs. Description of the radiographic findings of a fracture should identify the following aspects: the bone involved, the location of the fracture, the type of fracture, and the amount of displacement. Noting whether a fracture is diaphyseal or metaphyseal helps with decisions that affect healing. Other terms used to describe the location of a fracture within a bone include *proximal* or *distal*; *medial* and *lateral*; and *head, neck, shaft,* or *base*.

In the radiograph in Fig. 2-14, the fracture would be accurately described as a nondisplaced, nonangulated oblique fracture of the left distal fibula (or distal fibula metaphysis). Examples of other fractures and corresponding radiographic interpretations are presented in Figs. 2-15 to 2-17.

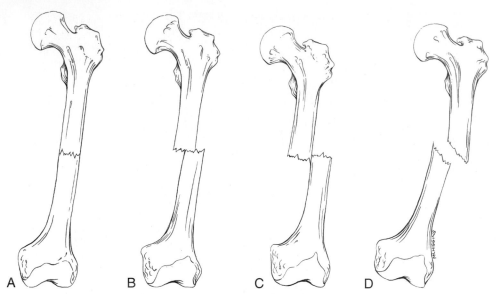

FIGURE 2-9 Apposition of midshaft fractures of the femur. **A,** End-to-end apposition. **B,** Fifty percent end-to-end apposition. **C,** Side-to-side (bayonet) apposition, with slight shortening. **D,** No apposition.

FRACTURE SELECTION

In the approach to a patient with a newly diagnosed fracture, emphasis should be placed on identifying patients who need prompt treatment and

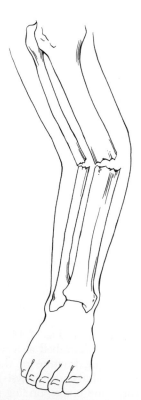

FIGURE 2-10 Apex medial angulation in a midshaft tibia and fibula fracture.

those who can have a splint applied and receive definitive treatment later. Primary care providers can manage a wide range of fractures and achieve good clinical results if they carefully select which fractures to manage based on general guidelines.

Referral Decisions

This decision is influenced by the nature of the fracture, the presence or absence of coexistent injuries, the characteristics of the patient, local practice patterns, and the expertise and comfort level of the primary care provider. The following guidelines can be used in making decisions regarding orthopedic referral:

1. Avoid managing any fracture that is beyond your comfort zone unless a more experienced provider is available to guide your management. The comfort of both the patient and the provider is often enhanced if the provider explains his or her experience with fracture management and lets the patient choose between referral and continuing under his or her care.
2. Identify patients with complicated fractures.
3. Strongly consider referring any patient who is likely to have difficulty complying with treatment.

Complicated Fractures Requiring Urgent Action or Consultation

A minority of fractures are complicated by conditions that require urgent action. The key to the management of these conditions is early recognition followed by prompt definitive treatment.

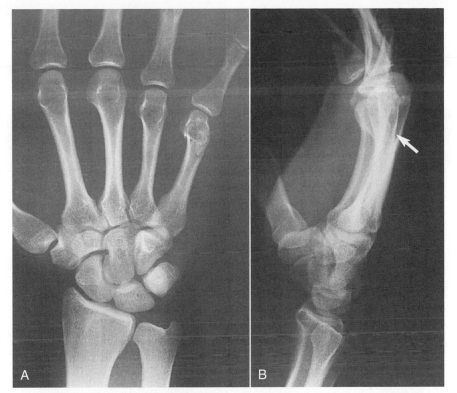

FIGURE 2-11 **A,** Anteroposterior view of a fifth metacarpal neck (boxer's) fracture. **B,** Lateral view showing apex dorsal angulation . The *arrow* points to the apex of the angle.

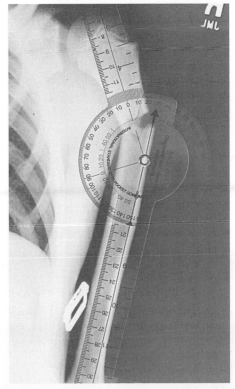

FIGURE 2-12 Use of a goniometer to measure degrees of angulation.

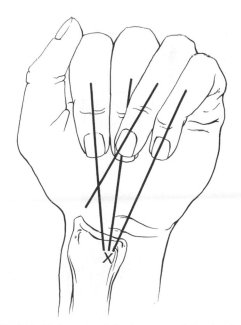

FIGURE 2-13 Rotational displacement of the ring finger. All fingers should line up on the same point on the distal radius.

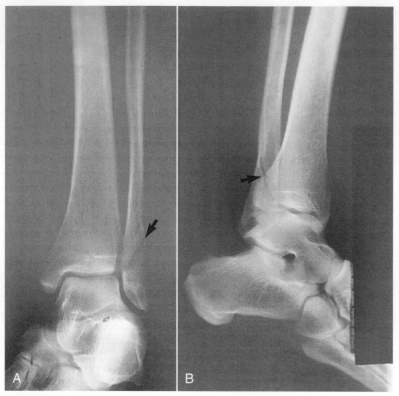

FIGURE 2-14 Nondisplaced, nonangulated oblique fracture of the distal fibula (*arrows*). **A,** Anteroposterior view. **B,** Lateral view.

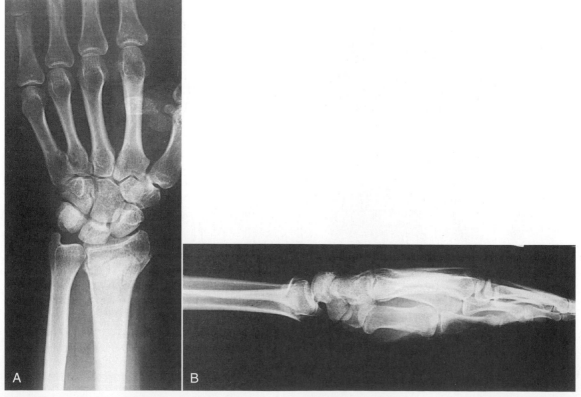

FIGURE 2-15 A, Anteroposterior and, **B,** lateral views of the wrist. Comminuted fracture of the distal radius with 3 mm of shortening and 10 degrees of apex volar angulation.

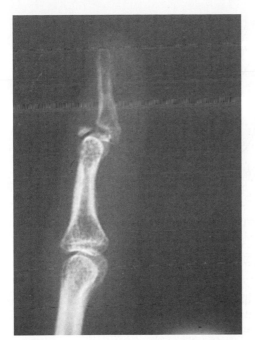

FIGURE 2-16 Lateral view of the finger. Avulsion fracture of the dorsal aspect of the distal phalanx involving approximately 30% of the articular surface. Visible are 4 mm of dorsal displacement of the fragment and volar subluxation of the distal phalanx at the distal interphalangeal joint.

Life-Threatening Conditions

Fortunately, life-threatening conditions are rare. When they do occur, they are almost always associated with major trauma or open fractures. Life-threatening conditions that may occur with fractures include hemorrhage, fat embolism, pulmonary embolus, gas gangrene, and tetanus.

The most common life-threatening condition associated with fractures is significant hemorrhage. Half of all pelvic fractures cause blood loss sufficient to require transfusion, and significant hemorrhage frequently occurs with closed femur fractures.

Fat embolism is much less common. It is usually associated with long bone or pelvis fractures in young adults or hip fractures in elderly adults. It generally develops 24 to 72 hours after the fracture, and symptoms include a classic triad of hypoxemia, neurologic impairment, and a petechial rash. In the early stages, fat embolism may be difficult to distinguish from pulmonary embolism. After respiratory distress occurs, patients develop confusion and an altered level of consciousness. The characteristic petechial rash, present up to half the time, is caused by the occlusion of capillaries by fat globules and is found on the head, neck, trunk,

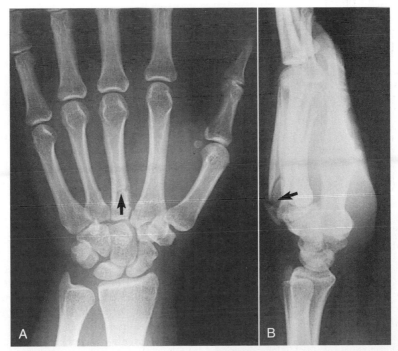

FIGURE 2-17 Anteroposterior (**A**) and lateral (**B**) views of the hand. Transverse fracture of the base of the third metacarpal with 20 degrees of apex dorsal angulation and 1 cm of dorsal displacement of the metacarpal at the carpometacarpal joint (*arrows*).

subconjunctiva and axillae. Overall mortality ranges from 5% to 15%.[5]

Patients with fractures are predisposed to venous thrombosis and therefore pulmonary embolism. Immobilization of limbs, decreased activity levels, and soft tissue injury contribute to the increased risk of venous thrombosis. Gas gangrene after a fracture is almost always associated with injuries that penetrate to muscle. This infection is marked by pain and wound drainage and typically progresses rapidly to local spread, toxemia, and death. Tetanus may also occur after open fractures and may involve local or generalized muscle spasm and muscle hyper-irritability.

Arterial Injury

Only a small percentage of fractures involve arterial injuries. However, such injuries can produce disastrous outcomes, such as loss of a limb or permanent ischemic contracture. Fortunately, when recognized early and treated appropriately, arterial injuries usually have a good outcome. Arterial injuries are most common in dislocations, fractures with penetrating injuries (e.g., gunshot wounds), and fractures of certain sites.[6] Arterial injury commonly accompanies displaced fractures and dislocations of the elbow and knee. A displaced supracondylar fracture is shown in Fig. 2-18. In such injuries, the proximal fragment often causes kinking and occlusion of the brachial artery (Fig. 2-19). When evaluating a supracondylar fracture, the physician should presume that an arterial injury is present until proved otherwise. Arterial injuries should be suspected in any patient with a

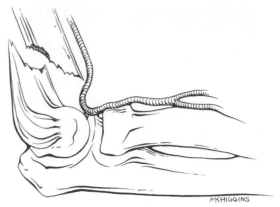

FIGURE 2-19 Injury to the brachial artery caused by a displaced supracondylar fracture.

knee dislocation. Some institutions routinely perform arteriograms on all knee dislocations regardless of a normal circulatory examination to detect initially asymptomatic intimal tears that can go on to develop complete occlusion.

Primary care providers can minimize the adverse outcomes of arterial injuries by following these guidelines:

1. **Assess circulation distal to the injury in all patients with a fracture or dislocation.** This is most often done by assessing the presence and strength of distal pulses. Slow capillary refill (greater than 3 seconds) and pallor are signs of arterial injury.

2. **Assess circulation as soon as possible after the patient seeks treatment.** Ideally, this would be done within minutes of an initial examination before radiographs are ordered. Signs of disrupted blood flow include skin mottling, a cool extremity, and decreased sensation.

3. When dislocations and displaced fractures are accompanied by an absent distal pulse and orthopedic assistance is not readily available, primary care providers should attempt such reductions promptly. In many cases, kinking of the artery rather than actual arterial injury impairs circulation. If the limb is pulseless, much is to be gained and little lost by attempted reduction. If no one with experience in reductions is available soon after radiographs are obtained, one or two gentle reduction attempts by the primary care provider would be appropriate. The reduction technique would differ from those of other reductions in which it is desirable to first reproduce the force that created the fracture, briefly exaggerating the deformity. In these cases, such a maneuver could cause additional vascular damage and should be avoided if possible.

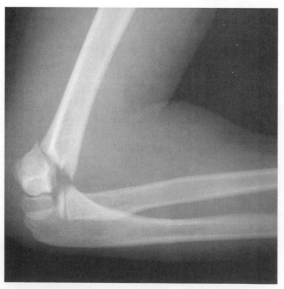

FIGURE 2-18 Displaced supracondylar fracture.

4. Repeat the vascular examination after any manipulation of the fracture site and whenever symptoms that suggest possible ischemia develop. Symptoms suggestive of limb ischemia include disproportionate pain, especially if limb immobilization and appropriate analgesia fail to relieve the pain. Ideally, ischemia would be detected at this early stage before permanent damage occurs. If ischemia is suspected, consultation should be considered even if pulses are present (see Compartment Syndrome, discussed later).
5. Document all vascular examinations in the medical record.

Nerve Injury

Many patients have mild paresthesia directly over the fracture site. This is most likely caused by local soft tissue edema. This paresthesia is benign and self-limited. Proximal humerus fractures, however, are an exception. Whereas most injuries to other nerves involve impaired nerve function distal to the fracture, paresthesia overlying the deltoid in these cases may actually indicate injury to the axillary nerve. For detection of nerve injuries, distal sensation should be assessed and documented in all fracture patients. When feasible, motor function should also be assessed, especially when a sensory deficit is suspected.

Nerve injuries are most common when a penetrating injury is present and in fractures near the elbow and knee. Dislocations of the hip, knee, and shoulder also have a high incidence of nerve injury. Most nerve injuries associated with fractures and dislocations are temporary neurapraxias caused by nerve stretching and resolve spontaneously with time. Nerve injuries associated with penetrating injury, open fracture, or complete loss of nerve function are likely to be more serious and require orthopedic referral. Open exploration and nerve repair are often necessary in such cases.

Compartment Syndrome

Compartment syndrome results when the pressure within a rigid fascial compartment prevents adequate muscle perfusion. It is most common in tibial and forearm fractures, where several such compartments exist. Soft tissue swelling within the fixed compartment causes increased pressure. As the pressure within the compartment increases, perfusion becomes impaired, leading to muscle ischemia and further swelling. Myonecrosis, ischemic nerve injury, and occlusion of arterial flow then occur. If left untreated, permanent ischemic contracture or loss of the limb may result.

The symptoms and signs of compartment syndrome change over time, so serial examination is important.[7] Pain is the most reliable early symptom, but it is not present in all cases. Typically, pain caused by compartment syndrome is disproportionate, deep, and poorly localized (analogous to the pain of cardiac ischemia). The presence of such pain, especially in a high-risk situation (e.g., crush injuries, fractures of the lower leg or forearm, and acute fractures treated with a circumferential cast), strongly suggests a compartment syndrome. Any of these symptoms may or may not be present in a given case. Paresthesia of the sensory nerve that passes through the compartment is another relatively early sign. Other symptoms and signs include pain that increases with passive stretch of the affected muscle, a firm "wood-like" feeling to the limb, and muscle weakness. When paralysis and pulselessness are present, permanent damage, loss of the limb, or both are likely.

To detect compartment syndrome early, the clinician must remain extremely alert to its potential occurrence, be aware of the early symptoms, and pursue further evaluation with compartment pressure measurement and orthopedic consultation in suspected cases. Interpreting the results of compartment pressure measurements can be complex because accuracy depends on proper calibration of the device, and needle placement and the pressure necessary to cause injury vary depending on the clinical scenario. Serial or continuous pressure measurements are usually more helpful than a single measurement.[8] Although there is no agreed upon compartment pressure threshold above which fasciotomy is indicated, this surgical procedure to decompress the affected compartments is the definitive treatment in the vast majority of cases.

Open Fractures

Open fractures are those in contact with the outside environment and require emergent orthopedic referral for irrigation, surgical debridement, and treatment with intravenous antibiotics to minimize complications. In obvious open fractures, exposed bone is clearly seen. In many open fractures, however, the bone edges pull back after breaking the skin and are no longer visible. To avoid missing these injuries, the clinician should suspect an open fracture whenever a break in the skin overlies a fracture. An open fracture exists whenever the hematoma around the bone ends communicates with the outside environment. Any break in the skin near a fracture should be carefully inspected and, if necessary, gently explored. Concern that the wound may communicate with the fracture hematoma warrants orthopedic consultation. Management of open fractures depends on the extent of soft tissue damage, the degree of wound contamination, and the overall health of the patient. Although they technically meet the definition of an open fracture, fractures of the distal phalanges with minor adjacent lacerations or nail bed injuries do not require emergent treatment by an orthopedist and can be managed by primary care providers.

Tenting of the Skin

Occasionally, severely angulated or displaced fractures produce enough pressure on the overlying skin to cause the skin to become ischemic. In such cases, the skin appears blanched and taut. If the pressure continues, the skin ultimately breaks down, converting a closed fracture into an open one. Prompt reduction is necessary in these situations. In most of these cases, delaying the reduction for 10 to 20 minutes while obtaining adequate anesthesia or orthopedic consultation does not adversely affect the outcome.

Significant Soft Tissue Damage

Some fractures are accompanied by severe injury to the adjacent muscle and skin. These injuries are prone to the development of compartment syndrome, infection, skin breakdown, and other complications. When considerable soft tissue damage is present, managing the soft tissue injury may be more difficult than managing the fracture itself. Early orthopedic consultation is recommended in such injuries to optimize management and prevent complications. Soft tissue damage of this extent is generally seen only in crush injuries.

Complicated Fractures That Often Require Referral

In addition to the injuries discussed earlier, other types of complicated fractures are likely to necessitate referral. These include fractures requiring reduction, multiple fractures, intraarticular fractures, fracture dislocations, epiphyseal plate fractures, and fractures with associated tendon injury. The referral rate for each type is highly dependent on the training and experience of the provider. Referral rates for complicated fractures managed in rural settings are shown in Table 2-1.

Perhaps the greatest variability in referral rate is seen with fractures requiring reduction. Many primary care providers have little experience with reductions and therefore refer all fracture patients. Other primary care providers reduce many fractures. The most common reductions performed by primary care providers involve the distal radius, metacarpals (fourth and fifth), fingers, and toes. Reduction techniques for these and other fractures are discussed in subsequent chapters.

Patients with multiple fractures are also more likely to require referral. When more than one bone is fractured, the fracture may be quite unstable (e.g., fractures of multiple adjacent metatarsals or fractures of both bones in the forearm or lower leg). In other cases, the treatment of one fracture may necessitate an alternative approach to treatment of the other. For example, a humerus fracture in a patient bedridden because of a femur fracture may require external traction rather than more traditional treatment.

Most patients with intraarticular fractures are referred. When a fracture extends to the joint surface, future degenerative joint disease is likely. This is particularly true if a step-off of more than 2 mm occurs or if the fracture fragment contains more than 25% of the joint surface. In estimating the amount of joint surface involved, the physician can imagine looking directly at the articular surface on end and visualizing the surface in three dimensions using information from all radiographic

Table 2-1	*Management of Complicated Fractures*			
	PATIENTS MANAGED BY FAMILY PHYSICIANS ONLY	PATIENTS MANAGED BY FAMILY PHYSICIANS WITH CONSULTATION	PATIENTS REFERRED	TOTAL NUMBER (% OF ALL FRACTURES)
Displaced fractures requiring reduction*	12	0	24[†]	35 (12)
Multiple bones fractured	27	0	8	35 (12)
Intraarticular	3	1	8	12 (4)
Fracture-dislocation	0	0	11	11 (4)
Open fracture	2[‡]	0	9	11 (4)
Epiphyseal plate fracture	2	3	5	10 (3)
Associated tendon injury	1	2	3	6 (2)
Possible nerve injury	0	1	1	2 (1)

From Hatch RL, Rosenbaum CI. Fracture care by family physicians. J Fam Pract 1994;38(3):238-244. Reprinted by permission of Appleton & Lange, Inc.
*Excludes fracture dislocations and hip fractures.
[†]In two cases, reduction was attempted unsuccessfully by the family physician before referral.
[‡]Both involved the distal phalanx of the finger. An additional six patients managed by the family practitioners had lacerations overlying the fracture site that did not extend to the periosteum.

views. Near-anatomic alignment is essential in the management of most intraarticular fractures.

Fracture dislocations are challenging to manage and often require operative repair. Essentially, all are managed by orthopedists. Similarly, fractures with a coexistent tendon injury are more challenging to manage, and the patients generally require referral.

Many fractures involving the physis in children heal well and do not require reduction. However, patients with these fractures are often referred because most primary care providers have limited experience managing these types of injuries and because future growth problems may develop at the fracture site. Guidelines for managing fractures in children are discussed separately at the end of the chapter.

Proper selection of which fractures to manage and which patients to refer is the key to successful fracture management. The remainder of this chapter includes guidelines for the acute and definitive care of uncomplicated fractures.

OVERVIEW OF ACUTE MANAGEMENT

Initial Assessment

Evaluation of a patient with a possible fracture begins with a focused history, including the cause of injury, presence of other injuries, previous injuries of the affected region, medical history, and allergies. The initial examination includes evaluating neurovascular status, inspecting for breaks in the skin, and assessing soft tissue injury. Palpation for areas of maximum tenderness allows the examiner to pinpoint likely fracture sites and order radiographs more appropriately. A bone may fracture in two places, or the adjacent joint may be injured, so it is important to palpate the entire bone and the joints above and below the fracture.

Knowledge of injury patterns associated with common causes of injury can also guide the examination. For example, inversion injuries of the ankle may cause fractures of the malleoli, the proximal fifth metatarsal, or the tarsal navicular bone. If patients have sustained such classic injuries, it is wise to palpate all of the bones that may be fractured.

Radiographic Studies

After urgent complications have been excluded and areas of point tenderness have been identified, appropriate radiographic studies are obtained. Three guidelines are helpful to consider:

1. Always obtain at least two views that differ by about 90 degrees. An AP view and lateral view are standard in the radiographic evaluation of most bones.

2. Radiographs should include the entire bone unless the physical examination allows the clinician to confidently rule out a fracture in the areas not seen on the radiograph. Consider obtaining radiographs of any adjacent bones or joints that are significantly tender.

3. Consider further radiographic views or other types of imaging whenever the physical examination strongly suggests a fracture but initial radiograph results are normal. Oblique views or special views (e.g., notch view of the knee) may prove helpful. As shown in Fig. 2-20, An AP view may appear quite normal, and the fracture is only revealed on the oblique view. A comparison view of the opposite, noninjured extremity can also confirm the presence of a fracture.

Immobilization

Virtually all acute fractures benefit from immobilization, which offers three benefits: it prevents loss of position, protects adjacent structures from additional injury, and provides considerable pain relief. Determining the appropriate duration and type of immobilization is the primary treatment decision for most fractures. Varying degrees of immobilization can be obtained by splinting, casting, internal fixation, external traction and fixation, or the use of a brace or sling. Only splinting and casting are considered here. The use of slings and braces is discussed in other chapters when these forms of immobilization constitute primary treatment for the fracture (e.g., clavicle and humerus).

To avoid an iatrogenic compartment syndrome, splinting is the preferred form of immobilization whenever additional swelling is expected. Additional swelling can be expected in all fractures that are less than 2 to 3 days old, especially if manipulation was required, soft tissue damage is present, or the patient is unlikely to comply with elevation. Under certain circumstances, casting may be indicated despite the likelihood of additional swelling (Table 2-2). If a cast is applied under such circumstances, it is strongly recommended that the cast

Table 2-2	Fractures Likely to Require Acute Casting: Unstable or Potentially Unstable Fractures
Fractures that required reduction
Fractures involving two adjacent bones (e.g., fractures of the midshaft of both the radius and ulna)
Segmental fractures
Spiral fractures
Fractures with strong muscle forces acting across the fracture site (e.g., midshaft fracture of the humerus or Bennett's fracture of the thumb)
Fracture dislocations

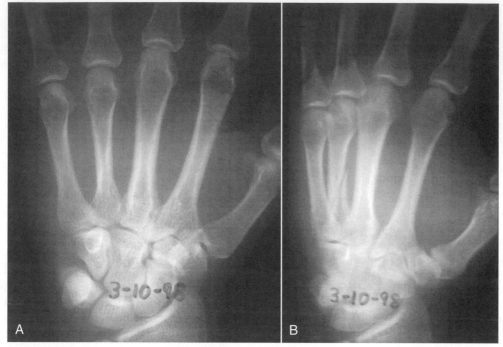

FIGURE 2-20 A, Anteroposterior view of the hand, which appears normal. **B,** Oblique view of the hand. An oblique fracture of the fourth metacarpal shaft is clearly seen.

be split and wrapped with an elastic bandage to keep it in position. Several days later, the bandage can be replaced with a layer of plaster or fiberglass to complete the cast.

Splinting is recommended in several other instances. If significant swelling is present, splinting is preferred. Otherwise, the cast will become loose and need to be replaced soon. Except in the situations listed in Table 2-2, casting is also likely to be a waste of effort whenever referral is planned because the consulting physician will often remove the cast to better assess and treat the patient. Splinting may be the preferred form of definitive care for some fractures, including most finger and toe fractures and metacarpal fractures (gutter splint). See the Appendix for a description of the stepwise method for applying various splints and casts.

Other Acute Measures

Pain relief and control of swelling are important goals of acute fracture treatment. Icing and elevation play important roles in achieving these goals. Initially, an ice pack should be applied for 20 to 30 minutes every 1 to 2 hours while the patient is awake. Applications can be decreased to three to four times a day by the second day and discontinued after 48 to 72 hours. The ice pack may be applied directly to the elastic bandage that secures the splint or to the cast. As much as possible, the patient should maintain the fracture site at or above

the level of the heart for an upper extremity fracture and above the hip for a lower extremity fracture. Compliance with elevation seems to improve when the provider explains that failure to keep the fracture site elevated will delay definitive treatment (e.g., casting) and increase pain. Even when immobilization, icing, and elevation are made optimal, analgesics are usually required for optimal pain relief. In many cases, acetaminophen or ibuprofen suffices. This is especially true in children with less severe fractures. Adults are more likely to require narcotic analgesics, especially if multiple or large bones are fractured.

In general, analgesics are needed for only the first 2 to 5 days after injury. If considerable pain is present despite usual doses of a narcotic, a fracture complication such as vascular injury, compartment syndrome, or infection may be present. In addition, a cast that presses too firmly against the skin may cause pain. This may be the result of excessive molding, improper cast shape, or indentations in the cast. High-pressure areas can lead to skin breakdown and ulceration.

Providers who frequently manage fractures find it helpful to provide patient information sheets that summarize acute treatment and warning signs of complications (go to Expert Consult for an electronic version of patient education handouts). Readers are invited to copy or modify this form for use in their practices.

Timing of the Initial Follow-up Visit

If referral is planned, discussing the case directly with the receiving physician improves communication and ensures appropriate timing of the referral. In general, orthopedists receiving a referral prefer to see the patient relatively soon (i.e., 1 to 3 days). Most patients managed by primary care providers are seen again approximately 3 to 5 days after the initial visit. At that time, swelling is likely to have subsided, and the patient is usually ready for casting. If a cast was applied to an acute fracture, a follow-up visit the next day is strongly recommended. This will allow the provider to split the cast if it is becoming too tight (or loosen the bandage if already split).

OVERVIEW OF DEFINITIVE CARE

Casting

Casting is the mainstay of treatment for most fractures. Casts help keep the fracture fragments in position until adequate healing can occur. It is important to note that some fractures do not require casting. For example, many fractures of the proximal fifth metatarsal and proximal humerus are treated without casting. In the application of a cast, it is helpful to follow certain guidelines. In deciding how to cast a fracture, the provider must choose which materials to use, what type of cast to apply, and how the extremity should be positioned. Casting should occur after swelling has decreased and stabilized, usually within 3 to 5 days

Cast Materials

Plaster and fiberglass are the primary materials used for casting. Each offers certain advantages and disadvantages. Plaster is considerably cheaper, has a very long shelf life, and is easier to work with. Many primary care providers prefer it, especially if they treat a relatively small number of fractures. Fiberglass is more durable and lighter. For these reasons, fiberglass is usually the material of choice for most clinicians.

Type of Cast

When choosing how to cast a fracture, it is crucial to determine which joints to include in the cast and how far to extend the cast. This varies according to the location and stability of the fracture and is discussed in detail for each fracture in the following chapters. Three principles merit discussion here. First, maximal immobilization cannot be obtained unless the joints both above and below the fracture are immobilized. This degree of immobilization is required for the majority of unstable or potentially unstable fractures. An unstable distal radius fracture requires a long arm cast, which immobilizes both the wrist and elbow joints. Second, if a bone is enclosed in a cast, the cast should usually include nearly the entire length of the bone. Short arm casts should extend nearly all the way to the elbow, enclosing nearly the entire length of the radius and ulna. Finally, immobilization of a joint should not be taken lightly. After immobilization, much time and effort are required to regain range of motion (ROM) and strength. This is especially true if the patient is older or if the duration of casting exceeds 8 to 10 weeks. The elbow and knee are particularly slow to regain function. For these reasons, long arm casts and long leg casts are often converted to short arm or short leg casts before healing is complete.

Positioning of the Extremity

In general, extremities are immobilized in the position of function. The wrist and hand, for example, are usually immobilized in a grasping position. The ankle and elbow are immobilized at 90 degrees. In some fractures, these guidelines must be violated to obtain an optimal outcome. The discussion of Colles' fractures in Chapter 6 illustrates this principle.

Confirming Fracture Position After Casting

Most fractures do not require repeat radiographs immediately after casting. Such radiographs are necessary only if the fracture required reduction or if the fracture may have lost its position (e.g., if the fracture is unstable or if excessive movement of the fractured extremity has occurred).

See the Appendix for stepwise instructions on how to apply various casts.

Follow-up Visits

Stable Fractures

Follow-up visits fall into four broad categories: initial cast checks, replacement of the cast, assessment for healing, and assessment of function after the cast is removed.

Cast checks

Some providers routinely schedule cast checks the day after a cast is applied. This maximizes the opportunity for early detection of casts that fit improperly or are too tight, allowing them to be replaced promptly before complications occur. However, a visit at this time is often inconvenient for the patient, especially if the fracture involves the lower extremity. For patients who are both cooperative and attentive, providing written instructions and calling the patient the day after casting should suffice. Patients reporting an uncomfortable cast should be seen as soon as possible to have the cast either replaced or adjusted (e.g., create a bivalve cast or cut a window in it). Scheduling the first return visit 3 to 5 days after casting offers advantages over next-day follow-up. If a cast will become loose, it is usually apparent within this time. Also, patients become used to the cast after several days and are more receptive to learning and initiating exercises of the affected extremity.

Replacing casts

When prolonged immobilization is required, casts often weaken and require replacement. Patients are generally seen approximately every 3 to 4 weeks to reassess the integrity of the cast. More frequent monitoring may be necessary in active children and for walking casts. In addition, certain fractures require different casts at different stages of healing. For example, many Colles' fractures are initially treated with a long arm cast followed by conversion to a short arm cast after partial healing has occurred.

Assessment of healing

Immobilization is generally continued until clinical union has occurred and the fracture site is strong enough to bear the stresses of daily activities. Longer immobilization generally increases the chance that this will occur. However, prolonged immobilization can lead to marked weakness and loss of ROM, leaving the patient with a long, difficult recovery. The approach to follow-up seeks to strike a balance between these considerations.

A follow-up visit is generally scheduled soon after union could be reasonably expected. At this visit, the cast is removed, and clinical healing is assessed by noting tenderness at the fracture site and ROM. A radiograph should be obtained to look for radiographic healing, keeping in mind that radiographic union lags clinical union by a few weeks.[9] Resolution of point tenderness and radiographic evidence of callus indicate that union has occurred. For some fractures (e.g., tibial shaft), it is also desirable to demonstrate stability to manual stress before discontinuing the cast. If significant tenderness remains or no callus is seen, the cast is replaced, and the patient is reassessed in 2 weeks. Predicting when union will occur is an inexact science. Hence, some patients are recasted several times before healing occurs. If no callus is seen 4 weeks after injury, repeat radiographs should be obtained every 2 to 4 weeks to document fracture union.

The duration of immobilization varies greatly among fractures. As a general rule, it is best to err on the side of longer immobilization for the lower extremity to maximize stability and shorter immobilization for the upper extremity to maximize ROM. If a longer period of immobilization is needed, a functional brace or splint that provides some immobilization and allows the patient to perform gentle ROM exercises out of the device is a good alternative to recasting.

Assessment of function after the cast is removed

Some amount of joint stiffness and loss of ROM are expected after immobilization of longer than 2 weeks. After the cast is removed, the patient should be instructed on how to perform stretching and strengthening exercises for the joints that have stiffened during cast treatment. Optimally, these exercises should be performed several times per day. A follow-up visit within 2 weeks after cast removal is necessary to document the return of normal motion and strength to the injured area. Patients who have continued pain, stiffness, or weakness should be seen every 2 to 4 weeks until return of normal function is achieved. Physical therapy should be considered for any patient who needs extra guidance and instruction in home exercises or anyone who is progressing very slowly in rehabilitation.

Unstable Fractures

Unstable fractures are much more likely to lose their position during treatment. In addition to the follow-up already described, they generally require extra visits to monitor the position of the fracture as well as more caution when assessing for healing.

Monitoring fracture position before healing occurs

The following scenario illustrates a fear common to many providers. A patient reports with a relatively straightforward fracture such as the one shown in Fig. 2-21. After an uncomplicated treatment course, follow-up radiographs reveal that the fracture has lost its position and healed with significant angulation (Fig. 2-22). Fortunately, such outcomes can be avoided if the provider identifies fractures that may lose their position and monitors their position before healing occurs. Radiographs obtained to monitor fracture position are taken without removing the cast. Table 2-2 lists some common unstable fractures that may require radiographic monitoring before healing.

The most unstable fractures require frequent monitoring. For example, midshaft fractures involving both the radius and the ulna in children may require radiographs as often as every 3 to 4 days until healing has occurred. In contrast, a distal radius fracture that required reduction generally requires monitoring at only one point before healing. In an adult, the optimum time to obtain such radiographs is 8 to 10 days after the injury. If the position is maintained at this time, it is unlikely to be lost. However, if the position has been lost, the fragments are still relatively mobile and can usually be

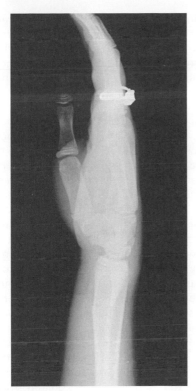

FIGURE 2-21 Transverse distal radius fracture with approximately 15 degrees of apex volar angulation. This amount of angulation is the maximum one would accept in this 12-year-old patient, whose angulation will most likely be corrected as she grows.

repositioned. In children, healing occurs more rapidly, and such follow-up films are best obtained 4 to 7 days after injury.

Assessment of healing

Assessment of healing in unstable fractures differs from that in stable fractures in one important regard: removing the cast before healing could allow an unstable fracture to lose position. To prevent this, the provider should obtain radiographs through the cast as the first step in assessing fracture healing. If callus is seen, the cast may be removed and healing assessed as noted earlier.

Stress Fractures

The term *stress fracture* is used to describe a type of fractures in which the bone composition is normal but the bone breaks after exposure to repeated overuse tensile or compression stress over time. This is in contrast to insufficiency fractures in which the bone composition is abnormal (e.g., osteoporosis) and the bone fractures when normal stress is applied. Stress fractures are classified as low risk or high risk based on the fracture site and the risk of complications, such as fracture propagation, nonunion, or displacement. Low-risk fractures

include those at the second through fourth metatarsal shafts, proximal humerus or humeral shaft, ribs, and pubic rami. High-risk sites are pars interarticularis of the lumbar spine, superior side of the femoral neck (i.e., tension side), anterior cortex of the tibia (i.e., tension side), tarsal navicular, and proximal fifth metatarsal.

Risk factors for stress injury to the bone include both extrinsic and intrinsic mechanical factors. Extrinsic factors include acute change in training routine (duration, intensity, frequency), footwear, and poor fitness level.[10,11] Intrinsic factors include bone mass, body composition, and biomechanical malalignment. A history of stress fractures is a predictor of future stress fractures in runners and military recruits. Especially in women, hormonal and nutritional factors influence the risk of stress fractures.[12] Delayed menarche, hypothalamic hypoestrogenic amenorrhea, and ovulatory disturbances place women at risk for stress fractures. Inadequate calcium, insufficient calories, and disordered eating are additional nutritional factors that adversely affect bone health. The combination of disordered eating, amenorrhea, and decreased bone density, termed the *female athlete triad*, puts women at particularly high risk for stress fractures.[13]

Clinical Presentation

The locations of stress fractures vary with the physical activity, but the vast majority of stress fractures

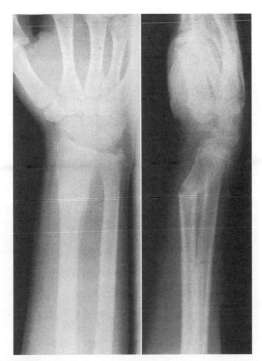

FIGURE 2-22 Follow-up radiograph taken 5 weeks after the radiograph shown in Fig. 2-21. Angulation has increased to 45 degrees, and abundant callus is present.

occur in the lower extremities. Most individuals report an insidious onset of pain that correlates with a change in equipment or training and is exacerbated by the offending activity. In the early stages, pain usually subsides shortly after exercise or activity. Most individuals with a stress fracture will have localized bony tenderness, and palpable periosteal thickening may be apparent, especially in persons with long-standing symptoms. Some persons have pain at the fracture site with percussion or vibration at a distance from the fracture, but this is an unreliable sign. Stress fractures of the femoral neck and navicular bone are often poorly localized. Joint ROM is usually maintained.

Imaging

Plain radiographs are indicated in the initial evaluation of a patient with a suspected stress fracture. Radiographic evidence of the fracture may not be present for weeks, and some fractures remain occult on plain films. Periosteal reaction may be the first clue to the presence of a fracture. Plain radiography is more likely to show a stress fracture in long bones such as the metatarsals, tibia, and fibula.

Although a triple-phase bone scan is highly sensitive in detecting stress fractures, it lacks specificity and can be falsely positive with shin splints. Because of these limitations, magnetic resonance imaging (MRI) has become the most useful radiographic modality in the evaluation of a suspected stress fracture when plain film results are negative.[14] MRI is also useful in distinguishing between shin splints and stress fractures and is better at differentiating pathologic fractures from stress fractures. Stress responses appear as edema in the bone: low signal on the T1-weighted sequences and higher signal (brighter) on T2-weighted and STIR (short tau inversion recovery) sequences (Fig. 2-23). MRI findings must be interpreted with caution, especially when no clear fracture is present, because isolated bone marrow edema is a nonspecific finding. The MRI appearance of stress response is similar to bone bruises, very early avascular necrosis, bone tumors, and osteomyelitis, but the clinical history usually allows distinction among these diagnostic possibilities. Stress responses of bone are distinguished from stress fractures by the absence of a fracture line that extends through the cortex into the medullary canal. The recovery time for a true stress fracture compared with that for a stress reaction can be similar, so the presence of the fracture line on MRI does not necessarily signal a longer symptomatic period.[15]

Ultrasonography is being used more extensively in the evaluation of overuse musculoskeletal conditions, and there are preliminary reports of its use in the diagnosis of lower extremity stress fractures.[16,17] It has not been adequately studied in enough different locations or in sufficient numbers to be recommended in the evaluation of a suspected stress fracture.

Indications for Orthopedic Referral

Patients with stress fractures at high-risk sites should be referred for possible operative management

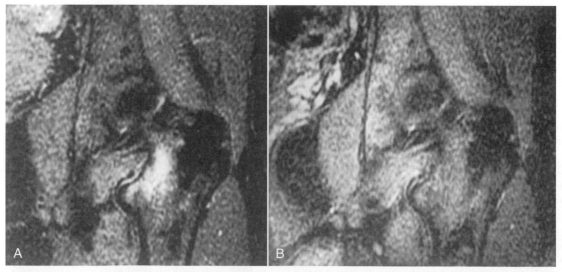

FIGURE 2-23 Stress response. Radiograph of the painful hip of a 28-year-old marathon runner. **A,** Coronal short tau inversion recovery (STIR) magnetic resonance image (MRI) of a focal area of increased signal in the region of the lesser tuberosity. The signal does not extend across the femoral neck, and no low signal intensity is apparent (e.g., *black line*). This distinguishes a stress response from a stress fracture. **B,** A coronal STIR MRI of virtual resolution of the previously identified bone edema. After 6 weeks of conservative management, the patient's symptoms resolved (*From Clin Sports Med 1997;16[2]:283.*)

because of the higher likelihood of nonunion and progression to complete fracture. Orthopedic referral should also be obtained for patients who cannot tolerate a lengthy rehabilitation process, when conservative treatment fails, and if follow-up imaging shows the fracture has extended or a nonunion has occurred.

Treatment

The treatment of stress fractures varies depending on the site (i.e., high or low risk). The goals of treatment include modification or reduction of activity to eliminate any pain, gradual rehabilitation of muscle strength and endurance, maintaining fitness, and reduction of risk factors as necessary. In general, early initiation of treatment leads to better outcomes. Typically, a period of 6 to 8 weeks of relative rest and refraining from the overuse stress is needed for bone healing. The rate of activity resumption should be modified based on symptoms and physical findings such as swelling and fracture site tenderness. Proper nutrition, including intake of adequate calories, calcium, and vitamin D, is essential for those with altered bone density and should be encouraged in all patients. A biomechanical evaluation to uncover factors contributing to overuse should also be performed.

The clinician should reevaluate the patient every few weeks during treatment. Pain should gradually resolve, so if symptoms persist after several weeks, compliance with the treatment should be evaluated. Those with persistent pain despite proper treatment may need more activity modification, further protection of the bone, and a more gradual rehabilitation program. After the diagnosis of a stress fracture is confirmed, follow-up imaging is rarely needed because clinical response to treatment is adequate to confirm healing for the vast majority of patients. Repeat imaging is reserved for those who fail to progress appropriately during the treatment period.

Return to Work or Sports

The time required to return to full work or competitive sports varies based on the bone affected, the length of symptoms, underlying bone health, and compliance with treatment. In general, 10 to 14 weeks are typically required for a full resumption of activity after a lower extremity stress fracture.

LATE FRACTURE COMPLICATIONS

Complex Regional Pain Syndrome

Complex regional pain syndrome (CRPS), an uncommon late complication of a fractured extremity, is the term used to describe a wide variety of regional, post traumatic, neuropathic pain conditions.[18] This syndrome was formerly known as reflex sympathetic dystrophy (RSD) because it was theorized that a pathologic sympathetically maintained reflex arc was responsible for the pain. CRPS has been subdivided into two types. Type I represents about 90% of the cases and corresponds to patients without a definable nerve lesion. In type II, a specific nerve lesion is present. The clinical features are identical, however. The pathogenesis of this disorder is unknown, and it can develop after a relatively minor injury. Fractures with associated soft tissue, nerve, or vascular injury may be at highest risk for this complication. Orthopedic consultation should be obtained for any patient in whom this condition is suspected.

Clinical Features

Most patients, but not all with CRPS, have an identifiable inciting injury, surgery, or vascular event (e.g., myocardial infarction or stroke) followed by pain, allodynia, hyperalgesia, abnormal vasomotor activity, and abnormal sudomotor (sweat) activity. Allodynia is disproportionately increased pain in response to a nonnoxious stimulus, and *hyperalgesia* refers to the disproportionate pain in response to mildly noxious stimuli. The quality of the pain is often burning and out of proportion to the initial injury. Symptoms of sympathetic dysfunction, such as color changes, temperature changes, and excessive sweating, typically wax and wane and may be late findings. Other symptoms include joint stiffness and swelling, muscle weakness, and dystonic movements. Patients with CRPS may adopt a protective posture of the extremity to guard against mechanical and thermal stimuli. Trophic changes occur much later in the course of CRPS. Nail and hair growth may be increased or decreased, brawny edema may be present, and contractures and loss of function may occur.

Diagnosis

No specific test is available to confirm the diagnosis of CRPS, and no pathognomonic clinical feature exists to identify the condition. Diagnostic testing is performed to exclude other conditions. Plain radiographs are helpful in the initial evaluation of a patient suspected of having CRPS to rule out other causes of pain in the extremity. The characteristic finding in CRPS is diffuse bone demineralization that begins near the joint and eventually involves the entire bone. Diffuse osteopenic changes are usually apparent several weeks after the onset of symptoms and become progressively more severe with time. As many as one third of patients with this condition have normal radiographs.

Specialized autonomic tests of resting sweat output or skin temperature may provide objective diagnostic help but are not widely available and require a specialist to perform the test.[19] These tests may be most useful in medicolegal cases requiring objective evidence of altered sympathetic nervous system function. Delayed bone scintigraphy will reveal increased uptake and thus increased vascularity after 6 weeks of symptoms and is most useful as a diagnostic tool in the early stages of the condition. Both bone scintigraphy and MRI have low sensitivity but high specificity for CRPS.[20] A regional sympathetic nerve block may be the most useful diagnostic and therapeutic test available. Quick and transient relief from pain and dysthesia after the nerve block are suggestive of CRPS.

Treatment

Prevention is the best treatment for CRPS, and recently vitamin C has been used to prevent CRPS after wrist fractures.[21] The earlier that treatment is initiated for CRPS, the better the prognosis for symptom relief. Successful treatment depends on a multidisciplinary approach.[22] Physical therapy to improve function, psychologic assessment, and counseling and patient education are key aspects of treatment. Adequate analgesia is necessary to allow the patient to participate fully in rehabilitation.

The medications that have been found to be useful for treating patients with CRPS include gabapentin, bisphosphonates, corticosteroids, nasal calcitonin.[23] Antidepressant medications are often helpful in treating those with neuropathic pain. Using an opioid is appropriate when pain is not controlled with other approaches such as ice, heat, nonnarcotic analgesics, or NSAIDs. Adjunctive treatment such as biofeedback, transcutaneous electrical nerve stimulation (TENS), splinting, or trigger point injections may also aid the patient.

If conservative measures fail, interruption of the abnormal sympathetic reflex can be considered, especially in patients with signs and symptoms of sympathetic dysfunction and a positive response to a diagnostic sympathetic nerve block. Other invasive treatments such as spinal cord stimulation, sympathectomy, and intrathecal analgesia should be reserved for patients with the most severe and refractory symptoms.

Osteomyelitis

Osteomyelitis after a fracture is considered chronic or nonhematogenous and is the result of a contiguous spread of infection from adjacent soft tissue, usually in the presence of an open fracture or after surgical fixation. Bacterial pathogens include *Staphylococcus aureus*, coagulase-negative staphylococci, and aerobic gram-negative bacilli, although chronic osteomyelitis is polymicrobial in more than 30% of cases. The long bones of the extremities are most often involved.

Clinical Presentation

The symptoms of chronic osteomyelitis are often insidious. Pain, low-grade fever, and localized swelling and erythema are typical. The external findings may be quite minimal. Drainage from a sinus tract is highly suggestive of osteomyelitis. With long-standing infection, the patient may experience loss of appetite and weight.

Blood culture results are usually negative in chronic osteomyelitis. The sedimentation rate is often elevated but is too nonspecific to be useful. White blood cell counts are only occasionally elevated in this condition. Cultures of the drainage from a sinus tract are often unrevealing and should not be used to determine antibiotic treatment. Bone biopsy is the only reliable means of accurately confirming the diagnosis and identifying the causative agent. Open biopsy yields superior results to percutaneous needle biopsy.[24]

The differential diagnosis for patients with suspected osteomyelitis after a fracture includes cellulitis, acute septic arthritis, gout, rheumatoid arthritis, and acute rheumatic fever. The radiographic findings typical of osteomyelitis help distinguish this condition from the more superficial cellulitis. Synovial fluid examination is helpful in distinguishing the acute arthropathies from osteomyelitis.

Imaging

The diagnosis of chronic osteomyelitis may be aided by plain radiographs, although their sensitivity and specificity are low. Typical findings include areas of radiolucency, irregular areas of destruction, periosteal thickening, and radiodense sequestra. Bone sclerosis is a late sign and indicates a long-standing infection. A triple-phase bone scan is highly sensitive and accurate in identifying osteomyelitis, but MRI is replacing radionuclide imaging because of its superior soft tissue resolution and ability to accurately define the extent and location of the infection.[25]

Treatment

Chronic osteomyelitis is often difficult to eradicate. Orthopedic referral is essential for all patients in whom this condition is diagnosed because surgical debridement is usually necessary. Management decisions depend on the location, causal organisms, and extent and duration of the infection. The optimal length of antibiotic therapy is not known but usually extends until debrided bone is covered by vascularized soft tissue. Prevention of osteomyelitis is of the utmost importance because of the difficulty in curing the infection after it is established. Meticulous irrigation and debridement of an open fracture to eliminate any wound contamination are paramount. Prophylactic antibiotics reduce the risk of osteomyelitis and should be given parenterally within 6 hours after open trauma and continued for 48 to 72 hours total or at least for 24 hours after wound closure.[26]

MANAGEMENT OF PEDIATRIC FRACTURES

Approximately 20% of children who seek injury evaluation have a fracture. Although the incidence of fractures varies by age, gender, and season of the year, the chance of a child's sustaining a fracture during childhood (birth to 16 years) has been estimated at 42% for boys and 27% for girls.[27] The most common injury sites in descending order of occurrence are fractures of the distal radius, hand (carpals, metacarpals, phalanges), elbow, clavicle, radial shaft, tibial shaft, foot, ankle, femur, and humerus.[28]

Management decisions for pediatric fractures differ from those for treatment of adult fractures for several reasons. In children's fractures, bone growth may be affected, abundant callus may form during healing, clinical healing is faster, fracture remodeling is more pronounced, children tolerate prolonged immobilization much better, and rehabilitation after immobilization is usually not needed. Fractures in children are generally less complicated and are more often treated by closed means, and nonunion is rare because of the abundant blood supply of growing bone. Certain fractures are much more common in children than adults or have characteristic patterns based on a childhood cause of injury or the unique features of growing bone. Knowledge of normal bone growth and development and the patterns of physeal injuries assists primary care providers in managing common pediatric fractures. It is beyond the scope of this book to discuss all fractures in children. Readers are directed to standard orthopedic fracture textbooks for more in-depth discussions of less common pediatric fractures.

Growing Bone

Anatomic Considerations

The major anatomic regions of growing bone include the epiphysis, physis, metaphysis, and diaphysis (Fig. 2-24). The epiphysis is a secondary ossification center at the end of long bones separated from the rest of the bone by the physis. The epiphysis is covered with articular cartilage or perichondrium. At birth, nearly all of the epiphyses are completely cartilaginous. Over time, they ossify

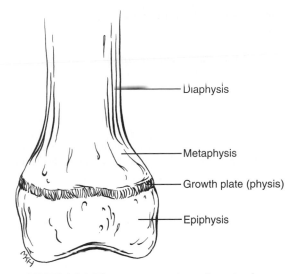

FIGURE 2-24 The anatomic regions of growing bone.

and thus become visible on radiographs. An apophysis is an epiphysis under tension at the site of a tendon insertion; it is not articular and does not participate in longitudinal growth. The tibial tuberosity where the patellar tendon attaches is one example of an apophysis. Apophyseal injuries do not interfere with growth and are typically overuse self-limited conditions in adolescents. The physis, or growth plate, contains cells that continuously divide and create new bone cells along the metaphyseal border, thereby adding to the length and girth of the bone. The metaphysis, which attaches to the physis, is the flared portion of bone at either end of the diaphysis (shaft). It begins at the portion of the bone where cortical bone diminishes and trabecular bone increases.

The rates of appearance of ossification centers and the subsequent rates of physeal closure vary depending on the bone. The relative lack of ossification of many epiphyses in young children and the radiolucency of growth plates can make fracture identification difficult. Although comparison views of the uninjured side need not be obtained in every case, they can assist clinicians in detecting fractures in skeletally immature patients when the source of injury and clinical examination suggest a fracture.

Differences Between Pediatric and Adult Fractures

Several factors contribute to the differences between fractures in children and adults. The attachment of the physis to the metaphysis is a point of decreased strength in the bone and becomes the site of injury after musculoskeletal trauma in children. Ligaments and tendons are relatively stronger than growing bone. With the same amount of injuring force, a child is more likely to fracture a bone, but an adult is more likely to tear a ligament, muscle, or tendon.

A child's periosteum is thicker, stronger, and more biologically active than that of an adult. The periosteum separates easily from the injured bone in children but is much less likely to be torn completely. A significant portion usually remains intact and functions as a hinge to lessen fracture displacement, and it serves as an internal restraint during closed reductions. The periosteum provides some tissue continuity across the fracture site, which promotes more rapid healing and stability.

The normal process of bone remodeling in children may realign malaligned fracture fragments, making near anatomic reductions less important in pediatric fractures than with adult fractures. Remodeling can be expected if the patient has 2 or more years of remaining bone growth, because mild angular deformities often correct themselves as the bone grows (Fig. 2-25). The potential for correction of fracture deformity is greater if the child is younger, if the fracture is closer to the physis, and if the angulation is in the same plane of motion as the nearest joint. The amount of remodeling is not predictable, so displaced fractures should still be reduced to achieve acceptable alignment. Rotational deformities are not usually corrected with bone remodeling.

Fractures in children may stimulate longitudinal growth of the bone. This increased growth may make the bone longer than it would have been if it had not been injured. Thus, some degree of fracture fragment overlap and shortening is acceptable and even desirable in certain fractures to counterbalance the anticipated overgrowth. This is particularly true for fractures of the femoral or tibial shaft.

Fracture Types

Growing bone in children has unique qualities that lead to different fracture types. A torus or buckle fracture occurs in response to a compressive force similar to the impacted fracture in an adult. This fracture usually occurs at the junction of the porous metaphysis, and the denser diaphysis is considered quite stable. A fracture of the shaft of a child's bone often results in a greenstick fracture, which involves a break of only one cortex. Immature bone has the ability to bow rather than break in response to applied force. This bowing is referred to as *plastic deformation* and typically occurs in long thin bones such as the ulna and fibula. If the deformity occurs in a young child (<3 years old) and is less than 20 degrees angulated, the deformity will usually self-correct.[29] Radiographic examples of fracture types unique to children are shown in Fig. 2-26 to Fig. 2-28.

Physeal Injuries

Injuries to the physis or growth plate constitute approximately 20% of all skeletal injuries in children. Girls tend to get growth plate injuries at an earlier age (9-12 years) compared with boys (12-15 years).[30] Damage to the physis can disrupt the speed of bone growth. A fracture through the physis results in a slower growth rate in the injured area while the remaining portion of the physis grows at its normal rate. This may cause angular deformities as the bone lengthens. The extent of growth plate disturbance is difficult to predict because disruption of the physis itself causes slowing, but injury near but not involving the physis may actually stimulate growth.

Most growth disturbance after a physeal injury is seen in a premature partial arrest of growth. The arrest is produced when a bone bridge or bar crosses the physis. As the uninjured physis grows, angular deformity occurs. Any fracture of a physis may result in a bone bar, but the size of the physis, its rate of growth, and its contour all affect bone bar production. Small uniplanar physes, such as in the phalanges and distal radius, are uncommon sites for bone bars, but the large irregular physes of the distal femur and proximal tibia account for the majority of bone bars.

The prognosis for physeal injuries is determined by several factors. The most important factors are the severity of injury (displacement, degree of comminution), the patient's age, the physis injured, and the radiographic type (discussed later). The severity of injury is the most important of these factors in determining prognosis. Physeal injury in a younger patient has a greater chance for growth disturbance and requires close monitoring. The site of injury affects the outcome. The distal femur and proximal tibia are prone to growth disturbance, and deformity is more likely at these sites because they contribute more longitudinal growth. The proximal radius and ulna and distal humerus contribute little to eventual bone length. Thus, growth arrest in these sites rarely causes deformity or length inequality.

Classification

Classification schemes for physeal injuries based on their radiographic configuration are designed to stratify injuries according to their relative risk of growth disturbance. The most often used scheme is the one put forth by Salter and Harris in 1963 (Fig. 2-29).[31] Type II fractures are by far the most common (accounting for approximately 50% of these injuries), followed in descending order by types I, III, IV, and V.

A type I injury is a disruption of the physis without injury to the epiphysis or metaphysis. The

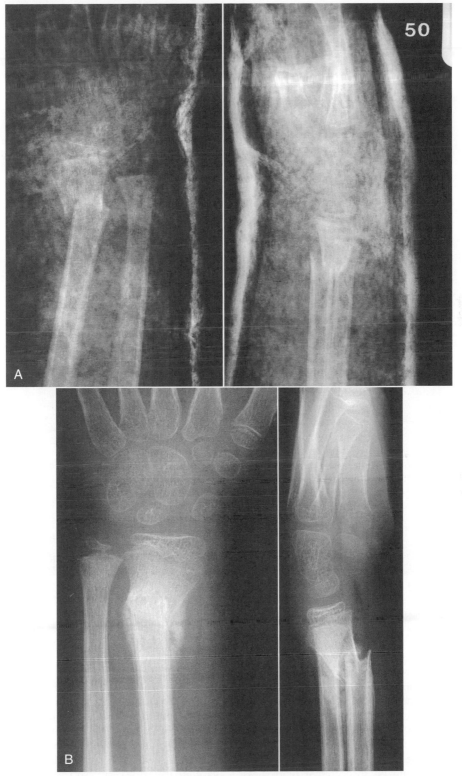

FIGURE 2-25 A, Six-year-old girl with an acute wrist injury. Radiograph of the wrist in plaster reveals a transverse fracture of the distal radius with lateral and dorsal translation and radial angulation of the distal fragment. The patient was treated with a long arm cast. **B,** Three weeks after injury. Prominent callus is present. The radial angulation is unchanged, and the dorsal angulation has increased. The patient had no tenderness over the fracture, and the cast was discontinued.

(Continued)

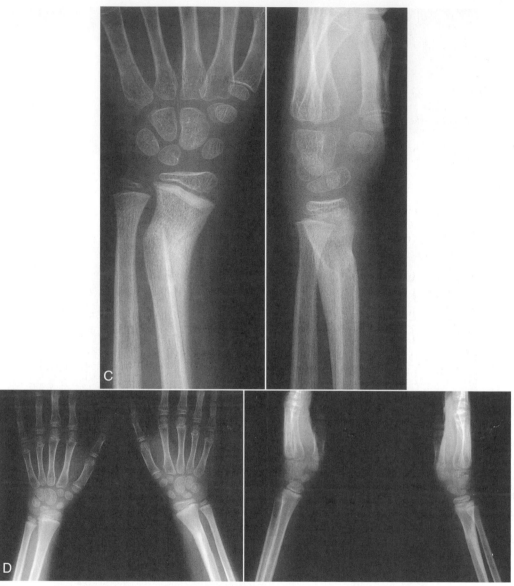

FIGURE 2-25, cont'd **C,** Two months after injury. The fracture shows further healing with decreased dorsal angulation and increased radial angulation. **D,** Six months after injury. Comparison radiographs show remodeling of the fracture with near anatomic alignment compared with the uninjured wrist. The fracture site is now barely visible.

separation usually occurs between the physis and metaphysis. These injuries can be difficult to detect when they are nondisplaced. The most common radiographic finding is widening of the physis, which may be apparent only on one view (Fig. 2-30). Comparison views of the uninjured side are often helpful in the diagnosis of these injuries. A type I fracture should be suspected if tenderness over the physis exists after an injury even if initial radiographs are normal. Type I fractures of the distal radius often result in displacement of the epiphysis (Fig. 2-31), and these injuries have a higher likelihood of physeal growth arrest.

Type II fractures are usually easily identified on routine radiographs (Fig. 2-32). These fractures course through a portion of the physis and then extend obliquely through the metaphysis. The periosteum on the side of the metaphyseal fragment often remains attached, which lends stability to fracture reduction and healing. Type II fractures vary greatly in severity, so the chance of impaired growth is variable. Factors leading to a more serious prognosis are an irregular and undulating physis (as in the distal femur or proximal tibia), fracture displacement, a large amount of the physis involved, and younger age of the child.

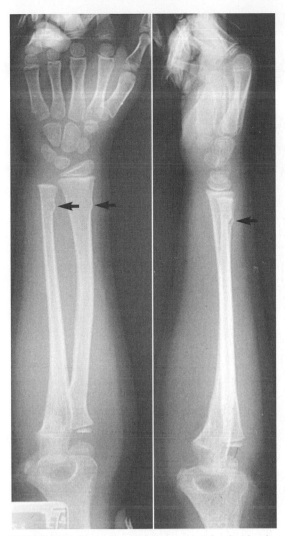

FIGURE 2-26 Torus (buckle) fractures of the distal radius and ulna (*arrows*).

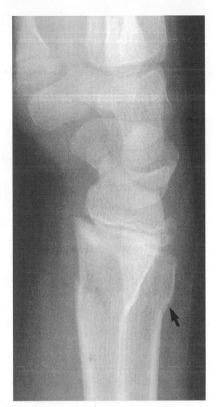

FIGURE 2-27 Lateral view of the wrist reveals a greenstick fracture of the radial metaphysis. A torus fracture of the ulna is also present (*arrow*).

A type III injury is an intraarticular fracture through the epiphysis that extends across the physis to the periphery (Fig. 2-33). In this type of fracture, a portion of the physis separates from its metaphyseal attachment. This type is more common when part of the physis begins to close in older children. Premature growth arrest frequently occurs after this injury, but bone length discrepancy is uncommon because the patient is often close to skeletal maturity. Angular deformity is unusual because the growth arrest is usually complete rather than partial. Treatment of type III fractures frequently requires open reduction because anatomic reduction of the articular surface is essential.

The fracture line in a type IV injury traverses the epiphysis, physis, and metaphysis (Fig. 2-34). These fractures are usually caused by axial loading

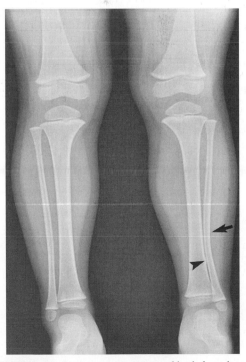

FIGURE 2-28 Anteroposterior view of both legs demonstrating plastic deformation of the left fibula (*arrow*). A torus fracture of the distal tibia is also apparent (*arrowhead*).

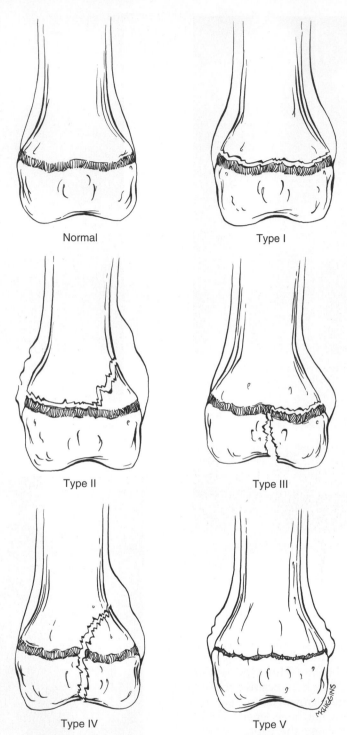

FIGURE 2-29 The Salter-Harris classification of physeal injuries.

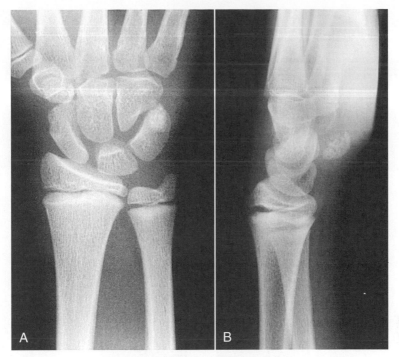

FIGURE 2-30 A Salter-Harris type I fracture of the distal radius. The anteroposterior view appears normal (**A**), but widening of the physis (**B**) is apparent in the injured radius on the lateral view.

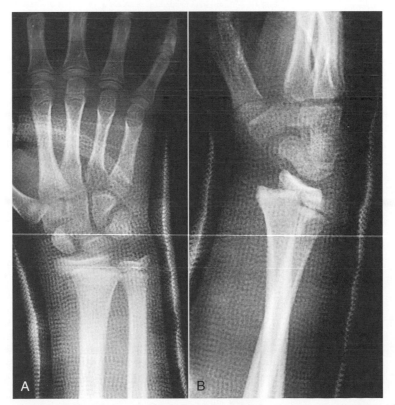

FIGURE 2-31 Anteroposterior (**A**) and, lateral (**B**) views of the wrist showing a type I fracture with dorsal and radial displacement of the distal radius epiphysis.

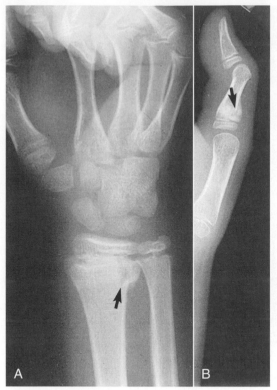

FIGURE 2-32 Examples of Salter-Harris type II fractures. **A,** Type II fracture of the distal radius (*arrow*). **B,** Type II fracture of the proximal phalanx of the thumb (*arrow*).

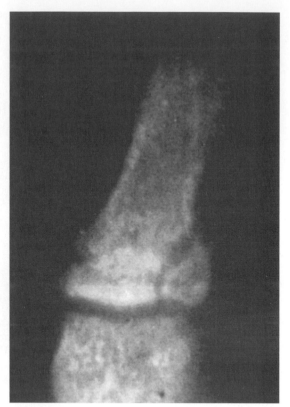

FIGURE 2-34 Type IV fracture of the distal phalanx.

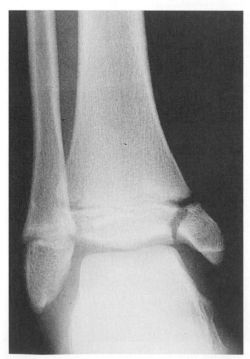

FIGURE 2-33 Type III fracture of the distal tibia.

or shear stress, and comminution is common. The risk of growth disturbance is highest in this type of fracture. Operative fixation to achieve anatomic reduction is nearly always required, and close follow-up to monitor for bone length discrepancies and angular deformities is essential.

Type V injuries are extremely rare, and some clinicians question whether or not this type even exists because it is diagnosed only in retrospect months or years after the original injury. In this type of injury, the physis sustains a crush or compression injury and is at great risk of growth arrest. These injuries initially have the same features as nondisplaced type I injuries: normal radiographs, tenderness over the physis, and some radiographic evidence of healing within 2 to 3 weeks. It is only when growth disturbance is discovered much later that a diagnosis can be made.

Clinicians have recently described a type VI fracture in which a portion of the physis has been removed or sheared off. Usually a portion of the accompanying epiphysis or metaphysis is also missing. These injuries are open fractures and most often result from gunshots or machinery trauma, such as that caused by a lawnmower or farm equipment. Premature closure of the exposed surface nearly always occurs, resulting in asymmetric bone growth.

Management of Physeal Injuries

In general, the risk of growth disturbance after a physeal injury increases as injuries progress from type I to type VI. Children with types III, IV, V, and VI fractures should be referred to an orthopedic surgeon for definitive care. Nondisplaced types I and II fractures can be managed effectively by primary care providers who adhere to general treatment principles. These fractures usually heal well with closed treatment. Both type I and type II fractures should be followed up long enough to ensure that normal growth resumes. The duration of follow-up varies depending on the severity of the injury and the age of the child. Three months may be adequate after a type I fracture, but at least 6 months are required after a type II fracture. Monthly radiographs should be obtained during this follow-up period. Type I fractures with displacement of the epiphysis, displaced type II fractures, or type II fractures involving a large portion of the physis, in a younger child, or involving the femur or tibia should prompt an orthopedic referral. Patients with displaced fractures requiring reduction should be referred as soon as possible because each day of delay makes reduction more difficult. Reduction maneuvers should be performed as gently as possible to reduce the risk of damage to the physeal cartilage, and repeated reduction attempts are best avoided.

Informing the patient and the parent about the possibility of growth disturbance after a physeal injury is essential. The likelihood of occurrence based on the Salter-Harris type and regardless of the treatment chosen should be explained. The need for consistent follow-up to monitor the growth of the bone radiographically should be emphasized.

Treatment Guidelines

Sedation and Analgesia

Proper sedation and analgesia are important in the management of fractures in pediatric patients. Sedation is often needed before a closed reduction is performed in a young child. Procedural sedation is generally used in the emergency setting, and effective and safe sedation requires the selection of appropriate drugs given in the appropriate doses on properly selected patients. The clinician must determine the appropriate level of sedation or analgesia (or both) required for a particular fracture procedure. Children receiving deep sedation should have an intravenous line; lighter levels of sedation accomplished through oral, nasal, or intramuscular routes may not require this.

Respiratory depression is always a concern when procedural sedation is performed, especially with a combination of sedative agents. Regardless of the intended level of sedation, the patient may move into a deeper state of sedation without warning. Respiratory rate, blood pressure, and oxygen saturation must be monitored vigilantly by qualified medical personnel. Before any attempt at sedation is made, the presence of resuscitation equipment and individuals trained in life support is required.

The choice of pharmacologic agents for procedural sedation in children should be based on the type of procedure, the patient's underlying medical condition, and the clinician's level of experience and comfort with the various agents. Sedative-hypnotic agents commonly used in the emergency department setting include benzodiazepines, ketamine, barbiturates, etomidate, and propofol. Midazolam is a short-acting benzodiazepine with a rapid onset of action and is widely used for pediatric sedation. Because midazolam has no analgesic activity, supplementation with opioids or regional anesthetic blocks is necessary. Close cardiorespiratory monitoring is essential because the combination of an opioid and benzodiazepine can lead to respiratory depression. A complete discussion of pediatric sedation is beyond the scope of this book, and readers are directed to reviews on the subject.[32,33]

Immobilization and Rehabilitation

Children tolerate prolonged immobilization much better than adults. Disabling stiffness or loss of ROM is distinctly unusual after pediatric fractures. After cast immobilization, physical therapy is rarely needed because children tend to resume their normal activity gradually without much supervision. Even though fractures of growing bones generally heal with a large callus, the new bone is still fibrous and not yet restored to its original strength. Depending on the child's activity level and age, a 2- to 4-week period of protection from collision or contact activities is usually prudent after immobilization is discontinued.

Fractures of Abuse

Physical abuse of children unfortunately occurs far too frequently in the United States. Fractures are the second most common injury after soft tissue injuries in physically abused children.[34] A majority of fractures in children younger than 1 year of age are caused by physical abuse, and abuse accounts for a significant portion of fractures in children younger than age 3 years.[35] In abused children who sustain a fracture, most have a single fracture with the most common locations being the femur, humerus, and skull.[36]

History

In the evaluation of a child with a musculoskeletal injury, the examiner must obtain a thorough history to assess the possibility that the injury was not accidental. The specifics surrounding the episode of trauma should be delineated and documented carefully. If possible, the child should be interviewed separately from the parent or caregiver. A nonjudgmental approach that includes asking open-ended questions and avoiding leading ones is best. Important questions include, "What exactly happened?" "Who witnessed the event?" and "Who discovered the injury?" The examiner should attempt to establish what the child was doing at the time of the injury, when the incident occurred, when health care was obtained, who is responsible for child care, and the current household circumstances. The caregiver or parents' telling of the history, reaction to the event, interaction with the child, and cooperation with the health care team should be observed carefully for signs of evasiveness, vagueness, or inconsistency in reporting the circumstances of the injury.

Knowledge of the usual causes for individual injuries and fractures and understanding of the developmental abilities of the child are essential in making a diagnosis of child abuse. The clinician should try to decide whether the reported trauma history is consistent with the severity or extent of the injury. Although it is not unusual for young children to fall, it is unusual for them to sustain a significant injury from the fall alone, and it is quite rare for an infant to sustain a fracture from a fall from a sofa or changing table.[37] Inconsistencies between the mechanism of injury described by the parent or caregiver and the child's injuries warrant a report to Child Protective Services.

Physical Examination

The physical examination of a child with a musculoskeletal injury should be thorough enough to detect evidence of abuse beyond a fracture. Suspicious burns or scars; retinal hemorrhages; bruises on the back of the head, buttocks, abdomen, cheeks, or genitalia; signs of neglect; lesions in various stages of healing; and different types of injuries coexisting all are findings that should raise suspicion of child abuse. Care should be taken in evaluating bruises in Southeast Asian children who may have been subjected to the cultural healing practice of "cupping" or "coining," which leaves circular lesions on the skin.

Imaging

The radiographic evaluation for suspected child abuse is based on the presenting complaints, physical findings and age of the child. The skeletal survey is considered the method of choice for global skeletal imaging in cases of suspected child abuse and is mandatory for all children younger than two years of age according to the American Academy of Pediatrics Section on Radiology.[38] The standard skeletal survey includes AP and lateral views of the skull and chest; lateral views of the spine; AP views of the pelvis, long bones of the extremities, and feet; and posteroanterior oblique views of the hands. The skeletal survey should be followed by additional detailed views of any site where abnormalities are detected. A repeat skeletal survey taken 2 weeks after the initial evaluation may increase the diagnostic yield and is recommended in high-risk cases. The second study may show fractures that were not apparent initially and may aid in determining the fracture age more precisely. If unchanged from the initial evaluation, the second survey may also suggest an explanation other than fracture for the original abnormalities and may lower the suspicion of abuse.[39]

Radionuclide bone scanning is more sensitive to plain radiography in the evaluation of suspected child abuse but has several disadvantages compared with the skeletal survey, including lower specificity, higher cost, frequent need for sedation, and inability to determine the age of the fracture. For these reasons, skeletal survey is the preferred first-line screening test.

Determining the fracture age based on the stages of fracture healing is often needed in the evaluation of child abuse. The progression of changes is as followed:

- First 7 to 10 days: Soft tissue changes
- 7 to 14 days: Periosteal new bone
- 2 to 3 weeks: Increased fracture gap caused by resorption of necrotic bone at the fracture edges
- 2 to 3 weeks: Soft callus
- 3 to 6 weeks: Hard callus

Fracture Patterns

No particular fracture pattern or location is pathognomonic of child abuse. Fractures suspicious for child abuse include any fracture of the femur in a child who is too young to walk, any fracture that is inconsistent with the history provided by the caregivers, any fracture that occurs in combination with nonskeletal injuries, any healing fracture for which there was a delay in seeking medical attention, and multiple fractures in various stages of healing. Fracture locations that are more suggestive of intentional injury in children include the skull (in children younger than 18 months of age), rib, sternum, scapula, spinous process, and metaphyseal corner.

REFERENCES

1. Dimitriou R, Tsiridis E, Giannoudis PV. Current concepts of molecular aspects of bone healing. *Injury.* 2005;36: 1392-1404.
2. Gaston MS, Simpson AH. Inhibition of fracture healing. *J Bone Joint Surg Br.* 2007;89:1553-1560.
3. Van Staa, TP, Leufkens HG, Abenhaim L, et al. Use of oral corticosteroids and risk of fractures. *J Bone Miner Res.* 2000;15:993-1000.
4. Dodwell ER, Latorre JG, Parisini E, et al. NSAID exposure and risk of nonunion: a meta-analysis of case-control and cohort studies. *Calcif Tissue Int.* 2010;87(3):193-202.
5. Mellor A, Soni N. Fat embolism. *Anaesthesia.* 2001;56: 145-154.
6. Schlickewei W, Kuner EH, Mullaji AB, Gotze B. Upper and lower limb fractures with concomitant arterial injury. *J Bone Joint Surg Br.* 1992;74:181-188.
7. Shadgan B, Menon M, O'Brien PJ, Reid WD. Diagnostic techniques in acute compartment syndrome of the leg. *J Orthop Trauma.* 2008;22:581-587.
8. Harris IA, Kadir A, Donald G. Continuous compartment pressure monitoring for tibia fractures: does it influence outcome? *J Trauma.* 2006;60:1330-1335.
9. Claes L, Grass R, Schmickal T, et al. Monitoring and healing analysis of 100 tibial shaft fractures. *Langenbecks Arch Surg.* 2002;387:146-152.
10. Jones BH, Thacker SB, Gilchrist J, et al. Prevention of lower extremity stress fractures in athletes and soldiers: a systematic review. *Epidemiol Rev.* 2002;24:228-247.
11. Rome K, Handoll HH, Ashford R. Interventions for preventing and treating stress fractures and stress reactions of bone of the lower limbs in young adults. *Cochrane Database Syst Rev.* 2005;(2):CD000450.
12. Callahan LR. Stress fractures in women. *Clin Sports Med.* 2000;19:303-314.
13. Nattiv A, Loucks AB, Manore MM, et al. American College of Sports Medicine position stand. The female athlete triad. *Med Sci Sports Exerc.* 2007;39:1867-1882.
14. Spitz DJ, Newberg AH. Imaging of stress fractures in the athlete. *Radiol Clin North Am.* 2002;40:313-331.
15. Yao L, Johnson C, Gentili A, et al. Stress injuries of bone: analysis of MR imaging staging criteria. *Acad Radiol.* 1998;5:34-40.
16. Banal F, Gandjbakhch F, Foltz V, et al. Sensitivity and specificity of ultrasonography in early diagnosis of metatarsal bone stress fractures: a pilot study of 37 patients. *J Rheumatol.* 2009;36:1715-1719.
17. Bodner G, Stockl B, Fierlinger A, et al. Sonographic findings in stress fractures of the lower limb: preliminary findings. *Eur Radiol.* 2005;15:356-359.
18. Stanton-Hicks M, Janig W, Hassenbusch S, et al. Reflex sympathetic dystrophy: changing concepts and taxonomy. *Pain.* 1995;63:127-133.
19. Schurmann M, Gradl G, Andress HJ, et al. Assessment of peripheral sympathetic nervous function for diagnosing early post-traumatic complex regional pain syndrome type I. *Pain.* 1999;80:149-159.
20. Schürmann M, Zaspel J, Löhr P, et al. Imaging in early posttraumatic complex regional pain syndrome: a comparison of diagnostic methods. *Clin J Pain.* 2007;23: 449-457.
21. Stevermer JJ, Ewigman B. Give vitamin C to avert lingering pain after fracture. *J Fam Pract.* 2008;57:86-89.
22. Stanton-Hicks MD, Burton AW, Bruehl SP, et al. An updated interdisciplinary clinical pathway for CRPS: report of an expert panel. *Pain Pract.* 2002;2:1-16.
23. Quisel A, Gill JM, Witherell P. Complex regional pain syndrome: which treatments show promise? *J Fam Pract.* 2005;54:599-603.
24. Howard CB, Einhorn M, Dagan R, et al. Fine needle bone biopsy to diagnose osteomyelitis. *J Bone Joint Surg (Br).* 1994;76(2):311-314.
25. Pineda C, Vargas A, Rodriguez AV. Imaging of osteomyelitis: current concepts. *Infect Dis Clin North Am.* 2006; 20:789-825.
26. Gosselin RA, Roberts I, Gillespie WJ. Antibiotics for preventing infection in open limb fractures. *Cochrane Database Syst Rev.* 2004;(1):CD003764.
27. Landin LA. Fracture patterns in children: analysis of 8,682 fractures with special reference to incidence, etiology and secular changes in a Swedish urban population 1950-1979. *Acta Orthop Scand Suppl.* 1983;202:1-109.
28. Wilkins KE, Aroojis AJ. The incidence of fractures in children. In: Beaty JH, Kasser JR, eds. Rockwood & Wilkins Fractures in Children. 6th ed. Philadelphia: Lippincott-Raven; 2006:5-20.
29. Mabrey JD, Fitch RD. Plastic deformation in pediatric fractures: mechanism and treatment. *J Pediatr Orthop.* 1989;9:310-314.
30. Peterson HA, Madhok R, Benson JT, et al. Physeal fractures: part 1. Epidemiology in Olmsted County, Minnesota, 1979-1988. *J Pediatr Orthop.* 1994;14:423-430.
31. Salter RB, Harris WR. Injuries involving the epiphyseal plate. *J Bone Joint Surg.* 1963;45(suppl A):587-622.
32. Mace SE, Barata IA, Cravero JP, et al. Clinical policy: evidence-based approach to pharmacologic agents used in pediatric sedation and analgesia in the emergency department. *Ann Emerg Med.* 2004;44:342-377.
33. Rodriquez E, Jordan R. Contemporary trends in pediatric sedation and analgesia. *Emerg Med Clin North Am.* 2002;20:199-222.
34. Kocher MS, Kasser JR. Orthopaedic aspects of child abuse. *J Am Acad Orthop Surg.* 2000;8:10-20.
35. Leventhal JM, Martin KD, Asnes AG. Incidence of fractures attributable to abuse in young hospitalized children: results from analysis of a United States database. *Pediatrics.* 2008;122:599-604.
36. King J, Diefendorf D, Apthorp J, et al. Analysis of 429 fractures in 189 battered children. *J Pediatr Orthop.* 1988;8:585-589.
37. Lyons TJ, Oates RK. Falling out of bed: a relatively benign occurrence. *Pediatrics.* 1993;92:125-127.
38. American Academy of Pediatrics, Section on Radiology. Diagnostic imaging of child abuse. *Pediatrics.* 2009;123:1430-1435.
39. Zimmerman S, Makoroff K, Care M, et al. Utility of follow-up skeletal surveys in suspected child physical abuse evaluations. *Child Abuse Negl.* 2005;29:1075-1083.

3

FINGER FRACTURES

Co-Author: Ryan C. Petering

Finger fractures are the most common types of fractures seen in primary care settings. Many of these fractures are sport or work related, but they may also occur in common activities of daily living such as housework, cleaning, and dressing. Finger fractures may be caused by blunt trauma, hyperextension, hyperflexion, or twisting forces. Distal phalanx fractures are the most common followed in frequency by proximal phalanx fractures and fractures of the middle phalanx. Most phalangeal fractures heal well without complication. Angulated or malrotation deformities can occur as a result of the numerous tendon attachments and muscle forces acting across fracture fragments. Knowledge of the typical deforming forces and evaluation of fracture stability are essential in the management of finger fractures.

See Appendix for stepwise instructions for gutter and thumb spica splints used in the treatment of finger fractures.

Go to Expert Consult for the electronic version of a patient instruction sheet named "Broken Hand or Wrist," which covers the steps of care from pain relief to rehabilitation exercises. This can be copied to hand out to patients to assist them during the treatment period.

DISTAL PHALANX FRACTURES

Anatomic Considerations

The extensor tendon splits at the midpoint of the proximal phalanx, forming the central slip that inserts on the middle phalanx and the lateral bands that reunite to insert at the dorsum of the base of the distal phalanx. The flexor digitorum profundus (FDP) inserts at the volar base of the distal phalanx. The FDP pulls the distal interphalangeal (DIP) joint into flexion when the extensor tendon is avulsed. Fibrous septa extend from the volar aspect of the distal phalanx to the skin. These fibrous septa support the distal phalanx, and thus most fractures in this location are stable.

Mechanism of Injury

Most fractures of the distal phalanx are caused by crushing injuries, which result in one of several fracture patterns: comminuted ("crushed eggshell"), transverse, or longitudinal (Fig. 3-1). Axial loads may also cause fractures of the distal phalanx. Frequently, distal phalanx fractures have associated extensive soft tissue injuries involving the tip of the finger, nail bed, or both. Avulsion fractures of the extensor and flexor tendons are discussed separately in the next section.

Clinical Presentation

The patient usually reports a crushing injury to the distal phalanx. On examination, the distal phalanx is tender and swollen. Range of motion (ROM) may be limited by swelling and pain. It is crucial to ensure active flexion and extension of the DIP joint to document tendon integrity. The nail may be torn, and the nail bed may be lacerated. If the nail is intact, a subungual hematoma may be present. In some cases, substantial amounts of soft tissue may be avulsed from the tip of the finger or the palmar tuft over the distal phalanx. In all distal finger injuries, it is important to document sensation to two-point discrimination (the normal discrimination distance is 5 mm).

Imaging

Three views of the distal phalanx are recommended: anteroposterior (AP), lateral, and oblique. Axial loads may cause either transverse or longitudinal fractures. The longitudinal fracture is usually stable, but the transverse fracture must be examined for angulation (Fig. 3-2). The nail bed can sometimes become lodged within a transverse distal phalanx fracture. Widening of the fracture site on the lateral view and avulsion of the root of the nail plate may indicate this complication. Fractures of the distal tip (tuft fractures) are often comminuted.

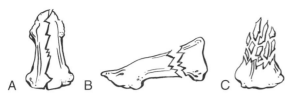

FIGURE 3-1 Distal phalanx fracture types. **A,** Longitudinal. **B,** Transverse. **C,** Comminuted or "crushed eggshell."

Indications for Orthopedic Referral

Emergent Referral

Open fractures, intraarticular fractures, tendon compromise, and fractures with vascular compromise should be evaluated by a specialist within 2 to 3 hours of injury.

Routine Referral

Angulated or displaced transverse fractures are often unstable and difficult to reduce because of interposition of soft tissue between the fracture fragments. If closed reduction is unsuccessful or reduction cannot be maintained with simple splinting, referral to an orthopedic surgeon for wire fixation is indicated.

Initial Treatment

Table 3-1 summarizes the management guidelines for distal phalanx fractures. The initial treatment of distal phalanx fractures should focus on management of the soft tissue injury and protective

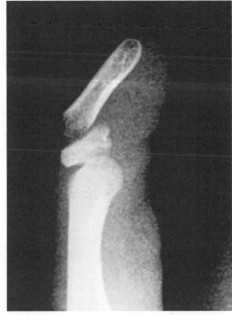

FIGURE 3-2 Angulated transverse fracture of the distal phalanx. *(From Browner BD, Jupiter JB, Levine AM, Trafton PG [eds]. Skeletal Trauma: Fractures, Dislocations, Ligamentous Injuries. Philadelphia, WB Saunders, 1992.)*

splinting. A U-shaped padded aluminum splint or fingertip guard should be anchored to the middle phalanx to provide protection for the tender distal phalanx and to maintain the DIP joint in extension. The splint should protect against blunt impacts to the fingertip during the healing period.

Table 3-1	*Management Guidelines for Distal Phalanx Fracture*
	INITIAL TREATMENT
Splint type and position	Protective aluminum splint, "U" shaped
	Distal interphalangeal joint in extension
Initial follow-up visit	1 to 2 weeks
Patient instruction	Keep finger elevated
	Avoid compressive tape or dressing
	FOLLOW-UP CARE
Cast or splint type and position	Same as above
Length of immobilization	3 to 4 weeks or until finger is no longer sensitive to impact
Healing time	4 to 6 weeks
Comminuted fractures may take several months for complete resolution of symptoms	
Follow-up visit interval	Every 2 to 4 weeks
Repeat radiography interval	Only need to repeat radiographs for persistent symptoms
Patient instruction	Continue active motion of PIP and MCP joints
	Nail deformity is possible
Indications for orthopedic consult	Angulated, open, or displaced transverse fractures
	Failed closed reduction
	Nonunion
	Severe persistent symptoms after 6 months

MCP, metacarpophalangeal; PIP, proximal interphalangeal.

Compressive circumferential taping of the distal phalanx should be avoided, especially in the case of a comminuted crush fracture. Elevation and ice should be used in the first 24 to 48 hours to reduce soft tissue swelling. The patient should be warned that these fractures may remain painful for months because of bleeding into the many fibrous septa in the finger pad.

Nail Bed Injury

A large or painful subungual hematoma that is less than 48 hours old should be drained. Beyond this time frame, the hematoma may be too clotted for drainage. Decompression of the hematoma is most easily achieved by burning a hole in the nail with a hot paper clip or cautery unit. Two or three holes may be needed for adequate drainage. If the pressure of a handheld drill or 18-gauge needle is too painful, digital nerve block should be considered when a subungual hematoma is drained. A large hematoma (i.e., a subungual hematoma involving more than 50% of the nail) associated with a distal phalanx fracture usually indicates an underlying nail bed laceration. No clear advantage is gained from removing an intact nail to repair a nail bed laceration.[1] The hematoma should be drained and the patient advised that there may be some deformity of the nail, although the intact nail usually lessens the deformity.

If the nail is avulsed, it should be removed and the nail bed repaired with absorbable interrupted sutures (6-0 or 7-0 chromic) under digital block anesthesia. The wound should be debrided of any nonviable or grossly contaminated tissue and thoroughly irrigated. The surrounding soft tissue injury should be loosely approximated. The cleansed nail should be placed back under the nail fold to splint the repair and to prevent adhesions from forming between the nail matrix and nail fold. Holes should be placed in the nail for drainage, and sutures should be placed laterally along the nail margins to prevent disruption of the germinal matrix of the nail. A sterile nonadherent dressing such as Vaseline gauze can be used as a substitute if the avulsed nail is unusable. The nail splint or gauze should remain in place for approximately 2 to 3 weeks until the new nail plate forms.

The use of prophylactic antibiotics after distal phalanx fractures complicated by nail bed laceration repair is controversial. A recent randomized controlled trial found no benefit with the addition of antibiotics to good wound care compared with placebo.[2] A first-generation cephalosporin antibiotics for 5 to 7 days should be considered if gross contamination has occurred, if the wound is more than 24 hours old, or if the patient is immunocompromised.

Follow-up Care

Most fractures of the distal phalanx, including comminuted tuft fractures, heal well with protective splinting for 3 to 4 weeks. The DIP joint should be immobilized, leaving the proximal interphalangeal (PIP) and metacarpophalangeal (MCP) joints free for ROM exercises. The splint should be used until the finger is no longer painful or sensitive to impact. Patients should be advised that some deformity of the nail is likely in the case of a nail bed injury, although the full extent of the deformity will not be apparent for 4 to 5 months.

Follow-up radiographs are not usually necessary because they do not alter management. However, repeat radiographs are recommended for evaluation of displaced transverse fractures that have undergone closed reduction or in patients who have severe symptoms despite splinting.

Return to Work or Sports

Patients with "crushed eggshell" or longitudinal fracture patterns may return to work or sports activities with adequate protection (e.g., "U"-shaped aluminum splint, volar splint) as long as pain is tolerable. Patients with transverse fractures should protect the finger until nontender because of the possible volar displacement of the distal fragment.

Complications

Delayed union can occur after a comminuted fracture of the distal phalanx. Nonunion is uncommon, but when present, it is usually caused by interposition of soft tissue between the fracture fragments. Patients with comminuted fractures may experience pain, hypersensitivity, or numbness and have difficulty with fine functions of the fingertip for several months.

Pediatric Considerations

Fractures of the distal phalanx in pediatric patients are usefully classified as extraphyseal or physeal. The management of extraphyseal fractures of the distal phalanx in children is similar to that in adults and is based on the stability of the fracture pattern and the status of the nail bed. Closed fractures with an intact nail bed are managed with splinting of the DIP joint and distal phalanx in extension for 3 to 4 weeks until clinical healing of the fracture site. The PIP joint should be left free for normal ROM. The patient may need protective splinting for contact activities for an additional 2 weeks. If the nail bed is lacerated, a digital nerve block is performed; the nail plate removed; and the nail bed debrided, irrigated, and repaired. Nail bed repair usually requires a fine absorbable suture material (e.g., 7-0 chromic). Unstable fractures (e.g., transverse fractures not reducible by closed means) should be referred to an orthopedic surgeon. Complications of distal phalanx fractures in pediatric patients include osteomyelitis and nail bed abnormalities. A patient with either of these complications should be referred to an orthopedic surgeon for definitive care.

Physeal injuries to the distal phalanx are discussed in the sections on mallet finger and jersey finger.

MALLET FINGER

This is the most common closed tendon injury of the finger. Mallet finger occurs more often in men than in women, but affected women are approximately 10 years older than men with this injury.[3] The long finger (third digit) is most commonly injured, followed by the ring finger, index finger, small finger, and thumb.

Mechanism of Injury

The so-called mallet finger injury is caused by avulsion of the extensor tendon from the dorsum of the base of the distal phalanx with or without an avulsed bony fragment. This injury results from forced flexion of the extended fingertip and can occur with sports (e.g., catching a ball) or with even minor household trauma (e.g., making a bed or dressing and undressing) (Fig. 3-3).

A zone of relative avascularity exists in the extensor tendon 11 to 16 mm proximal to the insertion of the terminal tendon at the dorsum of the distal phalanx. This zone of relative avascularity predisposes the patient to injury at this site and contributes to the complications and delays in healing seen with the mallet finger injury.

Clinical Presentation

The patient describes an injury consistent with forced flexion of the extended DIP joint and reports pain at the dorsum of the DIP. During physical examination, the patient has tenderness and swelling at the dorsum of the DIP and is unable

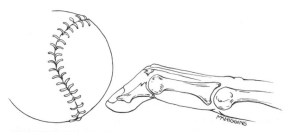

FIGURE 3-3 Mallet finger. Forced flexion of the distal interphalangeal joint causing avulsion of the extensor tendon.

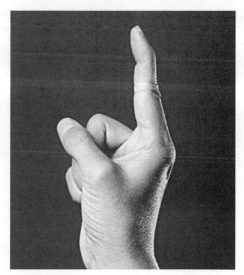

FIGURE 3-4 Mallet finger deformity.

to actively extend the DIP joint. Active extension at the DIP joint should be tested with all fingers in flexion. The typical mallet finger appearance is attributable to the unopposed flexor tendon at the DIP joint after the extensor tendon is avulsed (Fig. 3-4). Varying degrees of loss of extension indicate whether the tear of the tendon is partial or complete. Patients with partial tears have weak active extension and a loss of 5 to 20 degrees of extension ("extensor lag"). With a complete tendon rupture, the patient has total loss of active extension, and a 50- to 60-degree deformity or extensor lag is typical. The size of the bony avulsion does not necessarily correlate with the amount of extensor function lost.

Imaging

AP, lateral, and oblique views of the finger should be obtained. If radiographs show no apparent fracture, a pure tendon avulsion may have occurred. More commonly, a small fleck of bone may have been avulsed, which will be better visualized on the lateral view (Fig. 3-5). Occasionally, as much as one third of the articular surface is avulsed, and volar subluxation of the distal fragment is seen.

Indications for Orthopedic Referral

Because surgical treatment may result in infection or an unacceptably stiff DIP joint and splinting the finger produces results similar to surgery for acute mallet finger injuries, surgical intervention is reserved for special cases or particular fracture patterns.[4] Surgical referral should be considered for volar subluxation of the DIP joint (Fig. 3-6), inability to fully extend DIP passively, avulsion fracture involving greater than 30% of the articular

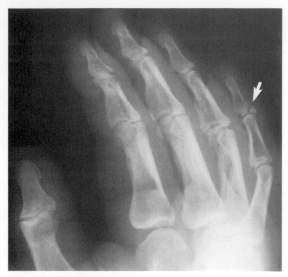

FIGURE 3-5 Minimally displaced mallet finger avulsion fracture of the fifth finger.

surface, or a "swan-neck" deformity (i.e., hyperextension of PIP joint or flexion of DIP joint).

Surgical treatment decisions should be individualized and take into account the time since the injury, the degree of loss of extension, the amount of functional disability, the ability of the patient to comply with conservative treatment, and the potential economic hardship of prolonged splinting in certain occupations.

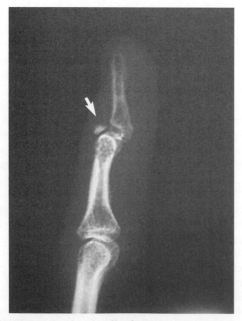

FIGURE 3-6 Displaced mallet finger avulsion fracture with volar subluxation of the distal phalanx.

Initial Treatment

Table 3-2 summarizes the management guidelines for mallet finger fractures. Most patients with mallet finger injuries should be treated conservatively with prolonged splinting of the DIP joint in slight hyperextension. Success rates for conservative treatment are similar to those for surgical treatment, and patient satisfaction with the outcome of treatment is good. Successful closed treatment requires careful attention to the details of treatment to avoid complications and loss of position.

The DIP joint should be splinted in slight hyperextension without causing pain. This can be done with a dorsally-placed padded aluminum splint, a volar unpadded splint, or a Stack splint (Fig. 3-7). The slightly hyperextended position of the DIP can be confirmed by inspection of the splinted finger from the lateral perspective. Overextension, which may lead to necrosis of skin over the DIP joint, should be avoided. Skin blanching while the splint is applied is a sign of overextension. It is important that the PIP joint is left free during splint application. Splinting has been shown to be effective for up to 3 months after injury. A Cochrane review did not find sufficient evidence that one type of splint was more effective than another.[5]

Follow-up Care

Nonsurgical treatment of the majority of mallet finger injuries is safe, effective, well tolerated, and cost efficient. Mallet finger injuries should be splinted in slight hyperextension continuously for 6 to 8 weeks. The patient must not let the DIP joint drop into flexion at any time during the period of continuous splinting and should be instructed to support the tip of the finger at all times when changing the splint (e.g., after bathing). The patient usually needs some assistance in changing or reapplying the splint because two hands are needed to hold this alignment and properly apply the splint. Compliance with these instructions should be assessed at each follow-up visit at 2-week intervals until healing has occurred.

After the continuous splint has been discontinued, nighttime splinting is recommended for an additional 2 to 3 weeks. Alternatively, a weaning period can be initiated in which the splint is removed three times daily to allow ROM exercises for the DIP joint and then replaced. If flexion of the DIP joint occurs at some point during the healing process, the time clock goes back to "day 1," and the 6-week splinting procedure should be restarted.

Complete radiographic healing of distal phalanx fractures often takes up to 5 months. Repeat radiographs should be obtained at the conclusion of

Table 3-2	Management Guidelines for Dorsal Avulsion Fracture ("Mallet Finger")
	INITIAL TREATMENT
Splint type and position	Dorsal padded aluminum splint, volar splint, stack splint
	DIP joint in slight hyperextension
Initial follow-up visit	2 weeks
Patient instruction	Do not attempt to flex DIP joint
	Get assistance with changing or retaping splint
	FOLLOW-UP CARE
Cast or splint type and position	Same as above
Length of immobilization	6 to 8 weeks followed by 2 to 3 weeks of nighttime-only splinting
Healing time	8 to 10 weeks
Follow-up visit interval	Every 2 weeks
	Assess compliance with continuous splinting
Repeat radiography interval	6 weeks after injury
	Every 1 to 2 months if the patient remains symptomatic
Patient instruction	Must keep DIP joint extension at all times
	Do not attempt to flex DIP joint
Indications for orthopedic consult	Volar displacement of distal phalanx
	Consider for displaced or more than 30% articular involvement
	Late mallet deformity after failed attempt at splinting
	Swan-neck deformity
	Inability to passively extend DIP

DIP, distal interphalangeal.

continuous splinting and then every 1 to 2 months if the patient remains symptomatic.

Return to Work or Sports

Patients with mallet finger injuries may return to work or sports with adequate protection of the

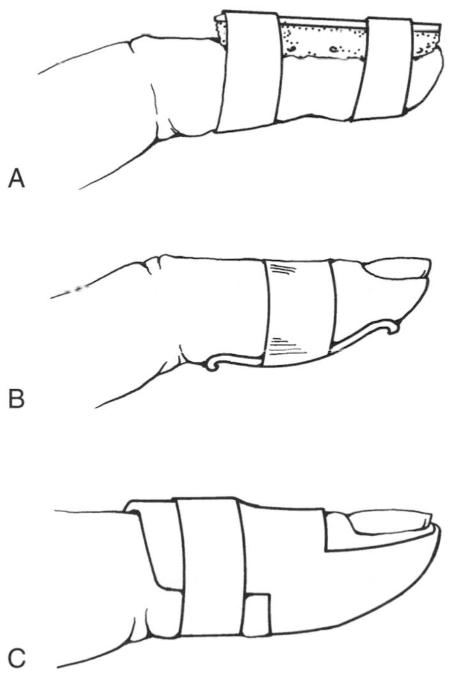

FIGURE 3-7 Mallet finger splints. **A,** Dorsal padded splint. **B,** Volar unpadded splint. **C,** Stack splint.

injury (i.e., splinting the DIP joint in slight hyperextension). After the period of mandatory splinting is completed (i.e., 6 to 10 weeks), further protective splinting or buddy taping may be needed for patients involved in occupations or sports that predispose them to reinjury for up to another 6 weeks.

Complications

Extensor Lag

Many patients initially have a slight to moderate extensor lag (i.e., lack of full extension of the DIP joint). After an appropriate trial of conservative therapy, some patients may continue to have a small extensor lag, especially if the patient sought treatment relatively late after injury. If the patient is not satisfied with some degree of extensor lag, another 6-week course of extension splinting may be performed with good results. However, only a minority of patients complain of difficulties with activities of daily living, and only a small percentage report work-related difficulties. Small degrees of extensor lag are a common complication of mallet finger injury but are surprisingly well accepted by most patients.

Late Mallet Finger

Although patients often seek treatment for the mallet deformity weeks or months after injury, many of these cases can be treated successfully up to 2 to 3 months after the initial injury. The patient should receive a trial of conservative therapy (i.e., splinting the DIP joint in slight hyperextension for

8 to 10 weeks). Patients must be warned about the poor prognosis for late-presenting mallet deformity because the longer the delay from injury to treatment, the less successful the result. Patients who have persistent symptoms after several weeks of splinting may benefit from operative repair. Left untreated, the mallet finger injury will progress to a swan-neck deformity of the finger (hyperextension of the PIP joint with flexion contracture of the DIP joint). A patient with this late sequela of an untreated mallet finger should be referred to an orthopedic surgeon.

Pediatric Considerations

In the pediatric age group, the mallet finger injury usually involves injury to the epiphysis at the base of the distal phalanx (Fig. 3-8). Whereas children younger than 12 years of age are likely to sustain a Salter-Harris type I or II injury, teenagers are more likely to sustain a true bony mallet finger injury (i.e., a displaced type III fracture) (Fig. 3-9). Follow-up care of nondisplaced pediatric mallet finger injuries requires splinting of the DIP joint in slight hyperextension for 4 to 6 weeks. It may be a challenge to get pediatric patients to adhere to continuous splinting. Casting or surgery should be considered if there is concern about adherence. Displaced fractures need to be reduced. Reduction requires digital nerve block with or without conscious sedation, gentle flexion of the distal phalanx to recreate the deformity, and extension of the distal fragment to restore bony congruity. The patient should be referred for surgical repair if closed reduction is unsuccessful or if the dorsal

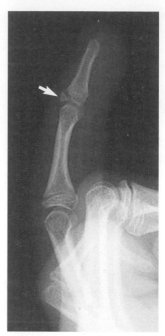

FIGURE 3-9 Pediatric mallet finger, type III fracture. (*From Thornton A, Gyll C. Children's Fractures: A Radiological Guide to Safe Practice. Philadelphia, WB Saunders, 1999.*)

fragment is greater than 50% of the articular surface. Some clinicians recommend alternating between dorsal and volar splints to avoid skin breakdown dorsally or temporary paresthesias volarly. Radiographs are checked weekly for the first 2 weeks and then every 2 weeks until healing occurs to monitor the patient for signs of loss of reduction or volar subluxation of the distal fragment. A variant of Salter-Harris types I and II fractures is a Seymour fracture, which includes avulsion of the proximal edge of the nail from the eponychial fold. This is considered an open fracture and should be treated as such. Management includes debridement, nail removal, irrigation, reduction as needed, nail replacement, and antibiotics.[6] Failure to recognize these fractures may result in substantial complications.

As in adult patients, extensor lag is a common complication in pediatric mallet finger injuries. Extension splinting can be continued but is less effective after the third or fourth month. However, extensor lag of up to 10 degrees is well tolerated by most patients.

FLEXOR DIGITORUM PROFUNDUS AVULSION (JERSEY FINGER)

Anatomic Considerations

The ring finger is most commonly injured (75% of FDP injuries) because of its exposed and vulnerable

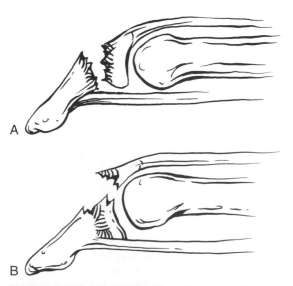

FIGURE 3-8 Pediatric mallet finger fracture patterns. **A,** Type I fracture with flexion of the distal fragment by the unopposed flexor digitorum profundus. **B,** Displaced type III fracture, a true "bony mallet."

position when the fingers are flexed.[7] Three types of FDP avulsion injury have been described[8] (Fig. 3-10).

Type I

In a type I injury, the tendon is retracted to the palm so that both vincula are ruptured with some loss of blood supply. The palm is tender at the lumbrical level. Radiographs show no fractures. Patients with this type of injury should be referred immediately because surgery must be undertaken within 7 to 10 days or tendon retraction, and scarring will be irreversible.

Type II

The most common type of FDP avulsion is the type II injury in which the tendon is avulsed and retracted to the level of the PIP joint. In this

injury, the long vinculum remains intact, so some blood supply is retained. Radiographs often show a small fleck of bone at the level of the PIP joint, which is best seen on the lateral view. The volar aspect of the PIP is tender and swollen, and the patient is unable to actively flex the DIP joint. Because the length of the tendon is largely preserved and some blood supply is maintained, the tendon can often be reinserted 2 to 3 months after injury. It is important to be aware that a type II injury can become a type I injury if the remaining vinculum gives way and the tendon is then retracted into the palm.

Type III

In a type III injury, a large bony fragment is avulsed from the volar aspect of the distal phalanx, which causes the tendon to be held at the level of the A-4

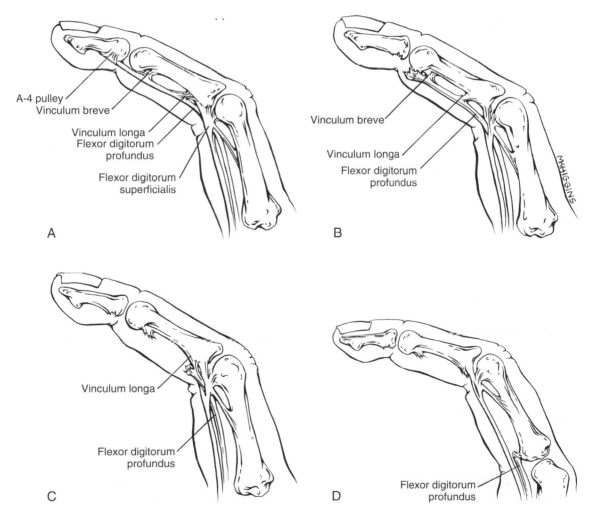

FIGURE 3-10 Types of flexor digitorum profundus (FDP) avulsion injuries. **A,** Normal anatomy. **B,** Type III injury. The vincula breve and longa are intact. The FDP is retracted to the distal interphalangeal joint. **C,** Type II injury. The vinculum breve is torn and the vinculum longa intact. The FDP is retracted to the proximal interphalangeal joint. **D,** Type I injury. The vincula breve and longa are torn. The FDP is retracted to the metacarpophalangeal joint.

pulley. In this injury, both vincula are intact, and blood supply to the tendon is preserved. Open reduction and internal fixation of the large bony fragment are required but can be performed as late as 2 to 3 months after injury.

Mechanism of Injury

The so-called jersey finger injury is caused by avulsion of the FDP tendon from the volar base of the distal phalanx and usually occurs as a player grabs another's jersey. The avulsion is caused by forced extension while the DIP joint is held in flexion.

Clinical Presentation

Avulsion of the FDP is an uncommon injury and is often missed on initial presentation or may go unnoticed for a number of weeks. The diagnosis is based on the typical mechanism of injury along with an inability to actively flex the DIP joint. FDP integrity is tested by stabilizing the PIP in extension by holding the middle phalanx and asking the patient to flex at the DIP joint. An inability to flex the DIP is consistent with FDP injury. The site of maximal tenderness may give a clue as to how far the tendon is retracted, but this is not always accurate.

Imaging

Lateral and oblique views are needed to identify an avulsed fragment of bone associated with an FDP avulsion. Good-quality radiographs and often a "hot light" are required to identify a small avulsed fleck of bone. The level at which the bony fragment is seen is quite variable, but it often becomes trapped near the middle phalanx and PIP joint.

Treatment

Prompt diagnosis and early referral are vital to treatment of patients with this injury. This injury is not amenable to outpatient management. The injured finger should be splinted with the DIP and PIP joints in slight flexion while the patient awaits referral to an orthopedic or hand surgeon. The timing of surgery can vary: for patients with type I injuries, immediate surgery is recommended; surgery may be deferred for several days to weeks for patients with type II or type III injuries.

Return to Work or Sports

The repaired tendon must be protected from disruptive forces for 6 to 12 weeks—approximately 12 weeks for type I injuries and 6 to 8 weeks for type II or III injuries. Early rehabilitation is important to obtain the best clinical result.

Complications

If the FDP is avulsed and retracted to the level of the palm (i.e., a type I injury), the tendon's blood supply may be interrupted, and bleeding into the tendon sheath may lead to fibrosis and scarring. Flexion deformities of the injured finger may result. Patients with type I injuries who seek treatment weeks to months after injury have a poor prognosis and may require arthrodesis, tenodesis, or a free tendon graft. The outcome of late surgical intervention for patients with type I injuries is poor, and no further treatment may be an appropriate choice for some patients. Surgically repaired FDP may lose some DIP extension; however, grip strength and DIP joint flexion are generally preserved.

Pediatric Considerations

Avulsion of the FDP is seldom seen in school-age children but does occur in adolescents. Unlike the common pattern in the adult, a fragment of the metaphysis and a variable amount of the physis is avulsed (Salter-Harris type IV) in adolescent patients. This fragment is tethered at the distal edge of the A-4 pulley (similar to the type III injury in adults). In this type of injury, the length of the tendon and its blood supply are preserved. The patient's DIP and PIP joints should be splinted in slight flexion and the patient referred promptly to a hand surgeon. Heavy sutures, mini-screws, and pullout wires have all been successful in bone-to-bone fixation. Pinning of the joint should be avoided to allow early ROM exercises for the DIP joint.

DISTAL INTERPHALANGEAL JOINT DISLOCATION

Pure dislocations and fracture dislocations of the DIP are uncommon injuries. They are nearly always dorsal and may be associated with open wounds. The most common mechanism of injury is hyperextension of the DIP joint. Fracture dislocations of the DIP joint nearly always involve avulsions of the extensor or flexor tendons, as discussed earlier.

Patients with a dorsal dislocation of the DIP joint have an obvious deformity of the fingertip. The dislocation is often reduced by the patient or someone else before seeking medical care. A lateral radiograph easily identifies this injury (Fig. 3-11).

Simple longitudinal traction under digital block anesthesia is usually all that is required to reduce the dislocation. Occasionally, hyperextension followed by traction and digital pressure is necessary. If the reduction is maintained with active ROM, the joint is considered stable. The DIP joint should be splinted in extension for 2 to 3 weeks. Open reduction is necessary for any dislocation that is irreducible.

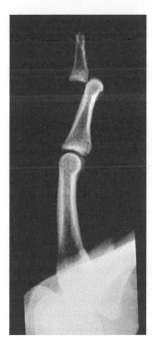

FIGURE 3-11 Dorsal dislocation of the distal interphalangeal joint.

MIDDLE PHALANX SHAFT FRACTURES (ADULT)

Anatomic Considerations

At the volar aspect of the PIP joint, the flexor digitorum superficialis (FDS) splits to allow the profundus tendon to pass between its two slips. The FDS inserts broadly along the volar surface of the middle phalanx. Thus, a fracture at the neck of the middle phalanx results in apex volar angulation as the proximal fracture fragment is pulled into flexion by the FDS (Fig. 3-12, A). A fracture at the base of the middle phalanx results in apex dorsal angulation as the distal fragment is pulled into flexion by the FDS (Fig. 3-12, B). Fractures

through the middle two thirds of the shaft of the middle phalanx may be angulated in either direction.

Mechanism of Injury

Fractures of the middle phalanx are usually caused by a direct blow to the dorsum of the phalanx. Less commonly, middle phalanx fractures may be caused by an axial load to the finger.

Clinical Presentation

The diagnosis is suspected with the typical history of a blow to the dorsum of the middle phalanx combined with tenderness and swelling on physical examination. Although malrotation is more commonly seen in proximal phalanx fractures, patients with middle phalanx fractures should be carefully evaluated for this complication. A rotational deformity should be suspected if not all fingers point to the radial styloid with the fingers in full flexion (See Fig. 2-13 in Chapter 2). If the patient is unable to flex the fingers fully because of pain, the symmetry in the planes of the fingernails while the fingers are semiflexed can be checked to determine malrotation. The uninjured hand should always be examined for comparison.

Imaging

Three views of the involved finger are required: AP, lateral, and oblique. Radiographs typically show a transverse fracture, most commonly at the neck or base. Oblique, spiral, and comminuted fractures are nearly always unstable (Fig. 3-13).

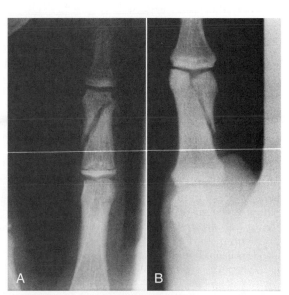

FIGURE 3-13 A, Oblique fracture of the middle phalanx. **B,** Oblique intraarticular fracture of the middle phalanx. Both of these fractures are unstable, and the patient should be referred to an orthopedic surgeon.

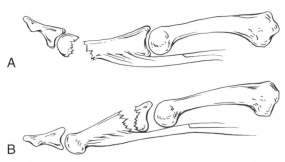

FIGURE 3-12 A, Middle phalanx neck fracture with apex volar angulation. **B,** Middle phalanx base fracture with apex dorsal angulation.

Rotational deformities can cause characteristic radiographic changes, including asymmetry of the diameters of the fracture fragments or a double shadow of the two condyles of the head of the middle phalanx on the lateral view.

Indications for Orthopedic Referral

Patients should be referred to an orthopedic surgeon if angulation cannot be corrected and maintained with closed reduction or if malrotation is present. Patients with oblique or spiral fractures should also be referred because of these fractures' inherent instability. Intraarticular fractures of one or both condyles of the middle phalanx at the level of the DIP joint virtually always need internal fixation to restore normal joint function, so these patients should also be referred.

Initial Treatment

Table 3-3 summarizes the management guidelines for middle phalanx shaft fractures.

Nondisplaced Fractures

Truly stable nondisplaced, nonangulated fractures of the middle phalanx may be treated with buddy taping. With this method of treatment, the injured finger is taped to the adjacent finger, and the patient is encouraged to move the finger as much as possible. A single layer of cotton gauze or cast padding between the fingers prevents skin maceration. This form of dynamic splinting minimizes joint stiffness.

Displaced or Angulated Fractures

Displaced or angulated fractures of the middle phalanx shaft may be successfully reduced by closed reduction, but care must be taken to ensure that the fractures remain stable after reduction. Longitudinal traction is applied while the patient is under digital block anesthesia. Manipulation of the distal fragment follows to bring it into alignment with the proximal fragment. Postreduction radiographs are mandatory. The finger should be immobilized in an ulnar or radial gutter splint, immobilizing the wrist in slight extension with the MCP joint at 70 to 90 degrees of flexion and the PIP and DIP joints in minimal (5 to 10 degrees) flexion. (See Appendix for description of how to apply a gutter splint.) The injured finger should be buddy taped to the adjacent finger during immobilization with cast padding between the fingers to prevent maceration of the skin. Separate volar and dorsal splints with the hand and fingers in the same position as described for a gutter splint can be used as an alternative to a gutter splint.

Table 3-3	*Management Guidelines for Middle or Proximal Phalanx Shaft Fractures*
	INITIAL TREATMENT
Splint type and position	Buddy taping for nondisplaced fractures
	Gutter splint after closed reduction
Initial follow-up visit	Within 7 to 10 days
Patient instruction	Keep hand elevated
	Maintain active ROM of uninjured fingers
	FOLLOW-UP CARE
Cast or splint type and position	Nondisplaced: buddy taping
	Stable after reduction: gutter
Length of immobilization	3 to 4 weeks for buddy taping
	4 weeks for splinting
Healing time	4 to 6 weeks
Follow-up visit interval	Every 1 to 2 weeks to assess joint motion and return to normal hand function
Repeat radiography interval	Within 7 to 10 days to check for alignment
	Every 1 to 2 weeks for reduced fractures
Patient instruction	Encourage active motion while buddy taped
	Active ROM exercises after splinting
Buddy taping protection during sports for 4 to 6 weeks after clinically healed	
Indications for orthopedic consult	Malrotation or uncorrected angulation
	Oblique or spiral fractures
	Intraarticular fractures of one or both condyles
	Loss of alignment at any time during immobilization

ROM, range of motion.

Follow-up Care

Nondisplaced Fractures

Patients with nondisplaced stable fractures treated with buddy taping should be reexamined within 7 to 10 days, and repeat radiographs should be taken to ensure that no angulation or displacement has occurred. Three to 4 weeks of buddy taping should be adequate for clinical healing. Follow-up radiographs are necessary only if clinical healing is prolonged or at any time during treatment if loss of fracture alignment is suspected. Patients should be seen every 1 to 2 weeks until healing occurs to assess joint motion and progress toward return of normal hand function.

Stable Fractures after Closed Reduction

Repeat radiographs should be taken within 1 week after closed reduction to check for alignment. Radiographs should be obtained with the finger in the splint. No more than 10 degrees of angulation is tolerable. If any rotation has occurred, the patient should be referred to an orthopedic surgeon for consideration of operative fixation. If alignment is maintained, the gutter splint should be continued for 4 weeks. Immobilization should not be continued during the several months it may take for complete radiographic healing to occur because prolonged immobilization can lead to disability. Active ROM exercises are started immediately after immobilization is completed to prevent joint stiffness. Patients should be seen every 2 weeks until they have regained normal finger function.

Return to Work or Sports

Patients with nondisplaced fractures can return to play or work after pain is controlled. After the initial period of immobilization, the patient should continue to wear protective splinting for 4 to 6 weeks during sports or occupational activities that may cause a reinjury to the middle phalanx. During treatment, buddy taping protection for nondisplaced fractures is acceptable during athletic activities. Patients with displaced fractures can return to noncontact, limited lifting activities after 3 to 4 weeks with protective splinting as above. Full activities should be delayed until radiographs demonstrate callus, which may take 6 to 12 weeks.

Complications

Malrotation is a common problem for patients with middle phalanx fractures. Although remodeling in the sagittal plane (i.e., flexion–extension) is extensive, no significant remodeling in the coronal plane (i.e., adduction–abduction) occurs at the middle phalanx. Malunion may also occur, especially if treatment is delayed. Failure to recognize an intraarticular fracture is common and may lead to poor healing and loss of function. Loss of motion at the PIP joint is a frequent complication.

MIDDLE PHALANX FRACTURES (PEDIATRIC)

Extraphyseal Fractures

Extraphyseal middle phalanx injuries (e.g., shaft fractures of the middle phalanx) in pediatric patients should be managed as outlined for adults. Neck and condylar fractures of the middle phalanx are usually unstable, and patients should be referred to an orthopedic surgeon.

Physeal Fractures

Anatomic Considerations

The unique anatomy of the immature hand affects the pattern of fractures seen. Understanding this anatomy is essential to detecting clinical findings, interpreting radiographic changes, and planning therapy for pediatric patients. The growth plate (physis) is situated uniformly at the base of all the phalanges. The volar plate originates from the neck of the proximal phalanx and inserts onto the epiphysis of the middle phalanx. The collateral ligaments of the PIP joint originate from the collateral recess at the neck of the proximal phalanx and insert onto both the epiphysis and the metaphysis of the middle phalanx. Some of the collateral ligament fibers also insert distally onto the volar plate. The central slip of the extensor tendon inserts onto the dorsum of the middle phalanx epiphysis, and the FDS has a long and broad insertion on the volar shaft and neck of the middle phalanx.

Mechanism of Injury

Two common physeal fracture patterns are seen. Avulsion of the central slip of the extensor tendon is caused by forcible flexion of the extended finger, resulting in avulsion of the epiphysis dorsally. Radial or ulnar deviation forces may cause lateral avulsion fractures because the distal portion of the collateral ligament avulses a small portion of the metaphysis at the base of the middle phalanx. A third fracture pattern is less common: in adolescents, axial load forces may cause a "pilon fracture" at the base of the middle phalanx.

Clinical Presentation

The patient describes the typical mechanism of injury: either forced flexion of the extended finger or radial or ulnar deviation forces applied to the finger. During physical examination, the patient has local tenderness and possibly slight ecchymosis. The child may refuse to move the digit actively and resist passive motion. Malrotation should be excluded by an examination of the plane of the nails in the semiflexed position.

Imaging

In the case of lateral avulsion fractures caused by radial or ulnar deviation forces, a small chip fracture is seen at the radial or ulnar aspect of the metaphysis at the base of the middle phalanx (extraphyseal injury or a type II fracture). In the case of forced flexion of the extended finger, the epiphysis at the base of the middle phalanx is displaced dorsally (type III fracture). In adolescent patients with axial load injuries, a pilon fracture (comminution of the epiphysis of the base of the middle phalanx) may result (Fig. 3-14).

Indications for Orthopedic Referral

Patients with irreducible dorsal avulsion fractures, pilon fractures, fractures involving more than 25% of the articular surface, fracture fragments displaced more than 1.5 mm, and neck or condylar fractures should be referred to orthopedic surgeons.

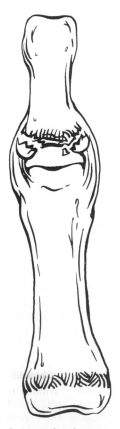

FIGURE 3-14 Pediatric "pilon fracture" at the base of the middle phalanx.

Initial Treatment

The PIP joint should be splinted in extension with a dorsal padded aluminum splint. The DIP and MCP joints should be left free for ROM. Patients with displaced avulsion fractures, intraarticular fractures, and pilon fractures should be splinted in a similar manner and referred to an orthopedic surgeon within a few days.

Follow-up Care

Avulsion Fracture of the Central Slip of the Extensor Tendon

Early follow-up is the key to recognizing and treating loss of reduction. The patient should be seen 7 to 10 days after initial treatment, and repeat radiographs should be obtained to confirm normal alignment. If reduction is intact, the PIP joint is splinted in extension with a dorsal padded aluminum splint. Immobilization should be limited to 3 to 4 weeks. Loss of reduction is more likely in older pediatric patients (i.e., patients who are closer to skeletal maturity). Patients with loss of reduction or an inability to maintain reduction should be referred for possible pin fixation.

Lateral Avulsion Fractures

Lateral avulsion fractures are usually stable and heal well. The patient should be seen after 7 to 10 days to confirm healing and normal alignment. After the initial visit, the patient can be seen every 1 or 2 weeks until the finger is no longer tender. Immobilization should be limited to 3 weeks, after which ROM exercises should be initiated.

PROXIMAL INTERPHALANGEAL JOINT INJURIES

The PIP joint of the finger is prone to injury, deformity, pain, and functional deficit. There is generally poor tolerance for prolonged immobilization of the PIP joint. It is important the clinician consider accurate anatomic diagnosis, rational splinting, and early active protected motion for best outcomes.

Anatomic Considerations

The PIP joint is a hinge joint, allowing only flexion and extension. It is stabilized by the bony architecture, the volar plate, and the collateral ligaments. The volar plate is a thick connective tissue structure that bridges the volar aspect of the PIP joint (Fig. 3-15). Its major function is to prevent hyperextension of the PIP joint. The flexor tendons pass superficially to the volar plate. The collateral ligaments originate on the proximal phalanx and insert at the middle phalanx; they prevent radial

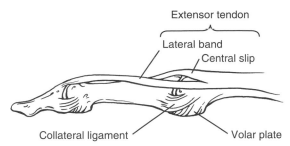

FIGURE 3-15 Lateral view of the proximal interphalangeal joint. The central slip passes directly over the joint, and the lateral bands pass around the joint. The thick fibrocartilaginous volar plate prevents hyperextension. Collateral ligaments prevent lateral motion of the joint.

or ulnar deviation of the PIP joint and are taut throughout the ROM of the joint. Some of the collateral ligament fibers attach directly into the volar plate. The central slip of the extensor apparatus passes dorsally across the PIP joint and inserts on the dorsum of the middle phalanx. The lateral bands arise from the extensor apparatus lateral and distal to the central slip. The triangular ligament is a fibrous stabilizer of the lateral bands as they fuse in the midline before insertion on the distal phalanx. Injury to the central slip of the extensor tendon and the triangular ligaments allows the lateral bands to slip volar to the longitudinal axis of the PIP joint, thus pulling the PIP into flexion. In this displaced position the lateral bands are under tension, which eventually leads to hyperextension of the DIP joint.

Volar Plate Injuries

Mechanism of Injury

Injury to the volar plate is caused by hyperextension of the PIP joint. Such an injury may be accompanied by dorsal subluxation or dislocation of the middle phalanx.

Clinical Presentation

The patient reports a hyperextension injury to the affected finger and complains of pain and swelling at the PIP joint. During examination, maximum tenderness is apparent at the volar aspect of the PIP joint. A digital nerve block may be necessary to detect any hyperextension laxity to passive stretch. The radial and ulnar collateral ligaments (UCLs) of the PIP joint must also be examined. If they are tender, stress should be applied to each collateral ligament to test function.

Imaging

Two views of the PIP joint are required: AP and lateral. A small avulsion fracture of the volar lip of the base of the middle phalanx is commonly seen

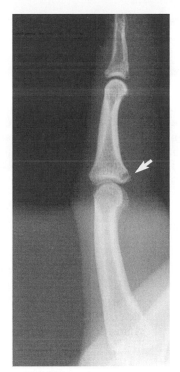

FIGURE 3-16 Nondisplaced avulsion fracture of the volar plate.

(Fig. 3-16). A dorsal PIP fracture dislocation often occurs when a larger amount of the volar lip is fractured. The larger fragment predisposes the PIP joint to volar instability when the joint is hyperextended, allowing the middle phalanx to displace dorsally (Fig. 3-17). Joint congruity should be carefully assessed on the lateral film. Parallel congruity between the dorsal base of the middle phalanx and the head of the proximal phalanx should be apparent. The presence of the "V" sign indicates joint

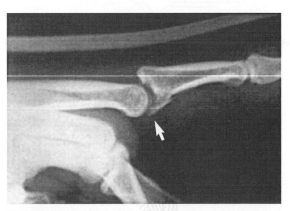

FIGURE 3-17 Volar plate avulsion fracture with dorsal subluxation of the middle phalanx. (*From Browner BD, Jupiter JB, Levine AM, Trafton PG [eds]. Skeletal Trauma: Fractures, Dislocations, Ligamentous Injuries. Philadelphia, WB Saunders, 1992.*)

subluxation (Fig. 3-18). One of the most common errors in treating volar plate injuries is failure to recognize the subluxation.

Indications for Orthopedic Referral

Surgical treatment is indicated for volar plate injuries in which the middle phalanx remains subluxated after closed reduction. If the fracture fragment involves more than 40% of the articular surface, internal fixation is usually required for adequate healing. Patients with fracture dislocations of the PIP joint should be referred to orthopedic surgeons.

Initial Treatment

Nondisplaced Fractures

Small nondisplaced avulsion fractures of the volar lip of the middle phalanx without subluxation can be treated with buddy taping or a dorsal finger splint with the PIP joint in slight flexion.

Fractures with Dorsal Subluxation

Dorsal subluxation of the middle phalanx often occurs when larger avulsion fracture fragments are present. This PIP joint dorsal subluxation may be reduced by flexing of the PIP joint while traction is applied. If postreduction radiographs reveal congruity of the articular surfaces and no subluxation of the middle phalanx (no "V" sign), the injured finger should be immobilized in a dorsal extension block splint (Fig. 3-19). The initial position of the PIP joint should equal the amount of flexion required to maintain the reduction, usually 45 to 60 degrees. The splint is secured only over the

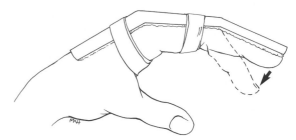

FIGURE 3-19 Dorsal extension block splint.

proximal finger to allow active flexion at the PIP joint. If any question arises about the presence of subluxation or if the primary care provider is uncomfortable with attempting closed reduction, the finger should be splinted in 20 to 30 degrees of flexion, and the patient should be referred for orthopedic management.

Follow-up Care

Nondisplaced Fractures

Nondisplaced avulsion fractures without subluxation should be buddy taped in slight flexion until pain resolves and then heal well. Active ROM exercises should be started after 1 week. Protective buddy taping during athletic activities should be continued for 6 to 8 weeks after the initial injury. Patients should be warned that the PIP joint will remain swollen for 6 to 12 months and that they can expect some permanent enlargement of the joint.

Fractures with Dorsal Subluxation

For fractures with dorsal subluxation, the patient should be reexamined at weekly intervals and a repeat lateral radiograph taken during each visit to document good alignment. If the reduction is maintained, the amount of flexion at the PIP joint is reduced by 10 to 15 degrees each week. Usually within 4 weeks, the PIP joint will be fully extended, and the splint can be discontinued. Patients should be encouraged to perform active flexion at the DIP and PIP joints during the entire period of splinting. If the radiographs reveal joint incongruity at any time, the patient should be referred to an orthopedic surgeon.

Return to Work or Sports

Patients may return to work or play while splinted; however, patients requiring manual dexterity may need modification of their work activity because the extension block splint interferes with hand function. After the initial treatment period, buddy taping protection should be applied for an additional 2 to 3 weeks or longer for patients who

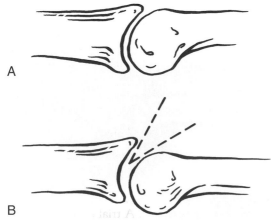

FIGURE 3-18 "V" sign of joint incongruity. **A,** Parallel congruity between the dorsal base of the middle phalanx and the head of the proximal phalanx. **B,** Incongruity of the joint with a resultant "V" between the two articular surfaces.

participate in sports or activities that may predispose them to reinjury.

Complications

Late complications of volar plate injuries include a stiff PIP joint, flexion contracture of the PIP joint caused by scarring of the volar plate, and symptomatic hyperextensibility of the PIP joint. Persistent laxity of the volar plate can lead to hyperextension of the PIP joint with compensatory flexion of the DIP joint, resulting in a swan-neck deformity of the finger. Failure to recognize and correct for subluxation associated with a volar plate injury may result in any of these complications.

Pediatric Considerations

Good outcomes can be achieved with conservative management in a dorsal aluminum extension block splint at 15-degree flexion applied for 10 days for stable volar plate fractures in children (volar plate only and volar plate with avulsion fracture without dislocation).[9] After 10 days in the block splint, buddy taping can be used as needed for sports.

Avulsion of the Central Slip of the Extensor Tendon (Boutonniere Injury)

Mechanism of Injury

The so-called boutonniere injury (i.e., "buttonhole" injury) is caused by disruption of the central slip of the extensor tendon, which is torn from the dorsal aspect of the middle phalanx when the extended PIP joint is forcibly flexed (Fig. 3-20). During the weeks after injury, the lateral bands of the extensor mechanism pull the PIP into flexion, which results in hyperextension at the DIP—the classic boutonniere deformity. A small dorsal avulsion fracture at the base of the middle phalanx may be associated with rupture of the central slip. Occasionally, disruption of the central slip is caused by dorsal dislocation of the middle phalanx.

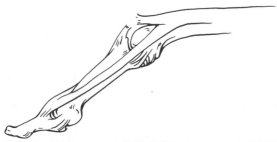

FIGURE 3-20 Rupture of the central slip of the extensor tendon, causing a boutonniere deformity.

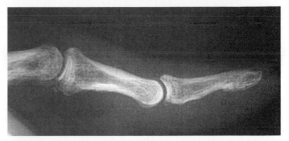

FIGURE 3-21 Boutonniere deformity that developed 1 month after an untreated intraarticular fracture of the middle phalanx with central slip injury. Note the flexion deformity of the proximal interphalangeal joint and the compensatory hyperextension of the distal interphalangeal joint.

Clinical Presentation

Patients with acute injuries of the type that causes boutonniere deformity do not exhibit typical symptoms until 4 to 6 weeks later (Fig. 3-21). Rather, during physical examination, the patient has swelling at the PIP joint and has tenderness at the dorsum of the PIP joint. The patient is unable to actively extend the PIP joint against resistance. If active ROM cannot be adequately determined because of pain, digital block anesthesia can be applied after sensory function is documented. Rupture of the central slip of the extensor tendon should be distinguished from the more typical "jammed" finger. Whereas a patient with a jammed finger has tenderness radially or ulnarly at the collateral ligament, a patient with the boutonniere injury has tenderness at the dorsum of the PIP joint and is unable to actively extend the PIP joint against resistance.

Imaging

Most boutonniere injuries involve the rupture of the central slip of the extensor tendon without an accompanying fracture. The lateral view is best for visualizing the small dorsal avulsion fracture that may occur in association with the boutonniere injury. If the dorsal fracture fragment is quite large, volar subluxation of the middle phalanx may occur.

Indications for Orthopedic Referral

Patients with a late-presenting boutonniere deformity probably require surgical correction, but successful results with nonoperative extension splinting can be obtained even when treatment is delayed for up to 6 weeks. A trial of splinting may be warranted even for patients with chronic boutonniere deformity because late surgical repair may yield poor results. Patients with boutonniere injuries associated with a large displaced dorsal avulsion fracture that limits passive ROM should be referred for open reduction and internal fixation.

Treatment

The PIP joint should be splinted in continuous full extension, most commonly with a dorsal padded aluminum splint. The DIP and MCP joints should be left free for adequate ROM. The patient should be reexamined at 2-week intervals until healing has occurred. Repeat radiographs are not necessary if a small nondisplaced dorsal avulsion fracture was present at the time of initial injury. Patients must be instructed to actively and passively flex and extend the DIP joint during the healing process because movement at the DIP joint helps bring the lateral bands closer to the midline and speeds healing of the triangular ligaments. The PIP joint should remain splinted in continuous extension for 6 weeks in extension followed by either nighttime splinting or buddy taping continuously for 3 to 4 additional weeks. Splinting is continued until full active extension at the PIP joint and full active flexion at the DIP joint are restored. Lack of adequate rehabilitation, even after correct diagnosis and treatment, may result in loss of normal active and passive flexion in the DIP joint.

Return to Work or Sports

Patients may return to work or play during the splinting period; however, patients requiring manual dexterity will have difficulty with the PIP extension splint. Patients at risk for repeat flexion injuries should wear a protective splint for 4 weeks after the initial 6-week treatment period.

Lateral Avulsion Fractures

Injury to the collateral ligaments of the PIP joint may result in a lateral avulsion fracture at the base of the middle phalanx. It is important to examine the PIP with the MCP in 90 degrees of flexion because an extended MCP will tighten the collateral ligaments. Small nondisplaced fractures heal with buddy taping. Early active motion should be encouraged. Buddy taping should be worn continuously for 3 weeks and for a maximum of 3 to 4 additional weeks during sports or activities that may stress the finger. Patients should be advised that they may have some residual soreness in the PIP joint for several months and some permanent fusiform enlargement of the joint as a result of scarring during the healing process.

Even when lateral deviation stress reveals joint opening, patients should receive a trial of buddy taping before consideration of surgical repair of a torn collateral ligament. Patients with large avulsion fractures, displaced fractures (>2 to 3 mm), or fractures involving more than 30% of the articular surface should be referred for open reduction and internal fixation.

Proximal Interphalangeal Joint Dislocation

Mechanism of Injury

Hyperextension of the PIP joint, usually the result of an axial load to the finger, causes dorsal dislocation of the PIP joint. Dorsal dislocations are the most common type. The PIP can also dislocate ventrally and laterally.[10] Fracture dislocation most often involves a fracture of the volar aspect of the PIP.

Clinical Presentation

Most commonly, the PIP dislocation has been reduced before a clinician sees the patient. The patient describes a hyperextension injury to the affected finger and reports pain and swelling at the PIP joint. Tenderness at the radial or ulnar aspect of the joint indicates injury to the collateral ligament; tenderness volarly indicates injury to the volar plate. Hyperextension stress may reproduce the patient's pain and also indicates injury to the volar plate. A digital nerve block may be necessary to detect any hyperextension laxity to passive stretch. Active and passive ROM of the PIP joint should be assessed; rupture of central slip of the extensor mechanism results in loss of active extension of the PIP joint.

Imaging

Three views of the injured finger should be obtained: AP, lateral, and oblique. Views of the whole hand should not be obtained because the key findings may be obscured by the other fingers. The most important radiograph is the true lateral view (Fig. 3-22). The radiograph should be examined carefully for a small avulsion fracture at the base of the middle phalanx. The oblique view is useful in detecting condylar fractures of the head of the proximal phalanx. The examiner must be sure that the patient has a simple PIP dislocation and not the much more serious PIP fracture dislocation, for which the patient should be referred.

Indications for Orthopedic Referral

Irreducible PIP joint dislocation (commonly caused by the volar plate, flexor tendons, or both lodging in the PIP joint) should be referred. Bayonet dislocations of the PIP joint involve both dorsal and radial or ulnar dislocation of the PIP joint; the deformity is obvious on both the AP and lateral projections. Patients with this injury should be referred to orthopedic surgeons for definitive treatment. Any patient who has an open dislocation of the PIP joint must be referred for joint debridement and primary repair of the volar plate.

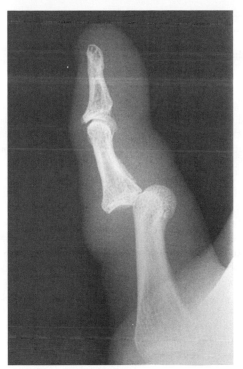

FIGURE 3-22 Dorsal dislocation of the proximal interphalangeal joint.

Patients with fracture dislocations of the PIP joint should likewise be referred for surgical therapy.

Initial Treatment

Reduction of the PIP dislocation can be performed using any of several techniques. The examiner should hold the proximal phalanx firmly and grasp the middle phalanx with the other hand. While applying traction, the examiner should gently hyperextend the PIP and then pull the PIP joint into flexion.

An alternative method of reduction is for the examiner to grasp the injured finger with both hands, applying the index fingers to the volar aspect of the proximal phalanx and the thumbs to the dorsum of the proximal phalanx. The examiner uses the thumbs to gently push the displaced middle phalanx up, out, and away from the head of the proximal phalanx and then gently flexes the PIP joint.

After reduction, the examiner should check for active extension at the PIP joint to determine whether the central slip of the extensor tendon is intact. The examiner should also check for tenderness at the volar aspect of the PIP joint. Tenderness at this spot may indicate injury to the volar plate or a small avulsion fracture of the volar lip at the base of the middle phalanx. Repeat radiographs should be obtained to rule out a small fracture of the volar lip of the base of the middle phalanx,

which may have been caused by the original injury or the reduction itself. It is important that all post-reduction PIP dislocations are imaged to rule out fracture, including those that are relocated before presentation. The PIP joint should be protected from further hyperextension stress by buddy taping the injured finger to the adjacent finger.

There is no consensus on management of fracture dislocations of the PIP. If greater than 30% of the volar articular surface is fractured, the patient should be referred for surgical fixation. Less than 30% articular surface fracture can be managed with dorsal extension block as described for volar plate injuries above.[11]

Follow-up Care

The finger with the injured PIP joint should be buddy taped to the adjacent finger for 3 to 6 weeks. Active ROM exercises should be started after 1 week. The patient should be warned that symptoms may persist for 12 to 18 months and that swelling of the PIP joint may be permanent.

Return to Work or Sports

Protective buddy taping during occupation- or sport-related activities should be continued for 6 to 8 weeks after the initial injury.

Complications

Irreducible dorsal dislocation of the PIP joint is relatively uncommon but may be caused by interposition of structures such as the volar plate, the flexor tendons, or both between the head of the proximal phalanx and the base of the middle phalanx. Recurrent dorsal dislocations of the PIP joint are rare and require orthopedic referral.

PROXIMAL PHALANX SHAFT FRACTURES (ADULT)

Anatomic Considerations

Proximal phalanx fractures are often unstable because of the numerous muscle and tendon attachments. Apex volar angulation typically is apparent with fractures of the proximal phalanx. The proximal fracture fragment (base of the proximal phalanx) is pulled into flexion by the interosseous muscles, and the distal fracture fragment is pulled into extension by the extensor apparatus (Fig. 3-23).

Mechanism of Injury

Fractures of the proximal phalanx are usually caused by a direct blow to the dorsum of the hand, resulting in a transverse fracture. These fractures are usually unstable. Twisting or torque applied to the proximal phalanx may cause oblique or spiral

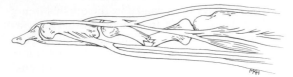

FIGURE 3-23 Apex volar angulation after fracture of the proximal phalanx.

fractures, which are prone to shortening or malrotation. Crush injuries may cause significant comminution of the fracture.

Clinical Presentation

The diagnosis may be suspected with a history of a direct blow to the dorsum of the proximal phalanx along with localized pain and swelling. During physical examination, the patient has tenderness at the dorsum of the proximal phalanx. Because malrotation is a frequent complication of proximal phalanx fractures, the examiner should check for malrotation by confirming that the fingernails are parallel in the semiflexed position and that all four fingers are directed toward the radial styloid in full flexion (Fig. 2-13 in Chapter 2). Malrotation up to 10 degrees is usually well tolerated, but malrotation greater than this may cause impaired hand function requiring surgical intervention and osteotomy. The injured hand should be compared with the uninjured hand to complete the diagnosis. As with all finger injuries, the examiner should confirm normal capillary refill and normal two-point discrimination at 5 mm.

Imaging

Three views of the injured finger are required: AP, lateral, and oblique. Typically, a transverse fracture through the proximal third of the proximal phalanx is seen. Radiographs should be carefully examined for angulation, shortening, and rotation. Volar angulation is best appreciated on the lateral view. A fracture involving 25 to 30 degrees of volar angulation may appear normal on AP radiographs, so the lateral radiographs must be reviewed carefully. The base of the injured proximal phalanx is often obscured by the other proximal phalanges. A transverse fracture through the neck of the proximal phalanx usually shows significant angulation (e.g., as much as 60 to 90 degrees of apex volar angulation). A rotational deformity should be suspected if the diameters of the fracture fragments appear asymmetric. Other fracture types include spiral or oblique fractures of the shaft of the proximal phalanx, condylar fractures at the head of the proximal phalanx, longitudinal

fractures, and avulsion fractures at the base of the proximal phalanx.

Indications for Orthopedic Referral

Fractures in which reduction cannot be maintained by closed means, angulated neck fractures, oblique or spiral shaft fractures, condylar fractures, and large displaced avulsion fractures at the base of the proximal phalanx require referral for pin fixation or open reduction and internal fixation.

Initial Treatment

Table 3-3 summarizes the management guidelines for proximal phalanx shaft fractures.

Fractures that require referral to an orthopedic surgeon should be immobilized in a radial or ulnar gutter splint with the MCP joints in 70 to 90 degrees of flexion and the PIP and DIP joints in slight flexion pending consultation.

Nondisplaced Transverse Fractures

A stable nondisplaced, nonangulated transverse fracture can be treated safely by buddy taping of the injured finger to an adjacent uninjured finger at both the proximal phalanx and the middle phalanx.

Angulated Transverse Fractures

Closed reduction of angulated transverse fractures can produce satisfactory results. A digital nerve block is recommended. When angulated transverse fractures of the proximal phalanx are treated, the controllable distal fragment must be brought into alignment with the uncontrollable proximal fragment. Because the muscles that exert deforming forces on the fracture site originate in the forearm, the wrist should be immobilized as well, usually in 30 degrees of extension (i.e., the so-called position of function).

Reduction Technique

For the purposes of reduction, the MCP and PIP joints should be flexed to 90 degrees. However, the PIP joint should never be immobilized in full flexion because it is prone to flexion contracture. The dorsally displaced distal fracture fragment is reduced volarly by application of pressure with the thumbs dorsally distal to the fracture line and application of counterpressure with the fingers volarly proximal to the fracture line. If the fracture is stable, a radial or ulnar gutter splint can be used to immobilize the finger. If the fracture reangulates with slight extension of the PIP joint, the fracture is unstable and requires internal fixation.

Fractures involving the ring or small fingers can be immobilized in an ulnar gutter splint. Fractures involving the index or long fingers can be immobilized in a radial gutter splint.

Follow-up Care

Nondisplaced Transverse Fractures

The patient should be seen 1 to 2 weeks after initial treatment to confirm healing and normal alignment. Normal extension without claw deformity should be confirmed, and malrotation should be ruled out by examination of the plane of the nails in the semiflexed position. Buddy taping should be continued until the patient has no tenderness at the fracture site, with protective buddy taping continued for 2 to 3 additional weeks for patients involved in occupation- or sports-related activities that could aggravate the injury.[12] Patients should be seen every 2 weeks until clinical healing has occurred, which is evident by absence of pain with palpation or motion.

Angulated Transverse Fractures

Careful clinical and radiographic follow-up is essential during the healing phase, for early detection of any fracture displacement, and to initiate corrective treatment. The patient should be seen 1 week after initial treatment, and repeat radiographs should be obtained to document normal alignment of the healing fracture. The patient should then be seen every 1 to 2 weeks for evaluation. Radiographs should be taken to confirm healing and document normal alignment.

Clinical healing of phalanx fractures occurs within 3 to 4 weeks. Immobilization of the phalanx usually should not exceed 3 weeks and should be followed by another 3 weeks of protected motion with buddy taping. Because radiographic healing of the phalanges ranges from 1 to 17 months and usually requires 5 months, immobilization of the injured finger should not be continued to the point at which bony healing is visible radiographically.

Return to Work or Sports

Displaced or angulated fractures that have been reduced should avoid high-risk activities during the initial immobilization. After the initial period of immobilization, the patient should continue to wear protective splinting for 4 to 6 weeks during sports or occupational activities that may cause a reinjury to the proximal phalanx. During treatment, buddy taping protection during athletic activities is acceptable for nondisplaced fractures.

Complications

Patients 50 years of age and older, those with associated tendon injuries, and those who have been immobilized for more than 4 weeks are more likely to have adverse outcomes such as joint stiffness and loss of joint ROM. Most fractures of the proximal phalanx involve some degree of volar angulation, which, if not detected and treated appropriately, may result in clawlike deformity of the finger. Lateral deviation (i.e., radial or ulnar deviation) usually complicates phalangeal fractures associated with significant bone loss, such as gunshot wounds or crush injuries. Oblique or spiral fractures of the shaft of the proximal phalanx can result in significant shortening; the distal spike of the proximal phalanx may impinge on the base of the middle phalanx, blocking flexion at the PIP joint. Patients with crush injuries, open fractures, and prolonged immobilization are at higher risk of developing tendon adherence. This is especially true of dorsal injuries caused by the broad surface contact between the dorsum of the proximal phalanx and the extensor aponeurosis. Joint stiffness is a common complication after proximal phalanx fracture, but an adequate rehabilitation program can prevent or correct this problem in most patients.

PEDIATRIC (PHYSEAL) FRACTURES OF THE PROXIMAL PHALANX

The proximal phalanx is the most commonly injured bone in pediatric hand fractures. Of these injuries, the most common is a Salter-Harris type II fracture at the base of the proximal phalanx of the fifth digit.

Anatomic Considerations

The growth plate (physis), located at the base of the proximal phalanx, is relatively unprotected at the MCP joint level. The physis of the metacarpals is at the base of the thumb metacarpal but at the distal portion of the index, long, ring, and small finger metacarpals. The collateral ligaments of the MCP joint originate and insert exclusively onto the epiphyses of these opposing bones. The relative strength of the ligaments compared with the growth plate preferentially directs forces through the physis.

Mechanism of Injury

Most physeal fractures of the proximal phalanx are caused by lateral deviation forces (i.e., radial deviation and ulnar deviation) combined with twisting or rotational forces.

Clinical Presentation

The patient describes radial or ulnar deviation of the injured finger, usually with some rotatory component as well. During physical examination, the patient has tenderness at the dorsum of the base of the proximal phalanx; the patient may also have tenderness at the radial or ulnar aspect of the base of the proximal phalanx. Evidence of malrotation should be sought by examination of the plane of the nails in the semiflexed position. As with all finger injuries, capillary refill and two-point discrimination at 5 mm should be confirmed by examination.

Imaging

Failure to recognize the extent of the patient's injury on initial radiographs is a common problem that can have significant influence on the ultimate outcome. Fig. 3-24 shows the three most common fracture patterns for physeal fractures of the base of the proximal phalanx. Extraarticular fractures are either a type II fracture or an "extra octave" fracture (Fig. 3-25), which involves a tension fracture on one side of the proximal phalanx, paired with a compression fracture on the opposite side. The intraarticular fracture is consistent with a type III or IV fracture; that is, the fracture line extends through the epiphysis (type III) or through both the metaphysis and the epiphysis (type IV).

Campbell's straight-line method can be used to detect subtle malalignment. A line is drawn through the centers of the long axis of the phalanges and metacarpals; normally, these lines should be collinear, but a fracture or dislocation will skew this relationship (Fig. 3-26).

Angulated fractures at the base of the proximal phalanx may be obscured by the other digits. Examination under fluoroscopy or use of tomograms may be helpful in this situation.

Indications for Orthopedic Referral

Patients with malaligned fractures, irreducible fractures, fractures unstable after attempted closed reduction, fractures involving more than 25% of the articular surface, or residual displacement of more than 1.5 mm should be referred to orthopedic surgeons for operative treatment. Intraarticular fractures of the base of the proximal phalanx (type

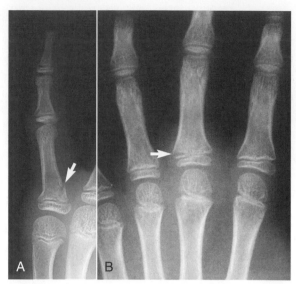

FIGURE 3-25 A, Nondisplaced type II fracture of the proximal phalanx. *(From Thornton A, Gyll C. Children's Fractures: A Radiological Guide to Safe Practice. Philadelphia, WB Saunders, 1999.)* **B,** Pediatric "extraoctave" fracture at the base of the proximal phalanx. The *arrow* points to the tension side of the fracture.

III or IV fractures) should be splinted and the patient referred promptly to an orthopedic surgeon.

Initial Treatment

Nondisplaced fractures can be splinted in the safe position (i.e., a gutter splint with the wrist in 30 degrees of extension, the MCP joints fully flexed, and the PIP and DIP joints in extension). Closed reduction can be attempted for displaced physeal fractures at the base of the proximal phalanx. A digital nerve block and conscious sedation are used before attempts at reduction. The MCP joint is fully flexed, and the proximal phalanx is used as a lever arm, pulling the finger in the opposite direction of the deformity, to reduce the fracture. Postreduction radiographs should be obtained to confirm alignment. Use of a hard object in the adjacent web space to assist reduction should be avoided because this technique may cause a neuropraxia injury to the digital nerve.

Follow-up Care

The patient should be seen 1 week after initial treatment to confirm that no loss of reduction has occurred. The splint is removed, and the patient is examined for signs of malrotation by inspection of the nails in the semiflexed position. Radiographs are repeated on this first follow-up visit to confirm that reduction has held. The gutter splint should remain on until clinical healing, usually within 3 to 4 weeks. Protected motion with buddy taping should be used for 2 additional weeks, particularly

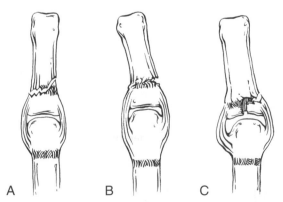

FIGURE 3-24 Physeal fracture patterns of the proximal phalanx. **A,** Extraarticular type II fracture. **B,** Extraarticular "extra octave" fracture with tension on one side and compression on the other. **C,** Intraarticular type III fracture.

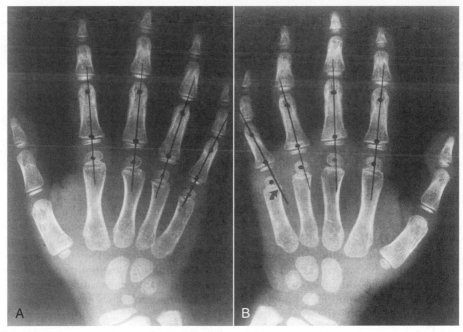

FIGURE 3-26 Campbell's straight-line method for detecting malalignment in pediatric proximal phalanx fractures. **A,** The long axis of the proximal phalanx should align with the long axis of the metacarpal as they do in this normal hand. **B,** If a fracture has occurred in the proximal phalanx, the axes will not be collinear (*arrow*). (*From Rockwood CA Jr, Green DP, Bucholz RW, Heckman JD [eds]. Rockwood and Green's Fractures in Adults, 4th ed, vol 1. Philadelphia, Lippincott-Raven, 1996.*)

for sports activities. Because these injuries occur close to the physis, remodeling usually takes places quickly in both the flexion–extension and abduction–adduction planes.

Complications

The age of the patient and the location of the fracture strongly influence the development of complications. Failure to correctly note the presence of an intraarticular fracture can have severe consequences for the function of a child's digit. Remodeling potential is usually good, especially in the flexion–extension plane and among children 10 years of age and younger. However, remodeling in the abduction–adduction plane is considerably less reliable. Because of the rapid healing of most pediatric fractures, exuberant callus formation can be seen among children for whom treatment is delayed, which often results in a malunion. Early degenerative changes are rare but may affect children who have sustained intraarticular fractures or who have joint sepsis. An angular deformity or loss of longitudinal growth can result whenever the fracture involves the physis.

DISLOCATIONS AND LIGAMENT INJURIES OF THE METACARPOPHALANGEAL JOINT

The MCP joint of the thumb is more exposed and anatomically more complex than the MCP joint of the other fingers. This influences injury patterns as

well as treatment. Hence, these two groups of injuries are discussed separately.

Dislocations of the Finger Metacarpophalangeal Joint (Excluding the Thumb)

Anatomic Considerations

The volar plate and collateral ligaments provide stability to the MCP joint. The collateral ligaments are lax when the joint is extended and tight when the joint is flexed. This is a crucial consideration. If the MCP is immobilized in extension, these ligaments shorten. This deprives the ligaments of the laxity needed for extension, leading to significant joint stiffness. Collateral ligaments are named with use of the radius and ulna as a frame of reference. For example, the collateral ligament of the second MCP that is on the side of the joint next to the third metacarpal is named the *ulnar collateral ligament* because it lies on the same side of the second MCP as the ulna. The direction of a MCP dislocation is determined by the direction the proximal phalanx has moved in relation to the metacarpal head.

Dorsal Dislocation

Dorsal dislocations are much more common than lateral dislocations. They are generally produced by hyperextension injuries that rupture the volar plate. Patients have a hyperextension deformity, pain, and swelling. Dorsal dislocations fall into two categories: simple and complex. It is important to distinguish between them because the treatment differs for each.

Simple Dislocations

Simple dorsal dislocations are actually subluxations; that is, the joint surface of the proximal phalanx is still partially in contact with the joint surface of the metacarpal. During physical examination, the proximal phalanx usually lies in 60 to 90 degrees of hyperextension. Radiographs typically show this angle as well as partial contact of the two joint surfaces. Simple dislocations can almost always be treated with closed reduction.

Complex Dislocations

In complex dislocations, the joint surfaces remain apart. The torn volar plate often lies between the two joint surfaces, preventing closed reduction. During physical examination, the phalanx lies in less hyperextension (typically 20 to 30 degrees). The presence of a dimple in the palm near the affected metacarpal head also suggests a complex dislocation. Radiographs reveal no contact between the two joint surfaces (best seen on the lateral view). The sesamoid lying between the joint surfaces of the phalanx and metacarpal is pathognomonic for a complex dislocation (Fig. 3-27).

Indications for Orthopedic Referral

Patients with the following conditions should be referred: dorsal dislocations associated with a fracture fragment that is displaced more than 2 mm or larger than 20% of joint surface, simple dislocations that cannot be reduced after two or three attempts, and complex dislocations that cannot be reduced on the first attempt and require prompt open reduction.

Treatment

Reduction should be performed with the patient's wrist and interphalangeal joints in flexion, which relaxes the flexor tendons and facilitates reduction. The joint should be hyperextended to 90 degrees. While the joint surface of the phalanx is pressed against the metacarpal head, reduction can be achieved by pushing the base of the phalanx into a flexed position. During the reduction maneuver, traction on the digit must be strictly avoided to prevent the joint space from opening and the volar plate from slipping into the joint, thus converting the injury into a complex dislocation. Successful reduction is usually accompanied by a palpable clunk. A wrist block may be necessary if pain prevents reduction.

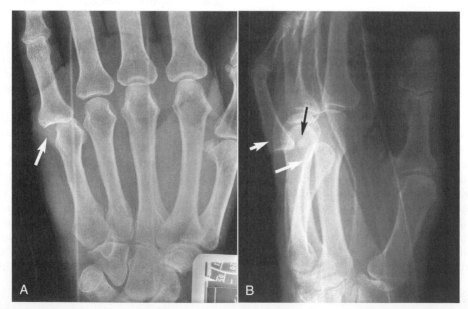

FIGURE 3-27 Complex dislocation of the fifth metacarpophalangeal joint. **A,** Anteroposterior view. **B,** Lateral view. On the lateral view, note that the proximal phalanx of the fifth finger (*short arrow*) lies nearly 1 cm above the fifth metacarpal head (*long arrow*), and no contact occurs between the joint surfaces of these two bones. Note that the phalanx lies at approximately a 20-degree angle to the metacarpal. A sesamoid bone can be seen lying directly between the ends of these two bones (*narrow arrow*). The latter is a pathognomonic sign of a complex dislocation.

One or 2 days after reduction, the affected finger should be buddy taped and ROM exercises begun. Alternatively, the finger may be splinted in 60 degrees of flexion for 7 to 10 days. Buddy taping and ROM exercises should be started as soon as the splint is removed and follow-up continued until ROM and function approach baseline. The patient should be referred to occupational therapy, an orthopedic surgeon, or both if recovery is slow or unsatisfactory.

Lateral Dislocation

This unusual injury is generally caused by a force that pushes the finger in an ulnar direction, injuring the radial collateral ligament (RCL). The finger MCP joints are protected by the adjacent fingers and metacarpals, making these injuries much less common than collateral ligament injuries of the thumb. Patients have tenderness over the collateral ligament and mild swelling. Radiographs may reveal an avulsion fracture. The patient should be referred if the avulsion is significant (displaced more than 2 mm or involving more than 20% of the joint surface); the injury occurred more than 10 to 14 days previously because prolonged symptoms are likely and steroid injections, surgery, or both may be needed; or gross instability is present because surgery may be the preferred treatment.

Acute injuries without significant avulsion fractures can be splinted in 50 degrees of flexion for 3 weeks. Buddy taping to the adjacent finger can be used for an additional 2 to 3 weeks to provide additional protection as ROM begins. Follow-up should be continued until ROM and function approach baseline. If recovery is unsatisfactory, the patient should be referred to an occupational therapist, an orthopedist or hand surgeon, or both.

Volar Dislocation

Volar dislocation is a rare, poorly understood injury and typically requires open reduction. All patients with volar dislocations should be referred to orthopedic surgeons.

DISLOCATIONS AND LIGAMENT INJURIES OF THE THUMB METACARPOPHALANGEAL JOINT

Avulsion Injuries to the Ulnar Collateral Ligament of the Thumb (Skier's Thumb or Gamekeeper's Thumb)

An abduction injury to the UCL of the MCP joint of the thumb, referred to as *gamekeeper's thumb* or *skier's thumb*, is a common injury of the hand, particularly in athletes. This injury often goes unreported but can cause significant disability if not detected and treated properly. An avulsion fracture at the insertion of the UCL at the base of the proximal phalanx often accompanies this injury.

Anatomic Considerations

Mediolateral stability of the MCP joint is provided by the UCL and RCL. The UCL is on the side of the thumb adjacent to the web space between the thumb and index finger. Originating from the metacarpal head, the UCL inserts on the lateral tubercle of the proximal phalanx. The UCL is lax when the MCP joint is extended and tight when it is flexed. The aponeurosis of the adductor pollicis is superficial to the UCL and may become trapped between the ends of the torn ligament. This interposition of soft tissue, the so-called Stener lesion, prevents primary healing in cases of complete rupture of the ligament and requires surgical repair (Fig. 3-28).

Mechanism of Injury

Injury to the UCL is usually caused by abduction stress to the thumb MCP joint combined with hyperextension. This may occur with a fall on an outstretched hand, which causes forced abduction of the thumb (e.g., a fall during skiing while holding a ski pole, the so-called skier's thumb injury).

Clinical Presentation

The patient describes the typical cause of injury as already mentioned and reports pain at the ulnar aspect of the MCP, which is exacerbated by abduction or extension of the thumb. During physical examination, the patient has acute tenderness at the ulnar aspect of the first MCP joint. The patient may also have mild to moderate swelling and ecchymosis at this site. Pinch strength may be decreased, especially in cases of complete rupture of the ligament. Sensation (e.g., two-point discrimination at 5 mm) and motor function should be assessed, but these are usually normal.

Stress testing the joint should be performed after radiographs have been obtained to rule out an associated avulsion fracture. Stress testing may displace an otherwise nondisplaced fracture fragment, if one is present. If no fracture is seen, ligamentous laxity should be tested by application of a radial (valgus) stress to the MCP joint at 30 degrees of flexion (Fig. 3-29). Testing valgus stability at 0 degrees may yield false-negative results because of the stabilizing force of the adductor aponeurosis. Normal ligamentous laxity of the MCP joint varies greatly from person to person; therefore, it is essential to examine the uninjured thumb and assess its laxity before testing the

Normal   Stener lesions

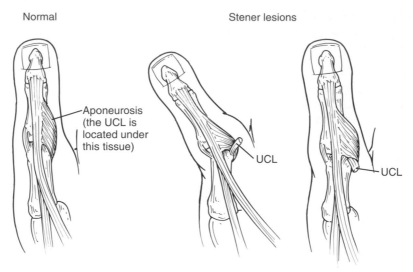

Aponeurosis
(the UCL is
located under
this tissue)

UCL

UCL

FIGURE 3-28 Stener lesion. When the ulnar collateral ligament is torn, the proximal end of the ligament displaces outside of the adductor aponeurosis.

injured thumb. Local anesthetic block may be necessary to control the patient's pain, allowing proper valgus stress testing and increasing diagnostic accuracy. An incomplete rupture is characterized by less than 30 degrees of valgus deviation or 0 to 15 degrees increased valgus deviation than the noninjured thumb. A complete rupture is characterized by 30 degrees of valgus deviation or 15 degrees of increased valgus deviation compared with the noninjured thumb.[13]

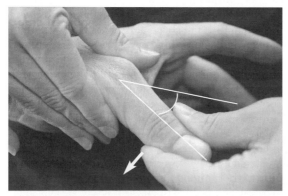

FIGURE 3-29 Evaluation of the stability of the ulnar collateral ligament (UCL). (1) Stabilize the first metacarpal with one hand. (2) Grasp the proximal phalange between two fingers. (3) Move the MCP joint into 30 degrees of flexion. (4) Apply a valgus force while keeping the metacarpal stable (move in the direction of the *arrow*). Compare the laxity to the noninjured thumb. A complete rupture is characterized by 30 degrees of valgus deviation or 15 degrees of increased valgus deviation compared with the noninjured thumb.

Hyperextension laxity and marked laxity in full extension are indicators of a complete ligament rupture. Ligament stability testing may be difficult in the acute setting because of pain and swelling, and a digital nerve block may be necessary to adequately test the UCL.

Imaging

AP, lateral, and oblique radiographs of the thumb are indicated for all patients with a significant thumb sprain because an associated avulsion fracture at the base of the proximal phalanx occurs in 20% of these cases (Fig. 3-30). The most common fracture types seen are a small fragment avulsed from the base of the proximal phalanx or a large intraarticular fragment involving 25% or more of the articular surface. Stress radiographs can also be used to assess stability when the physical findings are equivocal. Local anesthesia with a digital nerve block may be necessary to obtain adequate stress views. Magnetic resonance imaging is very sensitive in detecting Stener lesions.

Indications for Orthopedic Referral

Patients should be referred to orthopedic surgeons if they have fractures displaced more than 2 mm, fractures involving 20% or more of the articular surface, complete tears of the UCL (>35 degrees opening on valgus testing), concern for a Stener lesion, or symptomatic chronic injury. Surgical repair within 2 to 3 weeks of injury usually achieves better results than late reconstruction.

Initial Treatment

Table 3-4 summarizes the management guidelines for avulsion injuries to the UCL of the thumb.

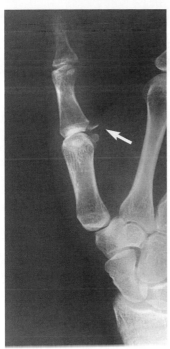

FIGURE 3-30 Avulsion fracture of the proximal phalanx of the thumb associated with an ulnar collateral ligament tear.

Nondisplaced avulsion fractures and UCL injuries without joint laxity do well with nonoperative treatment. They are best treated with a thumb spica cast or thumb spica splint (see Appendix for a stepwise description of how to apply these).

Follow-up Care

The thumb spica cast or splint should be continued for 3 to 6 weeks or until the patient has no thumb tenderness. The patient should be reevaluated every 2 weeks. The rehabilitation of this injury is similar for both surgical and nonoperative treatment. Rehabilitation exercises are started 3 to 4 weeks after initiation of therapy. They consist of flexion–extension ROM exercises for the thumb MCP joint, strengthening exercises for the forearm flexors, and strengthening of the extensors and intrinsic muscles of the hand used in pinch and handgrip.

Return to Work or Sports

For the prevention of excessive abduction, the thumb should be protected for 2 to 3 months after injury with a removable splint or by taping the thumb to the index finger.

Complications

When UCL ruptures are untreated or inadequately treated, scar tissue usually develops between the torn ends of the ligament, and the patient has chronic instability in the MCP joint. This leads to early degenerative changes, painful deformity of the joint, and decreased pinch strength. These patients should be evaluated by a hand surgeon for possible reconstructive surgery; options include tendon graft reconstruction, tendon transfer, tendon advancement, tenodesis, or arthrodesis in cases of extreme arthritis.

Table 3-4	Management Guidelines for Avulsion Injury to the Ulnar Collateral Ligament of the Thumb
	INITIAL TREATMENT
Splint type and position	Thumb spica splint with wrist in slight extension, thumb in slight abduction
Initial follow-up visit	Within 7 to 10 days
Patient instruction	Maintain active ROM at the thumb IP joint, MCP joints, and elbow
	FOLLOW-UP CARE
Cast or splint type and position	Thumb spica splint or cast with wrist in slight extension, thumb in slight abduction
Length of immobilization	4 to 6 weeks
Healing time	4 to 6 weeks
Follow-up visit interval	Every 2 weeks to assess joint motion and return to normal hand function
Repeat radiography interval	Not usually necessary unless patient reinjures hand
Patient instruction	Maintain active ROM at the thumb IP joint, MCP joints, and elbow
Buddy taping or splint protection during sports for 4 to 6 weeks after clinically healed	
Indications for orthopedic consult	Fracture displaced more than 2 mm
	Intraarticular fracture (>20% of articular surface)
Complete tear of ligament (greater than 35 degrees opening on valgus testing)	Concern for Stener lesion
	Symptomatic chronic injury

IP, Interphalangeal; MCP, metacarpophalangeal; ROM, range of motion.

Pediatric Considerations

The UCL rarely ruptures in children. A pediatric skier's thumb is more likely to involve a Salter Harris III intraarticular fracture at the base of the proximal phalanx of the thumb. These injuries require surgical fixation.

Radial Collateral Ligament Injury

RCL injuries of the thumb are less common than UCL injuries.[14] When an RCL injury is seen acutely, tenderness is maximal on the radial side of the joint (i.e., the side that is away from the other fingers). Radiographs should be obtained to rule out an associated fracture. Palmar subluxation on imaging is a sign of ligament instability.

Referral is indicated if a fracture fragment is displaced more than 2 mm, more than 3 mm of palmar subluxation, or greater than 30% gapping on stress testing, or if it involves more than 20% of the joint surface. Patients with chronic injuries, such as those who seek treatment more than 10 to 14 days after injury, should also be referred.

Unlike the UCL, delayed repair of complete RCL tears provides good results. Most patients with recent RCL injuries are candidates for conservative treatment even if the tear is complete. If radiographs show no fracture, the joint should be stressed in extension and 30 degrees of flexion to assess the degree of laxity. As described previously, pain and guarding may necessitate use of a digital block for this examination. If laxity is noted, the thumb should be immobilized for 3 to 4 weeks in a thumb spica cast with the MCP in slight flexion. ROM exercises should begin promptly after cast removal. Follow-up should continue until ROM and hand function approach the baseline. If recovery is slow, it may be beneficial to refer the patient to an occupational therapist, an orthopedic surgeon, or both.

Often RCL injuries are missed initially or the patient does not seek care until the symptoms become chronic. Patients with chronic RCL injuries have pain when using the thumb. Frequently, a prominence is noted on the radial side of the joint. Radiographs may show mild subluxation, and the joint will demonstrate laxity when stressed. Referral is recommended in these cases because steroid injection or surgery may be needed.

Dislocations of the Thumb

The thumb may dislocate laterally, dorsally, or volarly, similar to the other fingers. Diagnostic considerations and reduction technique are the same as already described for finger dislocations. Referral is indicated if a significant fracture is present or reduction fails. The thumb has no deep transverse metacarpal ligament holding the palmar

plate dorsally. Closed reduction of a thumb MCP dislocation is more likely to be successful than other digit dislocations. Once adequate anesthesia is achieved, the proximal phalanx is first hyperextended as far as possible on the metacarpal, and then the base of the proximal phalanx is pushed into flexion. Management differs after reduction. With the thumb it is important to assess lateral stability after reduction. If complete rupture of the UCL or RCL is detected, treatment proceeds as previously described for these injuries. If these ligaments are not completely torn, a thumb spica splint should be applied for 3 to 6 weeks with ROM exercises and regular follow-up afterward. The thumb usually regains stability, but the patient is likely to experience pain and tenderness for months after the injury. In some cases the volar plate fails to heal, producing chronic instability that requires surgical repair.

REFERENCES

1. Batrick N, Hashemi K, Freij R. Treatment of uncomplicated subungual haematoma. *Emerg Med J.* 2003;20:65.
2. Stevenson J, McNaughton G, Riley J. The use of prophylactic flucloxacillin in treatment of open fractures of the distal phalanx within an accident and emergency department: a double-blind randomized placebo-controlled trial. *J Hand Surg Br.* 2003;28(5):388-394.
3. Bendre A, Hartigan B, Kalainov D. Mallet finger. *J Am Acad Orthop Surg.* 2005;13(5):336-344.
4. Geyman JP, Fink K, Sullivan SD. Conservative versus surgical treatment of mallet finger: a pooled quantitative literature evaluation. *J Am Board Fam Pract.* 1998;11(5):382-390.
5. Handoll HH, Vaghela MV. Interventions for treating mallet finger injuries. *Cochrane Database Syst Rev.* 2004;(3):CD004574.
6. Cornwall R, Ricchetti ET. Pediatric phalanx fractures. *Clin Orthop Relat Res.* 2006;445:146-156.
7. Leggit JC, Meko CJ. Acute finger injuries: part II. Fractures, dislocations, and thumb injuries. *Am Fam Physician.* 2006;73(5):827-834.
8. Tuttle HG, Olvery SP, Stern PJ. Tendon avulsion injuries of the distal phalanx. *Clin Orthop Relat Res.* 2006;445: 157-168.
9. Weber DM, Kellenberger CJ, Meuli M. Conservative treatment of stable volar plate injuries of the proximal interphalangeal joint in children and adolescents. *Pediatr Emerg Care.* 2009;25:547-549.
10. Freiberg A, Pollard BA, Macdonald MR, Duncan MJ. Management of proximal interphalangeal joint injuries [review]. *Hand Clin.* 2006;22:235-242.
11. Calfee RP, Sommerkamp TG. Fracture-dislocation about the finger joints. *J Hand Surg.* 2009;34(suppl A):1140-1147.
12. Oetgen ME, Dodds SD. Non-operative treatment of common finger injuries. *Curr Rev Musculoskelet Med.* 2008;1:97-102.
13. Carlsen BT, Moran SL. Thumb trauma: Bennett fractures, Rolando fractures, and ulnar collateral ligament injuries. *J Hand Surg.* 2009;34(suppl A):945-952.
14. Patel S, Potty A, Taylor EJ, Sorene ED. Collateral ligament injuries of the metacarpophalangeal joint of the thumb: a treatment algorithm. *Strat Traum Limb Recon.* 2010;5:1-10.

METACARPAL FRACTURES

Co-Author: Charles W. Webb

Fractures of the metacarpals are the second most common type of fracture seen in a primary care setting. They are classified according to the anatomic location of the fracture: head, neck, shaft, and base. The neck and shaft are the most common fracture sites for the second through fifth metacarpals. Most first metacarpal fractures occur at the base. The treatment of fractures involving the first metacarpal differs from that involving fractures of the second through fifth metacarpals, because the biomechanics of the thumb are distinct from those of the other fingers. Management of fractures of the first metacarpal is discussed separately.

See Appendix for stepwise instructions for gutter and thumb spica splints and short arm casts used in the treatment of metacarpal fractures.

Go to Expert Consult for the electronic version of a patient instruction sheet named "Broken Hand or Wrist," which covers the steps of care from pain relief to rehabilitation exercises. This can be copied to hand out to patients to assist them during the treatment period.

METACARPAL HEAD

Anatomic Considerations

The head of the metacarpal is cam shaped; that is, the radius of the pivot point from the metacarpal to the phalanx is greater in flexion than in extension. This allows the collateral ligaments joining the metacarpal to the proximal phalanx to be relaxed in extension, permitting slight lateral motion, and to become taut in flexion (Fig. 4-1). If the metacarpophalangeal (MCP) joint is immobilized in extension, the collateral ligaments shorten, and the MCP joint becomes stiff. The metacarpal heads are weakly joined by the distal transmetacarpal ligament.

Mechanism of Injury

Fractures of the metacarpal head are usually caused by crush injuries or direct blows. The second metacarpal is the most likely to be injured, presumably because of its position as a "border metacarpal" and the fact that its base is fixed to the distal carpal row. Fractures of the first metacarpal head are rare.

Clinical Presentation

During examination, the MCP appears tender and swollen with poor range of motion (ROM), and pain is exacerbated by axial compression of the affected digit. The patient should be examined for any rotational deformity. Careful inspection of the soft tissue over the MCP joint is necessary to detect whether contact with a tooth has caused a small laceration. These lacerations can lead to serious infection if not treated with aggressive wound exploration and cleansing.

Imaging

A standard three-view hand series (anteroposterior [AP], lateral, and oblique) is usually adequate to diagnose a fracture of the metacarpal head. Occasionally, a 10-degree pronated or supinated lateral view is helpful. All metacarpal head fractures are intraarticular. Most are comminuted, and only infrequently is a two-part fracture observed. Fractures of the head are often combined with neck fractures (Fig. 4-2). Collateral ligament avulsion fractures may also be seen.

Indications for Orthopedic Referral

Patients with displaced and comminuted metacarpal head fractures should be referred to an orthopedist for surgical fixation.[1] If the comminution is severe, the patient may do just as well with splint immobilization followed by early active motion, but the consultant should decide between surgical and conservative treatment.

Initial Treatment

Table 4-1 summarizes the management guidelines for metacarpal head fractures. The acute management of these fractures should include ice, elevation, analgesics, and immobilization in a radial or ulnar gutter splint (**see Appendix for a stepwise description of how to apply a gutter splint**) or a

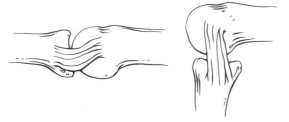

FIGURE 4-1 The collateral ligaments of the metacarpophalangeal joint are relaxed in extension but become taut in full flexion.

soft bulky hand dressing with the hand in a position of function. A position of function is with the wrist in 20 to 30 degrees of extension and the fingers and thumb in a slightly flexed position. The hand should be immobilized until the patient is seen by the orthopedist or returns for a follow-up visit in 1 week.

Follow-up Care

Nondisplaced fractures of the metacarpal head should be treated with a gutter splint for approximately 2 weeks (prolonged immobilization should be avoided). Repeat radiographs should be obtained

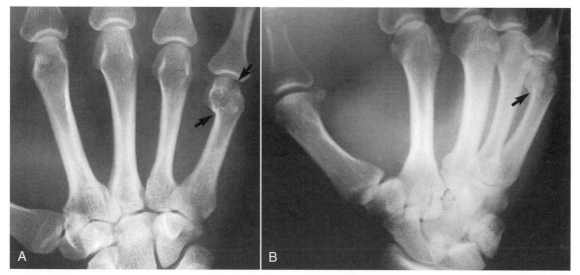

FIGURE 4-2 A, Anteroposterior view. **B,** Oblique view of the hand demonstrating a fracture of the fifth metacarpal head and neck (*arrows*).

Table 4-1	*Management Guidelines for Metacarpal Head Fracture*
	INITIAL TREATMENT
Splint type and position	Gutter splint: wrist, 30 degrees of extension; metacarpophalangeal, 70 to 90 degrees; proximal interphalangeal or DIP, 5 to 10 degrees; or bulky hand dressing
Initial follow-up visit	1 week
Patient instruction	Icing, elevation of hand above level of heart
	FOLLOW-UP CARE
Cast or splint type and position	Gutter splint
Length of immobilization	2 to 3 weeks
Healing time	4 to 6 weeks
Follow-up visit interval	Every 2 weeks
Repeat radiography interval	1 week after injury to check for alignment
	At completion of immobilization to document healing
Patient instruction	Begin active ROM exercises after immobilization
Indications for orthopedic consult	Displaced fractures
	Comminuted fracture

DIP, distal interphalangeal; ROM, range of motion.

within a week of injury to ensure that the fragments are not displaced, and active ROM exercises should be started after immobilization. Patients with displacement at any time during the healing process should be referred to an orthopedic surgeon.[2,3]

Complications

Chronic stiffness caused by tendon adhesions, collateral ligament shortening, or dorsal capsular contracture is the most common complication of these intraarticular fractures. Comminuted metacarpal head fractures may result in moderate to severe loss of ROM. Avascular necrosis can occur, especially after occult compression fractures from decreased blood flow to the fracture site.[4,5]

Return to Work or Sports

Fractures of the metacarpal head are difficult to treat, and rehabilitation efforts must be closely monitored to promote full ROM. The patient should begin ROM exercises at the MCP joint as early as possible, initially under the direct supervision of an experienced physical therapist or hand therapist. Early motion helps mold fracture fragments into an acceptable articular surface. Rehabilitation can then be advanced to help patients regain fine hand movements and functional grip strength. Patients may be ready to resume work 6 to 8 weeks after injury, but treatment must be individualized.[3,6]

Pediatric Considerations

Epiphyseal and physeal fractures of the fifth metacarpal head are not uncommon, especially among patients 12 to 16 years of age. When these injuries occur, they are most usually Salter-Harris type II fractures (Fig. 4-3); epiphyseal and physeal fractures of the second and third metacarpal heads rarely occur. Anatomic considerations are particularly important for injuries to the metacarpal head in this age group. The collateral ligaments at the MCP joint originate and insert almost exclusively on the epiphysis. The growth plate is thus relatively unprotected from injury, and a tense effusion can occur after fracture of the metacarpal epiphysis. This pressure can tamponade the vessels supplying the epiphysis, leading to necrosis and growth arrest.

The typical mechanism of injury is an axial load to the finger, usually accompanied by some rotational component. The dorsum of the child's hand should be examined carefully for significant swelling, which may not be immediately apparent. During physical examination, the patient's finger should be evaluated for malalignment because the "border digits" (i.e., the second and fifth metacarpals) are particularly prone to malalignment injuries. A small amount of displacement in the

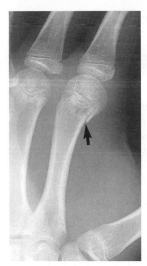

FIGURE 4-3 Salter-Harris type II fracture of metacarpal head (*arrow*). (*From Thornton A, Gyll C. Children's Fractures: A Radiological Guide to Safe Practice. Philadelphia, WB Saunders, 1999.*)

metacarpal head can cause significant malrotation of the distal portion of the finger.

Nondisplaced avulsion fractures caused by the collateral ligaments or minimally displaced type II fractures can be treated conservatively. The patient's hand should be immobilized for 2 to 3 weeks in an ulnar or radial gutter splint with the wrist in slight extension, the MCP joints in full flexion, and the proximal interphalangeal (PIP) and distal interphalangeal (DIP) joints in full extension. Active ROM exercises should be started after immobilization. Splinting for nondisplaced and minimally displaced fractures yields consistently positive results.

Displaced fractures should be splinted and the patients referred promptly for definitive treatment by orthopedic surgeons.

Intraarticular head-splitting Salter-Harris type II, type III, and type IV fractures are rare. As mentioned earlier, the rich blood supply of the epiphyseal and periphyseal areas can lead to avascular necrosis caused by intracapsular bleeding. The treating physician should consider aspiration of the MCP joint effusion to reduce the risk of pressure necrosis. Reducible but unstable fractures may require pin fixation, and displaced intraarticular fractures may require open reduction and internal fixation. In such cases, the referring physician may consider joint aspiration before referral.

METACARPAL NECK

Anatomic Considerations

The dorsal and volar interosseous muscles originate from the shafts of the metacarpals and act as flexors of the MCP joints. After a metacarpal neck fracture, the action of the interosseous muscles causes volar displacement of the metacarpal head (apex dorsal angulation). Some degree of angulation (20 to 40 degrees) of the neck can be accepted in the fourth and fifth metacarpals, because compensatory motion at the carpometacarpal (CMC) joint is available. The bases of the second and third metacarpals are practically fixed at the distal carpal row with virtually no motion. Thus, no angulation is tolerated in neck fractures of the second and third metacarpals.

Mechanism of Injury

Metacarpal neck fractures usually result from a direct axial force such that is caused by punching a solid object or wall with a clenched fist. The fifth metacarpal neck fracture is by far the most common hand fracture encountered and is referred to as a boxer's fracture.

Clinical Presentation

When a metacarpal neck fracture occurs, the dorsum of the hand is tender and swollen, sometimes quite significantly. The MCP joint is depressed because of the apex dorsal angulation of the fracture. If the angulation is severe (>40 degrees), the displaced metacarpal head may interfere with the normal function of the extensor apparatus, causing pseudoclawing. Hyperextension of the MCP joint and flexion of the PIP joint as the patient attempts to extend the finger (Fig. 4-4) confirm the presence of pseudoclawing.

Malrotation often accompanies a metacarpal neck fracture, and the patient should be examined carefully to detect this type of displacement. Malrotation occurs more commonly in the border metacarpals (i.e., the second and fifth metacarpals). With the fingers in a semiflexed position, the plane of the fingernails should be aligned; in the fully flexed position, the fingers should all point toward the distal radius. The hand must be examined for any evidence of teeth marks that may result from a punching injury because this is a source for infection and should be treated as an open fracture.[5,7,8]

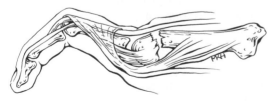

FIGURE 4-4 Comminution of the volar cortex in metacarpal neck fractures allows volar displacement of the metacarpal head. This may in turn disrupt the extensor mechanism, causing the so-called pseudoclawing phenomenon.

Imaging

Three views of the hand are usually adequate to visualize a metacarpal neck fracture (AP, lateral, and oblique views). The fracture is often comminuted on the volar side. The typical apex dorsal angulation should be measured on the lateral view (Fig. 4-5). The normal metacarpal neck angle is 15 degrees, so a measurement of 40 degrees of apex dorsal angulation represents true angulation of only 25 degrees.[2,8]

Indications for Orthopedic Referral

Patients with angulated or displaced fractures of the second or third metacarpal neck require referral for operative treatment. Patients who have metacarpal neck fractures with rotational malalignment must also be referred. If any degree of residual angulation is unacceptable to the patient, referral for internal fixation is indicated.

Initial Treatment

Table 4-2 summarizes management guidelines for metacarpal neck fractures. The best method of treating angulated fractures of the fourth or fifth metacarpal has not been universally established. Although reduction of these fractures is relatively easy, maintaining the reduction is often difficult. Virtually all neck fractures are inherently unstable because of deforming forces of the interosseous muscles and comminution of the volar cortex. The only position of the MCP joint that adequately holds the reduction is full extension. However, the MCP joint is prone to significant stiffness if held in extension for longer than 7 to 10 days. The risk of disabling loss of joint mobility outweighs the benefits of this positioning, so it is recommended to place the MCP joints in 70 to 90 degrees of flexion.

Fractures requiring that the patient be referred to an orthopedic surgeon should be immobilized in a radial or ulnar gutter splint with the MCP joints in 70 to 90 degrees of flexion and the PIP and DIP joints in slight flexion until the patient is seen by the consultant.

Nondisplaced Fractures (Second or Third Metacarpal) and Fractures with Mild Angulation (Fourth or Fifth Metacarpal)

Patients with nondisplaced fractures of the second or third metacarpal or mildly angulated fractures of the fourth (<30 degrees) or fifth (<40 degrees) metacarpal can have the injured hand immobilized in a radial or ulnar gutter splint. Several alternatives to rigid splint immobilization in the treatment of metacarpal neck fractures have been proposed in small trials, including elastic bandaging, functional taping, molded bracing, and

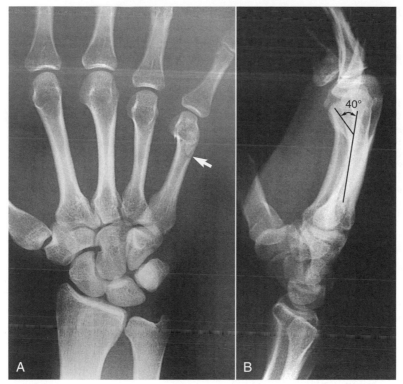

FIGURE 4-5 A, Anteroposterior view (*arrow*). **B,** Lateral view of a boxer's fracture. Forty degrees of apex dorsal angulation is observed on the lateral view.

functional treatment.[9-12] None of these treatments has been shown to be definitively superior to rigid splinting, but they are good alternatives to those who may not tolerate the stiffness associated with immobilization.

Fractures with Significant Angulation or Pseudoclawing (Fourth or Fifth Metacarpal)

An attempt at closed reduction is mandatory if pseudoclawing is apparent during physical examination. Patients with significant angulation (fourth

Table 4-2	Management Guidelines for Metacarpal Neck Fracture
	INITIAL TREATMENT
Splint type and position	Gutter splint: wrist, 30-degree extension; MCP, 70 to 90 degrees; PIP or DIP, 5 to 10 degrees
Initial follow-up visit	Within 4 to 5 days for second or third metacarpal
	Within 7 to 10 days for fourth or fifth metacarpal
Patient instruction	Icing, elevation
	FOLLOW-UP CARE
Cast or splint type and position	Gutter splint
Length of immobilization	3 to 4 weeks
Healing time	4 to 6 weeks
Follow-up visit interval	Every 2 weeks
Repeat radiography interval	At initial follow-up to check for angulation or malrotation
	Every 2 weeks to document position and healing
Patient instruction	Begin ROM exercises after immobilization (handgrip strengthening)
	Avoid contact sports for 4 to 6 weeks after immobilization or use orthotic protection
Indications for orthopedic consult	Angulated or displaced fractures of second or third metacarpal
	Malrotation
	Angulation unacceptable to patient after closed reduction
	Unable to hold reduction position
	Malunion with painful grip or pseudoclawing

DIP, distal interphalangeal; MCP, metacarpophalangeal; PIP, proximal interphalangeal; ROM, range of motion.

metacarpal >30 degrees, fifth metacarpal >40 degrees) but no pseudoclawing often benefit from closed reduction. However, they may also achieve good clinical healing from immobilization without reduction. Patients should be advised that residual angulation and deformity are likely despite closed reduction. The deformity is usually cosmetic and causes no functional impairment. Patients may decide against reduction if they accept these possible outcomes.

Other factors to consider in decision making regarding reduction include the amount of soft tissue padding in the palm (a petite hand may not tolerate as much residual deformity), occupational recreational demands of the hand (especially gripping or use of hand tools), and length of time from the injury to time of treatment.

Method of Reduction

Anesthesia can be administered by either a hematoma block at the site of the fracture or an ulnar nerve block at the wrist. For a hematoma block, a Betadine scrub of the skin is performed over the fracture site. The local anesthetic (5 to 8 mL of 1% lidocaine without epinephrine) is injected gradually by alternate injection, with half the volume of anesthetic injected initially. The blood from the hematoma is then withdrawn up to the original volume. The mixture of blood and lidocaine is repeatedly injected and reaspirated until the anesthetic is dispersed in the hematoma. The final aspirate should be equal to the original anesthetic volume so that the volume of fluid in the hematoma has not been increased.

A complete ulnar nerve block involves injections for both the ulnar nerve at the wrist and the dorsal sensory branch of the ulnar nerve. Performance of an ulnar nerve block begins with a sterile scrub of the skin over the ulnar side of the wrist. The provider palpates the pisiform bone, a prominence felt just beyond the distal wrist crease on the ulnar side of the wrist with the wrist in extension. Between 2 and 3 mL of 1% lidocaine without epinephrine is injected into the subcutaneous tissues just proximal to the pisiform bone between the proximal and distal creases of the wrist (Fig. 4-6). The dorsal sensory branch of the ulnar nerve is anesthetized by injection of a wheal of lidocaine around the ulnar aspect of the wrist to the dorsum of the ulnar styloid at the level of the distal wrist crease.

After adequate anesthesia has been achieved and plaster or fiberglass splints are ready for application, reduction can be attempted. If finger traps are available, they are helpful in disimpacting the fracture fragments before reduction.

The patient holds the elbow adducted to the side, the wrist is extended, and the MCP joint is

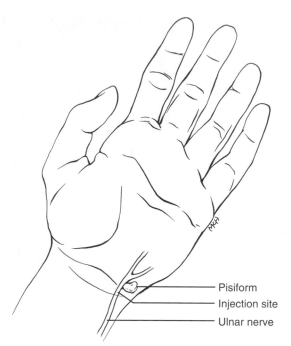

FIGURE 4-6 Correct needle position for an ulnar nerve block. Lidocaine is injected just proximal to the pisiform bone between the proximal and distal creases of the wrist.

Pisiform
Injection site
Ulnar nerve

flexed maximally. The examiner grasps the shaft of the flexed proximal phalanx and uses it as a lever arm to push the metacarpal head dorsally. At the same time, the examiner applies counterpressure just proximal to the fracture site at the dorsum of the metacarpal (Fig. 4-7).

Another reduction technique, the so-called 90-90 method, is also effective. With this method, the MCP, PIP, and DIP joints all are flexed to 90 degrees for the reduction maneuver only. Dorsally directed pressure is applied over the flexed PIP joint while at the same time a volar directed force is applied over the area of the fractured metacarpal (Fig. 4-8). After reduction, the hand should be immobilized in an ulnar gutter splint. The wrist should be positioned at 30 degrees of extension with the MCP joint at 90 degrees and the interphalangeal (IP) joints in extension (if using a gutter splint). A postreduction lateral view radiograph of the splinted hand should be taken to check for fracture alignment.

Follow-up Care

Nondisplaced fractures of the second or third metacarpal need follow-up radiographs within 4 to 5 days to look for angulation or malrotation. Any amount of change in position is an indication for prompt orthopedic referral. For fourth or fifth metacarpal fractures, repeat AP and lateral radiographs should be obtained within 7 to 10 days to evaluate whether the reduction position has been

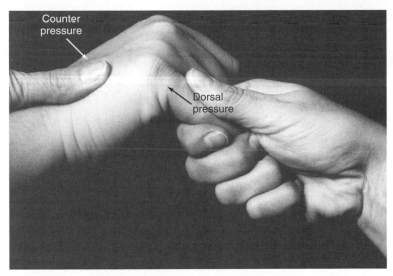

FIGURE 4-7 Method of reduction for metacarpal neck fracture. The metacarpophalangeal joint is flexed, and the proximal phalanx is used to help reduce the metacarpal neck fracture.

maintained. If the fracture is significantly more angulated than in the prereduction radiographs or the reduction has slipped back to its original position, orthopedic referral should be considered. If fracture alignment is maintained, the patient can be seen again in another 2 to 3 weeks.

Most metacarpal neck fractures heal after 4 weeks of immobilization. If compliance with a splint is a concern or the patient prefers a cast, the splint can be converted to a cast. A short-arm cast is applied with the wrist in 30 degrees of extension and MCP joints in 90 degrees of flexion. The cast

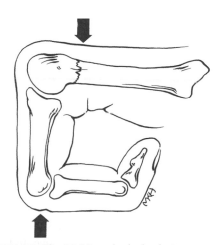

FIGURE 4-8 The 90-90 method of reducing a metacarpal neck fracture. The metacarpophalangeal, proximal interphalangeal (PIP), and distal interphalangeal joints all are flexed to 90 degrees. Dorsally directed pressure is applied to the flexed PIP joint while a volar-directed force is applied over the apex of the fracture.

extends to the palmar crease on the volar side and to the PIP joints on the dorsal side. If gutter splinting is used, PIP and DIP motion are begun when the splint is discontinued.

Complications

Stiffness of the MCP and PIP joints is not uncommon after a metacarpal neck fracture. The stiffness may be the result of prolonged immobilization, tendon adhesions, or interosseous muscle contracture. More aggressive hand rehabilitation under the supervision of a physical or occupational therapist will help the patient regain motion and function. Malunion with apex dorsal angulation can occur; the farther the fracture is from the MCP joint, the more likely it is that the deformity will cause a painful grip, a prominence of the metacarpal head in the palm, or pseudoclawing. Rotational malunion also occurs and is more common in the second and fifth metacarpals. Patients with a symptomatic malunion should be referred for consideration of a corrective wedge osteotomy.

Return to Work or Sports

After immobilization, the patient should begin ROM exercises of the MCP joint and handgrip strengthening (e.g., squeezing a rubber ball). Patients should avoid contact sports for 4 to 6 weeks after immobilization to reduce the risk of reinjury.[6]

Major determinants for return to sports participation include the fracture type and stability, as well as the athlete's sport and position played. The athlete may return to play after full or near-normal ROM has been achieved and clinical (although

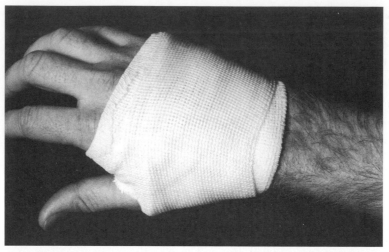

FIGURE 4-9 A fiberglass "glove cast" can be used to stabilize a metacarpal fracture while allowing early motion at the wrist.

not necessarily radiographic) evidence of fracture healing exists. This usually requires 4 to 6 weeks. Depending on the athlete's sports and position played, the athlete may return to play earlier with adequate external protection.

An alternative therapeutic option for athletes who wish to continue to compete during the period of immobilization is the so-called glove cast.[13] A fiberglass cast is applied just distal to the distal palmar crease of the wrist. The cast extends to the neck of the metacarpals and is circumferential across the dorsal and palmar sides of the hand, including the thenar aspect and the ulnar border (Fig. 4-9). This cast allows maximal finger and wrist function while still protecting the fracture site.

Pediatric Considerations

Pediatric patients with nondisplaced or minimally displaced metacarpal neck fractures should have the hand immobilized in an ulnar or radial gutter splint with the wrist in slight extension, the MCP joints in full flexion, and the PIP and DIP joints in extension.

For pediatric patients with a mildly displaced metacarpal neck fracture, closed reduction usually produces good results. Anesthesia is achieved with a hematoma block or ulnar nerve wrist block. After reduction, adequate padding is used, but overpadding should be avoided (two layers of cast padding are sufficient). Dorsal and volar plaster splints are used to hold the wrist in slight extension (the "position of function") and the MCP joints in maximal flexion. Significant stiffness rarely develops in children, so the PIP and DIP joints can be included in the splint and held at full extension. The patient should be reexamined at 5 to 7 days after reduction to ensure that reduction is

maintained. If alignment is maintained, the volar and dorsal splints are replaced with a gutter splint. If the splint is in good repair and is holding proper position, it can remain in place for 3 to 4 weeks.

METACARPAL SHAFT

Anatomic Considerations

Fractures of the metacarpal shaft may be transverse, oblique, or comminuted. Most transverse fractures result in apex dorsal angulation because of the pull of the interosseous muscles. Oblique fractures tend to shorten and rotate rather than angulate. Up to 5 mm of shortening can be accepted as long as no angulation or rotational malalignment is apparent. The third and fourth metacarpals tend to be more stable because of the splinting effect of the adjacent metacarpals and the transverse metacarpal ligaments (Fig. 4-10). Compared with neck fractures, much less angulation is tolerated in metacarpal shaft fractures. For any given angulation of the shaft, the deformity is more pronounced, and the likelihood of pseudoclawing is increased. The detection of rotational malalignment is critical in the management of metacarpal shaft fractures because even small degrees of malrotation cause significant overlap of the fingers when the MCP joint is flexed.

Mechanism of Injury

Transverse fractures are usually the result of a direct blow to the metacarpal. Oblique and spiral fractures are caused by a twisting force. Comminuted fractures result from significant trauma such as a crush injury or gunshot wound and are frequently associated with extensive soft tissue damage.

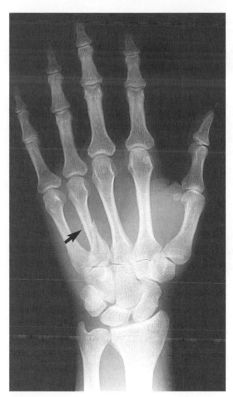

FIGURE 4-10 A stable oblique fracture of the fourth meta-carpal shaft with minimal shortening (*arrow*).

Clinical Presentation

During examination, the dorsum of the hand is tender and swollen. ROM is limited, especially flexion at the MCP joint. A rotational deformity must be detected early. With the fingers in a semi-flexed position, the plane of the fingernails should be aligned; in the fully flexed position, the fingers should all point toward the distal radius.

Imaging

Three views of the hand (AP, lateral, and oblique) are usually adequate to visualize metacarpal shaft fractures. Radiographs should be examined for shortening, angulation (Fig. 4-11), and comminution. A difference in the diameters between the two fracture fragments may indicate malrotation.

Indications for Orthopedic Referral

Indications for orthopedic referral include malrotation, shortening of more than 5 mm, inability to reduce dorsal angulation or maintain the reduction, displaced fractures, comminuted fractures, and more than one metacarpal fractured.

Initial Treatment

Table 4-3 summarizes management guidelines for metacarpal shaft fractures. Fractures that require referral to an orthopedic surgeon should be immobilized in a radial or ulnar gutter splint with the MCP joints in 70 to 90 degrees of flexion and the PIP and DIP joints in slight flexion while the patient awaits consultation.

Nondisplaced Fractures

Nondisplaced metacarpal shaft fractures can be immobilized in a radial or ulnar gutter splint. Regular icing and elevation of the hand above the level of the heart are essential to help reduce swelling in the first 48 hours. The patient should be advised of the importance of returning within 5 to 7 days for repeat radiographs to ensure correct alignment of the fracture.

Angulated Fractures

The same principles apply to the management of angular deformity in the shaft as those in the neck of the metacarpal. Only minimal angulation can be accepted in the second and third metacarpal shafts because of the lack of compensatory motion at the CMC joint. Angulation of more than 10 degrees in the second or third metacarpal or more than 20 degrees in the fourth or fifth metacarpal should be corrected. The more proximal the fracture, the less angulation that can be accepted.[14]

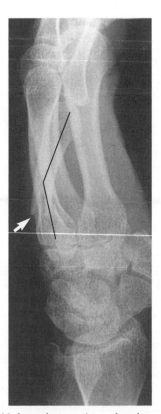

FIGURE 4-11 Lateral view. Apex dorsal angulation of a metacarpal shaft fracture (*arrow*).

Table 4-3	*Management Guidelines for Metacarpal Shaft Fracture*
INITIAL TREATMENT	
Splint type and position	Gutter splint: wrist, 30 degrees extension; MCP, 70 to 90 degrees; PIP or DIP, 5 to 10 degrees
Initial follow-up visit	Within 5 to 7 days
Patient instruction	Icing, elevation
FOLLOW-UP CARE	
Cast or splint type and position	Gutter splint
Length of immobilization	4 weeks
	Continue immobilization for another 2 weeks if no radiographic healing is apparent at 4 weeks (allow gentle ROM out of splint daily during this time)
Healing time	6 to 8 weeks
Follow-up visit interval	Every 2 weeks
Repeat radiography interval	At 5 to 7 days to check position
	Every 1 to 2 weeks to document position and healing
Patient instruction	Begin ROM exercises after immobilization
	Avoid contact sports for 4 to 6 weeks after immobilization or use orthotic protection
Indications for orthopedic consult	Malrotation
	Shortening >5 mm
	Inability to reduce dorsal angulation or maintain reduction
	Displaced fractures
	Comminuted fractures
	Fractures of more than one metacarpal

DIP, distal interphalangeal; MCP, metacarpophalangeal; PIP, proximal interphalangeal; ROM, range of motion.

Method of Reduction

A hematoma block at the site of the fracture is the simplest method of anesthesia and produces significant pain relief, although complete anesthesia is not always obtained. The technique for performing a hematoma block is described in the Initial Treatment section for metacarpal neck fractures.

A Bier block provides excellent anesthesia for closed reduction of hand fractures and is easily performed. A needle or intravenous catheter is inserted into a superficial vein on the hand. The arm is then elevated and exsanguinated by wrapping of an elastic bandage distally to proximally. A blood pressure cuff is applied to the upper arm and inflated to 250 mm Hg. Great care should be taken to ensure that the cuff does not deflate. A clamp can be used on the tubing to prevent an air leak. After the cuff is secure, the elastic bandage is removed. The arm is lowered to the level of the heart, and 20 to 40 mL of 0.5% lidocaine is injected. The needle or catheter is removed. Anesthesia of the arm is usually produced within 5 to 10 minutes. A second cuff can be inflated distal to the first cuff and the original cuff deflated to prevent pain from the tourniquet effect. The cuff should remain inflated for at least 20 minutes. If the cuff deflates before this time, the patient may receive a toxic dose of lidocaine into the general circulation. Drugs and equipment to treat a systemic reaction to lidocaine must be on hand. A

long-acting anesthetic such as bupivacaine should never be used for this type of regional block.

After adequate anesthesia has been achieved and plaster or fiberglass splints are ready for application, reduction can be attempted. If finger traps are available, they are helpful in disimpacting the fracture fragments before reduction. Traction should be maintained on the digit while volar directed pressure is applied over the apex of the fracture. After reduction, the hand should be immobilized in a gutter splint. The wrist should be positioned at 30 degrees of extension with the MCP joint at 90 degrees and the IP joints in extension. Splinting the injured finger and buddy taping it to an adjacent finger help maintain normal alignment.

An alternative method of reduction is also effective. The patient holds the elbow adducted to the side, the wrist is extended, and the MCP joint is flexed maximally. The examiner grasps the shaft of the proximal phalanx and uses it as a lever arm to push the metacarpal head dorsally. At the same time, the examiner applies counterpressure just proximal to the fracture site at the dorsum of the metacarpal (See Fig. 4-7).

A postreduction lateral view radiograph of the splinted hand should be taken to check for fracture position. If the result is unsatisfactory, a repeat attempt is advised. If closed reduction is unsuccessful, the patient should be referred for surgical fixation.

Follow-up Care

The patient should be seen within 5 to 7 days of initial treatment to obtain follow-up radiographs. If proper alignment has not been maintained, the patient should be referred to an orthopedic surgeon. If the fracture is stable, splint immobilization should be continued for 4 weeks. If no evidence of radiographic healing (no callus) is apparent at 4 weeks, the gutter splint should be continued for an additional 2 weeks with the patient being allowed to remove the splint a few times per day for gentle ROM exercises. Radiographic healing lags considerably behind clinical healing for transverse diaphyseal shaft fractures, but typically some callus is evident by 6 weeks (Fig. 4-12). Repeat radiographs should be obtained every 7 to 10 days to ensure continued stability. A new splint should be applied whenever the reduction of edema in the hand causes significant loosening. Active motion of the PIP and DIP joints after the gutter splint is discontinued.

Complications

The complications after metacarpal shaft fractures are the same as those listed for metacarpal neck fractures.

Return to Work or Sports

If participating in contact sports, the patient should wear a protective wrist splint over the fracture site for an additional 4 to 6 weeks to prevent reinjury. A useful alternative is the so-called glove cast as described previously for metacarpal neck fractures (See Fig. 4-9). This cast protects the fracture site but allows functional wrist and forearm motion. The patient may be referred to a hand or physical therapist for help regaining full ROM and normal grip strength.[6]

Pediatric Considerations

The management of children with metacarpal shaft fractures is similar to that of adults. These injuries tend to occur in older children and

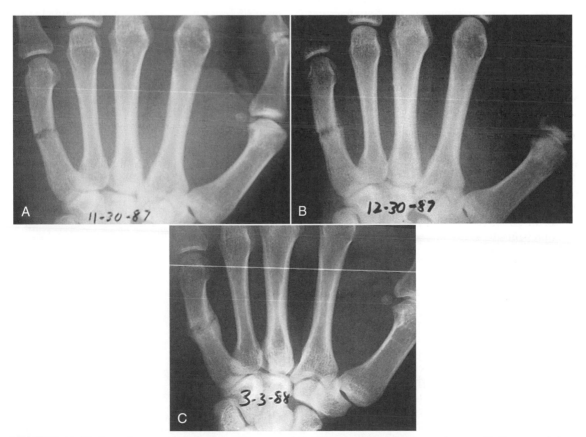

FIGURE 4-12 Healing of a transverse diaphyseal fracture of the fifth metacarpal. **A,** Original injury. **B,** One month later the amount of callus is minimal. **C,** Approximately 3 months after injury, adequate callus is apparent, although the fracture is far from being completely healed radiographically.

teenagers, and the usual cause of injury is a torsional force applied to the finger that leads to a spiral or oblique fracture of the metacarpal shaft. However, a transverse fracture pattern may result if the hand is stepped on. A dorsal blow causing a transverse fracture is uncommon in children.

The patient reports the typical mechanism of injury to the finger and complains of pain at the dorsum of the affected finger. When examined, the site of the fracture may show prominence in the dorsum of the hand. The patient should be examined for any sign of malrotation or shortening. With the fingers in a semiflexed position, the planes of the fingernails should be aligned; in the fully flexed position, the fingers should all point toward the distal radius.

Reduction and immobilization of these fractures are similar to those already outlined for adults. After closed reduction, the patient's hand is placed in dorsal and volar splints with the wrist in the position of function and the MCP joints in maximal flexion. The hand should be immobilized for 3 to 4 weeks.

It is important for the treating physician to be aware that, although pediatric metacarpal neck fractures show a great deal of remodeling, this is not true for pediatric metacarpal shaft fractures. Thus, careful reduction, postreduction radiographs, and confirmation of maintenance of reduction at follow-up are especially important when treating children and teenagers with this injury. A particular problem with this injury is the possibility that the periosteum may become interposed in the fracture site, particularly in spiral fractures of the metacarpal shaft, leading to malunion or delayed union. Patients with unstable fractures, irreducible fractures, or multiple metacarpal fractures should have a splint applied and be referred to an orthopedic surgeon. If the injury fails to respond to closed reduction, the patient may be treated with percutaneous pin fixation or with open reduction and internal fixation.

METACARPAL BASE

Anatomic Considerations

Fractures of the second and third metacarpals are rarely displaced owing to their relatively fixed position at the CMC joint. Fractures of the fourth metacarpal base are more often displaced or associated with a disruption of the CMC joint than fractures of the bases of the second and third metacarpals are. CMC joint dislocation or instability is most commonly associated with a fracture of the fifth metacarpal base because of the obliquely oriented sloping surface of the fifth CMC joint and the fact that the base is not stabilized on both sides.

The radial aspect of the base of the fifth metacarpal is attached to the fourth metacarpal and the hamate bone. In a typical fracture, the radial one fourth or one third of the base is avulsed and remains attached. The large metacarpal fragment is displaced dorsally by the pull of the extensor carpi ulnaris (Fig. 4-13). The motor branch of the ulnar nerve may be injured after fractures of the base of the fourth or fifth metacarpal, particularly if a crush injury is present.

Mechanism of Injury

Fractures of the base of the metacarpals usually result from two mechanisms of injury: a direct blow to the dorsum of the hand or a torsional force exerted on the digit. Punching or a fall on an outstretched hand are less common causes of base fractures.

Clinical Presentation

Tenderness and swelling at the base of the metacarpals are typical. If swelling is slight, a bony prominence may be detected in the area of the base of the injured metacarpal. Pain is increased with flexion and extension of the wrist. Checking carefully for rotational deformities is important because even slight rotation at the base is magnified at the fingertips. Active abduction and adduction of the fingers should be tested, because ulnar nerve injury

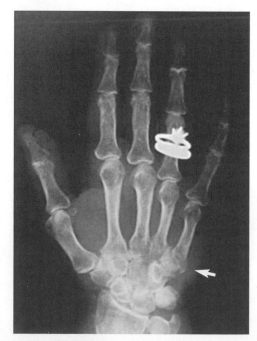

FIGURE 4-13 Comminuted fracture of the base of the fifth metacarpal with dorsal displacement of the metacarpal shaft. (*From Browner BD, Jupiter JB, Levine AM, Trafton PG [eds]. Skeletal Trauma: Fractures, Dislocations, Ligamentous Injuries. Philadelphia, WB Saunders, 1992.*)

can result in weakness of the intrinsic hand muscles. Ulnar nerve damage may be difficult to detect initially because of swelling or pain.

Imaging

A standard three-view hand series is required in the evaluation of fractures of the metacarpal base. Some of these fractures are subtle and require special views, computed tomography (CT), or magnetic resonance imaging (MRI) to confirm the diagnosis. Intraarticular fractures of the second metacarpal base are particularly difficult to detect radiographically. Careful inspection of the lateral view is essential to detect any dorsal displacement of the shaft, especially in fractures of the fifth metacarpal. The lateral view should also be closely examined for any subluxation or dislocation of the metacarpal base from the carpal row (Fig. 4-14).

Indications for Orthopedic Referral

Fractures of the base of the fifth metacarpal are inherently unstable and nearly always require pin fixation. Patients with malrotation or evidence of ulnar nerve damage should be promptly referred to an orthopedic surgeon. Subluxations or dislocations of the metacarpals at the CMC joint also require orthopedic referral.

Initial Treatment

Table 4-4 summarizes management guidelines for metacarpal base fractures. Patients with a fracture of the fifth metacarpal base should be immobilized with dorsal and volar splints with the wrist in 30 degrees of extension and the MCP joints free and referred to an orthopedic surgeon within 3 to 5 days.

Nondisplaced Fractures (Second, Third, and Fourth Metacarpals)

Nondisplaced fractures should be immobilized initially with dorsal and volar splints with the wrist in 30 degrees of extension and the MCP joints free. If the amount of swelling is stable and minimal, the patient can be placed in a short-arm cast. Ice should be applied regularly during the first 24 to 48 hours and the patient instructed to keep the hand elevated as much as possible.

Displaced Fractures (Second, Third, and Fourth Metacarpals)

Fractures of the metacarpal base with dorsal displacement should be reduced under regional anesthesia (see description of the technique for Bier block anesthesia in the Initial Treatment section for metacarpal shaft fractures). These fractures are reduced with volar-directed pressure over the apex

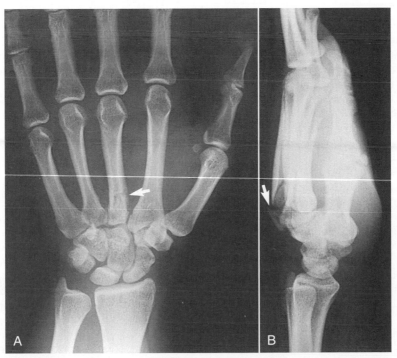

FIGURE 4-14 **A,** Anteroposterior view demonstrates a fracture of the base of the third metacarpal (*arrow*). **B,** Lateral view shows dorsal displacement of the shaft and dorsal subluxation of the metacarpal base from the carpal row (*arrow*).

Table 4-4	*Management Guidelines for Metacarpal Base Fracture*
	INITIAL TREATMENT
Splint type and position	Dorsal and volar splints
	Wrist, 30-degree extension; MCP, free
Initial follow-up visit	Within 5 to 7 days
Patient instruction	Icing, elevation
	FOLLOW-UP CARE
Cast or splint type and position	Short-arm cast; wrist, 30-degree extension
Length of immobilization	4 weeks
Healing time	6 to 8 weeks
Follow-up visit interval	Weekly for 3 weeks; then every 2 weeks
Repeat radiography interval	At 5 to 7 days to check position
	Weekly for a total of 3 weeks
Patient instruction	Begin ROM exercises after immobilization (flexion and extension of wrist and handgrip strengthening)
	Orthotic protection for 4 to 6 weeks after cast is removed
Indications for orthopedic consult	All fifth metacarpal base fractures
	Malrotation
	Ulnar nerve injury
	Subluxation or dislocation of CMC joint
	Inability to maintain reduction

CMC, carpometacarpal; MCP, metacarpophalangeal; ROM, range of motion.

of the fracture while longitudinal traction is applied to the affected digit. After reduction, the hand should be immobilized with dorsal and volar splints as described earlier. A postreduction lateral view of the splinted hand should be obtained to check for position. The goal of reduction is near anatomic alignment.

Follow-up Care

Patients with nondisplaced fractures or displaced fractures that have been reduced should be seen within 5 to 7 days for repeat radiographs and definitive casting. If there is redisplacement of the fracture fragments, the patient should be referred for consideration of operative treatment. Repeat radiographs should be performed weekly for the next 3 weeks to ensure stability of the fracture. Any change in position requires orthopedic referral.

A short-arm cast should be applied once swelling has decreased significantly, usually at the first follow-up visit. After the splint is removed, the function of the intrinsic muscles of the hand should be tested because ulnar nerve injury may have gone undetected initially. Cast immobilization should be continued for 4 weeks. After immobilization, the patient should begin rehabilitation exercises, including flexion and extension of the wrist and handgrip strengthening.

Complications

Unrecognized metacarpal base fractures may lead to chronic hand pain, and unrecognized displacement of fracture fragments may lead to symptomatic CMC joint arthritis. Ulnar nerve damage may cause paresis or wasting of the intrinsic muscles of the hand. Referral to a hand surgeon is advisable if any of these complications occur.

Return to Work or Sports

Orthotic protection of the fracture site should be used for an additional 4 to 6 weeks if the patient wants to participate in contact sports.

Pediatric Considerations

The base of the metacarpals is well protected by the bony congruence of the metacarpals and by the ligaments stabilizing the hand. Injuries in this area are uncommon in children and are usually the result of high-energy trauma such as a fall from height or a significant crush injury. Tenderness at the base of the metacarpals accompanied by a history of significant trauma should prompt suspicion of extensive soft tissue injury with or without a fracture at the base of the metacarpal. Occasionally, a dorsal blow or axial load may cause a fracture through the metaphyseal portion of the metacarpal base, leading to a small compression fracture that is usually stable. Patients with such a small compression fracture may be safely treated with immobilization in a gutter splint for 3 to 4 weeks or until the injury is nontender. Patients with a displaced fracture at the base of the metacarpal or in whom a fracture dislocation of the CMC joint is suspected should have the injury splinted and be referred promptly to an orthopedic surgeon for definitive treatment. Complications frequently include loss of reduction, malreduction of articular fragments, or late instability at the CMC junction.[1,3,8,15]

DISLOCATIONS OF THE CARPOMETACARPAL JOINT

Anatomic Considerations

Strong intermetacarpal and CMC ligaments secure the base of each metacarpal in place. Virtually no motion is possible at the third CMC. This allows the third metacarpal to serve the important biomechanical role of supportive strut for the hand. The most movable CMC joints are the fifth and the first. The ligaments of the first CMC are lax, allowing a wide ROM at this joint. Not surprisingly, these two joints (especially the first) are most likely to be unstable after dislocation. Important branches of arteries and nerves pass near the bases of several metacarpals, and these may be damaged at the time of injury. Examination of patients with possible CMC dislocations should therefore include a careful neurovascular examination of the hand and digits.

Mechanism of Injury

CMC dislocations are generally caused by high-force blows or by hitting an object with a clenched fist. Motorcycle accidents are common causes of dislocations of the first CMC.

Clinical Presentation

Because CMC dislocation injuries are generally caused by high forces, swelling may be marked and may obscure any deformity. These injuries are often missed initially. Maintaining extreme caution when assessing patients with injuries caused by high forces may help prevent this injury.

Imaging

Radiographic images required to view this injury are AP, lateral, and 30 degrees pronated lateral of the hand. If unable to visualize and dislocation is suspected or an occult fracture, then CT is recommended. When dislocated, the proximal metacarpal is almost always displaced dorsally. Often an associated fracture of one of the carpal bones occurs. CMC dislocations are easy to overlook on radiographs. When the injury is suspected, it is important to carefully examine the lateral view. Fig. 4-15 demonstrates a dorsal dislocation of the fourth metacarpal with an associated avulsion from an adjacent carpal. The AP view appears fairly normal apart from indistinct fourth and fifth CMC joint spaces. However, the displacement and avulsion can be observed on the lateral view. Special views are often needed to rule out a CMC

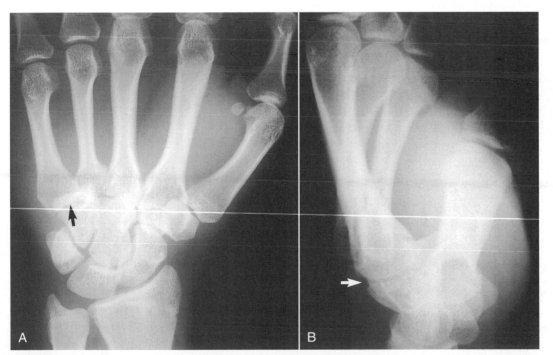

FIGURE 4-15 Dorsal dislocation of the carpometacarpal joint. **A,** Anteroposterior (AP) view reveals only a subtle abnormality: instead of a normal joint space at the base of the fifth metacarpal, double bone density can be seen indicating overlapping bones (*arrow*). **B,** On the lateral view, the proximal fourth metacarpal is dorsally displaced 4 to 5 mm, and an avulsion fracture from a carpal bone can be seen just proximal to it (*arrow*). Although the AP view suggests displacement of the fifth metacarpal as well, this cannot be observed on the lateral view.

dislocation. This is particularly true of the first CMC, for which a true AP view is usually required. MRI with longitudinal views may be needed to fully define the injury.

Indications for Referral

The reduction in CMC dislocations is often difficult to maintain, so patients with these injuries should be referred. Nearly all CMC dislocations, especially the first, require fixation. Even patients with chronic dislocations (those occurring more than 1 to 2 weeks earlier) should be referred because reduction may still be effective.

Initial Treatment

If this type of injury is suspected, it should be immobilized with a volar splint and referred to an orthopedic surgeon for reduction because most of these injuries require internal fixation.

Follow-up Care

Definitive treatment is reduction of the dislocation. This can be accomplished with adequate anesthesia (usually a Bier Block or axillary). Stability of the reduction is checked and if not stable, it requires a K-wire placement. Central dislocations of the CMC may require open reduction and internal fixation (ORIF) and pinning. If not treated in the first month, ORIF is required with clearing of the fibrous tissue before reduction and pinning.

Complications

Neurovascular injury is relatively common with CMC dislocations. Patients may have prolonged stiffness after injury, especially if the first CMC is involved.

Return to Sports or Work

The pins can be removed after 4 to 5 weeks and MCP motion initiated. After the pins are removed, a low-profile hand splint is made with emphasis on the MCP flexion. Return to sports occurs shortly after pin removal with bracing for contact or collision sports.

First Metacarpal Fractures (Adult)

Anatomic Considerations

The thumb is biomechanically quite different from the rest of the fingers, so fractures of the first metacarpal are distinct from those of other metacarpals. Most fractures of the first metacarpal occur at or near the base. The distinct fracture types involving the base are extraarticular, intraarticular, or epiphyseal (Fig. 4-16). Extraarticular fractures are the most common and are the easiest to treat.[15]

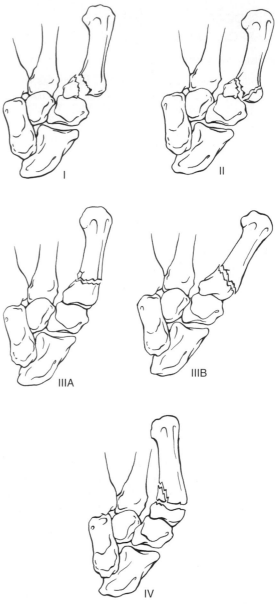

FIGURE 4-16 Four types of fractures of the base of the first metacarpal. Type I (Bennett's fracture dislocation) and type II (Rolando's fracture) are intraarticular. Type III fractures are extraarticular, either transverse (IIIA) or oblique (IIIB). Type IV fractures are seen only in children and involve the proximal epiphysis.

The type I fracture (Bennett's fracture dislocation) is characterized by a proximal fragment that remains attached to the trapezium by the volar ligament and a large metacarpal fragment that is pulled dorsally and radially by the abductor pollicis longus (Fig. 4-17). The type II fracture (Rolando's) is a comminuted fracture that may result in a "Y"- or "T"-shaped pattern at the base of the metacarpal. Often the base is severely comminuted. Unlike Bennett's fracture, no significant proximal

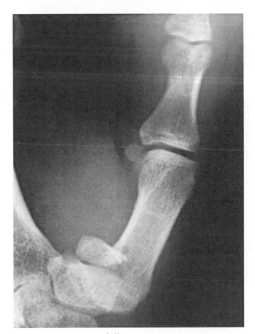

FIGURE 4-17 A typical Bennett's fracture-dislocation. A small fragment remains attached to the trapezium, and the larger metacarpal fragment is pulled dorsally and radially. (*From Browner BD, Jupiter JB, Levine AM, Trafton PG [eds]. Skeletal Trauma: Fractures, Dislocations, Ligamentous Injuries. Philadelphia, WB Saunders, 1992.*)

displacement of the larger metacarpal fragment occurs. Type II fractures are the least common of the thumb metacarpal fractures in adults and the most difficult to treat. Type I and type II fractures are intraarticular. Extraarticular fractures (type III) are either transverse or oblique. The type IV fracture is seen only in children and involves the proximal epiphysis of the thumb. Familiarity with these fracture types is important in the management of thumb fractures in primary care because distinguishing extraarticular fractures from the more complicated intraarticular fractures is essential.

Mechanism of Injury

Fractures of the base of the first metacarpal usually result from an axial load directed against a partially flexed thumb. This injury commonly occurs during a fistfight. A torsional force associated with a direct blow may cause a more oblique fracture. Other causes of injury include hyperabduction or hyperflexion of the thumb during a fall on the hand. The causes of injury for extraarticular and intraarticular fractures are the same.

Clinical Presentation

The patient typically has pain and swelling over the dorsum of the thumb and limited ROM of the MCP joint. Tenderness over the radial aspect of

the wrist or the anatomic snuffbox may indicate injury to the scaphoid, trapezium, or radial styloid.

Imaging

If a fracture of the thumb metacarpal is suspected, three views of the thumb should be obtained: true AP, lateral, and oblique views. The true AP view, taken with the hand in maximum pronation, delineates the CMC joint well. Oblique extraarticular fractures can sometimes be confused with Bennett's fractures, but close inspection of the radiograph should reveal whether or not the fracture line enters the joint (Fig. 4-18). Transverse extraarticular fractures often have some degree of apex radial angulation. Most occur in the proximal 25% of the metacarpal shaft. CT scanning is occasionally needed in the evaluation of intraarticular fractures to fully delineate the position of the fracture fragments and the CMC joint.

Indications for Orthopedic Referral

Mobility of the CMC joint is essential for normal hand function; therefore, restoring and maintaining good alignment of the articular surface are paramount in achieving adequate healing. For this reason, all patients with intraarticular fractures should be referred to orthopedic surgeons. Patients

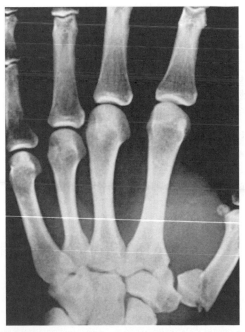

FIGURE 4-18 An oblique extraarticular fracture of the base of the thumb. Note that the fracture line does not enter the joint. This is an unstable fracture that is commonly confused with a Bennett's fracture. (*From Browner BD, Jupiter JB, Levine AM, Trafton PG [eds]. Skeletal Trauma: Fractures, Dislocations, Ligamentous Injuries. Philadelphia, WB Saunders, 1992.*)

with Bennett's fractures are usually treated with percutaneous pin fixation or open fixation if pin fixation fails. The treatment of a Rolando's fracture depends on the degree of comminution. Operative treatment is recommended if the fracture fragments are large enough to allow pin fixation. In cases of severe comminution, traction, external fixation, or brief immobilization with early ROM may remold the articular surface sufficiently to allow adequate mobility.

Extraarticular fractures are nearly always treated with closed means. If adequate reduction of an angulated fracture cannot be achieved or maintained, the patient should be sent to an orthopedist for consideration of pin fixation. Oblique fractures are generally more unstable after reduction, especially if the fracture line is steep.

Initial Treatment

Patients with intraarticular fractures should be placed in a thumb spica splint with the wrist in 30 degrees of extension and the thumb IP joint free and referred for definitive care.

Table 4-5 summarizes management guidelines for extraarticular fractures of the first metacarpal.

Nonangulated Fractures

Nonangulated extraarticular fractures should be treated in a short-arm thumb spica cast with the wrist in 30 degrees of extension and the thumb IP joint free. If the swelling is severe, a spica splint can be used until definitive casting at the first follow-up visit.

Angulated Fractures

Extraarticular fractures with more than 30 degrees of angulation should be reduced. A hematoma

block or Bier block (see description of the technique for Bier block in the Initial Treatment section for metacarpal shaft fractures) should provide adequate anesthesia. Closed reduction is accomplished by longitudinal traction, pressure over the apex of the fracture, mild pronation of the distal fragment, and extension of the thumb. Hyperextension of the MCP joint should be avoided during the reduction. After reduction, the thumb should be immobilized in a thumb spica cast and radiographs obtained. Because of the thumb's greater mobility, precise anatomic reduction is not necessary. Even 20 to 30 degrees of residual angular deformity is well tolerated and usually causes no detectable limitation of motion.[15]

Follow-up Care

Patients with nondisplaced fractures and those who have undergone closed reduction of an angulated fracture should be reevaluated at 1 to 2 weeks after injury and receive repeat radiographs. An earlier follow-up (within 3 to 5 days) is indicated for patients with oblique fractures and those with questionable alignment after reduction. If the fracture is angulated more than 30 degrees on the follow-up radiographs, a repeat reduction should be performed or orthopedic referral obtained. If the fracture position is stable, the thumb spica cast should be continued for a total of 4 weeks. Prolonged immobilization should be avoided to prevent excessive joint stiffness.

Complications

Complications are uncommon in cases of extraarticular fractures of the base of the thumb metacarpal. Residual angulation occasionally causes prominence

Table 4-5	*Management Guidelines for Extraarticular Fracture of Base of First Metacarpal*
	INITIAL TREATMENT
Splint type and position	Thumb spica splint
	Wrist, 30-degree extension; IP joint, free
Initial follow-up visit	Within 1 to 2 weeks
	Within 3 to 5 days if oblique fracture or alignment questionable
Patient instruction	Icing, elevation
	FOLLOW-UP CARE
Cast or splint type and position	Short-arm thumb spica cast
	Wrist, 30-degree extension; IP joint, free
Length of immobilization	4 weeks
Healing time	6 to 8 weeks
Follow-up visit interval	Every 2 weeks
Repeat radiography interval	At initial visit to check position
	Every 2 to 4 weeks
Patient instruction	Begin ROM exercises after cast is removed
Indications for orthopedic consult	Inability to achieve or maintain adequate closed reduction
	Oblique fractures
	Malunion with subluxation of CMC joint

CMC, carpometacarpal; IP, interphalangeal; ROM, range of motion.

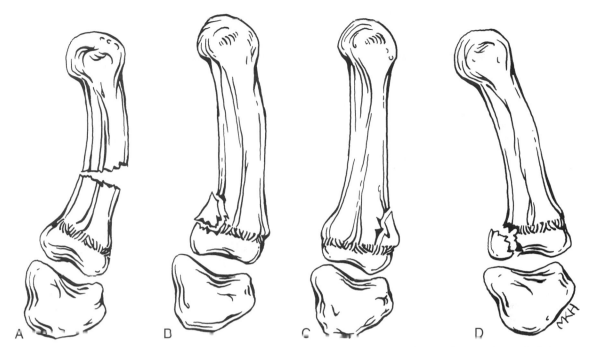

FIGURE 4-19 Classification of pediatric fracture patterns seen at the base of the thumb metacarpal. **A,** Shaft fracture. **B,** Salter-Harris type II fracture with a medial "metaphyseal flag." **C,** Salter-Harris type II fracture with a lateral "metaphyseal flag." **D,** Salter-Harris type III fracture (pediatric Bennett's fracture).

at the dorsum of the thumb and minimal loss of abduction. The most common complication of intraarticular fractures is painful arthritis. Malunion may predispose the patient to recurrent or chronic subluxation of the first CMC joint.

Return to Work or Sports

ROM exercises should be started after the cast is removed. Squeezing a plastic or foam ball can enhance both ROM and strength in the hand. Physical or occupational therapists may use flexible elastic bands or weblike material to further strengthen the thumb and promote full ROM. A removable flexible wrist splint incorporating the thumb and first MCP joint may provide some protection as the patient gradually returns to full use of the hand.[6]

First Metacarpal Fractures (Pediatric)

Physeal fractures of the thumb are common and are sometimes difficult to treat because of the deforming forces of the muscles and soft tissues that attach to the thumb metacarpal. Four different fracture patterns can be identified (Fig. 4-19). The most common pattern is a Salter-Harris type II fracture of the base of the thumb metacarpal with a metaphyseal flag medially (toward the ulnar side of the hand) (Fig. 4-20). The shaft is slightly displaced, usually with slight apex lateral angulation. The shaft of the thumb metacarpal is also subluxated proximally by the abductor pollicis longus.

Clinical Presentation

The patient has pain and swelling at the thumb, especially at the thenar eminence, and decreased thumb ROM. In particular, the examiner should evaluate radial abduction and palmar abduction of the thumb as well as thumb opposition. Malrotation of the thumb is difficult to assess but should be evaluated carefully; the thumb is usually perpendicular to the planes of the other nails in the fully flexed position.

Imaging

Three views of the hand (AP, lateral, and oblique) are required. Type II fractures of the medial base of the thumb metacarpal may appear reduced on the lateral view but are significantly displaced on the AP view. A hyperpronated view of the thumb is also recommended because it provides greater detail of the CMC joint.

Indications for Orthopedic Referral

Patients with irreducible or unstable type II fractures or type III or type IV fractures should be

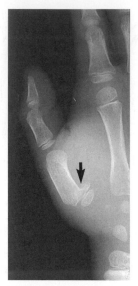

FIGURE 4-20 Salter-Harris type II fracture at the base of the thumb metacarpal. The most common pattern is shown here with a "metaphyseal flag" medially (toward ulnar side of the hand) (*arrow*). (*From Thornton A, Gyll C. Children's Fractures: A Radiological Guide to Safe Practice. Philadelphia, WB Saunders, 1999.*)

placed in a comfortable thumb spica splint and referred promptly to an orthopedic surgeon.

Initial Treatment

Table 4-6 summarizes management guidelines for nondisplaced Salter-Harris type II fractures at the base of the first metacarpal.

A pediatric patient with a nondisplaced or minimally displaced type II fracture at the base of the thumb can have the hand immobilized in a short-arm thumb spica splint or cast. The wrist is positioned in slight extension, and the thumb in slight abduction and extension.

A pediatric patient with a displaced fracture at the base of the first metacarpal should have the hand placed in a thumb spica splint and be referred to an orthopedic surgeon for definitive treatment.

Follow-up Care

The patient should be seen within 5 to 7 days to be sure the splint or cast still fits well. Repeat radiographs should also be obtained to ensure the fracture remains nondisplaced. ROM exercises at the thumb IP joint, elbow, and shoulder should be encouraged. The patient should be reexamined every 2 weeks until healing occurs, and the cast should be replaced if it becomes worn or loose. The patient's hand should remain immobilized for 4 to 6 weeks or until it is nontender.

Return to Sports

How soon a child may resume sports activities depends on the location and severity of injury, the hand and dexterity requirements of the sports, and the positions played. A child with a thumb metacarpal shaft fracture whose sport does not require great dexterity may return to play within 2 weeks if a protective thumb spica forearm splint or other protective equipment is worn. A child with an intraarticular or physeal injury whose sport demands greater dexterity may not be able to resume playing until the hand is completely or nearly nontender and has a full or near-normal ROM.

Complications

Nonunion is rare but can occur. Malunion is more common and may require osteotomy for

Table 4-6	Management Guidelines for Pediatric First Metacarpal Fractures: Nondisplaced Type II
	INITIAL TREATMENT
Splint type and position	Thumb spica splint
	Wrist, 30-degree extension; IP joint, free
Initial follow-up visit	5 to 7 days
Patient instruction	Icing and elevation of hand for 24 to 48 hours
	FOLLOW-UP CARE
Cast or splint type and position	Short-arm thumb spica cast
	Wrist, 30-degree extension; IP joint, free
Length of immobilization	4 to 6 weeks
Healing time	6 to 8 weeks
Follow-up visit interval	Every 2 weeks
Repeat radiography interval	At initial visit to check position; then every 2 to 4 weeks
Patient instruction	Maintain IP joint, elbow, and shoulder ROM
Indications for orthopedic consult	Irreducible or unstable type II fracture
	Type III or IV fracture
	Malunion with subluxation of CMC joint

CMC, carpometacarpal; IP, interphalangeal; ROM, range of motion.

correction. Intraarticular incongruity may cause pain, limited ROM, and early arthritis and may require operative repair.

REFERENCES

1. Light TR, Bednar MS. Management of intra-articular fractures of the metacarpophalangeal joint. *Hand Clin.* 1994;10:303-314.
2. Capo JT, Hastings H. Metacarpal and phalangeal fractures in athletes. *Clin Sports Med.* 1998;17(3):491-511.
3. Schupp CM. Sideline evaluation and treatment of bone and joint injury. *Curr Sports Med Rep.* 2009;8(3):119-124.
4. Green DP, Strickland JW. The hand. In: De Lee JC, Drez D Jr, eds. Orthopedic Sports Medicine: Principles and Practice. Philadelphia: WB Saunders; 2007:1393-1414.
5. Flinn SD. On-field management of emergent and urgent extremity conditions. *Curr Sports Med Rep.* 2006;5:227-232.
6. Jaworski CA, Krause M, Brown J. Rehabilitation of the wrist and hand following sports injury. *Clin Sports Med.* 2010;29:61-80.
7. Daniels JM, Zook EG, Lynch JM. Hand and wrist injuries: part I. Nonemergent evaluation. *Am Fam Phys.* 2004;69(8):1941-1948.
8. Leggit JC, Meko CJ. Acute finger injuries: part II. Fractures, dislocations, and thumb injuries. *Am Fam Phys.* 2006;73(5):827-834.
9. Statius Muller MG, Poolman RW, van Hoogstraten MJ, Steller EP. Immediate mobilization gives good results in boxer's fractures with volar angulation up to 70 degrees: a prospective randomized trial comparing immediate mobilization with cast immobilization. *Arch Orthop Trauma Surg.* 2003;123:534-537.
10. Braakman M, Oderwalk EE, Haentjens MH. Functional taping of fractures of the 5th metacarpal results in quicker recovery. *Injury.* 1998;29:5-9.
11. Harding IJ, Parry D, Barrington RL. The use of a moulded metacarpal brace versus neighbour strapping for fractures of the little finger metacarpal neck. *J Hand Surg (Br).* 2001;26:261-263.
12. Kuokkanen, HO, Mulari-Keranen, SK, Niskanen, RO, et al. Treatment of subcapital fractures of the fifth metacarpal bone: a prospective randomised comparison between functional treatment and reposition and splinting. *Scand J Plast Reconstr Surg Hand Surg.* 1999;33:315-317.
13. Toronto R, Donovan PJ, MacIntyre J. An alternative method of treatment for metacarpal fractures in athletes. *Clin J Sports Med.* 1996;6(1):4-8.
14. Mastey RD, Weiss AC, Akelman E. Primary care of hand and wrist athletic injuries. *Clin Sports Med.* 1997;16(4):705-724.
15. Peterson JJ, Bancroft LW. Injuries of the fingers and thumb in the athlete. *Clin Sports Med.* 2006;25:527-542.

CARPAL FRACTURES

Co-Author: Ryan C. Petering

Fractures of the carpal bones constitute approximately 6% of all fractures, but they are probably underdiagnosed. Scaphoid fractures are the most common fractures of carpal bones, accounting for more than 60% of all carpal injuries.[1] The complex anatomy of the wrist often makes diagnosis and treatment difficult. Overlooking a fracture or dislocation of a carpal bone can result in major complications and prolonged morbidity, so the clinician must maintain a high index of suspicion in the evaluation of wrist injuries.

See Appendix for stepwise instructions for short-arm and long-arm casts and splints used in the treatment of carpal fractures.

Go to Expert Consult for the electronic version of a patient instruction sheet named "Broken Hand or Wrist," which covers the steps of care from pain relief to rehabilitation exercises. This can be copied to hand out to patients to assist them during the treatment period.

SCAPHOID FRACTURES (ADULT)

Anatomic Considerations

The scaphoid lies at the radial aspect of the wrist and links the distal and proximal carpal rows (Fig. 5-1). The scaphoid is tethered to the proximal carpal row by strong volar ligaments: the radioscaphoid, scapholunate, and scaphocapitate. The scaphoid has a central indentation at its waist, which is crossed by the palmar radiocarpal ligament. The scaphoid serves as the principal bony block to excessive extension at the wrist and is therefore susceptible to fracture.

The blood supply to the scaphoid arises distally from branches of the radial artery (Fig. 5-2). The distal tuberosity of the scaphoid receives its blood supply from the anterior interosseous artery, and the proximal pole is completely dependent on the distal blood supply. Because of the vascular anatomy, fractures in the middle and proximal portion of the scaphoid are prone to nonunion at the fracture site and an increased incidence of avascular necrosis (AVN) of the proximal fracture fragment.

Mechanism of Injury

Scaphoid fractures are caused by two common types of injury: a longitudinally directed axial load, which usually results in a stable nondisplaced fracture, and a fall on the extended wrist, which places a tensile force at the volar scaphoid and a compressive force at the dorsal scaphoid.

Clinical Presentation

The patient reports the typical cause of injury, either an axial load to the wrist or a fall onto the extended wrist, and wrist pain. During physical examination, swelling is usually not present except in cases of fracture-dislocation. Wrist range of motion (ROM) is only slightly reduced, but pain is reproduced at the extremes of flexion and extension. Scaphoid compression tenderness, elicited by holding the patient's thumb and applying pressure along the axis of its metacarpal, is an accurate indicator of a scaphoid fracture. Point tenderness can be elicited at one of three common fracture locations: in the anatomic snuffbox (waist fracture); in the anatomic snuffbox with the wrist in ulnar deviation (distal tuberosity fracture); or just distal to Lister's tubercle, a small longitudinal bony prominence on the dorsal distal radius in alignment with the third metacarpal (proximal pole of the scaphoid). The tendons of the anatomic snuffbox are best demonstrated when the thumb is extended and the wrist is in a neutral position (Fig. 5-3).

Scaphoid fractures are often accompanied by unrecognized associated injuries. The same mechanism of injury may cause fractures of the distal radius, lunate, or radial head. Also, patients with scaphoid fractures may report symptoms suggesting injury to the median nerve, such as paresthesias of the palmar aspect of the thumb and second and third fingers.

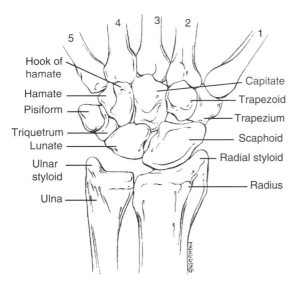

FIGURE 5-1 Schematic diagram of the carpal bones. Proximal row: scaphoid, lunate, triquetrum, pisiform. Distal row: trapezium, trapezoid, capitate, hamate.

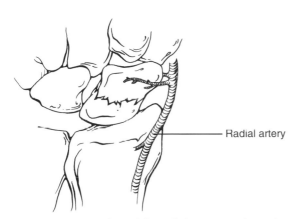

FIGURE 5-2 Branches of the radial artery supplying the scaphoid bone. The blood supply enters only the distal part of the scaphoid.

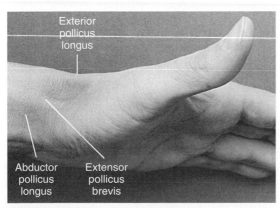

FIGURE 5-3 The anatomic snuffbox bordered by the tendons of the abductor pollicis longus and the extensor pollicis longus.

Imaging

Familiarity with the normal radiographic anatomy of the carpal bones assists the primary care provider in recognizing scaphoid fractures. The normal posteroanterior (PA) view of the wrist is shown in Fig. 5-4. Because of the similarity of their names, the positions of the trapezium and trapezoid are difficult to remember. Recalling that the trapezium articulates with the thumb may help in identifying these carpal bones. The three lines of Gilula should be found (Fig. 5-5). Disruption of one of these lines should alert the primary care provider to a fracture or carpal dislocation. On the lateral view of the wrist, the distal radius, lunate, and capitate line up along a longitudinal axis. The scapholunate angle is usually about 45 degrees, although a range of 40 to 60 degrees is considered normal (Fig. 5-6). Angles of more than 60 degrees indicate carpal instability and fracture displacement (Fig. 5-7).

If a scaphoid fracture is suspected, PA, lateral, and motion views (flexion–extension, radial deviation–ulnar deviation) of the wrist are recommended. Radiographs of the scaphoid often show no abnormalities in the acute setting, and negative radiograph results do not exclude the possibility of a scaphoid fracture. Fractures can be subtle and apparent on only one view (Fig. 5-8).

Fractures of the middle (waist) of the scaphoid are the most common (80%), followed by fractures of the proximal pole (15%), fractures of the distal tuberosity (4%), and fractures of distal articular surface (1%) (Figs. 5-9 and 5-10). The fracture may be stable or unstable; this is important because

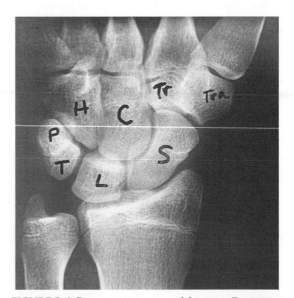

FIGURE 5-4 Posteroanterior view of the wrist. C, capitate; H, hamate; L, lunate; P, pisiform; S, scaphoid; T, triquetrum; Tra, trapezium; Tr, trapezoid.

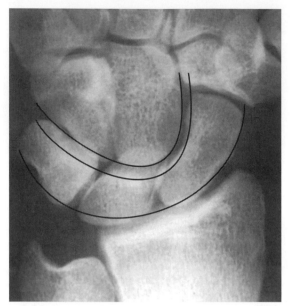

FIGURE 5-5 Lines of Gilula. Normal posteroanterior views of the wrist should reveal three contiguous lines. Lack of continuity of these lines may indicate dislocation, fracture, or instability of the carpal bones.

the rate of union and treatment options vary widely between stable and unstable fractures. A stable fracture is usually caused by impaction, is nondisplaced, has an intact cartilage envelope, and demonstrates incomplete separation of the two fragments. An unstable fracture is usually caused by a fall on the extended wrist, and demonstrates stepoff or angulation of 1 mm or more. Fractures of the scaphoid may be acute or a newly noted old fracture. An acute fracture shows a single fracture line, some degree of dorsal–radial comminution, and possibly dorsal angulation. A newly noted old scaphoid nonunion may show resorption at the fracture site (i.e., separation between fragments),

cystic changes, subchondral sclerosis, and displacement on both PA and lateral views (Fig. 5-11).

Radiographs should be examined for signs of ligament disruption and scapholunate dissociation, which can occur after a similar mechanism of injury. A gap of more than 2 mm between the scaphoid and lunate indicates a ligament disruption and is called the "Terry Thomas or David Letterman sign," named after celebrities who had a prominent space between their front teeth. This finding is best appreciated on a PA view of the slightly flexed fist (Fig. 5-12). Scapholunate dissociations are discussed separately at the end of this chapter.

Several clinicians have advocated use of magnetic resonance imaging (MRI) or computed tomography (CT) scan early in the evaluation of patients with clinical scaphoid fracture (trauma mechanism, snuff box tenderness, swelling) to avoid under- and overtreatment.[2-4] In addition to difficulty diagnosing scaphoid fractures, detecting displacement of 1 mm or more can be challenging on standard radiographs.[5] Because missed fractures and missed displaced fractures can lead to significant morbidity, it is reasonable to consider early advanced imaging in cases of suspected scaphoid fracture, especially in an athlete or laborer who would benefit from a more timely diagnosis. A bone scan also can be used 72 hours after the injury, but the lower specificity of bone scintigraphy has led to lower use of this modality.[6]

Indications for Orthopedic Referral

Patients with scaphoid fractures should be referred to an orthopedist if the fracture is displaced or angulated, if a nonunion develops after an adequate course of conservative therapy, or if AVN or scapholunate dissociation is suspected. Because of the higher risk of nonunion and AVN, the primary care provider should refer the patient for an orthopedic consultation or referral even for

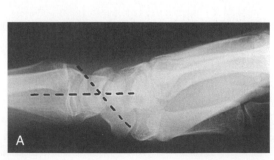

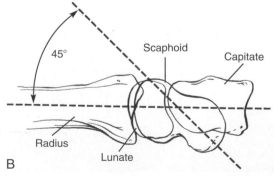

FIGURE 5-6 A, Lateral view of the wrist demonstrating the normal longitudinal alignment of the distal radius articular surface, lunate, and capitate and the normal axis of the scaphoid. **B,** The usual scapholunate angle is 45 degrees, with a normal range from 40 to 60 degrees.

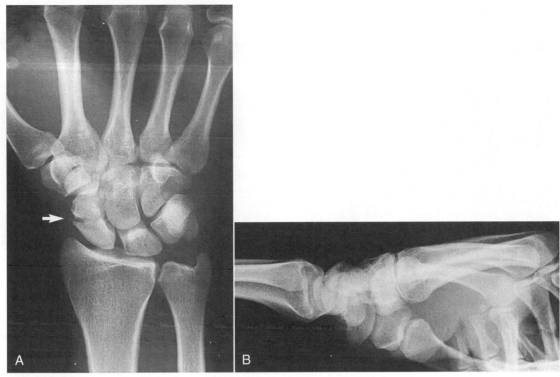

FIGURE 5-7 **A,** Posteroanterior view of the wrist demonstrating a middle third waist fracture of the scaphoid (*arrow*).
B, Lateral view showing volar displacement of the scaphoid and an abnormal scapholunate angle of 70 degrees.

nondisplaced scaphoid fractures because surgical management is often indicated (see below).

Initial Treatment

Table 5-1 summarizes management guidelines for suspected and nondisplaced scaphoid fractures.

The amount of swelling initially present after a scaphoid or suspected fracture is usually minimal. Therefore, a cast rather than a splint can usually be applied during the first visit. If the amount of swelling is moderate, a splint or bivalved cast should be used for immobilization.

Suspected Fracture with Radiographs That Show No Abnormalities

The precarious blood supply of the scaphoid makes healing problematic, and early appropriate immobilization is essential in obtaining a good result. Patients who have fallen on the extended wrist and have snuffbox tenderness should have the hand immobilized in a short-arm thumb spica cast or splint for 2 weeks even if initial radiographs show no abnormalities. The wrist should be placed in slight extension to prevent limited ROM when the

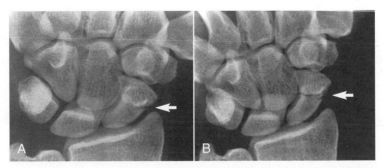

FIGURE 5-8 **A,** Posteroanterior view demonstrates a very subtle fracture line that could easily be overlooked (*arrow*).
B, The fracture line is much more apparent in the posteroanterior view in ulnar deviation (*arrow*). (*From Browner BD, Jupiter JB, Levine AM, Trafton PG [eds]. Skeletal Trauma: Fractures, Dislocations, Ligamentous Injuries. Philadelphia, WB Saunders, 1992.*)

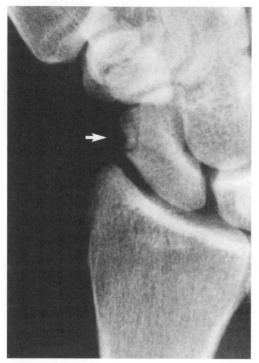

FIGURE 5-9 Nondisplaced fracture of the distal tuberosity (*arrow*).

cast is removed. The thumb is slightly extended and abducted, as if the patient is holding a small glass upright. The thumb interphalangeal (IP) joint should be free (i.e., the cast should end proximal to the flexure of the thumb IP joint). The first follow-up visit should be in 2 weeks.

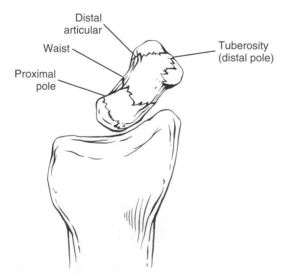

FIGURE 5-10 Common fracture patterns for the scaphoid.

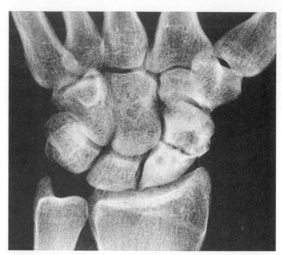

FIGURE 5-11 Typical sclerotic appearance of avascular necrosis after scaphoid fracture.

Nondisplaced Fracture

A recent systemic review and meta-analysis found surgical treatment of acute nondisplaced and minimally displaced scaphoid fractures resulted in significantly better patient-reported functional outcomes, greater patient satisfaction, better grip strength, shorter time to union, and earlier return to work than nonoperative care.[7] There were no significant differences between surgical

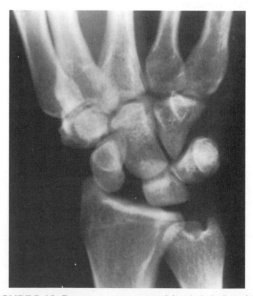

FIGURE 5-12 Posteroanterior view of the slightly flexed fist demonstrates a scapholunate dissociation, the "Terry Thomas or David Letterman sign." The gap between the scaphoid and lunate is larger than 2 mm, and the scaphoid appears foreshortened. (*From Browner BD, Jupiter JB, Levine AM, Trafton PG [eds]. Skeletal Trauma: Fractures, Dislocations, Ligamentous Injuries. Philadelphia, WB Saunders, 1992.*)

Table 5-1	*Management Guidelines for Suspected and Nondisplaced Scaphoid Fractures*
	INITIAL TREATMENT
Splint type and position	Suspected: short-arm thumb spica cast or splint
	Nondisplaced: distal third—short-arm thumb spica cast or splint (slight wrist extension)
	Middle or proximal—long-arm thumb spica cast or splint (slight wrist extension)
Initial follow-up visit	Suspected: 2 weeks
	Nondisplaced: 1 to 2 weeks
Patient instruction	Icing and elevation for 24 to 48 hours
	Maintain finger and shoulder ROM
	FOLLOW-UP CARE
Cast or splint type and position	Suspected: short-arm thumb spica cast
	Nondisplaced: distal third—short-arm thumb spica cast
	Middle or proximal—long-arm thumb spica cast for 6 weeks; then short-arm thumb spica cast for remaining weeks
Length of immobilization	Suspected: continue until diagnosis confirmed
	Nondisplaced: distal—4 to 6 weeks
	Middle—10 to 12 weeks
	Proximal—12 to 20 weeks
Healing time	Distal: 6 to 8 weeks
	Middle: 12 to 14 weeks
	Proximal: 18 to 24 weeks
Follow-up visit interval	Suspected: every 2 weeks until diagnosis confirmed
	Nondisplaced: every 2 to 3 weeks until radiographic union
Repeat radiography interval	Suspected: every 2 weeks until diagnosis confirmed
	Bone scan at 2 or 4 weeks from date of injury if plain films still show no abnormalities
	Nondisplaced: every 2 to 3 weeks until radiographic union
Patient instruction	Maintain finger, elbow, and shoulder ROM during immobilization
Indications for orthopedic consult	Consider for nondisplaced fractures because of high risk for poor healing
	Displaced fractures
	Nonunion
	Early signs of AVN

AVN, avascular necrosis; ROM, range of motion.

and conservative treatment with regard to pain, ROM, the rate of nonunion, infection, complications, or total treatment cost. Although the randomized controlled trials in this meta-analysis had some methodologic quality concerns, the acute surgical management of scaphoid fractures should be part of the management discussion with patients.

If nonoperative treatment is chosen, patients with a nondisplaced fracture of the middle third or proximal third of the scaphoid have improved healing times when treated in a long-arm thumb spica cast as opposed to a short-arm spica cast.[8] The elbow should be flexed to 90 degrees, the forearm in neutral pronation-supination, the wrist in slight extension, and the thumb in slight extension and abduction. The cast extends from the deltoid insertion on the arm to the proximal palmar crease on the palm. See the Appendix for stepwise instruction for how to apply a long-arm spica cast. A short-arm thumb spica cast can be used for a nondisplaced fracture of the distal third of the scaphoid. Early consultation with an orthopedist should be considered for proximal fractures because of the

risk of nonunion or AVN. The patient should be reevaluated within 1 to 2 weeks.

Displaced Fracture

A displaced fracture of the scaphoid should be immobilized in a long-arm thumb spica cast or splint. The patient should be referred promptly to an orthopedic surgeon.

Follow-up Care

Suspected Fracture with Radiographs That Show No Abnormalities

The patient should be reexamined with the wrist out of the cast after 7 to 10 days of immobilization. Repeat radiographs may demonstrate a fracture because immobilization has allowed demineralization of the fracture line. Patients with no tenderness in the anatomic snuffbox and radiographs that show no abnormalities at the time of the second visit can be dismissed safely. Patients whose radiographs appear normal but who have persistent point tenderness or scaphoid compression tenderness should either continue immobilization for 1 more week or have advanced imaging (CT scan, MRI or bone scan) to completely diagnose the injury. Patients with persistent tenderness and negative radiographs at 3 weeks from injury should be imaged with CT scan, MRI, or bone scan. Immobilization should continue as outlined for nondisplaced fractures if a fracture is present. Consultation with a hand specialist should be considered if the patient is still symptomatic and no fracture is seen with advanced imaging by 3 weeks after the injury.

Nondisplaced Fracture

The average duration of immobilization varies by fracture site: 4 to 6 weeks for distal tuberosity and distal third fractures, 10 to 12 weeks for middle third fractures, and 12 to 20 weeks for a proximal third fracture. If a long-arm cast is used initially, it should be continued for at least 6 weeks followed by a short-arm cast until the fracture is healed. Out-of-cast radiographs should be obtained every 2 to 3 weeks until evidence of radiographic union is present. If fracture healing is uncertain, CT scan or MRI should be used to confirm union. During each visit, patients should be encouraged to maintain active ROM of the fingers, thumb IP joint, and shoulder.

Return to Work or Sports

Because treatment of scaphoid fractures requires lengthy immobilization, wrist stiffness and forearm muscle atrophy are likely after the cast is removed. Referral to a physical therapist or occupational therapist is strongly encouraged to help the patient regain motion, strength, and function after cast immobilization. For athletes, the wrist should be protected in a rigid splint for sports activities until strength is 80% of the uninjured side and ROM is normal or near normal. The wrist should be protected for a minimum of 3 months after cast removal.

Complications

A concerning complication of scaphoid fractures is nonunion, which results from the precarious nature of the blood supply and movement at the fracture line. Incidence rates vary by fracture location and treatment but have been estimated to be approximately 10%.[9] Nonunion may be more common in missed scaphoid fractures with a delay in treatment.[10] In the long term, nonunion of a scaphoid fracture can lead to wrist arthritis. If a nonunion develops, the patient should be referred to an orthopedist. Often a further course of conservative therapy is attempted, but if it is unsuccessful, operative fixation, bone grafting, or both may be required.

Another serious complication is the development of AVN (Fig. 5-11). AVN is caused by interruption of the blood supply to the healing scaphoid and is strongly influenced by the anatomic site of the fracture line. AVN is estimated to occur in 13% to 50% of cases with the highest incidence in proximal fractures.[11] The incidence of AVN can be reduced by early recognition and proper immobilization of suspected scaphoid fractures, but it may occur even in cases managed appropriately. AVN results in destruction of the proximal fracture fragment, and this in turn causes significant arthritis of the wrist. Patients who demonstrate radiographic findings of AVN should be referred to an orthopedist for consideration of operative excision and bone grafting.

Other complications after a scaphoid fracture include paresthesias in the distribution of the median nerve and wrist instability caused by disruption of the suspensory ligaments between the scaphoid and the radius and carpals. Although most median nerve symptoms resolve spontaneously, signs of serious nerve injury may persist, including intractable pain, neurotrophic changes in the skin and bones, and atrophy of hand musculature. Patients with wrist instability initially seek treatment for wrist pain that resolves within a few weeks, but later a chronic dull aching pain develops in the dorsum of the wrist, which is worsened by repeated flexion and extension of the clasped hand.

Pediatric Scaphoid Fractures

Anatomic Considerations

The scaphoid is the most commonly fractured carpal bone among pediatric patients, just as it is with adults. However, the pattern of fractures seen is significantly different because of the immature nature of the carpal bones in children. Scaphoid fractures are uncommon in children because the physis of the distal radius usually fails first. At birth, the carpal bones are entirely cartilaginous, and ossification of the scaphoid begins at approximately 4.5 years of age in girls and 5.5 years of age in boys. The scaphoid ossifies eccentrically, starting distally and proceeding proximally. This process of progressive ossification produces different fracture patterns than are seen in adults. The incidence of scaphoid fractures increases throughout childhood and peaks at the age of 15 years. Fractures of the scaphoid are rare in children younger than 8 years old.[12]

Mechanism of Injury

Most scaphoid fractures in children are caused by falls from standing height or during sports-related activities such as biking or skateboarding. Some are caused by involvement in motor vehicle accidents or punching injuries. Because the carpal bones of children are incompletely ossified and therefore resilient, significant forces are usually required to cause a fracture. Other injuries often accompany scaphoid fractures in children, including fractures of the lunate or the distal radius or dislocation of the proximal carpal row. As is the usual pattern for young, skeletally immature patients, immature bones fail before the surrounding ligamentous attachments.

Clinical Presentation

The patient reports a fall on the extended wrist, usually from standing height. The patient also reports wrist pain and ROM limited by pain. Tenderness and some swelling in the anatomic snuffbox may be apparent during physical examination. Tenderness of the distal pole (at the anatomic snuffbox with the wrist in ulnar deviation) may also be elicited.

Imaging

If a scaphoid fracture is suspected on the basis of history, physical examination, or both, four views of the wrist are recommended: anteroposterior (AP), lateral, oblique, and pronation ulnar deviation. Although most pediatric scaphoid fractures are nondisplaced, many are incomplete and show disruption of a single cortex. Most pediatric scaphoid fractures involve the distal third of the bone. These include both extraarticular radial avulsion fractures unique to children and intraarticular fractures of the distal pole of the scaphoid, which can be either radial or ulnar. Middle third fractures constitute approximately one third of pediatric scaphoid fractures.

Pseudo-Terry Thomas Sign

In an injured child, the gap between the ossifying scaphoid and ossifying lunate may initially appear to be wide, leading to the incorrect diagnosis of a "Terry Thomas sign" or scapholunate dissociation. The scaphoid ossifies from distal to proximal, so the distance between the ossifying scaphoid and lunate bones appears to narrow as the child ages. Comparative views of the uninjured wrist are helpful in this situation, but carpal ossification is not perfectly symmetric.

Further Imaging

Because the carpal bones are largely cartilaginous and ossify as the patient grows, scaphoid fractures are often not seen on initial radiographs. The diagnosis may be delayed 1 to 2 weeks for many patients. MRI is often needed to confirm the diagnosis. CT or bone scan are reasonable alternatives.

Indications for Orthopedic Referral

Displaced fractures, nonunions, failed nonoperative treatment, and fractures associated with carpal injuries, and fractures of the proximal pole of scaphoid should be referred to orthopedic surgeons.

Initial Treatment

Table 5-2 summarizes management guidelines for pediatric scaphoid fractures.

In a child, an avulsion of the radial aspect of the distal scaphoid or a fracture of the distal third should be immobilized in a short-arm thumb spica cast or splint. The wrist should be immobilized in slight flexion and radial deviation. Patients with fractures at the waist of the scaphoid require immobilization in a long-arm thumb spica cast or splint. As with adults, pediatric patients with suspected scaphoid fractures and negative radiographs should be stabilized in thumb spica splint or cast and reevaluated in 2 weeks.

Follow-up Care

The patient should be seen again in 7 to 10 days. Repeat radiographs are necessary if the initial radiographs show no abnormalities. If the cast is loose or damaged, it should be replaced. If patients remain symptomatic at 2 weeks after the injury and no fracture has been seen on standard radiographs, advanced imaging should be obtained.

Children with an avulsion or distal-third fracture should remain in a short-arm thumb spica cast for 4 to 6 weeks. Patients with a nondisplaced scaphoid fracture should remain in long-arm thumb spica cast for 6 to 8 weeks. However, a fracture that has been left untreated for 10 days may require 10 weeks of cast immobilization: 3 to 6 weeks in a long-arm thumb spica cast followed by 3 to 7 weeks in a short-arm thumb spica cast.

Return to Sports

For athletes, the wrist should be protected in a rigid splint for sports activities until strength is 80% of the uninjured side and ROM is normal or near normal. The wrist should be protected for a minimum of 3 months after cast removal.

Complications

The most common complication among children and adolescents is failure to recognize the presence of a scaphoid fracture because of mild symptoms and radiographs that initially show no abnormalities. Nonunion is also a relatively common complication. Nonunion may be caused by neglect, misdiagnosis, or noncompliance with the treatment regimen. Most nonunions can be treated successfully with prolonged immobilization: 10 weeks

Table 5-2	*Management Guidelines for Pediatric Scaphoid Fractures*
INITIAL TREATMENT	
Splint type and position	Suspected: short-arm thumb spica cast or splint Nondisplaced: avulsion or distal third—short-arm thumb spica cast Middle third—long-arm thumb spica cast Wrist in slight flexion, slight radial deviation, leave thumb IP joint free
Initial follow-up visit	Suspected: 10 to 14 days Nondisplaced: 1 to 2 weeks
Patient instruction	Icing and elevation for 24 to 48 hours Maintain finger and shoulder ROM
FOLLOW-UP CARE	
Cast and splint type and position	Suspected: short-arm thumb spica cast Nondisplaced: avulsion or distal third—short-arm thumb spica cast Middle third—long-arm thumb spica cast for 6 weeks; then short-arm thumb spica cast for remaining weeks
Length of immobilization	Suspected: continue until diagnosis is confirmed Nondisplaced: avulsion or distal third—4 to 6 weeks Middle third fracture—6 to 8 weeks
Healing time	Avulsion or distal third: 6 to 8 weeks Middle third: 8 to 12 weeks
Follow-up visit interval	Suspected: every 2 weeks until diagnosis is confirmed Nondisplaced: every 2 to 3 weeks until radiographic union
Repeat radiography interval	Suspected: every 2 weeks until diagnosis is confirmed Bone scan at 4 weeks from injury if plain films still show no abnormalities Nondisplaced: every 2 to 3 weeks until radiographic union
Patient instruction	Maintain finger, elbow, and shoulder ROM during immobilization
Indications for orthopedic consult	Proximal pole fractures Displaced fractures Associated carpal fractures

IP, interphalangeal; ROM, range of motion.

are usually sufficient, but immobilization for up to 16 to 20 weeks may be necessary in some cases. Malunion can result if the unstable scaphoid fracture causes flexion of the scaphoid. Children are capable of significant remodeling in cases of a malunited scaphoid, and a trial of nonoperative therapy is warranted.

TRIQUETRUM FRACTURES

Anatomic Considerations

The triquetrum is part of the proximal carpal row and articulates with the lunate, to which it is attached by ligaments. During radial deviation of the wrist the triquetrum may articulate with the capitate. The pisiform bone often overlies the triquetrum, with which it articulates anteriorly. In close proximity to the triquetrum is the triangular fibrocartilaginous complex (TFCC), a confluence of structures just distal to the ulna that includes ligaments and an articular disk. The TFCC forms a strong support on the ulnar side of the wrist.

Mechanism of Injury

Fractures of the triquetrum are the second most common fractures among the carpal bones. The fracture can be caused by either hyperflexion or hyperextension of the wrist. With hyperextension

and ulnar deviation the hamate shears off the posteroradial aspect of the triquetrum. With hyperflexion, the dorsal radiotriquetral ligaments avulse their triquetral attachments. Avulsion or "chip" fractures are the most common form of fracture.[13] Fractures of the body of the triquetrum may be caused by a direct blow or occur in association with a perilunate dislocation. Injuries to the TFCC are common after a fall on the extended wrist combined with forearm torsion.

Clinical Presentation

The patient seeks treatment after falling on the outstretched arm, usually with the wrist extended and with ulnar deviation. Intense point tenderness 2 cm distal to the ulnar styloid is highly suggestive of injury to the triquetrum. When examined, the wrist may show little swelling or discoloration. Resisted wrist extension usually reproduces the patient's pain.

Imaging

Three views of the wrist are required: AP, true lateral, and oblique. A transverse fracture of the body of the triquetrum can usually be identified on a standard AP view. The AP view may not reveal a dorsal avulsion fracture because of the normal superimposition of the dorsal lip on the lunate. On the lateral view, a small fleck of avulsed bone may

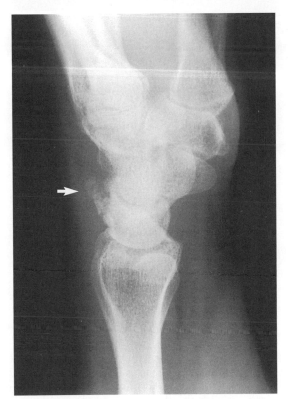

FIGURE 5-13 Lateral view of the wrist demonstrating an avulsion fracture of the dorsal surface of the triquetrum (*arrow*).

be seen dorsal to the proximal carpal row (Fig. 5-13). This small avulsion is often the only radiographic sign of a triquetral fracture. If a triquetral fracture is suspected clinically and routine radiographs show no abnormalities, a slightly oblique pronated lateral view projects the triquetrum dorsal to the lunate.[1]

Indications for Orthopedic Referral

Patients with markedly displaced fractures of the body of the triquetrum should be referred for operative treatment. Nondisplaced triquetral fractures routinely heal well without complication. Persistent pain despite proper treatment should alert the physician to the possibility of an unrecognized associated injury, such as a pisiform fracture, ligamentous disruption, or injury to the TFCC. If the patient has continued symptoms after conservative management, an orthopedist or hand specialist should be consulted.

Treatment

A volar splint is preferred immediately after injury to allow swelling to decrease. A short-arm cast with the wrist in the position of function (slight extension) should be placed after 3 to 5 days or once the swelling has decreased. Both the cast and splint should only extend to the distal palmar crease to allow flexion at the metacarpophalangeal joint. The wrist is examined out of the cast at 2-week intervals until healing occurs, usually within 4 weeks. Repeat radiographs are not necessary unless healing is delayed. Most patients with a transverse fracture of the body of the triquetrum require 4 to 6 weeks of immobilization in a short-arm cast.

Table 5-3 summarizes management guidelines for triquetrum fractures.

Return to Work or Sports

When immobilization is discontinued, the patient should be instructed regarding ROM exercises for the wrist, emphasizing extension, flexion, and ulnar and radial deviation. Athletes can usually participate in sports wearing a semirigid cast, with appropriate padding. If sports participation is not allowed while a cast is worn, the athlete can resume sports as soon as the injury is nontender.

Complications

Nonunion of a dorsal chip fracture of the triquetrum has been reported but is rare and usually does not cause persistent symptoms. Patients with a transverse fracture of the body of the triquetrum are more likely to experience symptomatic nonunion at the fracture site. Patients with evidence of nonunion on follow-up radiographs or with symptoms suggestive of wrist instability (dull aching wrist pain aggravated by repeated wrist flexion and extension) should be referred to an orthopedist.

Pediatric Considerations

Fractures of the triquetrum have been reported in children between the ages of 6 and 15 years, and the majority of fractures occur between the ages of 11 and 13 years. The injury generally results from hyperextension and ulnar deviation of the wrist, causing avulsion of a small flake of bone from the triquetrum. The patient usually reports a fall onto the extended wrist and complains of pain at the ulnar aspect of the dorsum of the wrist. During physical examination, the patient has tenderness 1 to 2 cm distal to the ulnar styloid. Three views of the wrist should be obtained: AP, lateral, and oblique. The typical avulsed flake of bone is usually most apparent on the lateral view. The patient should be treated in a short-arm cast for 3 to 4 weeks. Children with a fracture of the body of the triquetrum should be immobilized in a long-arm thumb spica cast for 6 weeks.

LUNATE FRACTURES

Anatomic Considerations

The lunate bone is part of the proximal carpal row and is well protected within the lunate fossa on the distal radial articular surface. It articulates with

Table 5-3	*Management Guidelines for Triquetrum Fractures*	
	INITIAL TREATMENT	
Splint type and position	Volar splint, wrist in slight extension	
Initial follow-up visit	2 weeks	
Patient instruction	Icing and elevation of hand for 24 to 48 hours	
	Maintain finger, elbow, and shoulder ROM	
	FOLLOW-UP CARE	
Cast and splint type and position	Short-arm cast, wrist in slight extension	
Length of immobilization	Dorsal avulsion: 2 to 4 weeks	
	Transverse body fracture: 4 to 6 weeks	
Healing time	4 to 6 weeks	
Follow-up visit interval	Every 2 weeks	
Repeat radiography interval	Dorsal avulsion: none	
	Transverse body fracture: every 2 weeks	
Patient instruction	Maintain finger, elbow, and shoulder ROM	
	Wrist exercises after cast removed—flexion, extension, ulnar-radial deviation	
Indications for orthopedic consult	Displaced body fractures	
	Associated injuries: pisiform fracture, ligament disruption, TFCC tear	
	Symptomatic nonunion after 6 weeks of immobilization	

ROM, range of motion; TFCC, triangular fibrocartilaginous complex.

the distal radius, the scaphoid, the capitate, and the TFCC. The blood supply of the lunate enters both dorsally and volarly, yet ischemic bony changes after lunate fracture are common and usually involve the proximal fracture fragment. Some patients seem predisposed to AVN of the lunate because of either abnormalities of blood supply or anatomic variations that place greater stress on the lunate, such as a slightly shorter ulna (i.e., negative ulnar variance). Ulnar variance is the length of the ulna relative to the radius on the PA view of the wrist. Negative ulnar variance occurs when the distal articular surface of the ulna is shorter than the radius (Fig. 5-14). Similarly, positive ulnar variance occurs when the ulna is longer than the radius. If the articular surfaces of the ulna and radius are at the same level, the condition is called *neutral ulnar variance.*

Mechanism of Injury

Most acute lunate fractures are caused by traumatic dorsiflexion of the wrist resulting from a fall on the extended wrist or a strenuous push of a heavy object. These fractures are often unrecognized initially and progress to AVN known as Kienbock's disease. Chronic compressive stress to the lunate may also lead to Kienbock's disease, with eventual lunate fracture and collapse.

Clinical Presentation

The patient usually reports pain in the wrist aggravated by motion after a fall on the extended wrist. Occasionally, patients seek treatment without any significant trauma to the wrist but with tenderness at the middorsum just distal to the radius. The

patient has tenderness at the dorsum of the wrist just distal to Lister's tubercle (a small longitudinal bony prominence on the dorsal distal radius in alignment with the third metacarpal). Tenderness may be accentuated by resisted extension of the third finger or compression along the axis of the third finger. The patient may not seek evaluation for days or weeks after an injury, thinking initially it was just a wrist sprain.

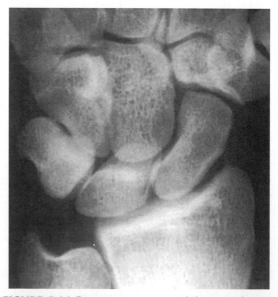

FIGURE 5-14 Posteroanterior view of the wrist showing negative ulnar variance. (*From Browner BD, Jupiter JB, Levine AM, Trafton PG [eds]. Skeletal Trauma: Fractures, Dislocations, Ligamentous Injuries. Philadelphia, WB Saunders, 1992.*)

Imaging

AP, lateral, and oblique views of the wrist are usually obtained, but the fracture line is often difficult to discern. On the AP view, it may be obscured by the concavity of the radial lunate fossa; on the lateral view, superimposition of other carpal bones may obscure a fracture. If a lunate fracture is suspected on clinical grounds, a CT scan or MRI is indicated to diagnose a fracture. Radiographs of patients who seek treatment after several weeks of symptoms should be examined for bony sclerosis, cystic changes, or collapse, which are signs of Kienbock's disease (Fig. 5-15).

Indications for Orthopedic Referral

Because of the potential for nonunion or AVN and the need for very close surveillance during the healing process to prevent these complications, all lunate fractures should be referred for orthopedic management.

Treatment

The patient should be immobilized in a double-sugar tong splint or a long-arm cast well molded over the wrist to compress the lunate area. The patient should then be referred to an orthopedist promptly for close follow-up. Most patients require several weeks of immobilization with radiographic studies at frequent intervals. Several retrospective studies have suggested better results with surgical management compared with conservative treatment.[14,15] The definitive surgical method for treatment of patients with Kienbock's disease is still debated. Ulnar lengthening or radial shortening has been used to decrease stress on the healing lunate. Other surgical procedures include lunate excision, prosthetic replacement, and intercarpal fusion.

Return to Work or Sports

After cast removal, the patient should start a physical therapy program that includes ROM and progressive strengthening exercises. The patient should wear a rigid splint for athletic activities until strength and ROM are similar to those of the uninjured wrist. The wrist should be protected for a minimum of 3 months after cast removal.

Pediatric Considerations

Acute lunate fractures are uncommon in children but have been reported. Nondisplaced avulsion fractures of the dorsal or volar horns of the lunate

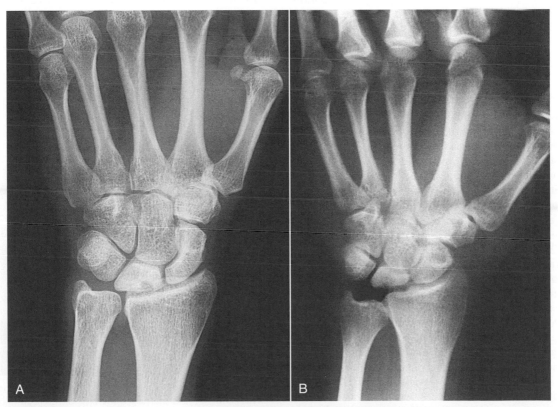

FIGURE 5-15 Radiographic appearance of avascular necrosis of the lunate (Kienbock's disease). **A,** Sclerosis and cystic changes in the lunate. **B,** The later stages of Kienbock's disease with sclerosis and collapse of the lunate. Note the presence of negative ulnar variance. Compare the appearance of the lunate with the normal lunate in Fig. 5-14.

usually heal well with cast immobilization. Truly nondisplaced transverse fractures of the body of the lunate usually heal well, especially among adolescents.

Kienbock's disease is uncommon in children but has been reported. Some children, especially younger children, have spontaneous revascularization with splint or cast protection. Surgical procedures to unload the lunate and allow protected revascularization have also been reported.

HAMATE FRACTURES

Hook of the Hamate

Anatomic Considerations

The hamate bone is situated at the ulnar aspect of the distal carpal row and articulates with the capitate, the triquetrum, and the fourth and fifth metacarpals. The "hook" of the hamate is a volar outcropping of bone that serves as part of Guyon's canal, which protects the ulnar nerve. The hook of the hamate protrudes volarly into the base of the hypothenar eminence and is attached to the piso-hamate ligament, the short flexor and opponens muscles of the fifth finger, and the transverse carpal ligament. In the presence of a fracture, these attachments exert deforming forces on the loose fragment and interfere with bone healing. The hook of the hamate is rather superficial in the palm and is susceptible to fracture. Because the ulnar nerve is close to the hamate hook, nerve injury has been associated with this fracture.

Mechanism of Injury

A fracture of the hook of the hamate is often a sports-related injury caused by blunt trauma to the ulnar base of the wrist from a bat, golf club, or racket. The injury usually occurs at the end of a swing. A fall on the extended wrist may also fracture the hamate. These fractures are often misdiagnosed, and patients may present with chronic pain in the hypothenar region.

Clinical Presentation

In cases of fracture of the hook of the hamate, the patient reports a sudden onset of pain in the palm proximal to the fifth finger, usually associated with a forceful swing with a bat, golf club, or racket. During examination, the patient has point tenderness in the palm over the hook of the hamate. To locate the hook of the hamate, the examiner places the IP joint of his or her thumb over the patient's pisiform bone and points the tip of the thumb toward the web space between the thumb and index finger. The hook of the hamate lies directly below the tip of the examiner's thumb in this position and can be palpated with deep pressure.

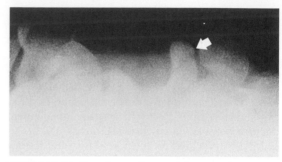

FIGURE 5-16 Carpal tunnel view of the wrist demonstrating a fracture of the hook of the hamate (*arrow*).

If the ulnar nerve is injured, the patient reports paresthesias in the fifth finger and ulnar aspect of the fourth finger, sensation to light touch and two-point discrimination may be impaired, and weakness of the intrinsic muscles of the hand may be detectable.

Imaging

Three views of the wrist are required: AP, lateral, and oblique. Radiographs may initially show no abnormalities, and comparison views of the uninjured wrist may be necessary. A carpal tunnel view, with the wrist maximally extended and the x-ray tube angled 25 degrees from the plane of the palm, usually demonstrates the fracture (Fig. 5-16). An oblique radiograph of the extended wrist with the forearm in supination may also be helpful in diagnosing this fracture. A CT scan of the wrist should be ordered if these views fail to show a fracture and clinical suspicion of hamate fracture is high (Fig. 5-17).

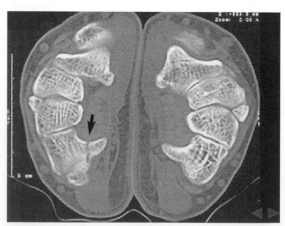

FIGURE 5-17 Axial computed tomography scan of both wrists shows a linear lucency at the base of the right hook of the hamate (*arrow*), representing a nondisplaced fracture. (*From Ouellette HA. The Teaching Files: Musculoskeletal. Philadelphia, WB Saunders, 2009.*)

Indications for Orthopedic Referral

Patients that fail conservative management, displaced hook fractures, and flexor tendon injuries and those electing immediate excision of fragment should be referred to orthopedics. There is some controversy as to the best definitive management of nondisplaced hook of the hamate fractures. If the fracture is diagnosed within 7 days of injury and there is no displacement, a trial of cast immobilization can be considered.[16] However, nonoperative therapy has a high failure rate and likely may result in prolonged recovery times. Failure to excise the fragment may lead to chronic hand pain and AVN of the fragment. The results of early excision of the avulsed hook of the hamate are generally excellent; however, there are risks of weakened grip strength, impaired sensation, and residual pain from ulnar nerve injury in Guyon's canal.[17]

Competitive athletes and patients who require heavy use of their hands for work often elect to proceed to immediate excision to avoid a trial of conservative therapy for 4 to 6 weeks that may fail and would result in another 4 to 6 weeks of time missed while recovering from surgery.

Treatment

In the acute setting, the wrist should be placed in a volar splint in slight extension. If nonoperative therapy is elected, a short-arm cast should be placed and should include the fourth and fifth metacarpophalangeal joints (in flexion) to prevent tendon shortening.[18] Casting may require between 8 and 12 weeks with frequent radiographs and examination to detect nonunion.

Return to Work or Sports

Athletes who undergo surgical excision of the avulsed hook of the hamate are usually able to return to sports 6 to 8 weeks after surgery. After excision, the patient is immobilized for 2 to 4 weeks, and aggressive rehabilitation is then instituted. The rehabilitation program should emphasize gentle ROM exercises and progressive strengthening of the wrist. Protective splinting should be used until the athlete has full nontender ROM and strength is 80% that of the uninjured wrist.

Body of the Hamate

Fractures of the body of the hamate are uncommon and are usually associated with other injuries to the hand. Dislocations at the carpometacarpal joint are frequent with hamate body fractures. During examination, the patient reports tenderness at the dorsum of the wrist just distal to the ulna. The fracture is usually readily apparent on routine radiographs. Patients with isolated, nondisplaced fractures can be treated safely in a short-arm cast

for 4 weeks. Patients with displaced fractures of the body of the hamate or hamate fractures with other associated fractures or dislocations should be referred for operative treatment.

Patients who are treated nonsurgically may return to work or sports immediately with the wrist protected in a semirigid synthetic cast. Patients treated surgically are restricted from sports participation until they have undergone 4 to 6 weeks of mobilization exercises. Protective splinting for athletic activities is continued for 3 months or until the injured wrist has normal or near-normal ROM and strength.

CAPITATE FRACTURES

The capitate is the largest of the carpal bones, centered within the distal carpal row. It is, therefore, usually well protected from injury and accounts for only 1% to 2% of carpal fractures. The distal capitate is covered with articular cartilage, and it articulates with the base of the third metacarpal. Proximally, the capitate articulates with both the lunate and the scaphoid; similar to the scaphoid, the proximal portion of the capitate has a tenuous blood supply, which makes it vulnerable to nonunion during the healing process. Fractures of the capitate are usually caused by high-energy trauma, such as a direct blow or crush injury. Isolated fractures of the capitate are rare; more commonly, fracture of the capitate is associated with other carpal fractures. Fractures of the capitate can usually be detected on the AP view, but initial radiographs may show no abnormalities. Oblique views of the wrist may be needed to detect fractures. Clinicians should have low threshold for CT scan because of the difficulty in imaging the capitate and concern for nonunion and AVN of fractures that have delayed diagnosis.

Patients with a nondisplaced or suspected fracture should be immobilized in a short-arm thumb spica cast for 6 to 8 weeks. Repeat evaluation and radiographs should be obtained 10 to 14 days after initial treatment. In cases of suspected capitate fracture, evaluation and radiographs should be repeated until symptoms resolve or a diagnosis is confirmed. Athletes who return to play during cast immobilization are at risk of fracture displacement, which may prolong healing and return to play time. Consider restricting these athletes from play while immobilized.

Patients with displaced fractures or multiple carpal injuries should be referred to an experienced orthopedic surgeon for definitive care. This type of injury is prone to nonunion and often requires open reduction and internal fixation with or without bone grafting.

Scaphocapitate Syndrome

A fracture unique to the capitate is the so-called scaphocapitate syndrome in which a high-energy injury to the hyperextended and radially deviated wrist causes a neck fracture of the capitate and a waist fracture of the scaphoid. With this injury, the proximal portion of the capitate may rotate 180 degrees. Recognition of this injury pattern and prompt referral for open reduction and internal fixation are essential for a good outcome.

Pediatric Considerations

Fractures of the capitate are the second most common carpal bone fracture in children but are often undiagnosed. Isolated capitate fractures may occur, but this fracture usually is associated with other carpal injuries. Capitate fractures are thought to result from impingement of the capitate on the dorsal lip of the lunate. The usual cause of injury is a fall on the outstretched hand or direct trauma to the dorsum of the hand (e.g., crush injury). High-energy trauma may also result in a fracture of the capitate (e.g., motor vehicle accident or fall from a height). In the case of a fall on the extended wrist, fracture of the neck of the capitate is often associated with concomitant fracture of the waist of the scaphoid, the so-called scaphocapitate syndrome.

During physical examination, the patient has tenderness at the dorsum of the hand just proximal to the base of the third metacarpal. Axial load of the third metacarpal may reproduce the patient's pain. The patient may not have painful wrist ROM. The examiner should also check for tenderness in the anatomic snuffbox because a scaphoid fracture may accompany a capitate fracture. Radiographs may show a fracture line through the neck of the capitate; less commonly, the fracture line passes through the body of the capitate. Radiographs with the wrist in distraction may demonstrate small osteochondral fragments in the midcarpal region indicative of an isolated capitate fracture. MRI is a useful diagnostic tool as well.

Closed treatment in a short-arm thumb spica cast for 5 to 6 weeks is usually successful. Cases of nonunion are usually associated with a delay in diagnosis and can be treated with open reduction and bone grafting. Patients with displaced fractures or fractures diagnosed weeks or months after injury should be referred to an experienced orthopedic surgeon; these fractures are prone to nonunion and often require open reduction and bone grafting. Patients with multiple carpal injuries should also be referred for definitive care.

PISIFORM FRACTURES

Fractures of the pisiform are uncommon and are usually nondisplaced. The pisiform is a sesamoid bone in the flexor carpi ulnaris tendon and is attached by ligaments to the triquetrum, the hamate, and the fifth metacarpal. Fractures of the pisiform are usually caused by a direct blow to the hypothenar eminence, and patients experience tenderness at that site. Routine wrist views may show no abnormalities, but the fracture is demonstrated by oblique views of the wrist with the forearm in 20 degrees of supination or by the carpal tunnel view. The fracture may be linear, comminuted, or avulsed. Most cases respond well to 4 to 6 weeks of immobilization in a short-arm cast. If symptomatic arthritis or nonunion develops, excision of the pisiform cures the condition.

TRAPEZIUM FRACTURES

Fractures of the trapezium account for fewer than 5% of all carpal fractures; however, they are significant because missed trapezium fractures cause thumb weakness and limited ROM and may remain painful for months. The trapezium forms a double-saddle articulation with the base of the thumb metacarpal. A direct blow to the adducted thumb can cause a vertical fracture through the body of the trapezium, and a fall on the extended wrist can cause an avulsion fracture of the trapezial ridge. Patients complain of local tenderness at the base of the thenar eminence. Pain intensifies with thumb motion or axial compression of the thumb.

Vertical fractures are best visualized on the AP view. Carpal tunnel views of the wrist are necessary to visualize the trapezial ridge fracture. As with other carpal fractures, early use of CT scan is advocated if there is no fracture seen despite high clinical suspicion. Most nondisplaced fractures heal after 4 to 6 weeks of immobilization in a short-arm thumb spica cast. Displaced fractures and articular surface fractures require surgical management. Early excision is recommended for small displaced bony fragments.

TRAPEZOID FRACTURES

Trapezoid fractures occur rarely. The usual mechanism of injury is a longitudinal force through the second metacarpal, which may result in a fracture with an associated dorsal dislocation of the trapezoid or metacarpal. Patients with a trapezoid fracture have localized tenderness over the dorsal hand near the base of the second metacarpal. These fractures are difficult to visualize on routine wrist radiographs and may require oblique views or CT scans for diagnosis. Nondisplaced fractures usually heal with 4 to 6 weeks of immobilization in a short-arm cast. Displaced fractures or fracture dislocations should be referred for operative treatment.[19]

CARPAL DISLOCATIONS

Dislocations of carpal bones are relatively uncommon. They merit consideration because they are easy to miss, and delays in diagnosis can adversely affect the outcome. Accurate characterization of the injury is difficult, and open repair is preferred in most cases. The emphasis of this section is on recognition of these injuries because referral is recommended in all suspected cases.

The primary considerations in the differential diagnosis are a mild sprain, carpal fracture, or fracture dislocation. Fracture dislocations can generally be detected if the physician carefully scrutinizes multiple radiographic views in all patients with known or suspected carpal dislocations. Special attention should be paid to the scaphoid and the distal radius because these are the most common sites of associated fractures.

Mechanism of Injury

Carpal dislocations usually result from a fall on an outstretched hand or from hyperextension injuries. Distinguishing mild carpal sprains from significant ligament injuries can be difficult. The force of the injury is a helpful clue, although patients with previous injuries or chronic stress of the ligaments (e.g., gymnasts and golfers) may rupture a carpal ligament with relatively minor trauma.

Clinical Presentation

The clinical presentation is highly variable. Patients generally report pain and swelling of the wrist, but it may be deceptively mild. Deformity ranges from absent to readily apparent. ROM is usually decreased, although it may be abnormal in only one direction (e.g., extension may be relatively normal while flexion is limited). The most reliable finding is point tenderness over the injured ligament(s). In the setting of trauma and wrist pain, this strongly suggests a significant ligament injury just as snuffbox tenderness strongly suggests a scaphoid fracture. Palpation over a displaced bone may reveal an abnormal fullness or stepoff. It may also produce a pop, click, or palpable movement of the bone. The displaced bone(s) may apply pressure to the median nerve and dysfunction or paralysis of this nerve may be present. Unfortunately, many significant carpal ligament injuries have none of these findings. Therefore, whenever point tenderness is present, the clinician should maintain a high index of suspicion for a carpal dislocation, fracture, or both.

Scapholunate Dissociations

The scapholunate interosseous ligament is the most commonly injured ligament of the wrist. Static or dissociative injuries have widened intercarpal spaces, gross instability, or both. Dynamic or nondissociative instability is not seen on standard radiographs but can be demonstrated with provocative examinations and stress radiographs. The history may be deceptive in that the injury often arises from very minor trauma, leading the patient, the physician, or both to interpret it as a minor sprain. This false sense of security may result in a prolonged delay in treatment that may lead to severe wrist degenerative joint disease. Detection of scapholunate dissociations can be enhanced if the physician maintains a high index of suspicion for this injury in any patient with wrist pain and tenderness over the scapholunate area even if the trauma was minor. The likelihood of this injury is enhanced if the patient has a history of repetitive wrist use (occupational or sports related) or if the patient experiences pain when making a fist.

An abnormally wide space between the scaphoid and lunate (>2 mm) is diagnostic (Terry Thomas or David Letterman sign; Fig. 5-12). Disruption of the lines of Gilula (Fig. 5-5) also are seen with dissociations. Views that stress the scapholunate joint may be required. In Fig. 5-12, a grip view (AP view of slightly flexed fist) was used to demonstrate this widening. Note also that the scaphoid in this view appears shortened with a ring-like density over its distal portion (compare with the normal scaphoid appearance shown in Fig. 5-14). The widened space may also be demonstrated on AP views with the hand in ulnar and radial deviation.

Perilunate Dislocation

Acute lunate and perilunate dislocations are rare but potentially devastating injuries of the wrist. Fig. 5-6 demonstrates the normal alignment of the lunate on a lateral view. The lunate should sit in the concavity of the distal radius, and the capitate sits in the concavity of the lunate. It should be possible to draw a straight line through these three bones, as shown in Fig. 5-6, B. Fig. 5-18, A, shows a lateral view of a perilunate dislocation. In this injury, the lunate remains in the concavity of the radius. However, the concavity of the lunate is empty, and the capitate sits dorsal to the lunate. It is impossible to draw a straight line through the three structures. The abnormality is far more subtle on the AP view (Fig. 5-18, B), but the triangular shape of the lunate is highly suggestive of a dislocation. Comparison to a film with a normal lunate position, such as Fig. 5-6, A, will help the clinician recognize this abnormal orientation of the lunate. This demonstrates an important principle: comparison views of the normal wrist can be helpful, especially for physicians who infrequently encounter carpal injuries.

In lunate dislocations, the lunate becomes dissociated from both the capitate and distal radius.

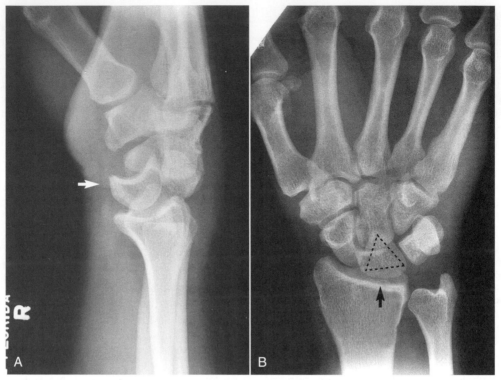

FIGURE 5-18 Perilunate dislocation. **A,** Lateral view, demonstrating misalignment of the capitate with the distal radius and lunate (*arrow*). **B,** Anteroposterior view, which appears deceptively normal unless compared with a normal wrist. Note the abnormal triangular appearance of the lunate (*arrow*).

On the lateral view, it loses its normal contact with both the radius and capitate. Fig. 5-19 demonstrates a lunate dislocation. In contrast to a perilunate dislocation, the rounded proximal surface of the lunate is not nestled in the concavity of the

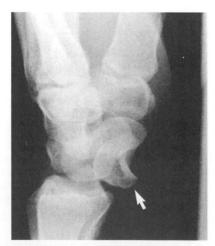

FIGURE 5-19 Lunate dislocation, lateral view. Note that the lunate has lost its normal relationship to the radius (*arrow*), but the capitate remains in a straight line with the radius. (*From Raby N, Berman L, DeLong G. Accident and Emergency Radiology: A Survival Guide. Philadelphia, WB Saunders, 1995.*)

radius. Instead, ligaments that hold the lunate to the radius have been disrupted, allowing the lunate to be displaced volarly. In addition, the capitate lies in a straight line with the radius in contrast to its dorsal displacement in perilunate dislocations (Fig. 5-18, A).

Imaging

Radiographic assessment of a patient with a possible carpal dislocation can be fairly complicated. Even readily apparent carpal dislocations are often overlooked on radiographs. This is partly attributable to the number and irregular shape of the carpal bones and the inherent difficulty in appreciating their proper anatomic alignment. Additional views or stress views are often necessary to detect significant ligament injury. Comparison views, an arthrogram, or MRI may also be necessary.

Treatment and Referral

Acute management of carpal dislocations should include a careful neurovascular examination with special attention to median nerve function. A neurologic or vascular deficit should prompt an emergent orthopedic consultation. Carpal dislocations without neurovascular compromise can be splinted in neutral position and discussed with an orthopedist. Some demand emergency orthopedic evaluation.

Static scapholunate injuries should be referred for surgical management. Dynamic scapholunate injuries may be initially treated with short-arm cast immobilization for 2 to 6 weeks depending on the severity of the injury. After nonoperative or operative management, a rehabilitation program with ROM exercises and strengthening exercises is crucial to return the wrist to full function.[20]

Because distinguishing mild sprains from significant ligament injuries can be difficult, referral is strongly recommended whenever the physician suspects a carpal sprain and is unable to reasonably exclude a significant ligament injury. Ideally, the patient should be splinted and seen in consultation within a few days to avoid the poorer outcome that can accompany delays in diagnosis. Because the evaluation and treatment of carpal dislocations are complicated, referring the patient to a hand specialist is best if one is available. Definitive treatment involves surgery in the vast majority of cases.

Complications

Complications are common after carpal dislocations. Median nerve palsy, reflex sympathetic dystrophy, AVN, and degenerative joint disease may occur. The lunate is especially susceptible to AVN after dislocation. Monthly radiographs for 6 months may detect the condition early enough to allow treatment before irreversible degenerative changes of the wrist occur.

REFERENCES

1. Geissler WB. Carpal fractures in athletes. *Clin Sports Med.* 2001;20(1):167-188.
2. Hansen TB, Petersen RB, Barckman J, et al. Cost-effectiveness of MRI in managing suspected scaphoid fractures. *J Hand Surg Eur Vol.* 2009;34(5):627-630.
3. Ty JM, Lozano-Calderon S, Ring D. Computed tomography for triage of suspected scaphoid fractures. *Hand (NY).* 2008;3(2):155-158.
4. Nguyen Q, Chaudry S, Sloan R, et al. The clinical scaphoid fracture: early computed tomography as a practical approach. *Ann R Coll Surg Engl.* 2008;90(6):488-491.
5. Bernard SA, Murray PM, Heckman MG. Validity of conventional radiography in determining scaphoid waist fracture displacement. *J Orthop Trauma.* 2010;24(7):448-451.
6. Yin ZG, Zhang JB, Kan SL, Wang XG. Diagnosing suspected scaphoid fractures. *Clin Orthop Relat Res.* 2010;468:723-734.
7. Buijze GA, Doornberg JN, Ham JS, et al. Surgical compared with conservative treatment for acute non-displaced or minimally displaced scaphoid fractures: a systematic review and meta-analysis of randomized controlled trials. *J Bone Joint Surg (Am).* 2010;92(6):1534-1544.
8. Gellman H, Caputo RJ, Carter V, et al. Comparison of short and long thumb spica casts for non-displaced fractures of the carpal scaphoid. *J Bone Joint Surg (Am).* 1989;71:354-357.
9. Prosser GH, Isbister ES. The presentation of scaphoid non-union. *Injury.* 2003;34:65-67.
10. Kawamura K, Chung KC. Treatment of scaphoid fractures and nonunions. *J Hand Surg.* 2008;33A:988-997.
11. Adams JE, Steinmann SP. Acute scaphoid fractures. *Orthop Clin North Am.* 2007;38:229-235.
12. Evenski AJ, Adamczyk MJ, Steiner RP, et al. Clinically suspected scaphoid fractures in children. *J Pediatr Orthop.* 2009;29:352-355.
13. Papp S. Carpal bone fractures. *Orthop Clin North Am.* 2007;38:251-260.
14. Salmon J, Stanley JK, Trail IA. Kienböck's disease: conservative management versus radial shortening. *J Bone Joint Surg (Br).* 2000;82:820-823.
15. Nakamura R, Watanabe K, Tsunoda K, Miura T. Radial osteotomy for Kienböck's disease evaluated by magnetic resonance imaging: 24 cases followed for 1-3 years. *Acta Orthop Scand.* 1993;64:207-211.
16. Whaln JL, Bishop AT, Linscheid RL. Non-operative treatment of acute hook of the hamate fractures. *J Hand Surg.* 1992;17A:507-511.
17. Scheufler O, Andresen R, Radmer S, et al. Hook of hamate fractures: critical evaluation of different therapeutic procedures. *Plast Reconstr Surg.* 2005;115:488-497.
18. Binzer TC, Carter PR. Hook of the hamate fracture in athletes. *Oper Tech Sports Med.* 1996;4:242-247.
19. Gruson KI, Kaplan KM, Pakisma N. Isolated trapezoid fractures: a case report with compilation of the literature. *Bull NYU Hosp Joint Dis.* 2008;66(1):57-60.
20. Lewis DM, Osterman AL. Scapholunate instability in athletes. *Clin Sports Med.* 2001;20(1):131-140.

6

RADIUS AND ULNA FRACTURES

Co-Author: Adam Prawer

Fractures of the distal radius are among the most common fractures, and of these, the most familiar pattern is the Colles' fracture, first described in 1814. Although Colles considered these to be stable fractures that usually enjoyed satisfactory outcomes, more modern experience has shown that these injuries require careful evaluation and treatment specific to the fracture pattern if they are to have good outcomes. Familiarity with the anatomy and natural history of distal radius fracture patterns is essential to managing or referring these fractures appropriately. Fractures of the radius and ulnar shaft are usually displaced and unstable, and most require operative treatment. Nondisplaced extraarticular fractures of the distal radius and isolated fractures of the ulnar shaft can be managed effectively by primary care providers. Those clinicians with additional experience in fracture reduction can safely manage displaced Colles' fractures with accurate assessment of fracture alignment and careful attention to follow-up care and rehabilitation. Fractures of the distal radius are common in children and adolescents and heal without difficulty in most cases.

See Appendix for stepwise instructions for a sugar-tong splint and short- and long-arm casts used in the treatment of radius and ulna fractures.

Go to Expert Consult for the electronic version of a patient instruction sheet named "Broken Hand or Wrist or Arm," which covers the steps of care from pain relief to rehabilitation exercises. This can be copied to hand out to patients to assist them during the treatment period.

DISTAL RADIUS FRACTURES (ADULT)

Anatomic Considerations

The distal radius has three separate articulations. The distal radial articular surface has two fossae, the scaphoid fossa and the lunate fossa, which articulate with the scaphoid and lunate in the proximal carpal row. The sigmoid notch is a concave groove that articulates with and stabilizes the distal ulna. The medial side of the distal radius is attached to the distal ulna, the triquetrum, and the lunate via the triangular fibrocartilaginous complex (TFCC). This complex is composed of the triangular fibrocartilage, the ulnocarpal meniscus, and the ulnolunate ligament. These attachments are responsible for ulnar styloid fractures that frequently accompany distal radius fractures.

Four anatomic measurements are important in the evaluation of distal radius fractures (Fig. 6-1). On the anteroposterior (AP) view, the slope of the distal radial articular surface, or radial inclination, is approximately 25 degrees, the radial length is approximately 1 cm from the tip of the radial styloid to an imaginary perpendicular line drawn from the distal ulnar articular surface, and the center of the radial joint surface should be 1 to 2 mm distal to the ulnar joint surface. The difference between the center of the radial joint surface and the ulnar joint surface is referred to as the *ulnar variance*. If the ulnar surface extends distal to the radial joint center, this is called a *positive ulnar variance*. This is abnormal and may interfere with normal wrist function. On the lateral view, the distal radius has a slight volar tilt of approximately 10 degrees. The median nerve and extensor pollicis longus tendon are in close proximity to the distal radius and may be injured in association with fractures in this location (Fig. 6-2).

Classification

Traditionally, the most common classification system of distal radius fractures is that introduced by Frykman in 1967[1] (Fig. 6-3). Types I and II are extraarticular fractures, types III and IV are intraarticular fractures involving the radiocarpal joint, types V and VI are intraarticular fractures involving the radioulnar joint, and types VII and VIII are intraarticular fractures involving both the radiocarpal and radioulnar joints. Even-numbered types indicate the presence of an ulnar styloid fracture in addition to the distal radius fracture. The Frykman classification is useful in describing

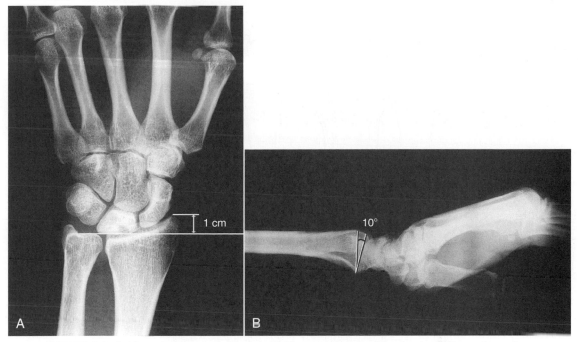

FIGURE 6-1 A, Normal average radial length. **B,** Normal volar tilt of the distal radial articular surface.

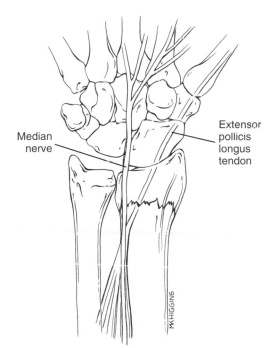

FIGURE 6-2 The median nerve or the extensor pollicis longus tendon may be injured in association with a distal radius fracture because of the close proximity of both to the bone.

fractures of the distal radius and evaluating the outcome of treatment. The higher the Frykman number, the greater the likelihood of poor results.

Signs of fracture instability include more than 20 degrees of dorsal angulation, marked comminution, and more than 10 mm of radial shortening. Stable fractures are usually extraarticular, with minimal to moderate displacement, and do not become redisplaced when reduced.

Mechanism of Injury

By far, the most common cause of distal radius fractures is a fall on an outstretched hand with the wrist in extension. Postmenopausal women incur 60% to 70% of all Colles' fractures. Another 10% to 15% are caused by violent injuries to younger patients in which the lunate is driven into the radius, causing a higher-force "die-punch" radius fracture.

Clinical Presentation

Patients report the typical cause of injury and complain of pain and swelling in the wrist. During examination, obvious swelling and ecchymosis of the wrist are apparent, especially dorsally. The displacement caused by a Colles' fracture has been called a "silver fork" deformity because of the gross appearance of the hand and wrist. The patient has point tenderness at the dorsal aspect of the wrist, and pain limits range of motion (ROM). Median nerve function should be tested by checking sensation at the volar aspect of the thumb and second

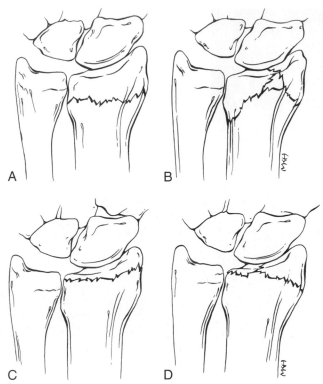

FIGURE 6-3 Frykman classification of distal radius fractures. Even-numbered types indicate the presence of an ulnar styloid fracture. **A,** Types I and II: extraarticular. **B,** Types III and IV: intraarticular involving the radiocarpal joint. **C,** Types V and VI: intraarticular involving the radioulnar joint. **D,** Types VII and VIII: intraarticular involving both the radiocarpal and radioulnar joints.

and third fingers. Capillary refill should take less than 2 seconds, and the radial pulse should be full. The scaphoid (anatomic snuff box) and other carpals should be palpated as well to seek evidence of associated carpal bone or ligament injuries.

Imaging

Three views of the wrist (AP, lateral, and oblique) are necessary in the evaluation of distal radius fractures. The AP view should be examined for the radial inclination, radial length, and ulnar variance (Fig. 6-1A), and the lateral view should be examined for the normal volar tilt of the distal radial articular surface (Fig. 6-1B). The radiocarpal and distal radioulnar joints should be examined for evidence that the fracture extends into the joint. High-risk features such as comminution, severe displacement, and more than 2 mm of articular surface stepoff should also be sought. Concomitant dislocation may indicate the present of either a Barton's or Hutchinson's fracture (discussed separately below). The Colles' fracture is an extraarticular fracture (Frykman types I and II) and usually occurs within 2 cm of the distal radial articular surface. In this fracture, the volar cortex fails in tension (sharp fracture), and the dorsal cortex fails

in compression (dorsal comminution). In a typical Colles' fracture, the distal fragment is displaced dorsally and proximally. The angle of radial inclination is decreased, the radial length is shortened, and the normal volar tilt is lost or reversed to a dorsal tilt (Fig. 6-4).

The radiographs should also be examined for associated fractures, particularly of the ulnar styloid, scaphoid, or lunate. Occasionally, disruption of the supporting ligaments of the wrist results in scapholunate dissociation, the so-called Terry Thomas sign, seen radiographically as a gap between the scaphoid and lunate (see Fig. 5-12).

Indications for Orthopedic Referral

Emergent Referral (Within 30 to 60 Minutes)

Patients with open fractures, acute neuropathy, tenting of the skin, compartment syndrome, or vascular compromise require emergent orthopedic referral. If specialist care is not promptly available, tenting or neurovascular compromise associated with a displaced fracture can generally be corrected by immediate closed reduction after adequate analgesia or local anaesthesia is achieved (discussed below).

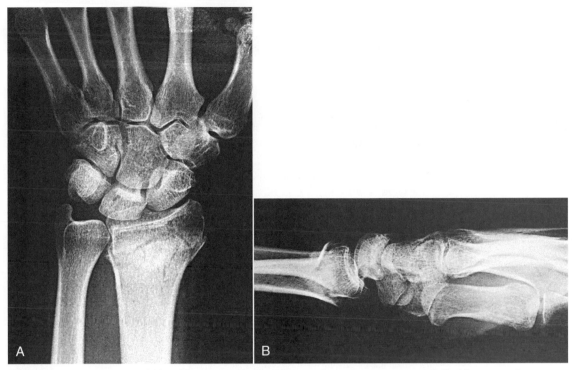

FIGURE 6-4 Anteroposterior (**A**) and lateral (**B**) views of the wrist demonstrating a typical Colles' fracture with comminution, radial shortening, and dorsal tilt of the radial articular surface.

Nonemergent Referral (Within 24 to 48 Hours)

If the fracture is displaced and the physician is uncomfortable performing the necessary reduction, the patient should be referred and have reduction performed within 24 hours (preferably). Physicians who are comfortable performing reductions can reduce and manage many distal radius fractures. However, certain distal radius fractures are inherently unstable and likely to lose position even if reduction can be achieved initially. These fractures are best treated by an orthopedic surgeon. There is a paucity of evidence regarding which specific radiographic and clinical features mandate surgical evaluation. Studies have illustrated that available systems tend to underestimate instability and should be used with caution.[2] Fractures with any of the following generally require referral: comminution, intraarticular extension, more than 20 degrees of dorsal angulation, displacement of more than two thirds the width of the radius, more than 5 mm of radial shortening or ulnar variance of more than 5 mm (i.e., ulnar joint surface >5 mm distal to the center of radial joint surface).[3,4] Other fractures that typically require operative fixation include fracture dislocations, fractures with associated injuries to carpal bones or ligaments, displaced intraarticular fractures (i.e., >2 mm stepoff on joint surface), fractures with large displaced ulnar styloid fragments, and fractures with palmar displacement (Smith's fracture, discussed below). Patient characteristics also influence the choice of operative or conservative treatment. "High-demand patients" (i.e., active patients whose dominant wrist is injured) are more likely to require surgery to obtain a satisfactory result. In elderly patients, particularly those at higher operative risk, it may be preferable to avoid surgery even if surgery would otherwise be strongly preferred for that particular fracture. This common practice has been validated in one small study of low-demand patients over the age of 70 years with unstable radius fractures. After nearly 5 years of follow-up, bony alignment was far better in the operative group, but functional and subjective outcomes were the same in both groups, and cast treatment was significantly less painful.[5]

Initial Treatment

Table 6-1 summarizes the management guidelines for distal radius (Colles') fractures.

The treatment of distal radius fractures should be individualized and modified by several key factors: fracture pattern, bone quality, patient's functional demands (i.e., age, hand dominance, occupation, hobbies, and activities), and associated injuries (e.g., median nerve compression, carpal fractures, and elbow fractures). Closed reduction and cast immobilization are still the standard treatments for stable fractures.

Table 6-1	*Management Guidelines for Distal Radius (Colles') Fractures*
INITIAL TREATMENT	
Splint type and position	Double sugar-tong splint Wrist in slight flexion and ulnar deviation, forearm in neutral position, elbow at 90 degrees
Initial follow-up visit	Nondisplaced: 3 to 5 days Displaced, reduced: 2 to 3 days
Patient instruction	Icing, elevation, ROM of fingers and shoulder
FOLLOW-UP CARE	
Cast or splint type and position	Nondisplaced: SAC, wrist in neutral position Reduced: LAC, wrist in slight flexion and ulnar deviation, forearm in neutral position, elbow at 90 degrees
Length of immobilization	Nondisplaced: 4 to 6 weeks LAC for 3 to 4 weeks followed by SAC until healed (total, 6 to 8 weeks) Elderly: LAC for 2 to 3 weeks followed by SAC until healed
Healing time	Nondisplaced: 6 to 8 weeks Reduced: 8 to 12 weeks
Follow-up visit interval	Nondisplaced: Every 2 to 3 weeks Reduced: Weekly until fracture stability ensured, then every 2 weeks until healed
Repeat radiography interval	Nondisplaced: At first follow-up visit, at 2 weeks, at 4 to 6 weeks Reduced: weekly for 3 weeks; then every 2 weeks if stable
Patient instruction	Finger and shoulder ROM exercises while immobilized Aggressive hand, wrist, and elbow rehabilitation after immobilization, especially in elderly adults
Indications for orthopedic consult	Intraarticular extension Severe comminution Inability to maintain reduction (younger patients and high-demand patients) Progressive symptoms of median nerve injury Early symptoms of reflex sympathetic dystrophy

LAC, long-arm cast; ROM, range of motion; SAC, short-arm cast.

Nondisplaced Extraarticular Fractures (Frykman Type I or II)

Patients with nondisplaced or minimally displaced extraarticular fractures can be treated initially with one of several splint types. The application of circumferential casts in the acute setting has been associated with an increased risk of ischemia and carpal tunnel syndrome and should not be performed unless the cast is bivalved. For nondisplaced fractures with no unstable features (see above), a well-molded "clamshell" splint should suffice. Indeed, one small study in adults[6] and several studies in children (see below) support use of a splint. A clamshell splint includes two separate components: a volar splint extending from near the elbow to the palmar crease plus a dorsal splint extending from near the elbow to the dorsal metacarpophalangeal (MCP) joints. To provide maximal stability, a well-molded sugar-tong splint could be used instead. It consists of a wrist and forearm splint that extends from the proximal palmar crease to the volar forearm around the elbow and back to the dorsum of the MCP joints. The elbow is flexed to 90 degrees, the forearm is placed in neutral pronation–supination, and the wrist is placed in neutral flexion-extension. See the

Appendix for a stepwise description of how to apply this splint. The patient should be advised to keep the arm elevated, begin active ROM at the shoulder and fingers immediately, and return for follow-up evaluation in 3 to 5 days.

Displaced Extraarticular Fractures (Frykman Type I or II)

Closed reduction of displaced extraarticular fractures can be attempted after adequate anesthesia. A hematoma block is adequate for most displaced fractures along with intramuscular or intravenous analgesia for the patient. Some patients require a Bier block or axillary nerve block (see Chapter 4 for a description of the hematoma block and Bier block techniques). Studies have compared different reduction techniques and found no difference in effectiveness.[7,8]

Reduction Method with Finger Traps

Traction is applied to the thumb and index and middle fingers with the elbow at 90 degrees of flexion and the forearm in neutral rotation. With a stockinette, 5 to 10 lb of traction is applied to the arm for at least 5 minutes before reduction is attempted (Fig. 6-5, A). The examiner's thumbs are placed on the dorsal aspect of the distal fracture slight pronation is often recommended to help prevent loss of position.[9] Splints that hold the wrist in greater than 15 degrees of volar flexion increase the risk of acute carpal tunnel syndrome[10] and complex regional pain syndrome (CRPS).[11] Using gently molded three-point control while shaping the splint helps maintain the reduction.

Reduction Method without Finger Traps

If finger traps are not available, closed reduction can be attempted with the help of an assistant (Fig. 6-6). The assistant holds the patient's elbow and provides countertraction. The forearm is supinated and held with the examiner's left hand while longitudinal traction is applied with the right hand and thumb to the distal fragment. The fracture is disimpacted by allowing dorsal angulation in the supinated position. Fracture reduction is accomplished by pronating the forearm and wrist. The pronation is done entirely with the right hand while the left hand remains stationary. The wrist is directed into ulnar deviation by this maneuver, which seems to correct radial and dorsal angulation of the distal fragment. After reduction, median nerve function should be tested and the arm splinted as previously described.

After reduction, postreduction radiographs are obtained. The goal of reduction is to restore normal length, alignment, and articular surface congruity. Adequate reduction requires no dorsal tilt to the distal radial articular surface, less than 5 mm of radial shortening, and less than 2 mm of displacement of fracture fragments. If these criteria are not met, a second attempt at closed reduction should be made. The patient should be instructed to keep the arm elevated, begin active ROM at the shoulder and fingers immediately, and return for follow-up evaluation in 2 to 3 days. If adequate reduction cannot be achieved by closed means, the patient should be referred to an orthopedic surgeon after the arm is splinted as previously described.

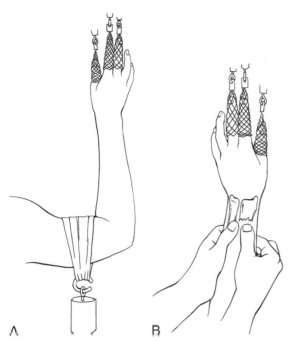

FIGURE 6-5 Colles' fracture reduction using finger traps. **A,** Finger trap traction position for closed reduction of a displaced distal radius fracture. **B,** The clinician's thumbs are placed on the dorsal aspect of the distal fracture fragment while the fingers are placed on the volar forearm just proximal to the fracture line. The distal fracture fragment is then pushed distally, volarly, and ulnarly.

fragment while the fingers are placed on the volar forearm just proximal to the fracture line. The distal fracture fragment is then pushed distally, volarly, and ulnarly to reduce the dorsal displacement and radial shortening common in Colles' fractures (Fig. 6-5, B). After reduction, median nerve function should be tested and a sugar-tong splint (described above) applied to hold the reduction. Splinting the wrist in 15 degrees of palmar flexion, 10 to 15 degrees of ulnar deviation, and

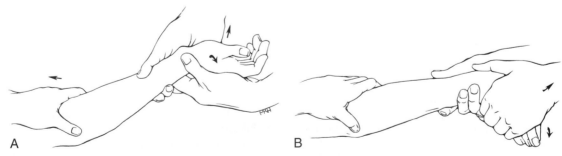

FIGURE 6-6 Colles' fracture reduction without finger traps. **A,** An assistant provides countertraction while the examiner applies traction with the right hand and thumb applied to the distal fragment. The forearm is supinated with the opposite hand, and the fracture is disimpacted while supination is maintained. **B,** The left hand remains stationary while reduction is accomplished with pronation of the forearm and wrist. The wrist is directed into ulnar deviation to correct radial and dorsal angulation.

Intraarticular Fractures (Frykman Types III to VIII)

If median nerve function is intact, the fracture should be stabilized in a sugar-tong splint and the patient referred to an orthopedic surgeon. If median nerve function is impaired, an attempt at closed reduction should be made with finger trap traction, and the patient's arm should be placed in a sugar-tong splint. The patient should then be referred urgently to an orthopedic surgeon.

Follow-up Care

Nondisplaced Extraarticular Fractures

Patients should be seen within 3 to 5 days to allow swelling to subside before definitive casting. The splint is removed, and neurovascular status is reconfirmed by checking the radial pulse, capillary refill at the fingers, and median nerve function. Repeat radiographs are obtained with the arm out of the splint to confirm that no loss of position has occurred. If the fracture remains nondisplaced or minimally displaced, a short-arm cast may be applied, extending from the distal palmar crease to within 2 inches of the antecubital fossa. The wrist is placed in neutral position, and the cast should permit full flexion at the MCP joints and at the elbow. Patients are instructed to maintain active ROM at the fingers, elbow, and shoulder, and they should return in 2 weeks for routine follow-up and repeat radiographs to check fracture alignment. Cast immobilization is continued for 4 to 6 weeks and may be discontinued when the patient no longer has tenderness at the fracture site. Repeat radiographs can be obtained at 4 to 6 weeks to document healing.

For patients 60 years of age and older, the period of immobilization should be as brief as possible, and the duration of remobilization (i.e., physical therapy to regain full ROM) should approximate the duration of immobilization. If the fracture is stable (determined by radiographs every 1 to 2 weeks), an acceptable alternative to cast immobilization is a cock-up wrist splint if the older patient is comfortable in this device. Use of the splint rather than a cast is more comfortable for patients and minimizes postimmobilization stiffness,[12] but selecting patients with stable fractures who agree to frequent follow-up is important in using this method of treatment effectively.

Comminution of the dorsal cortex commonly seen in Colles' fractures predisposes these fractures to loss of position and dorsal displacement of the distal fracture fragment. If displacement develops, the patient should be treated as described for displaced extraarticular fractures, bearing in mind that the fracture is very likely unstable unless loosening of the splint or cast contributed to loss of position.

Extraarticular Fractures After Closed Reduction

After closed reduction, the patient should be seen within 2 to 3 days. If swelling has decreased, the sugar-tong splint can either be wrapped more tightly to help maintain position or else a long-arm cast may be applied with the wrist and forearm in the position described above and the elbow at 90 degrees. The patient is seen again 1 week later, and repeat radiographs are obtained to check the position. If the reduction position has been lost, another reduction should be attempted. The patient should be examined and have radiographs taken every 1 to 2 weeks with the arm out of the cast and with a new, well-molded splint or cast applied. Loss of position should generally lead to orthopedic referral. Repeated closed reduction may be a reasonable alternative if loosening of the splint or cast allowed the displacement.

The total period of immobilization required for healing is usually 6 to 8 weeks. A sugar-tong splint or long-arm cast is used for the first 3 to 4 weeks, and a short-arm cast is used for the last few weeks of immobilization. Use of gently molded three-point control when applying splints and casts may help maintain the reduction. The patient should be converted to the short-arm cast when there is evidence of some radiographic healing and the fracture remains stable in an adequate position. For older patients, immobilization in a sugar-tong splint or long-arm cast should be for as brief a period as possible, usually no more than 2 weeks. Longer immobilization may cause wrist stiffness, and poor function may result.

Fracture site tenderness, swelling, ROM, and median nerve function should be checked during each visit. Radiographs should be examined for signs of dorsal displacement, volar angulation, and radial shortening. The patient should be instructed to maintain finger, elbow, and shoulder ROM daily. Finger exercises include full extension, full flexion, making a fist, opposing the thumb to each fingertip, claw exercises (flexion of the distal interphalangeal [DIP] and proximal interphalangeal [PIP] joints while the MCP joints are held in extension), flexion of the MCP joints with the PIP and DIP joints in extension, and abduction–adduction in the radioulnar plane. Shoulder exercises should include pendulum exercises and active elevation and rotation. When the cast is discontinued, full active ROM exercises are initiated; the duration of mobilization activities should approximate the duration of immobilization.

Return to Work or Sports

Return to work is dictated by the type of duty required and the degree of impaired ROM and strength. Patients returning to light duty and undemanding tasks can return to work immediately and pursue rehabilitation as already outlined. If the patient's occupation requires heavy labor and extensive use of the wrist and forearm, it is best to delay return to full duties until ROM at the wrist is maximized and strength is near normal. Modification of duties is another option for patients undergoing rehabilitation exercises. Wearing a protective volar splint during contact and collision sports activities may be useful in the first month after the immobilization cast is removed.

Complications

Fractures of the distal radius are associated with several complications, including malunion, hand stiffness, post traumatic arthritis, unrecognized associated injuries, tendon or nerve injury, compartment syndrome, and CRPS. Because of the dorsal comminution seen in distal radius fractures, malunion is a common complication. The distal radial fragment tends to be displaced dorsally, leading to limited wrist ROM and arthritis. Stiffness of the wrist is a common complication of distal radius fractures, particularly for patients older than 60 years. For these older patients, prolonged immobilization should be avoided, and cast immobilization should be as brief as symptoms allow.

Unrecognized associated injuries often complicate distal radius fractures. These include injuries to the wrist ligaments and carpal bones. Fractures of the ulnar styloid occur in nearly half of distal radius fractures. Small fractures of the distalmost part of the ulnar styloid are not clinically significant, but fractures across the base of the ulnar styloid may cause instability at the distal radioulnar joint (DRUJ).

Compression neuropathy most commonly affects the median nerve, although the radial and ulnar nerves may also be injured in distal radius fractures. Symptoms of median nerve injury include pain out of proportion to the injury, paresthesias in the volar aspect of the thumb and second and third fingers, and weakness of thumb opposition. Early symptoms of median nerve injury are usually caused by marked fracture displacement, stretching during the fall itself, edema or hematoma in the area of the carpal tunnel, swelling resulting from efforts at reduction, and compression resulting from cast placement and improper splint or cast position (>15 degrees of wrist flexion). Late symptoms of median nerve injury are more likely the result of volar displacement of the fracture fragment or nerve compression by excessive callus formation. Mild nonprogressive paresthesias may be observed, but unrelenting pain or signs of motor loss are indications for urgent carpal tunnel release and exploration of the median nerve.

CRPS after a distal radius fracture is associated with physical inactivity after cast immobilization. In the first few weeks after injury, burning shoulder pain and swelling of the hand and fingers develop. During the next few weeks, swelling decreases, but the pain persists. The severity of the pain prevents joint motion, and during the next 3 to 6 months, a "frozen" hand, shoulder, or both develop. Early skin changes include redness and swelling followed by dystrophic skin changes and mottling. Early recognition of the syndrome and prompt initiation of physical therapy measures may alleviate or reverse CRPS. CRPS can usually be prevented by substantial ROM exercises during the entire treatment period.

Smith's Fracture

Smith's fracture of the distal radius, sometimes referred to as the reverse Colles' fracture, is an uncommon and usually unstable fracture in which the distal radial fragment is displaced volarly and proximally (the so-called garden spade deformity). The cause of injury is usually a direct blow to the dorsum of the wrist. Less commonly, cyclists may sustain this fracture if they are thrown over the handlebars. During examination, the patient demonstrates fullness at the volar aspect of the wrist caused by volar displacement of the distal fracture fragment and has a dorsal prominence at the distal end of the proximal fragment. Extension of the wrist accentuates the deformity. Radiographs show a fracture of the distal radius, usually cortex to cortex through the metaphysis, with volar displacement of the distal radial fragment (Fig. 6-7). The fracture may be extraarticular or intraarticular or may be part of a fracture dislocation of the wrist.

Most Smith's fractures should be referred to an orthopedic surgeon, but a primary care provider skilled in fracture reduction techniques may attempt closed reduction if the fracture is extraarticular (Frykman type I or II). The anesthesia and distraction techniques (finger traps or countertraction) are the same as described for a Colles' fracture. While maintaining traction, the fingers of both hands support the proximal forearm fragment. The thumbs are placed on the volar aspect of the wrist and are used to push the distal fragment dorsally. The patient is placed in a single or double sugar-tong splint with the elbow flexed to 90 degrees, the forearm in neutral pronation–supination, and the wrist in slight extension. Postreduction radiographs are taken, and the same criteria for acceptable reduction as with the Colles' fracture are used. Severe comminution, intraarticular extension, and inability to maintain the reduction by closed means are indications for orthopedic referral. The same close follow-up with

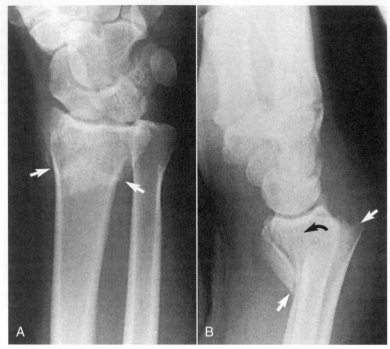

FIGURE 6-7 A, Anteroposterior view of the wrist demonstrating an impacted extraarticular distal radius fracture (*arrows*). **B,** Lateral view shows volar displacement of the distal fragment typical of a Smith's fracture (*arrows*). (*From Mettler FA Jr. Essentials of Radiology. Philadelphia, WB Saunders, 1996.*)

serial examinations, repeat radiographs, and regular cast changes as outlined earlier in the treatment of reduced Colles' fractures should be used in the management of Smith's fractures.

Barton's Fracture

Barton's fracture is a fracture dislocation of the distal radius in which either the volar or dorsal aspect of the distal radial articular surface is sheared off with disruption of the radiocarpal joint. It is usually caused by violent direct injury to the wrist. Seventy percent of Barton's fractures occur in young male laborers or motorcyclists. Barton's fractures are extremely unstable and require open reduction and internal fixation (ORIF). The key to treating these intraarticular fracture dislocations is anatomic reduction by surgical means and stabilization of the wrist joint. Initial treatment should consist of immobilization in a double sugar-tong splint with the wrist in neutral position and prompt referral of the patient to an orthopedic surgeon.

Hutchinson's Fracture

Hutchinson's fracture (also called chauffeur's fracture) is an intraarticular fracture dislocation in which the radioscaphocapitate ligament avulses a fragment of the radial styloid. It is often associated with carpal bone and ligament injuries. The most

common mechanism involves a firm blow to the radial styloid, which may be achieved by falling backward on an outstretched hand with ulnar deviation. Hutchinson's fractures require surgical repair.

DISTAL RADIUS FRACTURES (PEDIATRIC)

Fractures of the radius are common among children and adolescents. Fractures of the distal radial metaphysis are the most common and account for approximately 62% of these injuries. Another 14% of radius fractures among children involve the distal radial physis.

Metaphyseal Fractures

The metaphysis is particularly vulnerable because the cortex of the distal radius is thin, and the metaphysis extends more proximally in children than in adults. This anatomy leads to fractures unique to children, including torus fractures and greenstick fractures. Torus fractures are simple buckle fractures of the cortex caused by an axial force applied to the immature bone (Fig. 6-8). A typical greenstick fracture is caused by a severe bending force applied to the distal radius that causes a compression fracture (buckling or plastic bending) at the dorsum of the distal radius; the volar surface (i.e., the tension side) is typically disrupted (Fig. 6-9). Most metaphyseal fractures of

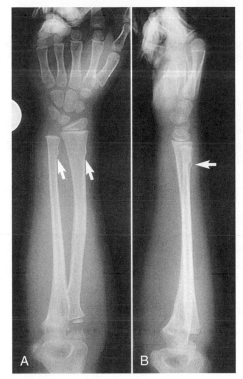

FIGURE 6-8 Torus (buckle) fractures of the distal radius (**A**) and ulna (**B**).

During physical examination, the patient has tenderness at the dorsum of the distal radius. Dorsal displacement of the distal fracture fragment may be disguised by soft tissue swelling. Capillary refill and radial pulses are usually normal, but median or ulnar nerve injury may be present because the nerves have been stretched. Paresthesias in the median nerve distribution are more likely if the fracture is significantly angulated or if significant swelling occurs at the fracture site. A complete examination of the elbow and wrist is essential because distal radius fractures may be associated with ipsilateral supracondylar or scaphoid fractures.

Imaging

AP and lateral views of the wrist are usually adequate to determine the type of fracture and the amount of displacement. For older children and adolescents, three views of the wrist should be ordered (AP, lateral, and oblique). It is important for the examining physician to distinguish torus-buckle fractures and greenstick fractures from "complete" fractures involving both cortices. Torus fractures of the distal radius metaphysis are nondisplaced because of the strong intact periosteum, which maintains alignment (Fig. 6-8).

the distal radius occur between the months of May and August and affect children between the ages of 9 and 14 years. Most distal radius fractures coincide with peak growing spurts for children (i.e., 11 to 12 years of age in girls and 13 to 14 years of age in boys). The distal metaphysis is at risk because of the relative porosity of the bone during peak periods of growth. The nondominant hand is involved in slightly more than half of all cases, and 70% of cases involve boys.

Mechanism of Injury

The patient usually sustains a fall on the extended wrist, causing tension on the strong volar intercarpal and radiocarpal ligaments. As with most injuries involving children and adolescents, the ligaments remain intact, but the bone fails, leading to fracture. A simple fall may result in a nondisplaced fracture, but a fall in conjunction with forward momentum (e.g., while the patient is riding a bicycle or inline skating) may produce displaced fractures. If the patient sustains a fall from a height, displaced fractures and concomitant fractures (e.g., supracondylar or scaphoid fractures) are more commonly seen.

Clinical Presentation

The patient usually describes a fall on the extended wrist and reports pain and swelling at the wrist.

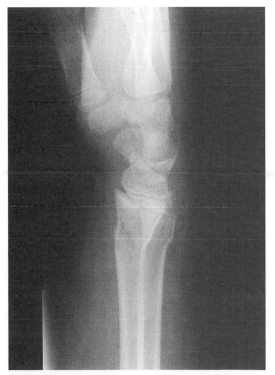

FIGURE 6-9 Lateral view of the wrist showing a greenstick fracture of the distal radius with 15 degrees of apex volar angulation. A torus fracture of the ulna is also present.

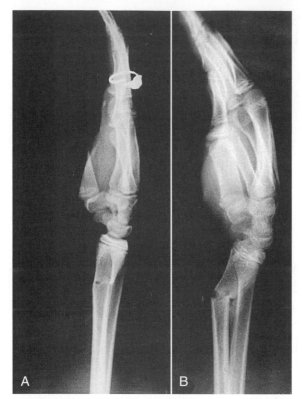

FIGURE 6-10 A, Greenstick fracture of the distal radius with 15 degrees of apex volar angulation. **B,** Follow-up radiograph taken 5 weeks later shows that the fracture is now complete and the angulation has increased to 30 degrees despite cast immobilization. Closer monitoring of fracture position during the healing phase might have prevented the late angulation.

Greenstick fractures usually show compression of the dorsal cortex and apex volar angulation (Fig. 6-9). The dorsal cortex usually remains intact but may undergo plastic deformation, and the volar cortex is usually disrupted. Less commonly, greenstick fractures show apex dorsal angulation with compression of the volar cortex. Late displacement or reangulation can result from greenstick fractures (Fig. 6-10). The most common pattern for a complete fracture is bayonet apposition with the distal fragment displaced proximally (Fig. 6-11). Distal radius fractures are rarely isolated and are frequently associated with an ulnar fracture, as seen in Figs. 6-8, 6-9, and 6-11. Intraarticular fractures are uncommon.

Indications for Orthopedic Referral

Emergent Referral (Within 30 to 60 Minutes)

As with adults, patients with open fractures, acute neuropathy, tenting of the skin, compartment syndrome, or vascular compromise require emergent orthopedic referral. If specialist care is not promptly available, tenting or neurovascular compromise associated with a displaced fracture can generally be corrected by immediate closed reduction after adequate analgesia or local anaesthesia is achieved.

Nonemergent Referral (24 to 48 Hours)

Operative repair of distal radius fractures in children is seldom indicated because the outcomes from nonoperative management are so good. Conditions that should prompt an orthopedic referral include displaced fractures that the physician is not comfortable reducing, Salter-Harris type III to V fractures, displaced Salter-Harris type I and II fractures, and severe local soft tissue injury. Patients with unstable greenstick fractures or complete fractures that are not amenable to closed reduction should also be referred. Failure to achieve an adequate reduction by closed methods should also prompt referral.

Treatment

Torus Fractures

Most patients can be safely treated using only a removable volar splint. Several studies have compared casting with splinting.[13-15] Treatment with splinting alone not only had no adverse impact on healing but also resulted in faster return of function. Casting does have an advantage in that casted patients appear to experience less pain. For this reason, it may be desirable to apply a cast at the first follow-up visit (3 to 5 days after injury) if significant discomfort persists after initial splinting. Ibuprofen is recommended for pain control. In children with distal forearm fractures, it not only provided better relief than acetaminophen with codeine but also caused much fewer side effects and allowed children to be more active.[16]

Torus fractures heal well with virtually no complications after immobilization for 2 to 4 weeks. Repeat radiographs to document healing are not necessary unless the child is not clinically healed after 4 weeks of casting. The patient is reexamined at 2 to 3 weeks after the initial injury; if the patient has no tenderness at the fracture site, immobilization is discontinued and ROM at the wrist is encouraged. The child should begin using the wrist for daily activities, and ROM exercises of the wrist can be performed if the wrist is a bit stiff after immobilization. Protection with a volar splint during vigorous activity for an additional 2 weeks is advisable to reduce the risk of reinjury.

Greenstick Fractures

Greenstick fractures have a greater chance of losing position and are typically treated by initial sugar-tong splinting for 2 to 3 days followed by a short or long-arm cast. Care must be taken in the

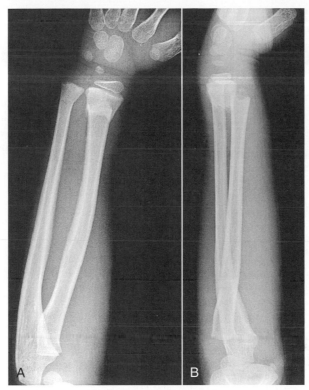

FIGURE 6-11 Anteroposterior (A) and lateral (B) views of the forearm showing complete fracture of the distal radius with bayonet apposition, shortening and volar displacement of the proximal radius shaft, and a greenstick fracture of the distal ulna metaphysis.

evaluation of greenstick fractures to ensure that only one cortex is involved (see Fig. 6-19). If both cortices are disrupted, the risk of angulation is much greater, and good immobilization and close follow-up is more important.

One can accept more dorsal angulation than lateral angulation because dorsal angulation remodels more readily. In addition, the more skeletally mature the child, the less remodeling will occur and the less angulation one can accept. Thus, although reduction is recommended for boys younger than 9 years of age with more than 20 degrees of dorsal angulation or 15 degrees of lateral angulation, less angulation is acceptable in older boys and in girls.[17] The acceptable angulation is 5 degrees less for each increase of 2 to 3 years, and when boys reach 13 years of age, dorsal angulation should not exceed 5 degrees, and lateral angulation should be 0 degrees. Acceptable angulation in girls is 5 degrees less than for boys of the same age because they are more skeletally mature at any given age. Patients should be referred if the primary care provider is uncomfortable with reduction procedures or uncertain whether reduction is necessary. Conscious sedation is usually needed for young children, and Bier block anesthesia is effective in older children. (See Chapter 4 for a

description of the Bier block anesthesia technique.) Traction is usually not needed. To correct apex volar angulation, the practitioner places the thumbs over the dorsal wrist and pushes the displaced fragment distally and volarly. Placing the thumbs over the volar wrist and pushing the displaced fragment distally and dorsally is the reduction maneuver used to correct apex dorsal angulation.

After reduction, a well-molded long-arm cast is applied using gently molded three-point control (Fig. 6-12). The ulnar aspect of the cast is split or the cast bivalved to allow for any swelling that may develop. The elbow is flexed to 90 degrees, the forearm is placed in neutral rotation, and the wrist is held in neutral flexion–extension. The patient is instructed to keep the arm elevated to minimize swelling and to maintain finger and shoulder ROM. Plaster is preferable to fiberglass in the treatment of these fractures because it spreads more easily to allow for expansion after reduction. Repeat radiographs should be taken at 5 to 7 days (5 days for younger children). If fracture alignment is still acceptable, the cast is closed and immobilization continued for 4 weeks. If the fracture has significantly reangulated, a repeat closed reduction should be attempted. Serial radiographs every 1 to

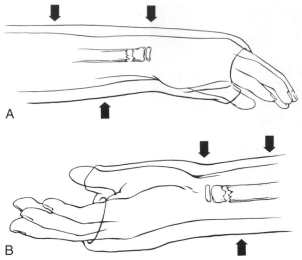

FIGURE 6-12 Three-point molding for radial metaphyseal fractures. **A,** For apex volar fractures, pressure is applied on the dorsal aspect of the cast and counterpressure is applied on the volar side just proximal to the fracture site. **B,** For apex dorsal fractures, pressure is applied on the volar side, and counterpressure is applied dorsally just proximal to the fracture site.

2 weeks should be taken to follow fracture alignment.

After 4 weeks of cast immobilization, the cast may be removed if there is clinical and radiographic evidence of healing. The patient is then placed in a volar splint for protection during "activity hours" for an additional week, and the splint may then be discontinued. Physical therapy is seldom necessary for patients in this age group.

Some amount of reangulation during the healing process is common, and parents and patients should be forewarned that this may occur and that it does not represent inadequate treatment. If the child has at least 5 years of growth remaining, up to 30 degrees of angulation in the dorsal–volar plane will usually remodel to an acceptable position. The acceptable amount of angulation is decreased by 5 degrees per year of growth remaining for those with less than 5 years of projected growth.

Complete Fractures

Complete fractures of the distal radius in children are nearly always angulated and have some degree of distraction of the fracture fragments. They have a higher chance of losing position during treatment and refracture after treatment. In general, these fractures should be immobilized in a sugar-tong splint with the elbow at 90 degrees, and the patient should be referred to an orthopedic surgeon for closed reduction and definitive care.

Complications

The most common bony complication is residual angulation. Most fractures remodel to produce an acceptable functional and cosmetic result. Some loss of forearm rotation may occur. Complications that are common in adult distal radius fractures (loss of wrist motion and distal radial joint dysfunction) are almost unheard of in pediatric fractures.

Other complications include concomitant fractures (supracondylar or carpal, particularly the scaphoid), median nerve injury (from improper immobilization or too-vigorous reduction and manipulation), compartment syndrome and refracture after premature discontinuation of protection.

Physeal Fractures

The physis of the distal radius is the most commonly injured physis among children. The peak age for sustaining this injury is 9 to 10 years of age in girls and 13 to 14 years of age in boys.

Anatomic Considerations

The distal radial epiphysis appears at the age of 1 year and unites by the age of 18 years. When the patient falls on the extended wrist, the periosteum ruptures at its thinnest site at the volar metaphysis but remains intact dorsally. The dislodged periosteum can be trapped between the fracture fragments volarly, preventing closed reduction. At the same time, the intact dorsal periosteum can help stabilize the fracture after reduction. Fractures of the distal radial physis rarely occur in isolation; a metaphyseal fracture of the distal ulna or avulsion of the ulnar styloid may also occur.

Mechanism of Injury

Most commonly, complete fracture of the distal radius in a child is caused by a fall onto the extended wrist. The physis fails in tension at the volar aspect of the distal radius, and a triangular fragment involving the distal metaphysis develops on the dorsal aspect of the distal radius.

Clinical Presentation

The patient usually describes a fall onto the extended wrist as well as pain and swelling at the dorsum of the wrist. During physical examination, the patient has tenderness at the dorsum of the distal radius. Dorsal displacement of the physis may not be well visualized because of swelling but is palpable.

Imaging

A nondisplaced type I fracture of the distal radius physis can be difficult to detect radiographically (Fig. 6-13). The presence of the pronator fat pad

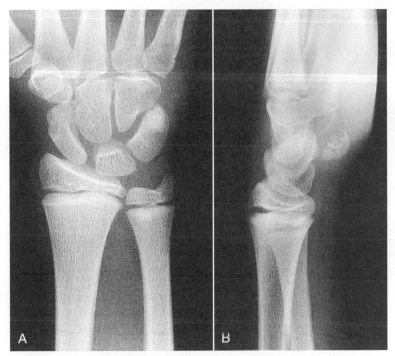

FIGURE 6-13 A Salter-Harris type I fracture of the distal radius. The anteroposterior view (**A**) appears normal but widening of the physis is apparent in the injured radius on the lateral view (**B**).

along the volar aspect of the distal radius on the lateral view (Fig. 6-14) is a reliable sign of an occult fracture, although its absence does not rule out a fracture. If there is marked localized tenderness over the physis, the patient should be treated for a physeal injury even if radiographs are normal.

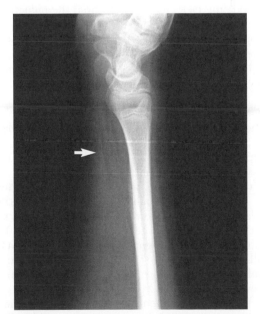

FIGURE 6-14 Lateral view of the wrist demonstrating the normal position of the pronator fat pad (*arrow*). Volar displacement of this fat pad would suggest an occult fracture.

In a type II physeal fracture, the metaphyseal fragment is most often located on the dorsal aspect of the radius. If the epiphysis is going to become displaced, it usually occurs dorsally (Fig. 6-15, A), although volar displacement occurs 10% of the time. Angulation of more than 25 degrees and more than 25% displacement of the epiphysis from the physis require reduction.

Indications for Orthopedic Referral

The conditions that should prompt an orthopedic referral include failure to achieve an adequate reduction by closed methods and all Salter-Harris type III and IV fractures. Closed reduction of displaced physeal fractures must be done promptly and gently, and repeat attempts at manipulation are not advisable. Patients should be referred to an orthopedic surgeon for closed reduction unless the primary care provider is experienced in the treatment of these injuries.

Initial Treatment

Nondisplaced or Suspected Fractures

Nondisplaced fractures can be treated initially with a short-arm splint or bivalved cast. The child with physeal tenderness but normal radiographs should have the arm immobilized for 2 weeks as though a fracture were present and then reevaluated. If repeat radiographs show callus formation, immobilization should be continued for an

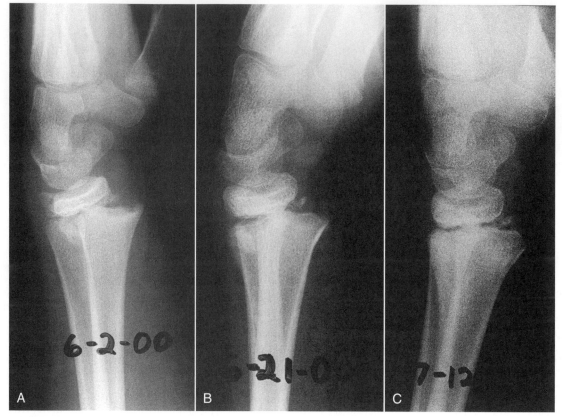

FIGURE 6-15 A, Type I fracture of the distal radius with half shaft dorsal displacement of the epiphysis. **B,** After 3 weeks in a long-arm cast, the fracture shows interval healing with decreased dorsal displacement. C, Six weeks after the injury, the dorsal displacement of the radial epiphysis has nearly resolved.

additional 2 weeks. If the radiographs are normal at the 2-week visit, a physeal injury is unlikely, and the cast can be discontinued.

Displaced Fractures

Displaced physeal fractures should be reduced as soon as possible by an experienced clinician. The longer the delay in reduction, the greater the chance of formation of a fibrous clot across the fracture site. If this occurs, a greater force must be applied to obtain an adequate reduction, which puts the physis at greater risk of injury and subsequent growth arrest. If a child is treated more than 3 days after the injury, manipulation of the fracture may cause more harm than good.

Closed reduction with the aid of finger traps for countertraction is an effective method of treating displaced physeal fractures of the distal radius. Traction is applied after adequate relaxation and analgesia are achieved, and the clinician can usually reduce the fracture by pushing the displaced epiphysis distally and volarly with the thumb (Fig. 6-16). If at least 50% apposition of the fracture fragments occurs after reduction and the child has at least 1 year of growth remaining,

normal alignment should be achieved through remodeling (see Fig. 6-15). To hold the reduction, the patient can be placed in a well-molded long-arm cast with the wrist in slight flexion and the forearm in neutral pronation–supination. The cast is bivalved to allow for any swelling that may develop.

Follow-up Care

The patient is seen in 1 week and in-cast radiographs are obtained. If fracture alignment is maintained, the splint is converted to a cast or the bivalved cast is closed. The patient should be examined every 1 or 2 weeks, and immobilization for 4 to 6 weeks is usually adequate for healing. A volar splint may be worn for 1 or 2 more weeks for both comfort and protection and to allow ROM and strengthening exercises as the child returns to full activity. Follow-up radiographs at 4 to 6 months and 1 year are essential to document normal growth.

If fracture alignment has not been maintained, repeat manipulation is not recommended because of the risk of injury to the growth plate. At this point, the injury should be splinted and the patient

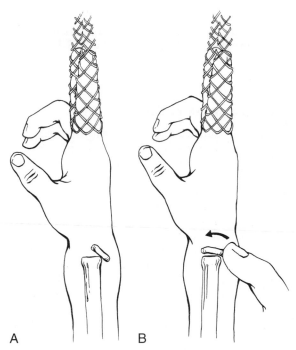

A   **B**

FIGURE 6-16 Method of closed reduction of a displaced epiphysis. **A,** The fingers are placed in finger trap traction. **B,** If the fracture does not reduce with traction alone, direct pressure should be applied over the fracture site in a distal and volar direction.

referred to an orthopedic surgeon for definitive treatment.

Complications

Common early complications after fracture involving the distal radial physis include soft tissue diastasis of the fracture, compartment syndrome, carpal tunnel syndrome, and associated supracondylar fracture. Wide separation of the fracture fragments on radiographs, difficulty achieving closed reduction, or both indicate that soft tissues such as periosteum, tendons, or nerves may be interposed between the fracture fragments. In this case, the patient must be referred to an orthopedic surgeon for open reduction of the fracture. Pain out of proportion to the perceived injury may also indicate that compartment syndrome has developed. If compartment syndrome is suspected, compartment pressures must be checked and fasciotomy considered.

Carpal tunnel syndrome may be caused by direct injury to the median nerve or be indirectly caused by swelling in or near the carpal tunnel. If paresthesias in the median nerve distribution persist, open release of the carpal tunnel may be necessary. Patients with an associated supracondylar fracture are particularly prone to redisplacement of the distal radius physis; patients with a supracondylar

fracture in addition to a displaced fracture of the distal radial physis should be referred to an orthopedic surgeon for pin restraint on physeal motion.

FRACTURES OF THE SHAFT OF THE RADIUS (ADULT): GALEAZZI'S FRACTURE

Anatomic Considerations

Solitary fractures of the radius at the junction of the middle and distal thirds were described by Galeazzi in 1934 and are typically complicated by subluxation or dislocation at the DRUJ. Instability at the DRUJ may be apparent initially or may develop during healing as a result of several deforming forces that act on the distal forearm. Gravity can aggravate dorsal angulation of the distal radial fragment and thereby cause subluxation of the DRUJ. The pronator quadratus rotates the distal radial fragment toward the ulna and exerts both palmar and proximal distracting forces. The brachioradialis and thumb abductors and extensors cause radial shortening and injury to the TFCC and can contribute to instability of the DRUJ. These are unstable fractures and have been termed "fractures of necessity," indicating that almost all cases require ORIF of the radius and repair of the DRUJ.

Mechanism of Injury

A fall on the extended, pronated wrist is the most common cause of a Galeazzi's fracture. A direct blow to the dorsolateral aspect of the wrist may also cause a radial shaft fracture at the junction of the middle and distal thirds of the radius, but this injury leaves the DRUJ intact and may therefore respond to closed treatment.

Clinical Presentation

Patients usually present with pain, swelling, and deformity of the wrist. Neurologic symptoms are uncommon. During physical examination, tenderness and swelling at the distal radius and tenderness at the DRUJ are apparent. In some cases, the distal radial fragment is angulated dorsally, which is apparent on examination. Although most Galeazzi's fractures are closed, an open fracture may occasionally result from a small puncture wound caused by the distal aspect of the proximal radial fragment.

Imaging

Radiographs should include the entire length of the radius and ulna as well as the wrist and elbow joints. AP and lateral radiographs are usually sufficient. On the AP view, a transverse or short oblique fracture at the junction of the middle and distal thirds of the radius is apparent. Findings suggestive of disruption of the DRUJ include a widening of the DRUJ on the AP view, fracture of the base of the ulnar styloid, radial shortening of more than 5 mm, and dislocation of the radius relative to the ulna on the lateral view (Fig. 6-17). On the lateral view, the radius shows apex dorsal angulation, and the distal ulna is displaced dorsally.

Treatment

Open fractures and neurovascular compromise require emergent referral. The midforearm is a high risk area for compartment syndromes. The physician should maintain a high index of suspicion for compartment syndrome and check compartment pressures if suggestive symptoms develop (e.g., disproportionate pain, paresthesia). Surgical treatment of Galeazzi's fractures is required because of the deforming forces outlined earlier and instability at the DRUJ. After neurovascular and radiographic evaluation, the patient's arm is placed in a well-molded double sugar-tong splint and referral to an orthopedic surgeon is made within 1 or 2 days. Anatomic reduction of the distal radius and

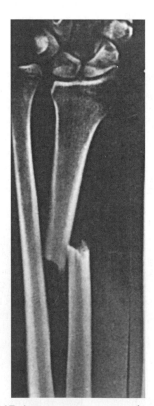

FIGURE 6-17 Anteroposterior view demonstrating a Galeazzi's fracture. Note the shortening of the radius and the widened distal radioulnar joint. (*From Browner BD, Jupiter JB, Levine AM, Trafton PG [eds].* Skeletal Trauma: Fractures, Dislocations, Ligamentous Injuries. *Philadelphia, WB Saunders, 1992.*)

DRUJ is necessary for satisfactory results in treating Galeazzi's fractures. ORIF with a dynamic compression plate and screws is the usual surgical procedure. Repair of the TFCC and stabilization of the DRUJ are also essential for a satisfactory outcome.

Return to Work or Sports

After cast immobilization is completed, patients should begin supervised physical therapy to regain normal or near-normal ROM and strength. Patients with undemanding occupations may resume work immediately while continuing rehabilitation. Patients involved in heavy labor should be offered light duty or delay returning to work until ROM and strength are near normal. Patients engaged in sports in which falls are possible should use a protective cylindrical splint on the forearm for 1 month after cast immobilization is completed.

Complications

The most common complication of Galeazzi's fracture is dorsal angulation of the radial fracture and subluxation of the DRUJ. Patients with nonunion or malposition may seek treatment weeks after injury, and these patients also require surgical correction. Infection may develop after open fractures.

Pediatric Considerations

Galeazzi's fracture is uncommon among children. As with adults, the injury is caused by a fall onto an outstretched hand, usually in combination with forced pronation. Although a fracture of the radial shaft is as obvious with children as with adults, the injury to the DRUJ may be overlooked with children. During physical examination, the patient has tenderness at the radial aspect of the radial shaft at or slightly distal to the midshaft. The patient may also have tenderness between the distalmost portion of the radius and ulna at the DRUJ.

As with most forearm injuries in children, it is important to see both the wrist and the elbow on radiographs; therefore, AP and lateral radiographs of the radius and ulna should be obtained. A transverse fracture of the radial shaft is obvious and usually occurs at the junction of the middle and distal thirds of the shaft. The distal radial fragment is usually displaced toward the ulna, but dorsal, volar, or even radial displacement can occur. Dislocation of the DRUJ is also present, although subluxation of that joint may not be obvious, and the ulnar styloid may be avulsed.

Children with Galeazzi's fracture are treated differently than adults. The recommended treatment for children is attempted closed reduction, which is best attempted under general anesthesia. Therefore, after the diagnosis of Galeazzi's fracture has been made, the patient's arm should be splinted in a sugar-tong splint with the forearm in neutral pronation–supination and the wrist in neutral flexion–extension. The patient should then be referred promptly to an orthopedic surgeon for definitive care.

Common complications among patients sustaining Galeazzi's fracture include malunion, nerve injury, subluxation of the radioulnar joint, or loss of the normal bowing of the radius. Angulation of 10 degrees or less usually produces good functional results; however, if the radial shaft fracture is angulated more than 10 degrees, loss of pronation and supination can be expected. If the radial shaft fracture heals with loss of the normal bowing of the radius, the functional length of the radius is increased, and incongruity of the DRUJ can result.

FRACTURES OF THE SHAFT OF THE RADIUS (PEDIATRIC)

Fractures of the proximal radial shaft are uncommon because the bone is strong proximally, and overlying muscles provide protection from injury. However, just distal to the middle of the radial shaft, the bone changes from a cylindrical to a more triangular shape; at the same time, the muscular protection becomes tendinous, exposing the midshaft to possible fracture. Fractures of the shaft of the radius account for 20% of all radius fractures in children. Of these radial shaft fractures, 75% occur in the distal third, 18% in the middle third, and 7% in the proximal third. Diaphyseal bone is stronger than metaphyseal bone, which is why fractures of the shaft are less common than fractures of the distal metaphysis. Shaft fractures are more common among younger children because as a child matures, the weaker bone shifts distally. Most radius shaft fractures in girls occur between ages 5 and 6 years. The incidence for boys peaks at age 9 years and again at ages 13 to 14 years.

Mechanism of Injury

The typical cause of injury is a fall onto an outstretched hand.

Clinical Presentation

The patient usually describes a fall on the extended or flexed wrist and reports pain and swelling at the wrist. A family member may notice some deformation of the forearm. The immediate postinjury deformity is usually the position into which the fracture tends to drift after swelling has subsided. The elbow should be examined carefully to rule out injury to the proximal ulna, dislocation of the radial head (i.e., Monteggia type IV lesion), or both.

Imaging

AP and lateral radiographs of the radius and ulna should be obtained, including both the proximal and distal radioulnar joints. Fractures are usually oblique (Fig. 6-18) or transverse (Fig. 6-19). The transverse fractures should be examined closely to determine if one (greenstick) or both cortices (complete) are involved (Fig. 6-19). Malrotation or plastic deformation of the radius can be determined by observing a break in the smooth curve of the radius or any sudden change in the width of the cortex. The position or rotation of the proximal fragment can be determined by the position of the radial tuberosity on the proximal radius. The tuberosity is medial in supination, is posterior in neutral pronation–supination, and is lateral in pronation. Comparison views of the uninjured forearm may be necessary to rule out or confirm rotation. Any angulation should be noted carefully; even minimal angulation can be accompanied by significant rotation. The elbow should be examined carefully to rule out injury to the proximal ulna, dislocation of the radial head, or both.

The ability of the fracture to remodel depends on the age of the patient, the location of the

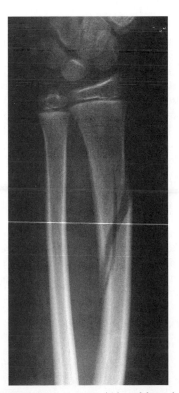

FIGURE 6-18 Anteroposterior (A) and lateral (B) views of a nondisplaced oblique fracture of the distal third of the radial shaft.

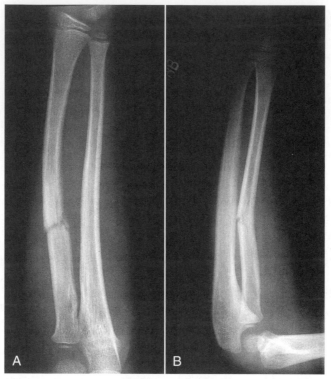

FIGURE 6-19 Anteroposterior (AP) (**A**) and lateral (**B**) views of the radius. On the AP view, it appears that this is a complete fracture. Closer inspection of the lateral view reveals an intact volar cortex, which indicates that this is a greenstick fracture. Approximately 15 degrees of apex dorsal angulation is present.

fracture site, and the degree of angulation. Younger children with more distal lesions and lesser degrees of angulation are more likely to remodel well and retain forearm rotation without cosmetic defect. For children 8 years of age and younger, 15 degrees of angulation and 45 degrees of rotation can be accepted. For children ages 8 to 15 years, 10 degrees of angulation and 30 degrees of rotation are acceptable.[18]

Indications for Orthopedic Referral

Patients with radius shaft fractures should be referred if the fracture is significantly angulated (>15 degrees in children younger than age 8 years and >10 degrees in children older than age 8 years), is significantly rotated, is severely comminuted, or is associated with nerve injury or compartment syndrome.

Initial Treatment

Nondisplaced Fractures

Patients with a nondisplaced radius shaft fracture should be placed in a well-molded sugar-tong splint with the elbow at 90 degrees of flexion. The patient should return in 1 week for radiographs to check alignment and for definitive casting.

Displaced Fractures

Patients with displaced fractures need fracture reduction, usually through closed methods. The patient should be placed in a well-molded sugar-tong splint with the elbow at 90 degrees of flexion and referred to an orthopedic surgeon for definitive care.

For clinicians without ready access to orthopedic referral or those with fracture reduction experience, closed reduction may be safely attempted for displaced fractures. Intravenous sedation is usually sufficient when incomplete greenstick fractures are being reduced. When one radial cortex remains intact, either full pronation or full supination will restore normal alignment.

When the distal fragment is displaced dorsally (i.e., apex volar angulation), a pronation force must be applied to achieve reduction. Apex volar greenstick fractures are reduced by fully pronating and flexing the wrist while gently correcting the angulation. When the distal fragment is displaced volarly (i.e., apex dorsal angulation), a supination force must be applied to achieve reduction. Apex dorsal greenstick fractures are reduced by fully supinating and extending the wrist while gently correcting the angulation. After reduction has been achieved, a sugar-tong splint is applied with the elbow flexed to 90 degrees.

For patients with complete fractures, an important principle must be observed: the reducible distal fragment must be brought into alignment with the irreducible proximal fragment.

The distal fragment may be in any position, but the position of the proximal fragment is determined by the deforming forces of the muscles involved. In this situation, some component of rotation must always be corrected.

Follow-up Care

The patient is seen in 1 week after initial treatment, and the splint is removed. If the fracture fragments are still in good alignment, a well-molded long-arm cast is applied. Significant loss of reduction requires remanipulation, and the patient should be promptly referred to an orthopedic surgeon for definitive care. The long-arm cast is continued for 6 weeks followed by an additional 6 weeks in a protective functional brace or splint to prevent refracture.

Return to Sports

Refracture is a major concern after radius shaft fracture, so contact and collision sports should be delayed until bone healing is complete (usually 10 to 12 weeks). As previously noted, the patient is in a long-arm cast for 6 weeks and then in a protective functional brace or splint for an additional 6 weeks. This prolonged immobilization requires the patient to undergo intensive physical therapy to regain full ROM. Physical therapy can be started when the patient's arm is placed in the functional brace. More aggressive rehabilitation, especially strength training, should begin after the brace is discontinued.

Complications

Because of the deforming forces acting on the shaft of the radius, complications after fracture are common and include refracture, malunion, synostosis, compartment syndrome, and nerve injury. The refracture rate after fracture of the radial shaft is approximately 5% even when radiographic healing is present. Greenstick fractures are especially prone to refracture, and treatment usually requires ORIF. If malunion develops within 4 weeks of initial injury, remanipulation and repeat reduction may be attempted. If malunion occurs 8 or more weeks after initial injury, corrective osteotomy may be required. However, it is best to delay the osteotomy for 4 to 6 months.

Nerve injury after fracture of the radial shaft is fairly common and may involve the ulnar nerve, median nerve, or posterior interosseous nerve (a branch of the radial nerve). Symptoms are usually transitory and resolve spontaneously. Patients with suspected neurapraxia should be observed; if no improvement is seen by 8 weeks after injury, surgical exploration and nerve release may be considered.

BOTH-BONE FOREARM FRACTURES (ADULT)

Anatomic Considerations

The radius and ulna are of approximately equal length and are bound distally by the capsule of the wrist joint, by the anterior and posterior radioulnar ligaments, and by the TFCC. They are bound proximally by the annular ligament and by the capsule of the elbow joint. The ulna acts as a relatively fixed strut around which the radius rotates in pronation and supination. The interosseous membrane is an important supporting structure in the forearm with fibers originating on the radius and inserting distally and obliquely on the ulna. The central portion of the interosseous membrane is thickened and provides longitudinal support to the shaft of the radius.

The radius and ulna are surrounded by muscle groups whose pull results in characteristic fracture displacement depending on the site of the fracture in relation to the supinators and pronators of the forearm (Fig. 6-20). Fractures of the proximal third (proximal to insertion of the pronator teres) result in supination of the proximal radius from the unopposed action of the supinator and the biceps tendon. Fractures of the middle third (distal to the insertion of the pronator teres) remain in neutral rotation because the muscles do not act across the fracture line, and the action of the supinators balances the action of the pronators. Fractures of the distal third of the forearm are usually stabilized by the broad pronator quadratus, but the action of the brachioradialis muscle may cause angulation of the distal radius.

Mechanism of Injury

Fractures of the radius and ulna are high-energy injuries and most commonly occur in motor vehicle accidents. Occasionally, a direct blow with a stick or club, a fall from a height, or a fall during athletic competition fractures both the radius and ulna.

Clinical Presentation

Patients complain of pain and swelling at the site of the fractures. Occasionally, nerve involvement causes symptoms of paresthesias, paresis, or loss of function. During examination, an obvious deformity is usually present. Motor and sensory function of the radial, median, and ulnar nerves should be documented and the radial pulse and

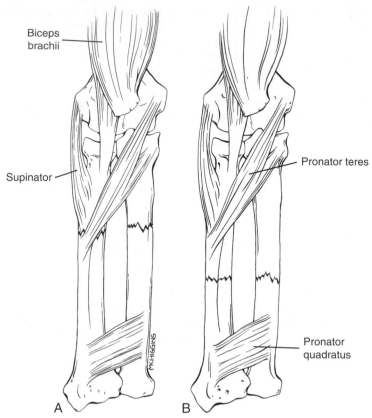

Biceps
brachii

Supinator

Pronator teres

Pronator
quadratus

A   B

FIGURE 6-20 Deforming forces acting on forearm fractures. **A,** Fractures of the proximal third result in supination of the proximal radius from the unopposed action of the supinator and the biceps tendon. **B,** Fractures of the middle third remain in neutral rotation because the action of the supinators balances the action of the pronators.

distal capillary refill assessed. Crepitus should not be elicited because this maneuver may cause further soft tissue injury. Open fractures should not be probed because this may cause deeper contamination. The forearm is at high risk for developing compartment syndrome. The physician should maintain a high index of suspicion for compartment syndrome and check compartment pressures if suggestive symptoms develop (e.g., disproportionate pain, paresthesia).

Imaging

Radiographs should include the entire length of the radius and ulna, including the wrist and elbow joints. AP and lateral views are usually sufficient. The level of the fracture depends on the cause of injury and the amount of force sustained. High-energy injuries are usually comminuted or segmental and involve severe soft tissue injuries as well. Low-energy injuries are usually transverse or short oblique in orientation. Fractures should be evaluated for the amount of displacement or "offset" and degree of angulation, shortening, and comminution. Most fractures are angulated more than 10 degrees or displaced by more than 50% of the shaft

width (Fig. 6-21). The nutrient foramen of the radius is seen on AP views of the forearm at the junction of the proximal and middle thirds of the radius and may be confused with a fracture; however, it is not seen on the lateral or oblique views.

Indications for Orthopedic Referral

Fractures of the radius and ulna are complex and difficult to treat successfully. Patients with these fractures should be referred in cases of displacement, angulation, comminution, shortening, rotation, compartment syndrome, nerve injury, open fracture, infection, or nonunion. Patients with nondisplaced fractures that develop displacement despite appropriate cast immobilization should also be referred.

Initial Treatment

Nondisplaced Fractures

Nondisplaced fractures of the radius and ulna are rare in adults. Treatment consists of immobilization in a bivalved long-arm cast with the wrist in slight extension, the forearm in neutral rotation,

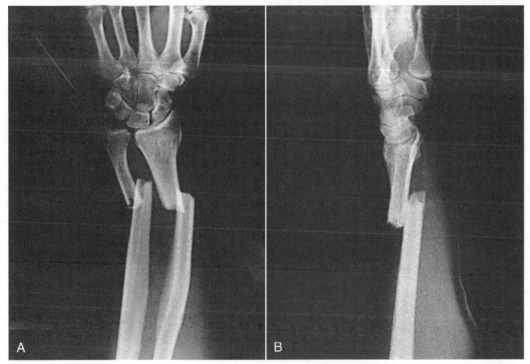

FIGURE 6-21 Anteroposterior (**A**) and lateral (**B**) views of transverse fractures of the distal third of both the radius and ulna with apex radial angulation and bayonet shortening. *(From Browner BD, Jupiter JB, Levine AM, Trafton PG [eds]. Skeletal Trauma: Fractures, Dislocations, Ligamentous Injuries. Philadelphia, WB Saunders, 1992.)*

and the elbow at 90 degrees flexion. The cast should extend from the proximal palmar crease to the deltoid insertion. A wire or plaster loop should be incorporated into the radial aspect of the cast just proximal to the level of the fractures and the cast suspended from the patient's neck with a sling through this loop (Fig. 6-22). This keeps the cast firmly against the ulna and helps prevent angulation of the fractures during healing. These are unstable fractures, and displacement can occur despite proper technique.

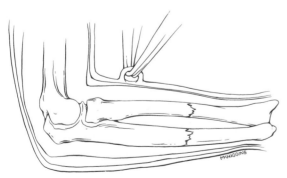

FIGURE 6-22 Long-arm cast with a loop placed proximal to the radius and ulna fracture sites keeps the cast firmly against the ulna and helps prevent angulation of the fractures during healing.

Displaced Fractures

Displaced fractures of the radius and ulna should be splinted and the patient referred within 24 to 48 hours to an orthopedic surgeon for definitive care. If the patient has neurologic or vascular compromise, closed reduction should be attempted before referral if immediate orthopedic assistance is not available. The arm is suspended in finger traps through the thumb and index and middle fingers, and countertraction is applied through the distal humerus. The level of the fracture is palpated along the subcutaneous aspect of the ulna and gently reduced, and a sugar-tong splint is applied and molded while the arm is still suspended. The patient is then referred urgently to an orthopedic surgeon.

Follow-up Care

Nondisplaced Fractures

Patients should be seen 1 week after injury, and repeat AP and lateral radiographs with the arm in the cast should be obtained and examined for any sign of displacement. The patient should be referred if the fracture becomes displaced. If alignment is maintained, patients should be seen weekly and in-cast radiographs obtained weekly for 1 month and then every 2 weeks until healing has occurred (usually 12 to 16 weeks). Follow-up radiographs should be compared with initial radiographs to detect any developing displacement. The long-arm cast should be reapplied 2 weeks and 4 weeks after the injury and every 4 weeks thereafter to maintain adequate immobilization as swelling decreases and muscle atrophy occurs. Diligent finger and shoulder ROM exercises three times daily should be encouraged. After the cast is discontinued, forearm, elbow, and wrist ROM and strengthening exercises should be started. Physical therapy referral is usually necessary because of the prolonged immobilization.

Displaced Fractures

Closed reduction may be attempted in selected cases, but poor results are common. Operative treatment is indicated for nearly all displaced fractures. External fixation may be appropriate in some cases, and surgical alternatives include plate fixation and intramedullary nail fixation.

Return to Work or Sports

Recovery after both-bone forearm fractures is more prolonged than for simpler fractures of the upper extremity. When cast immobilization is completed, patients should begin supervised physical therapy to regain normal or near-normal ROM and strength. Patients with undemanding occupations may resume work immediately while continuing rehabilitation. Patients involved in heavy labor should be offered light duty or delay returning to work until ROM and strength are near normal. Patients engaged in sports in which falls are possible should use a protective cylindrical splint for 1 month after cast immobilization is completed.

Complications

Fractures of the radius and ulna are high-energy injuries, and complications are common. Further treatment may be needed if nonunion, infection, nerve injury, compartment syndrome, radioulnar synostosis (bony fusion), or refracture occurs. Nonunion is most commonly seen if infection occurs, if closed reduction does not achieve adequate reduction, or if open reduction fails to achieve adequate fixation. Osteotomy and bone grafting may be necessary to correct nonunion of the forearm. Open fractures or closed fractures treated with open reduction are at risk for infection, presumably because of wound contamination and the significant degree of soft tissue injury seen in these fractures.

Nerve injury is relatively uncommon in closed fractures of the radius and ulna, but it may occur with open fractures or major trauma such as gunshot wounds or near-amputation. Early signs of compartment syndrome include deep, boring pain

out of proportion to the injury, pain with passive extension of the fingers, palpable induration of the flexor compartment, decreased sensation in the fingers, and loss of forearm muscle function. Treatment involves early and wide fasciotomy from the elbow to the wrist with delayed closure of the wound with or without skin grafts.

Radioulnar synostosis is a relatively uncommon complication usually seen in the setting of severely comminuted fractures of the radius and ulna. If the position of the forearm is functional, no treatment is necessary. If the position is nonfunctional, osteotomy to create a more functional position should be considered. Refracture is more likely after high-energy fractures or crush injuries, if adequate compression and reduction were not achieved, or if the original fracture site remains radiolucent.

BOTH-BONE FOREARM FRACTURES (PEDIATRIC)

Both-bone forearm fractures are less common than fractures of the distal radius or the elbow. The majority occur in the distal third of the radius and ulna shafts. Fractures in the proximal third of the radius and ulna are rare because the bones are stronger in this area and protected by muscle. Both-bone forearm fractures are described by the degree of completion, the direction of deformity, and the level of the fracture. The degree of completion is defined as plastic deformation, greenstick, or complete.

Mechanism of Injury

The usual cause of injury is a fall on an outstretched hand. Greater force is required to fracture through the diaphysis than is the case for distal radius (metaphysis) fractures.

Clinical Presentation

Deformity, swelling, and crepitus over the fracture site are quite obvious if the radius and ulna fractures are significantly displaced. Children with minimally displaced fractures may have only mild tenderness and swelling.

Imaging

AP and lateral radiographs of the entire radius and ulna, including the elbow and wrist, are essential for an accurate diagnosis of these injuries. The radiographs should be examined for degree of completion, presence of angulation, and any rotational displacement (Fig. 6-23). Indications of fracture rotation are a sudden change in the width of the cortex and a break in the smooth curve of the radius.

The recommendations for acceptable alignment for both-bone forearm fractures vary. It is impossible to predict the amount of remodeling in each

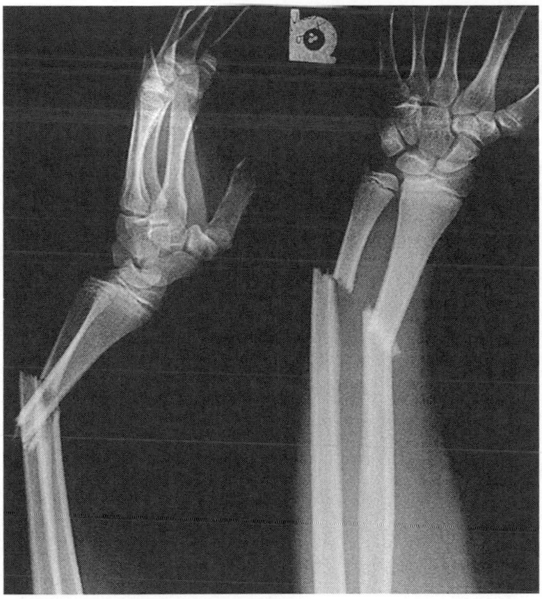

FIGURE 6-23 Complete transverse both-bone forearm fracture with 40 degrees of apex dorsal angulation, 20 degrees of apex ulnar angulation, and shortening of the radius and ulna with complete off-ending (0% apposition).

individual case. Generally speaking, younger children have a better chance of correcting fracture angulation, and the closer the fracture is to the growth plate, the greater the chance of remodeling. For children 8 years of age and younger, 15 degrees of angulation and 45 degrees of rotation can be accepted. For children ages 8 to 15 years, 10 degrees of angulation and 30 degrees of rotation are acceptable.[18] Overriding of the fracture fragments with bayonet apposition is acceptable as long as satisfactory alignment exists. Residual angular or rotational deformity often causes limitation of pronation and supination. Despite this loss of motion, functional impairment is uncommon.

Treatment

Because it is difficult to determine proper alignment and maintain a reduction of two parallel bones with rotary and angulatory forces acting on each, patients with displaced fractures should be referred to an orthopedic surgeon for definitive care. Nondisplaced or minimally displaced fractures of the radius and ulna shafts are treated with a long-arm cast with the forearm in neutral position for 6 to 8 weeks. Attaching a sling to a loop placed proximal to the level of the fracture can help prevent fracture displacement (see Fig. 6-22). Radiographs should be repeated weekly for the first 3 weeks to ensure no change in fracture alignment has occurred. If the fracture position remains stable after 3 weeks, radiographs can then be obtained every 2 weeks until the fracture is healed.

FRACTURES OF THE ULNAR SHAFT

"Nightstick" Fractures

As the name implies, isolated fractures of the ulnar shaft are usually caused by a direct blow. Patients with this fracture have point tenderness over the ulnar shaft and forearm swelling. Radiographs of the entire ulna, including the wrist and elbow, should be obtained. These fractures can be treated conservatively if at least 50% apposition of fragments and less than 10 degrees of angulation are apparent (Fig. 6-24). Nondisplaced or minimally displaced fractures initially can be treated for 7 to 10 days with a posterior splint until swelling decreases. The splint extends from the middle upper arm to the dorsum of the MCP joints with the wrist in slight extension, the forearm in neutral position, and the elbow at 90 degrees of flexion. The patient's arm can then be placed in a plaster sleeve or functional brace for the next 4 to 6 weeks

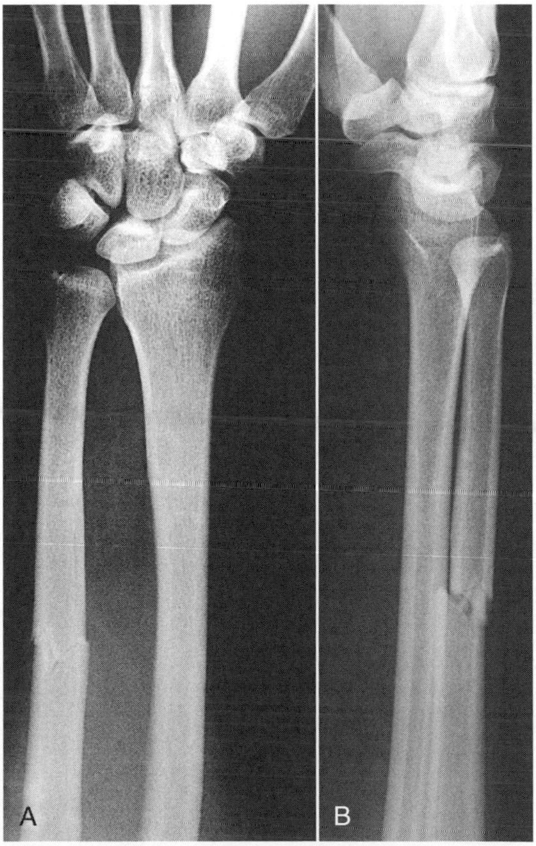

FIGURE 6-24 Anteroposterior (**A**) and lateral (**B**) views of a minimally displaced isolated fracture of the ulnar shaft.

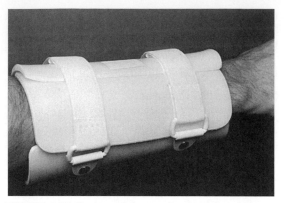

FIGURE 6-25 Functional forearm brace used in the treatment of isolated fractures of the ulnar shaft. The brace allows full motion of the elbow and wrist.

(Fig. 6-25). This type of bracing stabilizes the forearm while allowing free ROM at the wrist and elbow. If the patient still has marked pain with supination and pronation at the first follow-up visit, the posterior splint can be continued until symptoms subside. Weekly radiographs should be obtained for the first 3 weeks to detect any displacement that might necessitate referral. Exercises to strengthen the forearm and wrist are initiated after immobilization. Patients with comminuted or displaced fractures should be referred for open reduction and internal fixation.

Table 6-2 summarizes the management guidelines for nondisplaced isolated fractures of the ulnar shaft.

MONTEGGIA'S FRACTURES (ADULT)

Monteggia's classic description is a fracture of the proximal third of the ulna with anterior dislocation of the radial head. This fracture dislocation (type I) is the most common form of Monteggia's lesion (55% to 78%). A type II lesion is a fracture of the ulnar diaphysis with posterior angulation and posterior or posterolateral dislocation of the radial head (10% to 15%). Type III is a fracture of the ulnar metaphysis with lateral or anterolateral dislocation of the radial head (7% to 20%). Type IV is a fracture of both the radius and ulna at the proximal third of the forearm with anterior dislocation of the radial head (<5%).

Mechanism of Injury

The most common cause of injury is a fall on an outstretched, extended, and pronated elbow. With the hand planted on the ground, the weight of the body exerts an external rotation force on the forearm, causing even greater pronation. A direct blow to the posterior aspect of the proximal ulna can cause the same injury.

Clinical Presentation

The symptoms and signs of injury vary with the type of Monteggia's lesion encountered. In type I lesions, the radial head is palpated in the antecubital fossa, the forearm is shortened, and the diaphyseal fracture of the ulna is angulated anteriorly. Radial nerve neurapraxia is common, particularly injury to the posterior interosseous nerve. Patients may demonstrate loss of thumb extension or may

Table 6-2	*Management Guidelines for Nondisplaced Isolated Ulnar Shaft Fractures*
	INITIAL TREATMENT
Splint type and position	Posterior splint with elbow at 90 degrees
Initial follow-up visit	Within 7 to 10 days
Patient instruction	Icing, elevation of elbow
	Continue ROM of fingers and shoulder while in splint
	FOLLOW-UP CARE
Cast or splint type and position	Forearm plaster sleeve or functional brace
	Continue use of posterior splint until pronation and supination are no longer painful
Length of immobilization	4 to 6 weeks
Healing time	6 to 8 weeks
Follow-up visit interval	Weekly for first 3 weeks; then every 2 weeks until healed
Repeat x-ray interval	Weekly for 3 weeks; then at 6 weeks to document union
Patient instruction	Maintain active ROM at fingers, elbow, and shoulder
	Forearm and wrist strengthening after immobilization
Indications for orthopedic consult	>50% displacement
	>10% angulation
	Comminution
	Open fracture

ROM, range of motion.

report paresthesias to the dorsum of the thumb and second and third fingers.

Imaging

Radiographs should include the entire length of the radius and ulna, including the wrist and elbow joints. AP and lateral radiographs are usually sufficient, but occasionally additional radiocapitellar views may be needed to demonstrate dislocation of the radial head. The diaphyseal or metaphyseal ulna fracture is usually obvious and is typically nondisplaced or minimally displaced (Fig. 6-26). The ulna fracture may be angulated anteriorly or posteriorly. Dislocations of the radial head are often missed, sometimes owing to spontaneous reduction. A line drawn through the radial shaft and radial head should bisect the capitellum of the humerus if the radial head is not dislocated (McLaughlin's line). Although isolated fractures of the proximal ulna can occur, a high index of suspicion is necessary to diagnose a Monteggia's fracture dislocation in a timely manner.

Treatment

Recognition of the seriousness of the lesion and early referral for surgical management are essential in the treatment of fractures of the proximal ulna with radial head dislocation. After a Monteggia's fracture has been identified, the patient should be immobilized in a double sugar-tong splint and promptly referred to an orthopedic surgeon. ORIF of the ulna fracture is required, and this usually results in reduction of the radial head as well. If

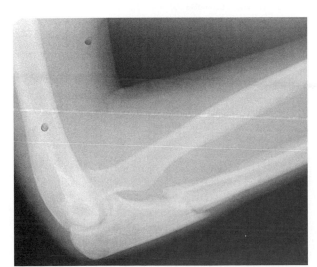

FIGURE 6-26 Lateral view of the elbow demonstrating a proximal ulna fracture and anterior dislocation of the radial head (type I Monteggia's fracture). Note that a line drawn through the radial shaft and head would not bisect the capitellum of the humerus.

the radial head is fractured, excision of the radial head may be necessary. Immobilization is discontinued after 6 weeks, and active ROM exercises are initiated.

Complications

The complication most commonly seen in association with Monteggia's lesion is neurapraxia of the radial nerve, particularly the posterior interosseous nerve. The prognosis for spontaneous recovery is excellent, and nerve exploration is not indicated. Heterotopic calcification around the elbow may occur and is aggravated by passive ROM exercises. When heterotopic calcification occurs, excessive immobilization should be avoided and active ROM exercises encouraged. Surgical excision is not recommended because recurrence is common. When nonunion occurs, it is usually associated with delayed presentation or missed diagnosis and must be treated with ORIF and bone grafting. Redislocation or subluxation of the radial head and loss of reduction of the ulna fracture may occur from inadequate open reduction or improper postoperative immobilization.

MONTEGGIA'S FRACTURES (PEDIATRIC)

As in adults, Monteggia's fracture in children is a fracture of the proximal third of the ulna accompanied by dislocation of the radial head. Although ORIF is indicated for the treatment of Monteggia's fracture in adults, attempted closed reduction is the procedure of choice for children.

Classification

Type I lesions are characterized by fracture of the proximal ulna with anterior angulation and anterior dislocation of the radial head. Type I lesions are usually caused by a fall on the extended hand and forced pronation of the forearm. Type II lesions demonstrate fracture of the ulna with posterior angulation and posterior dislocation of the radial head. Type III lesions show fracture of the ulna with lateral angulation and lateral dislocation of the radial head. Type IV lesions are rare among children but are similar to a type I lesion in which the shaft of the radius is also fractured.

Clinical Presentation

The patient usually describes a fall onto the outstretched hand and reports pain and loss of motion at the elbow. During physical examination, the elbow is tender and ROM is limited because of pain. Swelling may be minimal during initial treatment but markedly increases days after injury. The angulated fracture of the ulna or the dislocated radial head may be visible on inspection or palpable. Injury to the posterior interosseous nerve (a branch of the radial nerve) is common; therefore, sensation to the dorsum of the thumb and index and middle fingers should be checked. Motor function should be assessed as well (e.g., abduction of the thumb).

Imaging

Close examination of both the wrist and elbow joints is extremely important; therefore, AP and true lateral radiographs of the radius and ulna should be obtained. The Monteggia's lesion may be missed on the AP projection but is clearly visible on the lateral view. If it is not apparent whether the radial head is dislocated or not, comparison views of the uninjured radius and ulna should be obtained. In all projections, the axis of the radial neck should align with the midpoint of the radial head, which should be aligned with the humeral capitellum.

Indications for Orthopedic Referral

Although closed reduction is the procedure of choice for Monteggia's lesions among children, this reduction is best attempted under general anesthesia in the operating room. Therefore, after the diagnosis of Monteggia's fracture has been made, the patient should be referred immediately to an orthopedic surgeon for definitive care.

Treatment

The patient should be placed in a sling or sugartong splint in the position of maximum comfort and referred immediately to an orthopedic surgeon. The surgeon will usually attempt closed reduction under general anesthesia. If closed reduction is successful, the patient is placed in a long-arm cast for 4 to 6 weeks. If the ulna fracture is unstable, the radial head is irreducible, or reduction cannot be maintained, ORIF is indicated.

Return to Sports

After immobilization is complete, ROM and strengthening exercises are initiated. Return to sports may be considered after ROM is near normal and strength is at least 80% compared with the uninjured arm. A protective forearm splint may be worn for the first 1 or 2 months after return to sports.

Complications

As would be expected from the severity of this injury, complications are common. Elbow ROM may be limited, especially pronation and supination, although some loss of terminal flexion and extension may also be seen. ROM is better preserved among children who experience successful closed reduction. Associated fractures at the wrist may be overlooked at the time of injury; the

examining physician should always examine both the elbow and wrist joint carefully with this potential complication in mind. Occasionally, the ulna fracture fails to heal or the radial head demonstrates persistent or recurrent dislocation. In such cases, ORIF may be required. Heterotopic ossification may be seen in some patients, especially among those whose reduction was delayed. However, because this soft tissue calcification seldom interferes with function, it should be left alone. Synostosis between the proximal ulna and the radial shaft may occur; this complication does interfere with pronation–supination but usually recurs after resection. Compensatory motion at the shoulder minimizes the effect of this uncommon complication. As mentioned earlier, injury to the posterior interosseous nerve is a common complication of the Monteggia's fracture because of neurapraxia or axonotmesis to the nerve when the radial head becomes dislocated. Normal function may return by 8 to 12 weeks. Some clinicians recommend electromyography at 4 and 8 weeks after injury to assess function and recovery. If no improvement is seen by 8 weeks, surgical exploration should be considered.

WRIST DISLOCATIONS (RADIOCARPAL JOINT)

Dislocations of the wrist usually occur in conjunction with a fracture. The most common fracture dislocation patterns of the wrist are Barton's, Hutchinson's (chauffeur's) and die-punch fracture dislocations.

Pure dislocations of the radiocarpal joint are rare. When they do occur, the hand may be displaced in an ulnar (most common), dorsal, or volar direction. Patients with pure wrist dislocations generally have visible deformity, swelling, and point tenderness along the radiocarpal joint. Wrist dislocations should be viewed as orthopedic emergencies because neurovascular compromise is often present. Reduction should be performed expeditiously under appropriate analgesia or anesthesia with a neurovascular examination made before and after the reduction. Although reduction is not usually complicated, maintaining an acceptable position is difficult without open repair. Hence, essentially all wrist dislocations should be evaluated by an orthopedist even if postreduction position and neurovascular status appear excellent.

Occasionally, the hand will return to a normal or near-normal position before the patient seeks care. During examination, these patients have swelling and radiocarpal tenderness but no deformity. Their radiographs may appear normal. These patients are at risk for chronic radiocarpal instability, which may interfere with many activities. Referral should be considered for any patients who may have such injuries, especially if prominent swelling and poor active ROM are apparent. Referral should also be considered if normal hand and wrist function is slow to return.

REFERENCES

1. Frykman G. Fracture of the distal radius including sequelae shoulder-hand-finger syndrome, disturbance in the distal radio-ulnar joint and impairment of nerve function. A clinical and experimental study. *Acta Orthop Scan.* 1967; 108(suppl):3.
2. Jeong GK, Kaplan FT, Liporace F, et al. An evaluation of two scoring systems to predict instability in fractures of the distal radius. *J Trauma.* 2004;57:1043-1047.
3. Lafontaine M, Hardy D, Delince P. Stability assessment of distal radius fractures. *Injury.* 1989;20:208-210.
4. Altissimi M, Mancini GB, Azzara A, Ciaffoloni E. Early and late displacement of fractures of the distal radius. The prediction of instability. *Int Orthop.* 1994;18:61-65.
5. Arora R, Gabl M, Gschwentner M, et al. Comparative study of clinical and radiologic outcomes of unstable Colles type distal radius fractures in patients older than 70 years: nonoperative treatment versus volar locking plating. *J Orthop Trauma.* 2009;23:237-242.
6. Grafstein E, Stenstrom R, Christenson J. A prospective randomized controlled trial comparing circumferential casting and splinting in displaced Colles fractures. *CJEM.* 2010;12:192-200.
7. Earnshaw SA, Aladin A, Surendran S, Moran CG. Closed reduction of Colles fractures: comparison of manual manipulation and finger-trap traction: a prospective, randomized study. *Bone Joint Surg [Am].* 2002;84:354-358.
8. Handoll HHG, Madhok R. Closed reduction methods for treating distal radial fractures in adults. *Cochrane Database Syst Rev.* 2003;(1):CD003763.
9. Fernandez DL. Closed manipulation and casting of distal radius fractures. *Hand Clin.* 2005;21:307-316.
10. Dresing K, Peterson T, Schmit-Neuerburg KP. Compartment pressure in the carpal tunnel in distal fractures of the radius. A prospective study. *Arch Orthop Trauma Surg.* 1994;113:285-289.
11. Placzek JD, Boyer MI, Gelberman RH, et al. Nerve decompression for complex regional pain syndrome type II following upper extremity surgery. *J Hand Surg Am.* 2005; 30:69-74.
12. Millet PJ, Rushton N. Early mobilization in the treatment of Colles' fracture: a 3 year prospective study. *Injury.* 1995;26:671-675.
13. Abraham A, Handoll HH, Khan T. Interventions for treating wrist fractures in children. *Cochrane Database Syst Rev.* 2008;(2):CD004576.
14. Davidson JS, Brown DJ, Barnes SN, Bruce CE. Simple treatment for torus fractures of the distal radius. *J Bone Joint Surg Br.* 2001;83:1173-1175.
15. Plint AC, Perry JJ, Correll R, et al. A randomized, controlled trial of removable splinting versus casting for wrist buckle fractures in children. *Pediatrics.* 2006;117:691-697.
16. Drendel AL, Gorelick MH, Weisman SJ, et al. A randomized clinical trial of ibuprofen versus acetaminophen with codeine for acute pediatric arm fracture pain. *Ann Emerg Med.* 2009;54:553-560.
17. Waters PM. Distal radius and ulna fractures. In: Beaty JH, Kasser JR, eds. Rockwood and Wilkins' Fractures in Children. 5th ed. Philadelphia: Lippincott Williams & Wilkins; 2001:415.
18. Price CT, Mencio GA. Injuries to the shafts of the radius and ulna. In: Beaty JH, Kasser JR, eds. Rockwood and Wilkins' Fractures in Children. 5th ed. Philadelphia: Lippincott Williams & Wilkins; 2001:453.

7

ELBOW FRACTURES

Elbow fractures in adults and children are among the most complex of all fractures. The higher complication rate and need for near-anatomic reduction in these fractures necessitate orthopedic referral in most cases. Primary care providers play an important role in the prompt diagnosis of elbow fractures that need referral and in the treatment of nondisplaced fractures with splinting and early motion. Knowledge of normal elbow anatomy and radiographic alignment is essential in detecting displacement of fracture fragments, especially with intraarticular injuries. Encouragement of early motion to prevent joint stiffness is important in the successful management of any elbow fracture.

Elbow fractures represent approximately 10% of all fractures in children. The diagnosis and management of these injuries are complex, and most fractures should be managed by an orthopedist. The large amount of nonossified cartilage around the elbow makes detection of fractures difficult. Elbow fractures in children can lead to neurovascular injury, which further complicates management.

Go to Expert Consult for the electronic version of a patient instruction sheet named "Broken Elbow," which covers the steps of care from pain relief to rehabilitation exercises. This can be copied to hand out to patients to assist them during the treatment period.

RADIAL HEAD AND NECK

Radial head and neck fractures are common and account for approximately one third of all elbow fractures in adults. Most occur in middle adulthood (age 30 to 40 years). Other upper extremity injuries are frequently associated with radial head fractures.[1]

Anatomic Considerations

The radial head is a thick, disk-shaped end of the proximal radius with a shallow concavity for articulation with the capitellum of the distal humerus (Figure 7-1). The neck is the narrowed area just

below the head, and the tuberosity is a medial prominence just distal to the neck. A fall on an outstretched hand directs a longitudinal force from the wrist to the elbow, resulting in compression of the radial head against the capitellum. The radial head also articulates medially with the lesser sigmoid (radial) notch of the ulna. The annular ligament arises from the lateral collateral ligament complex, encircles the radial head, and attaches to the radial notch. This strong ligament prevents displacement of the radial head from its articulation with the ulna.

The radial head moves with forearm rotation as well as flexion and extension. It can be palpated in the depression about 1 inch distal to the lateral epicondyle with the elbow flexed to 90 degrees. It is medial and posterior to the wrist extensor muscle group. As the patient pronates and supinates the forearm, the radial head can be felt to rotate under the examiner's thumb (Figure 7-2).

Mechanism of Injury

Fractures of the radial head and neck most commonly occur as a result of a fall on an outstretched hand. In general, the severity of the fracture is proportional to the force applied during the fall. A valgus compressive force or direct trauma to the elbow may also fracture the radial head. Radial head fractures may occur in association with other fractures, dislocations, or soft tissue injuries, and detection of these associated injuries is important for proper treatment.

Clinical Presentation

The patient with a radial head or neck fracture has swelling over the lateral elbow and limited range of motion (ROM), especially in forearm rotation and elbow extension. Pain increases with passive rotation. Point tenderness over the radial head is the most reliable finding. A careful neurovascular examination with particular attention to radial nerve function (tested using the thumb's up sign) is essential.

If the patient has significantly restricted elbow motion, it is most often attributable to joint

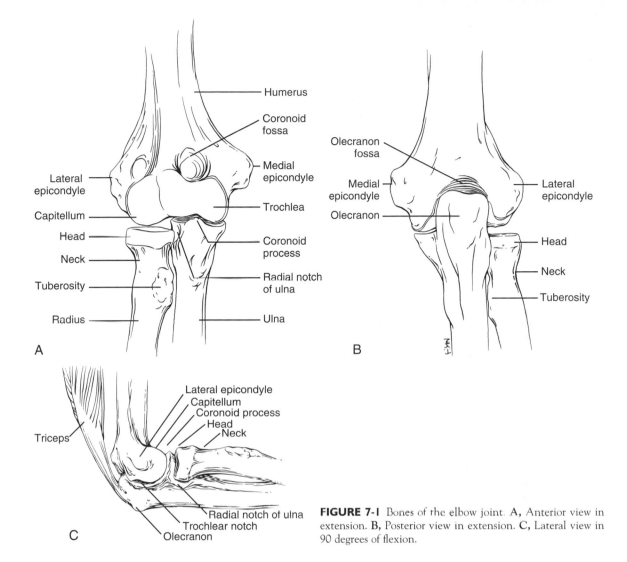

Humerus
Coronoid fossa
Medial epicondyle
Trochlea
Coronoid process
Radial notch of ulna
Ulna
Lateral epicondyle
Capitellum
Head
Neck
Tuberosity
Radius

A

Olecranon fossa
Medial epicondyle
Olecranon
Lateral epicondyle
Head
Neck
Tuberosity

B

Lateral epicondyle
Capitellum
Coronoid process
Head
Neck
Triceps
Radial notch of ulna
Trochlear notch
Olecranon

C

FIGURE 7-1 Bones of the elbow joint. **A,** Anterior view in extension. **B,** Posterior view in extension. **C,** Lateral view in 90 degrees of flexion.

distension and pain from a hemarthrosis, but occasionally a displaced fracture fragment causes a mechanical block to motion. Aspiration of the hemarthrosis and instillation of local anesthetic for pain relief are often necessary to perform a better evaluation of joint motion. The technique for joint aspiration is as follows:

1. Prepare the lateral elbow using sterile technique.
2. Visualize an imaginary triangle connecting the radial head, the lateral epicondyle, and the olecranon (Figure 7-3).
3. Anesthetize the skin.
4. Insert an 18-gauge needle on a 20-mL syringe through the joint capsule at the center of the triangle. Aspirate as much blood as possible.
5. Change syringes and instill 3 to 5 mL of a half-and-half mixture of 1% bupivacaine and 1% lidocaine without epinephrine.

After the procedure, detecting severe crepitation or complete blockage of motion through full extension and flexion indicates the presence of displaced fragments.

If the patient has significant wrist pain, central forearm pain, or both, an acute longitudinal radioulnar dissociation with disruption of the distal radioulnar joint (the so-called Essex-Lopresti fracture) may have occurred.

Imaging

Anteroposterior (AP) and lateral views of the elbow are usually sufficient to detect a radial head or neck fracture. A radiocapitellar view, an oblique view with the forearm in neutral rotation and the x-ray beam angled 45 degrees cephalad may be needed to visualize a fracture. These fractures can be quite subtle, with the only clue to their presence being a fat pad sign[2] (Figure 7-4). The fat pad sign occurs when the capsule around the elbow joint is

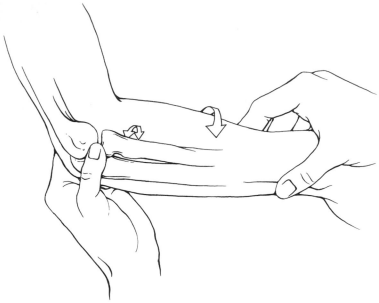

FIGURE 7-2 Palpation of the radial head just distal to the lateral epicondyle. Rotation of the forearm will rotate the radial head under the examiner's thumb.

distended by an intraarticular hemarthrosis. A small oval anterior fat pad may be a normal finding, but a sail-shaped lucency in front of the joint indicates a joint effusion (Figure 7-5). A lucency behind the joint indicates a posterior fat pad and is always abnormal. A fracture of the radial neck does not necessarily give rise to a fat pad sign because it is extraarticular.

Fracture patterns seen include damage to the articular surface, depression of the head, and angulated fractures of the head or neck (Figure 7-6). The radiographs should be examined closely to detect fragments lying free within the joint. These

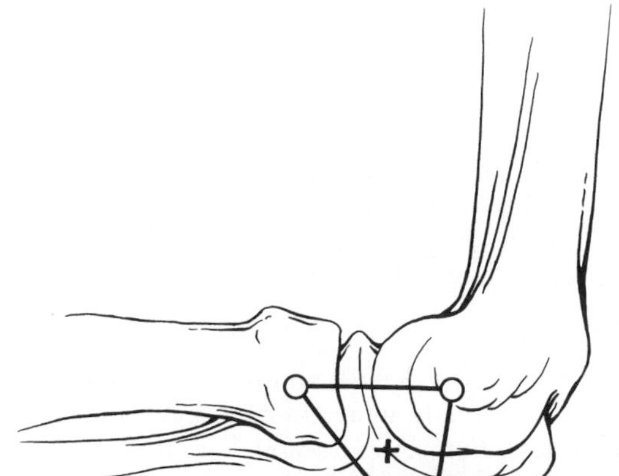

suggest chip fractures of the capitellum because radial head fracture fragments are rarely displaced proximally.

Radial head fractures are usually classified according to a modified Mason classification, which adds a fourth category to the original scheme to account for those fractures associated with an elbow dislocation.[3,4] The classification is based on the amount of head involvement and the degree of displacement:

Type I: Fissure or marginal sector, nondisplaced
Type II: Marginal sector, displaced
Type III: Comminuted involving entire head
Type IV: Fracture with associated elbow
    dislocation

Computed tomography (CT) may be needed to fully assess fracture displacement or comminution when surgery is being considered.

Indications for Orthopedic Referral

Emergent Referral

Emergency orthopedic referral should be obtained for any patient with an open fracture, elbow fracture dislocation, or any evidence of neurovascular injury.

Nonemergent Referral

Patients with fractures that are displaced more than 2 mm, involve more than one third of the articular surface, are angulated more than 30 degrees, are depressed more than 3 mm, or are severely comminuted should be referred for consideration of operative management. The presence

FIGURE 7-3 Proper needle placement for joint aspiration is at the center of the triangle formed by the radial head, lateral epicondyle, and olecranon.

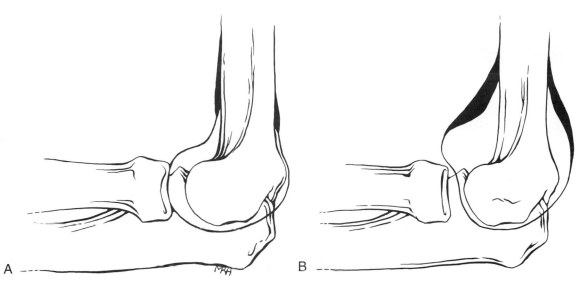

FIGURE 7-4 A, Position of the normal anterior fat pad. **B,** A joint effusion associated with a fracture displaces the anterior and posterior fat pads away from the humerus.

of any mechanical block regardless of the radiographic appearance of the fracture requires referral.

The criteria for open reduction of radial head and neck fractures vary. The factors that influence treatment choice include the amount of displacement; presence or absence of mechanical block; associated injuries such as radioulnar dissociation, elbow dislocation, or fracture of the coronoid; and the anticipated demand on the elbow. Excision of the radial head was formerly common in the management of radial head fractures, but this method of treatment has come under greater scrutiny, especially in younger, more active patients.

The treatment of type II fractures remains controversial because both nonoperative and operative approaches can produce satisfactory results.[5] The majority of type II and IV fractures require surgery, which often entails radial head resection and prosthetic replacement.

Initial Treatment

Table 7-1 summarizes management guidelines for fractures of the radial head and neck.

Dramatic pain relief can be provided by aspiration of blood from the elbow joint and instillation of a local anesthetic as described previously. Relieving the hemarthrosis may also allow the patient to

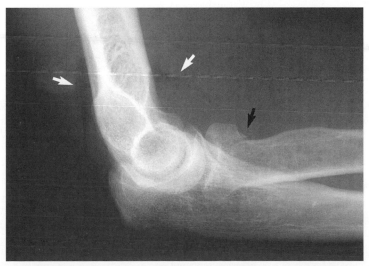

FIGURE 7-5 Anterior and posterior fat pads associated with a radial head fracture (*white arrows*). Note the triangular or sail shape of the anterior fat pad. The *black arrow* points to a subtle radial neck fracture.

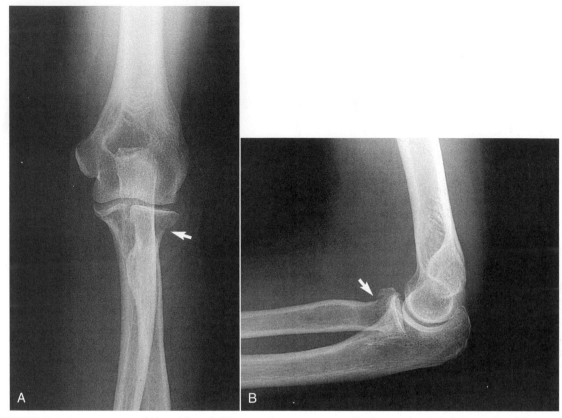

FIGURE 7-6 Anteroposterior (**A**) and lateral (**B**) views showing a minimally depressed and slightly angulated fracture of the radial head (*arrows*).

Table 7-1	*Management Guidelines for Radial Head and Neck Fractures*
	INITIAL TREATMENT
Splint type and position	Long-arm posterior splint
	Elbow in 90 degrees of flexion
	Consider aspiration of hemarthrosis
Initial follow-up visit	Within 1 week
Patient instruction	Icing and elevation in first 48 hours
	Forearm rotation as soon as pain permits
	FOLLOW-UP CARE
Cast or splint type and position	Sling for comfort only
Length of immobilization	1 week
Healing time	8 to 10 weeks to restore motion
Follow-up visit interval	Every 2 weeks to assess return of normal elbow motion
Repeat radiography interval	At first visit to check position or look for signs of initially occult fracture
Patient instruction	Active ROM exercises (forearm rotation, flexion, and extension) at least three to four times each day
	Physical therapy referral if no or little progress
	Some loss of extension expected
Indications for orthopedic consult	Fracture dislocation
	Mechanical block to motion
	>2 mm displacement
	>One third of the articular surface involved
	>3 mm depression
	>30 degrees of angulation
	Severe comminution

ROM, range of motion.

begin moving the elbow sooner.[6] Patients with nondisplaced fractures of the head or neck or those awaiting consultation with an orthopedist should have the arm immobilized in a long-arm posterior splint with the elbow at 90 degrees. They should be instructed to apply ice to the elbow and elevate it for the first 48 hours. The patient with a nondisplaced fracture should begin forearm rotation out of the splint as soon as pain permits, usually within the first few days. The patient should be seen in 1 week.

Follow-up Care

During the first follow-up visit, the posterior splint should be discontinued and the patient given a sling for comfort only. Repeat radiographs should be obtained to look for any further displacement of the fracture fragments or to look for evidence of a fracture if only a fat pad sign was visible initially.

Rehabilitation

Active ROM exercises, including forearm rotation, flexion, and extension, should be performed at least three or four times per day. Achieving maximum degrees of motion is preferred over trying to increase the number of repetitions. The patient should be advised that pain and stiffness will be present for several weeks, but most patients can expect good to excellent function after 2 to 3 months of rehabilitation. Patients who fail to make gradual progress in gaining elbow motion should be considered for physical therapy referral. Some loss of extension (10 to 15 degrees) is common but generally does not affect function.

Return to Work or Sports

Early return to work and daily activities is advisable to maximize function. The patient can participate in activities as tolerated after the initial weeks of immobilization in the posterior splint and sling. Work and sports activities will be limited by relative weakness of the forearm muscles caused by the injury, and activities requiring strength should be modified accordingly. Contact and collision sports should be avoided until the individual has normal strength and close to normal ROM. It may take 1 to 2 months to achieve the last 15 to 20 degrees of elbow extension, and most individuals will have good function despite this lack of full extension. Additional protection or bracing is not necessary for returning to sports.

Complications

The majority of patients with a nondisplaced fracture of the radial head or neck have a good clinical outcome. Mild limitation of extension or forearm rotation is the most common complication. Painful arthritis is an uncommon result. Some radial head fractures have an associated osteochondral fracture of the capitellum that was not detected on initial radiographs. This associated injury often leads to an increased incidence of osteoarthritis and joint stiffness and pain. Radial head excision can be complicated by proximal migration of the radius, elbow instability, distal radial–ulnar joint pain, or decreased forearm strength.

Pediatric Considerations

Radial Head and Neck Fractures

Radial head and neck fractures represent a small percentage of all elbow fractures in children. The low rate of fracture probably results from the large amount of cartilage in the radial head in skeletally immature children. The usual cause is a fall on an outstretched hand with valgus force applied across the radiocapitellar joint. Fractures of the radial neck usually occur through the physis (Salter-Harris type I or II) or just distal to the physis. The radial head can be angulated (usually apex ulnar angulation) or translocated after these injuries (Figures 7-7 and 7-8). Other injuries, such as elbow dislocation, fractures of the olecranon, or avulsion of the medial epicondylar apophysis, may be associated with radial head and neck fractures.

If the angulation of the radial head is less than 30 degrees and less than 4 mm of translocation is apparent, the fracture can be treated with a brief period of sling immobilization and early ROM exercises started 7 to 10 days after injury. Healing time is usually 3 to 4 weeks, and children generally need a shorter time to return to full elbow motion than adults. Displaced fractures should be immobilized in a posterior splint and the patient referred to an orthopedist for closed or open reduction. Residual tilt of the radial head is better tolerated than translocation of the head.

Radial Head Subluxation (Nursemaid's Elbow)

Go to Expert Consult for a video on how to perform a reduction maneuver for a radial head subluxation. Radial head subluxation, also known as nursemaid's elbow, is one of the most common elbow injuries in children, typically occurring between ages 1 and 4 years, with a peak incidence between 2 and 3 years of age.[7] The usual cause of injury is sudden longitudinal traction on the arm with the elbow extended such as that occurs when a child is pulled up by the arm. This force causes the annular ligament, which tethers the radial head to the adjacent ulna, to slip proximally and become interposed between the radius and the capitellum. Before the age of 3 years, the radial head is smaller than the diameter of the annular ligament and more easily slips out from beneath it when longitudinal force is applied to the arm.

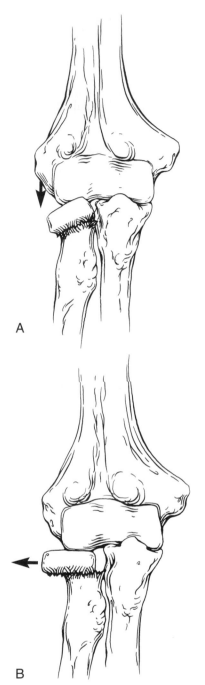

FIGURE 7-7 Displacement patterns of pediatric radial neck fractures. **A,** Apex ulnar angulation. **B,** Translocation.

After a radial head subluxation, the child reports pain and stops using the affected arm. The arm is usually held with the elbow in a slightly flexed and pronated position or with the elbow fully flexed. Any attempt to move the arm is resisted, and pain is most often elicited with supination. Radiograph results are often normal and not helpful before reduction unless the history

and examination are confusing or the mechanism of injury is other than a pull or twisting trauma. Radiographs should be obtained if reduction is unsuccessful.

Reduction of radial head subluxation does not require any analgesia or sedation and can be performed in the office. Supination/flexion and hyperpronation are the two techniques for reduction and both are effective. A systematic review found that reduction on the first attempt was more likely with hyperpronation though the evidence quality was low.[8] The method most commonly used is the supination/flexion method. This is performed by supination of the forearm followed by one smooth motion of flexion and pronation of the elbow while pressure is applied over the radial head (Figure 7-9). In the hyperpronation method, the examiner supports the child's arm at the elbow with one hand, grips the child's distal forearm with the other hand, and hyperpronates the forearm while pressure is applied over the radial head. A sudden release of resistance and the sensation of a pop signify reduction of the radial head. Usually within minutes, the child is comfortable and begins using the arm again. It may take up to 24 hours for the child to move the elbow normally. Immobilization is not necessary after this injury. If the child has not resumed normal activity after 24 hours, the parents should be advised to return to the office for a reevaluation of the injury, including radiographs. Prolonged symptoms and an irreducible subluxation indicate the need for orthopedic referral.

Recurrence of this injury is common, occurring in one quarter to one third of children, and should not be a cause for concern as long as the injury is reducible each time. Rarely does recurrent subluxation result in any permanent sequelae. To reduce

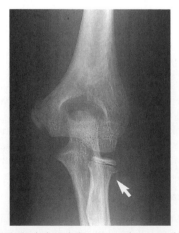

FIGURE 7-8 Radial neck fracture with minimal apex ulnar angulation. These subtle fractures are easily missed. (*From Thornton A, Gyll C. Children's Fractures: A Radiological Guide to Safe Practice. Philadelphia, WB Saunders, 1999.*)

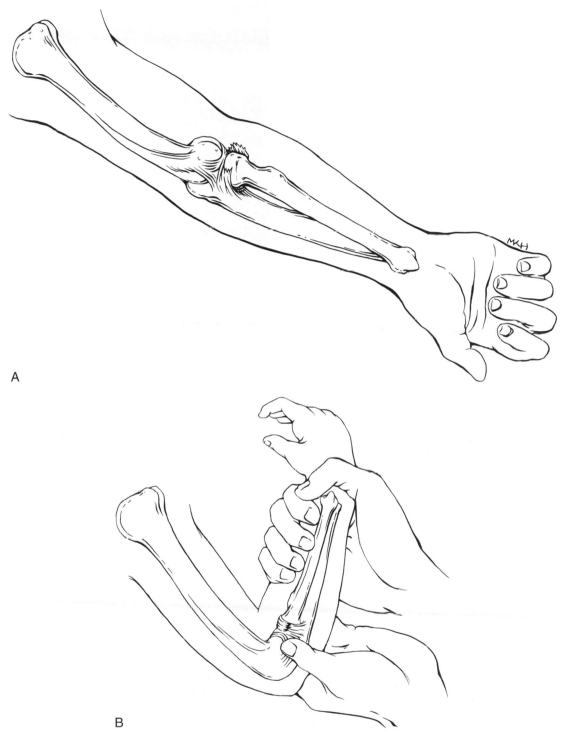

A

B

FIGURE 7-9 Supination/flexion reduction technique for a radial head subluxation. **A,** The forearm is extended and supinated. **B,** The elbow is then flexed and pronated while pressure is applied over the radial head.

the chance of reinjury, parents should be advised after the first episode to avoid lifting their child by the wrist. With time, as the radial head becomes larger and at less risk of subluxation, the child outgrows this condition, usually by age 4 or 5 years.

OLECRANON

Anatomic Considerations

The olecranon process and coronoid process together form the trochlear notch, which articulates with the trochlea of the distal humerus and provides bony stability for flexion and extension of the elbow (see Figure 7-1, C). The triceps muscle inserts by a broad tendinous expansion on the posterior aspect of the olecranon. The ulnar nerve lies in the groove between the olecranon process and the medial epicondyle and may be injured in association with a fracture of the olecranon (Figure 7-10).

The olecranon process is nearly subcutaneous, with only the olecranon bursa and triceps aponeurosis covering it. This superficial position makes it more susceptible to direct trauma. Most fractures are intraarticular, and near-anatomic alignment is necessary to ensure full ROM of the elbow. The amount of fracture displacement present often depends on the integrity of the triceps attachment and the force of the pull of the triceps muscle.

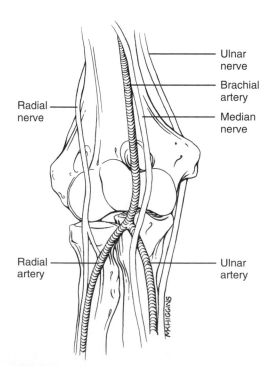

FIGURE 7-10 Neurovascular structures of the elbow.

Radial nerve

Radial artery

Ulnar nerve

Brachial artery

Median nerve

Ulnar artery

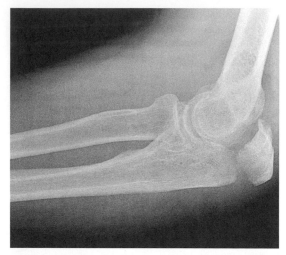

FIGURE 7-11 Fracture of the olecranon with significant posterior displacement of the proximal fragment.

Mechanism of Injury

Most fractures of the olecranon occur as a result of direct trauma to the point of the elbow during a fall or from an object striking the elbow.[9] These fractures are usually comminuted. An indirect force from a fall on a partially flexed elbow may result in a transverse or oblique fracture caused by forceful contraction of the triceps muscle.

Clinical Presentation

The patient has swelling and tenderness over the olecranon. Because most of the fractures are intraarticular, a hemarthrosis develops and limits ROM. The patient may be unable to actively extend the elbow against gravity if the triceps muscle is significantly injured. Documenting neurologic function of the arm and hand is essential because ulnar nerve injuries may accompany comminuted fractures of the olecranon.

Imaging

A true lateral view of the elbow is best for delineating fractures of the olecranon. Fracture patterns observed include avulsion, transverse, oblique, and comminuted. The radiographs should be examined carefully for the amount of displacement, extent of articular surface involved, and degree of comminution (Figure 7-11). Any fracture with less than 2 mm of displacement and no change in position with gentle flexion to 90 degrees and extension against gravity is considered nondisplaced and stable.

Indications for Orthopedic Referral

All displaced fractures of the olecranon require open reduction with internal fixation (ORIF), because closed reduction rarely achieves the near-anatomic alignment of the articular surface needed for a good functional result. If the patient is unable to actively extend the elbow, which indicates loss of triceps function, an orthopedic surgeon should be consulted.

Initial Treatment

Table 7-2 summarizes management guidelines for nondisplaced fractures of the olecranon.

Initially, the patient should be immobilized in a long-arm posterior splint with the elbow in 60 to 90 degrees of flexion and well molded posteriorly. A standard arm sling can be used to support the arm. Patients with displaced fractures should be referred within 3 to 5 days to an orthopedic surgeon. Those with nondisplaced stable fractures should be seen within 5 to 7 days.

Follow-up Care

At the first follow-up visit, repeat radiographs should be taken without the splint to make certain that displacement has not occurred. If the fracture remains stable, the patient can begin gentle supination and pronation exercises. A sling or a removable posterior splint can be used for comfort during the healing period. Flexion and extension exercises are started at 2 weeks. Motion should be limited to 90 degrees of flexion until there is radiographic evidence of fracture healing. Many patients benefit from working with a physical therapist during the rehabilitation period to ensure that they are progressing appropriately. Muscle strengthening, especially of the triceps muscle, is begun when

adequate bone healing has occurred (usually by 6 weeks). The fracture should be reevaluated radiographically at 2 and 4 weeks to check for fracture alignment and healing. Fracture union is usually present 6 to 8 weeks after injury, but complete return of elbow ROM may take up to 12 weeks.

Return to Work or Sports

The patient can participate in activities as tolerated after 2 to 3 weeks of immobilization in the posterior splint and sling. Work and sports activities will be limited by relative weakness of the arm muscles caused by the injury, and activities requiring strength should be modified accordingly. Patients may return to vigorous use of the arm 2 to 3 months after injury. Contact and collision sports should be avoided until the individual has normal strength and close to normal ROM. Wearing an elbow pad during contact or collision sports is advisable if the individual has slight tenderness over the fracture site despite good motion and strength. Loss of motion is a common finding, but most individuals will have good function despite this lack of full extension.

Complications

Complications of olecranon fractures include limited ROM, posttraumatic arthritis, nonunion, heterotopic ossification, and ulnar nerve injury. Loss of full extension is a common finding but only rarely causes significant loss of function. Poorer results occur if less than 2 mm of fracture offset could not be achieved during treatment.[9] The

Table 7-2	*Management Guidelines for Nondisplaced Olecranon Fractures*
	INITIAL TREATMENT
Splint type and position	Long-arm posterior splint
	Elbow in 90 degrees of flexion
	Collar and cuff or arm sling for support
Initial follow-up visit	Within 5 to 7 days
Patient instruction	Icing, elevation
	FOLLOW-UP CARE
Cast or splint type and position	Removable posterior splint or sling for comfort
Length of immobilization	2 to 3 weeks
Healing time	6 to 8 weeks for fracture union
	8 to 10 weeks to restore motion
Follow-up visit interval	Every 2 weeks
Repeat radiography interval	At 1, 2, and 4 weeks
	Check for any displacement
Patient instruction	Forearm rotation within 1 week of injury
	Flexion and extension at 2 weeks
	Some loss of extension is expected
	Flexion >90 degrees to be avoided until radiographic healing is apparent
Indications for orthopedic consult	>2 mm displacement
	Any change in fracture position with flexion and extension
	Inability to actively extend the elbow against gravity

numbness or paresthesias that accompany ulnar nerve injury nearly always disappear over time.

Pediatric Considerations

Injury to the physis of the olecranon is exceedingly rare, partly because the triceps tendon inserts on the metaphysis distal to the physis. Isolated metaphyseal fractures of the olecranon are relatively rare in children. They are usually associated with other fractures around the elbow. They may result from a fall on the elbow in a flexed or extended position; flexion injuries are the most common. Most flexion injuries are nondisplaced (Figure 7-12) and can be treated with 3 weeks of splint immobilization with the elbow in no more than 70 degrees of flexion. Radiographs should be taken within 7 days of the injury to ensure that no significant displacement of the fracture fragment has occurred. Displaced fractures should be splinted in partial extension and the patient referred to an orthopedic surgeon.

Coronoid Process

The coronoid process is a triangular projection of the anterior surface of the olecranon that forms the anterior portion of the trochlear notch (see Figure 7-1, A and C). Fractures of the coronoid process rarely occur in isolation and are associated with an elbow dislocation with spontaneous relocation almost half the time.[10] A sudden forceful contraction of the brachialis muscle may result in an avulsion fracture that appears as a small chip on the lateral view. Coronoid process fractures associated with a dislocation are usually more impacted against the trochlea of the distal humerus. Injury to the coronoid process may result in elbow instability that complicates healing and functional recovery. The presence of an associated fracture of the radial head leads to poorer outcomes.[10]

Patients with a fracture of the coronoid process have tenderness over the antecubital fossa and swelling around the elbow. The strength of the radial pulse should be checked with the elbow in 90 degrees of flexion to be sure it does not diminish in this position. The fracture is best seen on the lateral view. Regan and Morrey classified these fractures into three types: type I fractures involve the tip, type II fractures involve less than 50% of the height of the coronoid, and type III fractures involve more than 50% of the coronoid height.[11]

Patients with type I fractures of the coronoid process should have long-arm posterior splint immobilization with the elbow at 90 degrees and the forearm in full supination. Follow-up radiographs should be obtained at 1 week to ensure proper alignment. After 3 weeks of immobilization, diligent ROM elbow exercises should be started. A sling can be used for comfort during the rehabilitation period. Patients with type II or III fractures should be referred to an orthopedic surgeon for surgical repair.

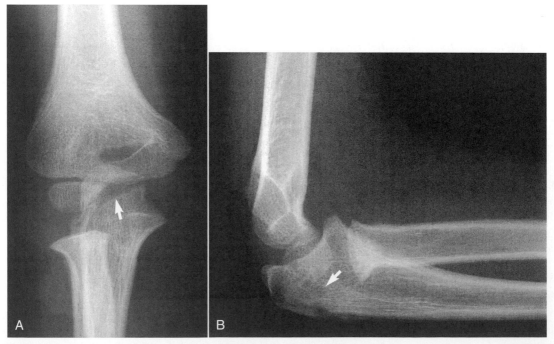

FIGURE 7-12 Anteroposterior (**A**) and lateral (**B**) views showing a nondisplaced fracture of the olecranon metaphysis (*arrows*).

DISTAL HUMERUS (ADULT)

Approximately 30% of adult elbow fractures involve the distal humerus.[12] In younger adults, fractures typically result from high-velocity injuries; older individuals are more likely to sustain a fracture from a fall from standing height. Most distal humerus fractures in adults are intercondylar. Fractures of the lateral epicondyle are exceedingly rare. Transcondylar fractures, although quite similar to supracondylar fractures, differ by their location within the joint capsule and their much smaller distal fracture fragment.

Anatomic Considerations

The distal humerus can be considered as two columns of bone with separate medial and lateral compartments (condyles). Each condyle has a non-articulating portion, called the epicondyle, and an articulating portion. The medial articulating portion is called the trochlea, and the lateral portion is the capitellum (see Figure 7-1, A). The coronoid fossa is a very thin section of bone that connects the two condyles. The epicondyles serve as points of origin for muscle groups of the forearm. The forearm flexors originate at the medial epicondyle, and the extensor muscle group originates at the lateral epicondyle. The epicondyles are the terminal points of the supracondylar ridges, which also serve as points of attachment for forearm muscles. The action of these various muscle groups surrounding the distal humerus results in fracture displacement and makes closed reduction more difficult.

The median nerve crosses the elbow over the anteromedial aspect, and the radial nerve courses over the anterolateral aspect of the joint. The ulnar nerve courses posterior to the medial epicondyle in the cubital tunnel. The brachial artery crosses the mid-anterior portion of the distal humerus and divides into radial and ulnar branches at the level of the proximal radial ulnar articulation (see Figure 7-10).

Fractures of the distal humerus are classified according to their location. Fractures may occur above the level of the condyles (supracondylar), at the level of the condyles (transcondylar), between the condyles with intraarticular extension (intercondylar), through the condyles (condylar), or through the epicondyles (Figure 7-13).

Supracondylar and Transcondylar Fractures

Mechanism of Injury

The vast majority of supracondylar and transcondylar fractures are of the extension type and result from a hyperextension injury to the elbow during a fall on an outstretched arm. A direct blow

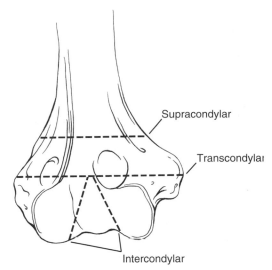

FIGURE 7-13 Distal humerus fracture locations.

to the elbow may also result in a fracture. Flexion-type fractures constitute only 2% to 4% of supracondylar fractures. Transcondylar fractures are more common in older adults, who have fragile bones.

Clinical Presentation

If the patient is seen soon after the injury, before marked swelling obscures bony landmarks of the elbow, the displaced distal fragment can often be palpated posteriorly. More commonly, the patient has significant swelling and pain, making palpation less effective. When examined, a supracondylar fracture may be confused with a posterior elbow dislocation.

A careful neurovascular examination is essential in the evaluation of supracondylar fractures because of the increased risk of brachial artery and nerve injury (see Figure 2-19). Signs of brachial artery injury include nonpalpable pulses at the wrist or cyanotic nail beds. Injury to any of the three major nerves may be associated with supracondylar fractures. Radial nerve injury is the most common. An inability to perform a thumb's up sign and decreased sensation over the dorsal web space of the thumb suggest radial nerve injury. Median nerve function is tested by performing an "OK" sign and sensory check of the palmar aspect of the index finger. An inability to spread the fingers against resistance and decreased sensation of the little finger indicate ulnar nerve injury.

Marked swelling of the forearm or palpable induration of the forearm flexors and pain on passive extension of the fingers may indicate an acute volar compartment syndrome (Volkmann's ischemia), necessitating emergency fasciotomy.

Imaging

AP and lateral views are adequate to diagnose supracondylar and transcondylar fractures. The following fracture patterns may be seen:

1. Nondisplaced: transverse fracture line seen on the AP view
2. Minimally displaced: apex anterior angulation of less than 20 degrees on the lateral view
3. Moderately displaced: medial or lateral displacement of the distal fragment
4. Markedly displaced: fracture line extends obliquely downward from the posterior humerus to the anterior humerus with the distal fragment displaced posteriorly and proximally; angulation or rotation is possible (Figure 7-14).

The anterior humeral line is useful in detecting displacement or angulation of the distal fragment (Figure 7-15). This line is drawn on the lateral radiograph along the anterior surface of the humerus through the elbow. Normally, this line transects the middle third of the capitellum. In an extension-type supracondylar fracture, the line transects the anterior third of the capitellum or falls entirely anterior to it.

Indications for Orthopedic Referral

Emergent Referral

Patients with fractures associated with limb-threatening vascular compromise should be referred to an orthopedic surgeon immediately. While awaiting consultation, patients should have long-arm posterior splint immobilization with the elbow in a position that does not impede distal blood flow.

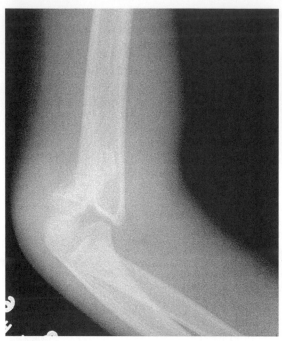

FIGURE 7-14 Displaced supracondylar fracture. The lateral view demonstrates an oblique fracture through the distal humerus with posterior displacement of the distal fragment.

Nonemergent Referral

Truly nondisplaced or minimally displaced supracondylar and transcondylar fractures without neurovascular compromise can be managed by the primary care provider. All other fractures require orthopedic management. Geriatric patients with osteopenic bone present unique challenges for the orthopedic surgeon. Fracture union, rather than motion, becomes a priority, and open reduction

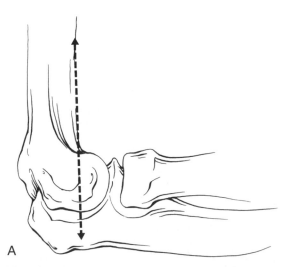

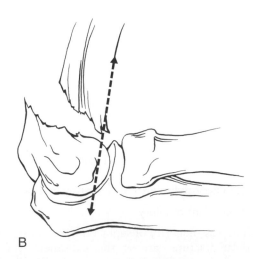

A   B

FIGURE 7-15 Anterior humeral line. **A,** Normally, this line transects the middle of the capitellum. **B,** In an extension-type supracondylar fracture, the line transects the anterior third of the capitellum or falls entirely anterior to it.

and internal fixation is often preferred to a total elbow replacement.

Initial Treatment

Table 7-3 summarizes management guidelines for nondisplaced supracondylar or transcondylar fractures of the distal humerus.

Patients with a nondisplaced supracondylar fracture should be placed in a long-arm posterior splint with the elbow in 90 degrees of flexion and the forearm in neutral rotation. The distal pulses should be checked after splint application; if the pulses are absent, the elbow should be extended to a point where they return. During the first 7 to 10 days, frequent checks of neurovascular function are necessary. The patient should be instructed to watch for signs of vascular and nerve compromise and be told to return immediately if they occur. Ice and elevation are crucial in reducing the swelling to prevent further impairment of neurovascular function. The patient should be reexamined within 24 to 48 hours.

Follow-up Care

Provided the patient has no neurovascular compromise, immobilization in a posterior splint should be continued. At 2 weeks, the patient may remove the splint while performing gentle ROM exercises, including flexion, extension, and forearm rotation. Use of the splint should be continued until adequate callus forms, usually within 6 weeks. After the splint is removed, more vigorous exercises should be performed to regain elbow motion.

Patients who fail to make gradual progress in gaining elbow motion or those who need extra assistance and supervision should be referred to a physical therapist. Repeat radiographs should be taken every week for the first 2 to 3 weeks to ensure continued fracture alignment. Orthopedic consultation is indicated if displacement occurs or if any signs of nerve or vascular injury develop.

Return to Work or Sports

Because the elbow may be immobilized for up to 6 weeks after a supracondylar fracture, an additional 1 to 3 months may be required to regain normal motion and function of the elbow. Patients can return to work as tolerated during the period of immobilization and rehabilitation as long as they are able to adapt their work activities to the restrictions imposed by a relatively weak and inflexible elbow. Work and sports activities will be limited by relative weakness of the forearm muscles caused by the injury, and activities requiring strength should be modified accordingly. Physical therapy is advisable for those who seek a more accelerated course to return to work or sports. Some loss of extension (10 to 15 degrees) is common but generally does not affect function.

Complications

Stiffness and loss of elbow motion are the most common complications after a supracondylar fracture. Minimizing the length of immobilization and assessing closely the patient's compliance and progress with rehabilitation help reduce the risk of

Table 7-3	*Management Guidelines for Nondisplaced Supracondylar or Transcondylar Fractures*
INITIAL TREATMENT	
Splint type and position	Long-arm posterior splint
	Elbow in 90 degrees of flexion, neutral forearm rotation
	Check distal pulses after splint applied
Initial follow-up visit	Within 24 to 48 hours
Patient instruction	Icing, elevation
	Carefully explain signs of neurovascular compromise
FOLLOW-UP CARE	
Cast or splint type and position	Long-arm posterior splint
	Elbow in 90 degrees of flexion, neutral forearm rotation
Length of immobilization	6 weeks or until adequate callus is present
Healing time	8 to 10 weeks to restore motion
Follow-up visit interval	Every 2 to 3 days for the first 7 to 10 days to check neurovascular status
	Every 1 to 2 weeks to assess healing and rehabilitation progress
Repeat radiography interval	Weekly for first 2 to 3 weeks; then every 2 weeks until callus is evident
Patient instruction	Gentle elbow ROM out of the splint at 2 weeks
	More active ROM exercises after splint is discontinued
	Loss of full extension expected
Indications for orthopedic consult	Neurovascular compromise
	Displaced fractures

ROM, range of motion.

a poor functional result. Neurovascular injuries may accompany the injury or may develop later. Delayed complications include Volkmann's ischemic contracture (brachial artery compromise resulting in wasting of the forearm and hand muscles), varus or valgus angulation, and nerve palsies.

Intercondylar Fractures

Mechanism of Injury

The most common cause of intercondylar fractures is a direct blow to the elbow, driving the olecranon into the distal humerus and disrupting the condyles. The position of the elbow at the time of the injury and the action of surrounding muscle groups determine the type of displacement. Intercondylar fractures are often associated with significant soft tissue injury, and open fractures may occur.

Clinical Presentation

When examined, the patient has marked soft tissue swelling and holds the forearm in pronation. Because of proximal migration of the ulna that occurs after an intercondylar fracture, the injured forearm may appear shortened. Crepitus or movement is felt when the condyles are pressed together between the thumb and index finger. Neurovascular injury is uncommon.

Imaging

By definition, all intercondylar fractures are intraarticular. The medial and lateral condyles are displaced in a **T** or **Y** configuration. T fractures have a single transverse line through the condyles, and Y fractures have two oblique lines through the humeral columns. In both of these configurations, the condyles are separated from the humeral shaft and may be rotated.

The classification criteria devised by Riseborough and Radin are most commonly used to guide the management of intercondylar fractures[13] (Figure 7-16). Four fracture types are seen:

Type I: nondisplaced between the capitellum and trochlea
Type II: separation of the capitellum and trochlea without rotation of the fragments in the frontal plane
Type III: separation of the fragments with rotation
Type IV: severe comminution of the articular surface with wide separation of the fragments

Indications for Orthopedic Referral

Type I fractures are uncommon but can be managed by primary care providers. Patients with all other types of intercondylar fractures should be referred to an orthopedic surgeon. The most important

prognostic factor for a good outcome is the degree of displacement of the intraarticular component. Cast immobilization, traction, collar and cuff sling, ORIF, and total elbow replacement are all used in the management of displaced intercondylar fractures.

Treatment

The treatment of nondisplaced intercondylar fractures is the same as outlined earlier for nondisplaced supracondylar fractures. Because the risk of neurovascular injury is much lower, the patient does not need as many follow-up visits in the first 7 to 10 days. It is still essential to advise patients about the signs of vascular and nerve compromise and instruct them to return immediately if such signs occur. The patient can be seen weekly for the first 3 weeks and every 2 weeks thereafter if healing and return of motion are proceeding as expected.

Return to Work or Sports

The guidelines for return to work or sports after an intercondylar fracture are the same as outlined for supracondylar fractures.

Complications

Complications after intercondylar fractures include loss of elbow motion (especially extension), nonunion or malunion, and symptomatic arthritis.

Condylar Fractures

Mechanism of Injury

Fractures of the lateral condyle result from an adduction and hyperextension force on the extended elbow or a direct blow over the posterior aspect of the flexed elbow. Medial condyle fractures can result from a fall on an outstretched arm with the elbow in varus position or a fall on the point of the elbow. Fractures of the lateral condyle are more common than those involving the medial condyle. Condyle fractures may be associated with fractures of both bones of the forearm.

Clinical Presentation

Patients usually seek treatment for swelling, limited ROM, and tenderness over the injured condyle. Crepitation with motion is often present. Forearm rotation accentuates the movement of the fractured lateral condyle, and elbow extension increases the movement of the medial condyle fragment. Signs of ulnar nerve injury may accompany medial condyle fractures.

Imaging

Two views of the elbow are adequate for diagnosing condylar fractures. The key to classifying fractures

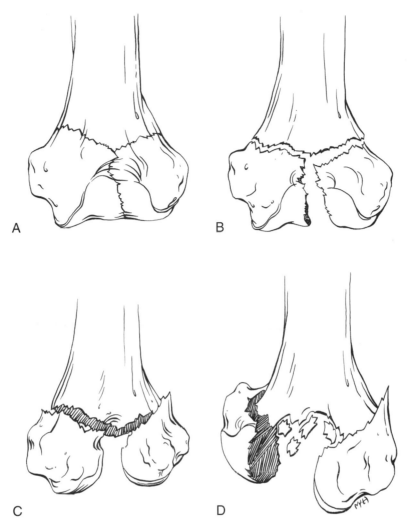

FIGURE 7-16 Intercondylar fracture types. **A,** Nondisplaced through the capitellum and trochlea. **B,** Separation of condyles without rotation. **C,** Separation with rotation. **D,** Comminuted with wide displacement.

appropriately is the position of the lateral trochlear ridge in relation to the fracture line. Fractures are classified as Milch type I or II (Figure 7-17). In type I fractures, the lateral trochlear ridge remains attached to the proximal humeral shaft, and the joint maintains mediolateral stability (Figure 7-18, A). In type II fractures, the lateral trochlear ridge is part of the fractured condyle. In these fractures, the radius and ulna may be displaced in a mediolateral direction if the collateral ligaments are torn.

Indications for Orthopedic Referral

Displaced type I fractures (Figure 7-18, B) and all type II fractures require operative treatment to restore the joint surface and normal elbow stability. Isolated fractures involving just the articular surfaces of the distal humeral condyles are extremely rare, but patients with these injuries should also

be referred to an orthopedic surgeon for open treatment.

Treatment

Aspiration of the joint hemarthrosis as described in the Clinical Presentation section for radial head fractures relieves patient discomfort. Patients with a type I nondisplaced fracture of the lateral or medial condyle should have immobilization in a long-arm posterior splint with the elbow in 90 degrees of flexion. For a lateral condyle fracture, the forearm is placed in supination and the wrist slightly extended to relieve extensor muscle forces on the fracture fragment. For a medial condyle fracture, the forearm is placed in pronation and the wrist slightly flexed to relieve the action of the muscles that originate on the medial epicondyle. Repeat radiographs should be taken every 3 to 5

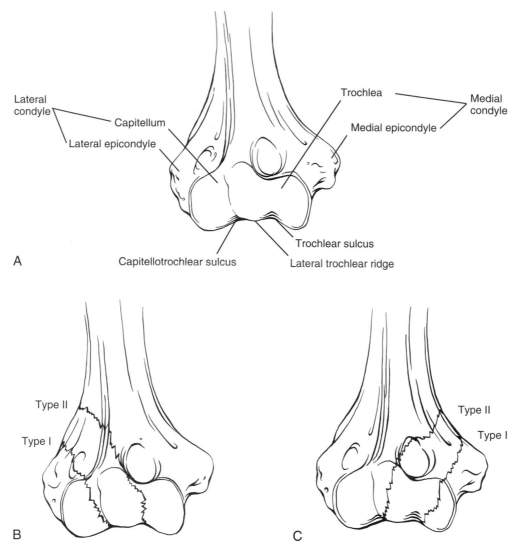

FIGURE 7-17 Milch condylar fracture types. **A,** Anterior view of the distal humerus. **B,** Lateral condyle fractures. In type I fractures, the lateral trochlear ridge remains intact. In type II fractures, the lateral trochlear ridge is a part of the fractured condyle, which may allow the radius and ulna to become displaced laterally. **C,** Medial condyle fractures. Type I fractures are stable with the lateral trochlear ridge intact. In type II fractures, the lateral trochlear ridge is a part of the fractured medial condyle, which may allow the radius and ulna to become displaced medially.

days in the first 2 weeks and then weekly thereafter to ensure that no late displacement of the fracture fragments has occurred. Orthopedic consultation should be obtained if any question about fracture alignment arises or if even slight displacement occurs.

Splint immobilization should be continued until some fracture healing is evident on the radiographs, but patients should begin gentle ROM exercises with the arm out of the splint after 2 weeks. More active motion exercises are begun after the splint is discontinued. Physical therapy may help the patient restore normal elbow function earlier or faster than a home exercise program.

Return to Work or Sports

The guidelines for returning to work or sports after a condylar fracture are the same as outlined for supracondylar fractures.

Complications

Condylar fractures may be complicated by limited joint motion, cubitus valgus (lateral condyle) or varus (medial condyle) deformity, posttraumatic arthritis, and ulnar nerve palsy.

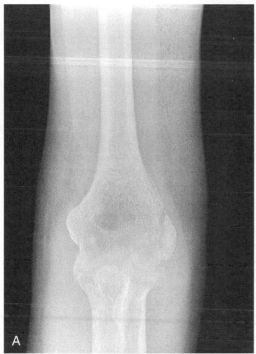

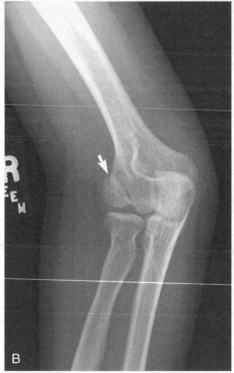

FIGURE 7-18 Type I fractures of the lateral condyle: non-displaced (**A**) and displaced (**B**) (*arrow*).

Medial Epicondyle Fractures

Mechanism of Injury

Isolated epicondylar fractures in adults are uncommon and usually result from a direct blow. Medial epicondyle fractures are much more common than lateral epicondyle fractures. In children, a medial epicondyle fracture occurs as an avulsion fracture associated with a posterior dislocation.

Clinical Presentation

Patients with a medial epicondyle fracture have localized swelling, tenderness, and crepitus over the medial epicondyle. Pain may be accentuated with elbow and wrist flexion or forearm pronation. Ulnar nerve function must be assessed because of the close proximity of the nerve to the epicondyle.

Imaging

The medial epicondyle is extracapsular, so the fat pad sign is usually absent. Fractures of the medial epicondyle may become displaced anteriorly and distally as a result of the action of the forearm flexor muscles. If the medial epicondyle can be seen in the lateral view, it is trapped within the joint.

Indications for Orthopedic Referral

Patients with displaced epicondylar fractures or those with intraarticular entrapment should be referred to an orthopedic surgeon for consideration of operative repair. Patients with evidence of ulnar nerve injury should also be referred. Closed reduction and short-term immobilization, open reduction with fixation, and excision of the fracture fragment are possible treatment options for displaced fractures.

Treatment

Patients with a nondisplaced isolated fracture of the medial epicondyle should have long-arm posterior splint immobilization with the elbow and wrist flexed and the forearm pronated. The splint is worn for 10 to 14 days, after which it is discontinued and active motion exercises are begun. Return of joint motion may take several weeks to months. Complications include limited motion, nonunion, ulnar nerve symptoms, and wrist flexor muscle weakness. Patients with nonunion associated with persistent symptoms should be referred to an orthopedist for possible excision of the fracture fragment.

DISTAL HUMERUS (PEDIATRIC)

More than half of all pediatric elbow fractures are supracondylar, and these combined with lateral condyle and medial epicondyle fractures make up more than 80% of elbow fractures in children.[14] The average age for supracondylar fractures is 5 to 8 years, and twice as many boys as girls sustain this fracture. The lateral condyle fracture is the second most common elbow fracture overall but the most common physeal elbow injury. It occurs most often in children 4 to 7 years of age. Medial epicondyle fractures make up approximately 10% of pediatric elbow fractures and occur more commonly in boys, and the typical age range is 9 to 14 years.

Anatomic Considerations

Knowledge of normal bony development and the neurovascular anatomy of the pediatric elbow are essential to recognition and treatment of elbow injuries in children. In newborns, nearly the entire elbow joint is cartilaginous (nonossified) and thus not visible on radiographs. The sequence of the process of ossification of the various growth centers can be memorized by use of the mnemonic "Come Read My Tale Of Love," which stands for the capitellum, radial head, medial epicondyle, trochlea, olecranon, and lateral epicondyle. Ossification of these growth centers occurs in a two year progression at approximately 1, 3, 5, 7, 9, and 11 years of age, respectively.

The brachial artery courses superficial to the brachialis muscle along the anteromedial aspect of the humerus. This artery is especially prone to injury after a supracondylar fracture with posteromedial displacement of the fragments. Additionally, the brachial artery may be tethered to the sharp edge of the proximal fracture fragment, thereby increasing the risk of brachial artery injury during movement of the injured arm or fracture manipulation. Fortunately, because of the extensive collateral circulation present at the elbow, it is rare for ischemia of the arm to occur from complete occlusion of the brachial artery.

Because of their close proximity, median nerve injury often accompanies brachial artery impingement (see Figure 7-10).

The radial nerve runs between the brachialis and brachioradialis muscles before crossing the elbow and penetrating the supinator muscle. The ulnar nerve crosses the elbow posterior to the medial epicondyle. The median and radial nerves are at risk of injury after supracondylar fractures after elbow hyperextension. The ulnar nerve is susceptible to injury when a supracondylar fracture with elbow hyperflexion or a direct blow to the posterior aspect of the elbow occurs.

Clinical Presentation

Important aspects of the clinical examination of children with elbow injuries include careful observation of the child's movement of the injured arm,

a thorough neurovascular examination, and a complete examination of the wrist and shoulder to detect associated injuries. Very young children are unable to give a history or tell the location or character of their symptoms. Active or passive ROM testing should be delayed until radiographs are obtained to rule out a displaced fracture. The vascular examination should include palpation of the brachial and radial pulses (injured and uninjured limb) and an assessment of capillary refill in the fingers. Pain in the forearm rather than the elbow, pain with passive finger extension, and a cool hand are signs of vascular insufficiency. A Doppler ultrasound study should be ordered if any doubt exists about the integrity of the blood supply. The following maneuvers test the integrity of nerve motor function while minimizing elbow movement to prevent injury from displaced fragments:

- "OK" sign: median nerve (anterior interosseus nerve branch)
- Thumb's up sign: radial nerve
- Finger spread against resistance: ulnar nerve

An examination of the following sites, using two point discrimination will evaluate peripheral nerve sensation:

- Palmar aspect of index finger: median nerve
- Thumb dorsal web space: radial nerve
- Little finger: ulnar nerve

In addition to a careful neurovascular examination, the elbow should be closely inspected for any break in the skin that might indicate an open fracture.

Imaging

Before obtaining radiographs, the practitioner should immobilize the elbow with medial and lateral splints to prevent potential injury from sharp fracture fragments during positioning for the radiographs. The best position for splinting is with the elbow flexed 20 to 30 degrees ("splint it where it lies"), which places the least tension on neurovascular structures. Initial AP and lateral views to diagnose a displaced fracture can be obtained in this position. Both elbow and forearm views should be obtained because forearm fractures can accompany supracondylar fractures. Definitive radiographs in the proper positions can be obtained after this initial screen after the patient is more comfortable and has received appropriate acute treatment.

Fractures and displacement of nonossified portions of the elbow are difficult to detect radiographically. Comparison views and additional oblique views are especially helpful in evaluating pediatric elbow injuries. Knowledge of some basic landmarks on the lateral view is essential when reviewing elbow radiographs. The anterior humeral line, drawn parallel to the anterior edge of the humerus, should course through the middle third of the capitellum (Figure 7-15). The radiocapitellar line, drawn through the axis of the radial shaft, points directly to the capitellum in all views. Disruption of these normal anatomic relationships indicates a displaced fracture. The fracture line may not be apparent in a nondisplaced supracondylar fracture, and a positive fat pad sign may be the only clue to an occult fracture[15] (see Figure 7-4).

Supracondylar Fractures

Mechanism of Injury

The weakest part of the elbow joint is the supracondylar area where the humerus flattens and flares. Children are more susceptible than adults to fractures in this location, because the hypermobile joint capsule allows the elbow to hyperextend during a fall on an outstretched arm. The most common type of supracondylar fracture is the extension type in which the hyperextended position drives the olecranon into the supracondylar portion of the humerus, resulting in a fracture. The nondominant arm is most commonly injured.

Clinical Presentation

Children with a supracondylar fracture have marked pain and swelling of the elbow with obvious deformity of the elbow joint if the fracture is significantly displaced. Nondisplaced fractures may have minimal swelling. Injury of the median, radial, or anterior interosseous nerve is possible, so careful testing of motor and sensory function is essential (as described above). Nerve injury after a supracondylar fracture is usually a temporary neurapraxia that disappears within 2 to 3 months.[16] The brachial artery is at risk of injury from the displaced fracture fragments, but vascular injury requiring surgical intervention is rare. Patients with normal initial neurovascular examination results warrant regular repeated evaluation, especially after movement of the affected extremity, splinting, or fracture reduction. Compartment syndrome of the forearm can complicate this fracture especially when a forearm fracture is also present. The clinician must be alert to the signs of increasing pressure such as unrelenting pain, severe swelling, and paresthesia.

Imaging

Supracondylar fractures in children are classified as type I (nondisplaced or minimally displaced), type II (displaced distal fragment with an intact posterior cortex), or type III (displaced with no contact between fragments). The anterior humeral line is abnormal in the vast majority of even minimally displaced supracondylar fractures (Figure 7-19). Displaced supracondylar fractures are easily seen on the lateral view (Figure 7-20).

Treatment

Emergent consultation (within 30 to 60 minutes) with an orthopedic surgeon should be obtained for any child with signs of vascular insufficiency or acute compartment syndrome. In addition, prompt orthopedic referral is indicated for type II or III fractures, fractures with neurovascular compromise, and open fractures. Most supracondylar fractures in children need surgical intervention because most are displaced. Nondisplaced (type I) fractures are immobilized initially in a sugar tong splint with the forearm in neutral rotation and the elbow at 90 degrees for 5 to 7 days followed by 2 weeks in a long-arm cast with the same arm positioning. Radiographs at 3 weeks after injury should reveal callus formation in the supracondylar area. At this point, the cast is discontinued, and active ROM exercises should be started. Less than optimal healing is more likely in cases of incomplete reduction, severe displacement, and extensive soft tissue damage. Supracondylar fractures can be complicated by malunion, most commonly a varus angulation of the elbow with loss of full extension (gun stock deformity). This rarely creates a functional impairment but may be of cosmetic concern.

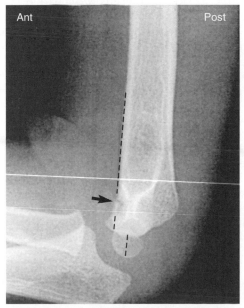

FIGURE 7-19 An incomplete supracondylar fracture (*arrow*). Note the posterior displacement of the capitellum from the anterior humeral line. Often this is the only clue to the presence of a supracondylar fracture. (*From Mettler FA Jr. Essentials of Radiology. Philadelphia, WB Saunders, 1996.*)

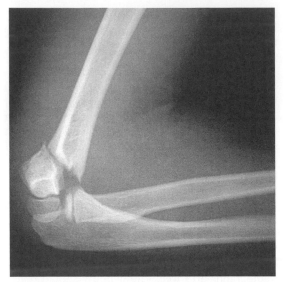

FIGURE 7-20 Supracondylar fracture in a skeletally immature individual (open physes). The lateral view demonstrates an oblique fracture through the distal humerus with posterior displacement of the distal fragment, anterior displacement of the humeral shaft, and apex anterior angulation.

Vascular injury and primary swelling from the injury can lead to the development of compartment syndrome within 12 to 24 hours, which may progress to Volkmann's ischemic contracture if not treated in a timely manner. This is characterized by fixed flexion of the elbow, pronation of the forearm, flexion at the wrist, and joint extension of the metacarpal–phalangeal joint.

Lateral Condyle Fractures

Wrist extensor muscles and the lateral collateral ligament attach to the lateral condyle. With a fall on an outstretched hand combined with a varus force, the lateral condyle may be avulsed. Patients report lateral elbow pain and swelling and decreased ROM. The most characteristic finding is localized swelling over the lateral distal humerus. In contrast to supracondylar fractures, neurovascular injury rarely complicates these fractures. The most common pattern is a Milch type II fracture in which the fracture line begins in the distal humeral metaphysis and extends just medial to the capitellar physis into the joint (Figure 7-21). In this type of fracture, there is potential elbow instability because the radius and ulna can displace laterally with the fragment. See Figure 7-17 for a description of the Milch classification of condylar fractures.

Because the fracture is intraarticular, open reduction is required to restore normal alignment in displaced fractures. Nondisplaced or minimally displaced (<2 mm) fractures can be treated acutely

with a posterior splint with the forearm in neutral position and the elbow at 90 degrees. To look for any displacement, the practitioner should order repeat radiographs to be taken in 3 to 5 days with the arm out of the splint and the elbow in full extension. If the fracture remains nondisplaced, the splint is reapplied, and radiographs are repeated in another 3 to 5 days. If no displacement is apparent, a long-arm cast should be applied for 3 weeks or until radiographic healing is evident. Close follow-up with weekly radiographs is essential because of the potential for late displacement in these fractures. Six to 12 weeks of immobilization is typical for clinical healing to occur. Growth arrest and nonunion are the most common complications and can result in a cubitus varus or valgus deformity. Cubitus valgus deformity can cause a late ulnar nerve palsy resulting from overstretching.

Medial Epicondyle Fractures

The medial epicondyle is the point of insertion of the forearm flexors and the ulnar collateral ligament. After a fall on an outstretched hand with valgus stress, a tear in the collateral ligament may occur in adults, but the relatively weaker medial epicondyle in children may avulse. Injuries resulting from a fall are often associated with an elbow dislocation with a spontaneous relocation. The

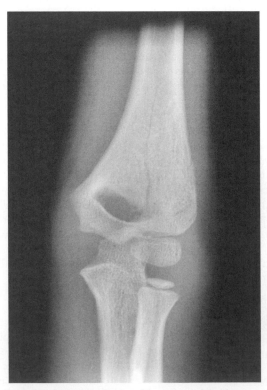

FIGURE 7-21 Nondisplaced lateral condylar fracture.

ulnar nerve lies just posterior to the epicondyle and can be injured if the fracture fragment becomes displaced. If the elbow is dislocated, the avulsed bony fragment can be dislodged and become trapped in the joint. Patients with these injuries should be referred to an orthopedic surgeon because of the increased likelihood of elbow instability and the possibility of ulnar nerve damage and bony fragments in the joint. If the elbow has not been dislocated and no ulnar nerve injury is apparent, nondisplaced medial epicondyle fractures can be treated with 2 to 3 weeks of immobilization in a posterior elbow splint (neutral forearm). Joint stiffness can be avoided by starting early ROM exercises out of the splint (once or twice daily for 10 to 15 minutes) within the first week after injury.

Little League Elbow

Little League elbow, or pitcher's elbow, is the term for a group of elbow overuse stress injuries in young athletes who throw. Medial symptoms are caused by repetitive valgus extension overload on the elbow. This excessive tension can result in a traction apophysitis of the medial epicondyle, a medial epicondyle avulsion fracture (Figure 7-22), and compression of the lateral structures (radial head and capitellum), resulting in osteochondritis dissecans (OCD). Medial epicondyle apophysitis occurs generally during childhood, and adolescents are at greater risk of an avulsion fracture or OCD. Risk factors for elbow injuries are regularly pitching with arm fatigue, competitively pitching for more than 8 months a year, and averaging more

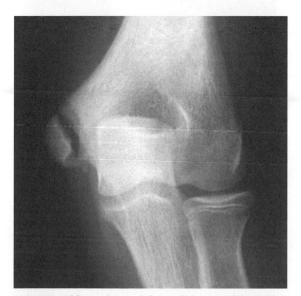

FIGURE 7-22 Avulsion of the medial epicondyle in association with a throwing injury in an adolescent. (*From Mercier LR. Practical Orthopedics, 5th ed. St. Louis, Mosby, 2000.*)

than 80 pitches per appearance.[17] The American Academy of Pediatrics recommends that measures should be used to prevent these injuries in young pitchers, including restriction of the amount of pitching (e.g., limiting pitches per game, months per year spent pitching); instruction in proper throwing techniques; avoidance of pitching when the arm hurts or is fatigued; and education of coaches, parents, and children about early warning signs.[18]

The usual symptoms are pain, popping, or giving way when the person throws. Young patients may not seek care until they are unable to throw because of the pain. Examination of the elbow reveals point tenderness over the medial epicondyle and pain with resisted flexion and pronation. No radiographic changes are associated with medial apophysitis. Avulsion of the medial epicondyle can be difficult to diagnose on radiographs unless it is widely displaced. Comparison views of the uninjured elbow may help. Magnetic resonance imaging may be necessary to detect OCD.

Treatment of medial apophysitis always involves complete rest from throwing until the elbow tenderness disappears (usually 3 to 6 weeks). A minimally displaced (<2 mm) medial epicondyle avulsion fracture is treated with a posterior elbow splint for 4 to 6 weeks. The patient should be referred to an orthopedic surgeon if the apophysis is more widely displaced. Early ROM exercises out of the splint can be started after the patient can perform them without pain (typically 1 to 2 weeks). If OCD is present, the joint may have to be protected for several months to allow the joint surfaces to heal and to prevent the formation of a loose body. If a loose body is present, surgical removal is indicated.

After treatment, return to throwing should be accomplished through a planned progressive rehabilitation program. Prevention is the key to management of Little Leaguer's elbow. Limiting pitching to approximately 100 pitches per game or practice is a sensible guideline for coaches to follow to protect their young players from overuse injury. Teaching young players proper pitching techniques to prevent excessive valgus stress may also reduce this overuse injury of the elbow.

ELBOW DISLOCATION

The elbow is the third most common location for a dislocation after dislocations of the shoulder and fingers. Elbow dislocations occur in a young active population and are often associated with sports injuries. Elbow dislocations are classified according to the position of the ulna relative to the humerus after injury (Figure 7-23). Posterior dislocations are more common than anterior ones. Pure lateral or

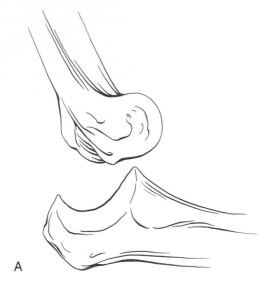

A

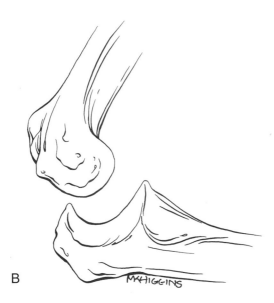

B   M K HIGGINS

FIGURE 7-23 Posterior (A) and anterior (B) elbow dislocations.

medial dislocations are rare. The usual cause of a posterior elbow dislocation is a fall on an out-stretched arm with the elbow hyperextended. Varus or valgus stress at the elbow at the time of injury may cause medial or lateral displacement of the radius and ulna. Anterior dislocations occur after a blow to the posterior forearm with the elbow flexed, which drives the olecranon forward.

Commonly associated injuries include brachial artery injury and nerve injury. Damage to the median, ulnar, and radial nerves has been reported after elbow dislocations. Radial nerve injury is rare. The median nerve may be stretched or become entrapped within the joint. Valgus displacement puts the ulnar nerve at risk for injury. It is imperative that the neurovascular status of the patient's hand and forearm be assessed before and after any attempt at reduction.

Patients with a posterior dislocation usually report severe pain with a foreshortened forearm held in flexion and prominent olecranon posteriorly. Swelling and deformity are apparent, and the elbow may appear similar to that seen after a supracondylar fracture. After an anterior dislocation, the arm is shortened, and the forearm is elongated and supinated. The patient usually holds the arm in full extension. AP and lateral radiographs of the elbow confirm a suspected dislocation. Radiographs should be examined closely for the presence of associated fractures, especially those involving the medial epicondyle or coronoid process (Figure 7-24).

Because of the increased risk of arterial or nerve injury, closed reduction of an elbow dislocation must be performed promptly. If orthopedic consultation is not immediately available, the primary care provider should attempt reduction.

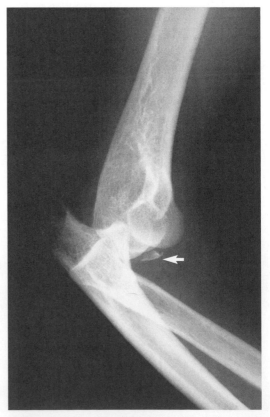

FIGURE 7-24 Posterior dislocation of the elbow with a small fracture fragment (*arrow*). The donor site could not be determined from the plain films but is probably from the medial epicondyle or the coronoid process.

Posterior Dislocation: Closed Reduction

Reduction is performed after administration of intravenous sedation and analgesia to achieve adequate pain relief and muscle relaxation. The simplest reduction maneuver involves countertraction on the humerus (posterior pressure from the front) while longitudinal traction is applied on the wrist and forearm. Distal traction is continued as the elbow is flexed. Downward pressure on the proximal forearm may be needed to disengage the coronoid from the olecranon fossa. If this method fails, the patient should be placed in a prone position with the elbow hanging off the side of the stretcher or table. A small pillow or rolled towel should be placed under the humerus just proximal to the elbow joint. A 5- or 10-lb weight is then hung from the wrist or gentle longitudinal traction is applied. After several minutes, the elbow dislocation should become reduced. Forward pressure on the olecranon may be necessary to accomplish reduction in this position.

Anterior Dislocation: Closed Reduction

The method of closed reduction of an anterior dislocation is essentially the reverse of the maneuver for a posterior dislocation. After the muscles are adequately relaxed, posterior and downward pressure is applied to the forearm while anterior pressure from behind is applied to the distal humerus.

Postreduction Follow-up

After reduction for either a posterior or an anterior dislocation, the elbow should be gently flexed and extended to test the stability of the joint and ensure that no mechanical block to motion exists. Documenting the neurovascular examination is essential. Postreduction radiographs should be closely examined for any associated fractures. The elbow should be immobilized in a posterior splint with the elbow in 90 degrees of flexion, and the patient should be referred to an orthopedic surgeon within 2 to 3 days. The patient should be made aware of the signs of neurovascular compromise or compartment syndrome and told to return immediately if they occur.

REFERENCES

1. van Riet RP, Morrey BF, O'Driscoll SW, Van Glabbeek F. Associated injuries complicating radial head fractures: a demographic study. *Clin Orthop Relat Res.* 2005;441:351-355.
2. O'Dwyer H, O'Sullivan P, Fitzgerald D. The fat pad sign following elbow trauma in adults: its usefulness and reliability in suspecting occult fracture. *J Comput Assist Tomogr.* 2004;28:562-565.
3. Mason ML. Some observations on fractures of the head of the radius with a review of one hundred cases. *Br J Surg.* 1954;42:123-132.
4. Johnston GW. A follow-up of one hundred cases of fracture of the head of the radius with a review of the literature. *Ulster Med J.* 1962;31:51-56.
5. Akesson T, Herbertsson P, Josefsson PO. Primary nonoperative treatment of moderately displaced two-part fractures of the radial head. *J Bone Joint Surg [Am].* 2006;88(suppl A):1909-1914.
6. Dooley JF, Angus PD. The importance of elbow aspiration when treating radial head fractures. *Arch Emerg Med.* 1991;8:117-121.
7. Schunk JE. Radial head subluxation: epidemiology and treatment of 87 episodes. *Ann Emerg Med.* 1990; 19(9):1019-1023.
8. Krul M, van der Wouden JC, van Suijlekom-Smit LW, Koes BW. Manipulative interventions for reducing pulled elbow in young children. *Cochrane Database Syst Rev.* 2009;7(4):CD007759.
9. Hak DJ, Golladay GJ: Olecranon fractures: treatment options. *J Am Acad Orthop Surg.* 2000;8:266-275.
10. Adams JE, Hoskin TL, Morrey BF, Steinmann SP. Management and outcome of 103 acute fractures of the coronoid process of the ulna. *J Bone Joint Surg [Br].* 2009;91(suppl B):632-635.
11. Regan W, Morrey BF. Classification and treatment of coronoid process fractures. *Orthopedics.* 1992;15:845-848.
12. Pollock JW, Faber KJ, Athwal GS. Distal humerus fractures. *Orthop Clin North Am.* 2008;39:187-200.
13. Riseborough EJ, Radin EL. Intercondylar "T" fractures of the humerus in the adult: a comparison of operative and nonoperative treatment in twenty-nine cases. *J Bone Joint Surg.* 1969;51A:130-141.
14. Lins RE, Simovitch RW, Waters PM. Pediatric elbow trauma. *Orthop Clin North Am.* 1999;30(1):119-132.
15. Skaggs DL, Mirzayan R. The posterior fat pad sign in association with occult fracture of the elbow in children. *J Bone Joint Surg (Am).* 1999;81:1429-1433.
16. Villarin LA, Belk KE, Freid R. Emergency department evaluation and treatment of elbow and forearm injuries. *Emerg Med Clin North Am.* 1999;17(4):843-848.
17. Olsen SJ, Fleisig GS, Dun S, Loftice J, Andrews JR. Risk factors for shoulder and elbow injuries in adolescent baseball pitchers. *Am J Sports Med.* 2006;34(6):905-912.
18. American Academy of Pediatrics. Committee on Sports Medicine and Fitness. Risk of injury from baseball and softball in children 5 to 14 years of age. *Pediatrics.* 2001;107(4):782-784.

8

HUMERUS FRACTURES

Humerus fractures constitute 2% to 4% of the fractures encountered in primary care and are relatively uncommon in children and young adults. When they do occur in these age groups, fractures generally result from severe trauma, and most often involve the distal humerus. As patients age, the incidence of humerus fractures increases dramatically. Proximal fractures predominate among older patients and are usually associated with osteoporosis and less severe trauma. Certain humerus fractures, primarily proximal fractures, have relatively few complications and thus are commonly managed by primary care providers.

This chapter discusses proximal and midshaft fractures. Accurate assessment, guidelines for referral, and management of more straightforward humerus fractures are emphasized. Fractures of the distal humerus are discussed separately in Chapter 7.

ANATOMIC CONSIDERATIONS

Several nerves and arteries lie close to the humerus. These may be damaged at the time of injury or during manipulation of the fracture. The axillary nerve and artery, posterior brachial plexus, and radial nerve are most prone to injury. Fortunately, such injuries are unusual unless considerable displacement is present.[1] The relationship of these structures to the proximal humerus is shown in Figures 8-1 and 8-2. Lower on the humerus, the neurovascular bundle runs along the medial border of the biceps. The radial nerve is in close proximity to the humerus shaft at the junction of the middle and distal thirds of this bone. Thus, angulated fractures of the distal third of the shaft often injure this nerve. A displaced shaft fracture with anterior angulation may damage the median or ulnar nerve.

The proximal humerus is divided into four sections: the anatomic neck (widened articular surface of the humeral head), surgical neck (constriction distal to the humeral head and tuberosities), greater tuberosity (superior aspect of the humeral head), and lesser tuberosity (anterior aspect of the humerus).

Fractures of the proximal humerus may disrupt the blood supply to the humerus head. Branches of the axillary artery enter the humerus distal to the anatomic neck and travel proximally to supply the head. Fractures of the anatomic neck often disrupt these vessels and are at high risk for avascular necrosis (AVN) of the humerus head. Displaced fractures of the proximal humerus may cause injury to the axillary or suprascapular nerve.

A number of tendons insert on or pass over the proximal humerus. The four rotator cuff tendons insert near the humerus head. The supraspinatus, infraspinatus, and teres minor muscles insert on the greater tuberosity, and the subscapularis inserts on the lesser tuberosity. Up to 40% of patients with a proximal humerus fracture may have an associated rotator cuff tendon tear.[2] The tendon of the long head of the biceps passes through the bicipital groove on the anterior aspect of the proximal humerus. The action of the rotator cuff muscles can displace bone fragments. Fractures through the bicipital groove occasionally lead to future problems by interfering with the function of the long head tendon.

PROXIMAL HUMERUS FRACTURES (ADULT)

Proximal humerus fractures make up 4% to 5% of all fractures.[3] Approximately 75% of proximal humerus fractures occur in those older than the age of 60 years, and they are three times more common in women because of their greater risk of altered bone density.[4,5]

Mechanism of Injury

Most proximal humerus fractures result from a fall onto an outstretched hand. This mechanism is especially common in older adults. Direct blows, such as falling onto the shoulder, are another common cause. Violent muscle contractions, such as those produced by seizures, may also fracture the humerus.

Clinical Presentation

Patients with proximal humerus fractures generally complain of diffuse shoulder pain, which may be

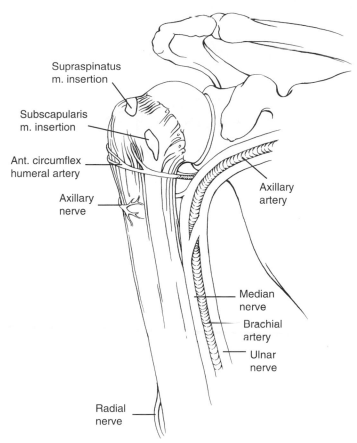

Supraspinatus
m. insertion

Subscapularis
m. insertion

Ant. circumflex
humeral artery

Axillary
nerve

Axillary
artery

Median
nerve

Brachial
artery

Ulnar
nerve

Radial
nerve

FIGURE 8-1 Anterior view of the proximal humerus.

considerable. They tend to hold the injured arm against the side and resist movement. In most cases, swelling develops early, and by the second or third day, a large ecchymosis may be apparent. The fracture site is usually point tender, but overlying structures and diffuse swelling make the fracture difficult to pinpoint during examination. Gross deformity of the shoulder and drooping of the arm are rarely caused by an isolated fracture; they suggest the presence of a dislocation.

A check of neurovascular status should be performed, including peripheral pulses and nerve function. Although it is difficult to distinguish muscle weakness caused by nerve injury from that caused by pain in the acute stages, the clinician should be on the lookout for injury to the axillary nerve (i.e., deltoid muscle weakness, decreased sensation over the mid-deltoid region). Injury to the suprascapular nerve results in weakness of the subscapularis muscle (internal rotation weakness).

Differential Diagnosis

Although the signs and symptoms of a shoulder dislocation may be similar to those of a proximal fracture, shoulder deformity or drooping is often evident in dislocations. Two views of the shoulder (anteroposterior [AP] and either a transscapular or axillary view) will confirm a dislocation by revealing that the humeral head has lost its normal relationship to the glenoid fossa (Figure 8-3). A more detailed discussion of shoulder dislocations, including additional radiographic examples, is presented at the end of this chapter.

Rotator cuff tears may also be difficult to differentiate clinically from fractures. However, radiographs of patients with rotator cuff tears are normal unless a fragment of bone was avulsed along with the tendon. Acromioclavicular (AC) separations also produce pain and decreased mobility of the shoulder, but tenderness is localized to the AC joint in these injuries.

Imaging

Shoulder Radiography

Most shoulder series include two AP views with the upper arm in internal and external rotation. These views alone are often insufficient to identify or adequately characterize proximal humerus fractures. Furthermore, patients with fractures generally resist rotation of the humerus, making it

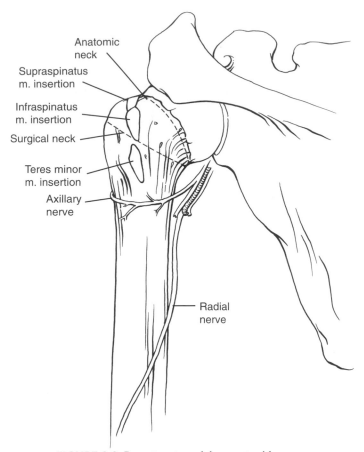

- Anatomic neck
- Supraspinatus m. insertion
- Infraspinatus m. insertion
- Surgical neck
- Teres minor m. insertion
- Axillary nerve
- Radial nerve

FIGURE 8-2 Posterior view of the proximal humerus.

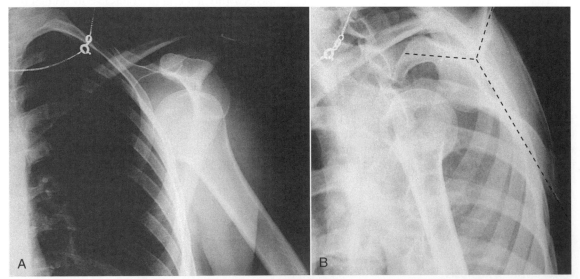

FIGURE 8-3 Anteroposterior (**A**) and transscapular or "Y (**B**) views showing an anterior dislocation of the humerus. On the transcapular view, note that the scapula resembles a "Y" (*dashed lines*). The humeral head should overlie the branch point of the "Y." Note that it instead lies anterior and inferior to this point. See Figure 8-4, B, for an example of the normal positioning of the humerus.

impossible to obtain two views at 90 degrees in this way. A trauma series is the preferred way to assess this region (Figure 8-4). Alternatively, a standard shoulder series augmented with either a transscapular or an axillary view is often adequate to rule out significant displacement and dislocation. A computed tomography (CT) scan is recommended if the plain radiographs are difficult to interpret or to delineate the extent of displacement to aid in preoperative planning.

Fracture Patterns

The majority of proximal humerus fractures are impacted and have little or no displacement or angulation. Frequently, multiple fragments are present. The most common fracture sites are the surgical neck and greater tuberosity. Lesser tuberosity fractures are uncommon, and anatomic neck fractures are rare.

Because proximal fractures may have a combination of elements, a wide variety of fracture patterns can occur. Several classification systems have been used to describe these often complicated patterns. These systems stratify fractures by risk and can be used to guide therapy.

The Neer system can be valuable in selecting fractures appropriate for primary care management.[6,7] Although the parameters were selected somewhat arbitrarily, the Neer classification has withstood the test of time and is still the most widely used. It is based on accurate identification of the four major fragments of the proximal humerus and how many of these fragments are displaced. The four fragments described in the Neer classification are the greater tuberosity, lesser tuberosity, head, and shaft (Figure 8-5). Most primary care providers are likely to manage only Neer one-part fractures, which include all nondisplaced proximal fractures. Regardless of the number of cleavage lines, fractures are classified as nondisplaced if no segment is displaced more than 1 cm or angulated more than 45 degrees. If all of the fracture fragments are nondisplaced, the injury is considered to be a one-part fracture because the fragments are in continuity and are held together by soft tissue. Examples of Neer one-part fractures are shown in Figures 8-6 to 8-8.

Approximately 50% of proximal humerus fractures are one-part or minimally displaced fractures.[3,8,9] The remaining proximal humerus fractures are significantly displaced and are classified as two-part, three-part, or four-part fractures. If one fragment is displaced or angulated from the remaining intact proximal humerus according to the criteria previously stated, the injury is classified as a two-part fracture. If two fragments are individually

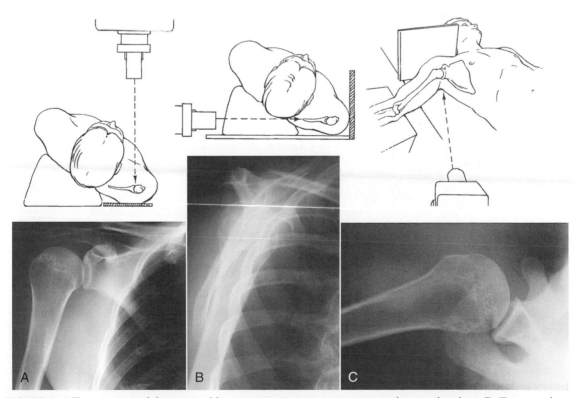

FIGURE 8-4 Trauma series of the proximal humerus. **A,** Anteroposterior view in the scapular plane. **B,** Transscapular or "Y" view. **C,** Axillary view.

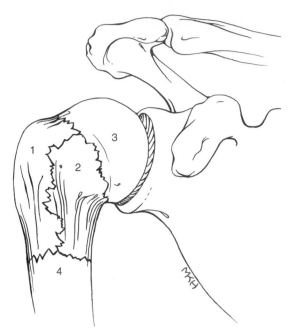

FIGURE 8-5 The four parts of the proximal humerus referred to in the Neer classification: 1, greater tuberosity; 2, lesser tuberosity; 3, head; and 4, shaft.

displaced from the proximal humerus but the humeral head remains in contact with the glenoid, it is considered a three-part fracture. Four-part fractures have three or more displaced fragments combined with the humeral head dislocated from the glenoid. Familiarity with the Neer system can help the primary care provider correctly identify proximal humerus fractures and improve communication with orthopedists at the time of referral.

Indications for Orthopedic Referral

Emergency referral is indicated for open fractures and those with neurovascular compromise. Patients with fractures that involve the anatomic neck should also be referred to an orthopedic surgeon because of the high risk of AVN.

Although systematic reviews comparing nonoperative and operative treatment of displaced fractures have found insufficient evidence to determine the optimal intervention for these fractures, treatment decisions for displaced fractures (two, three, and four part) should be left to the orthopedic surgeon.[10,11] If the fracture is determined to be stable by the surgeon (i.e., acceptable cortical contact between the shaft and head fragments and minimal tuberosity displacement), nonoperative treatment can lead to good outcomes.[12]

Somewhat surprisingly, patients often tolerate proximal humerus angulation of 25 to 45 degrees with minimal adverse effect on shoulder and arm function. This is largely the result of the extreme mobility of the shoulder joint, which is able to compensate well for angulation. Patients who are athletic or very active are less likely to tolerate the angulation. For such patients, consultation may be advisable whenever angulation approaches or exceeds 20 degrees. Consultation should also be considered when fractures involve the bicipital groove, because fractures in this area may interfere with proper functioning of the tendon of the long head of the biceps.

Initial Treatment

Table 8-1 summarizes management guidelines for proximal humerus fractures.

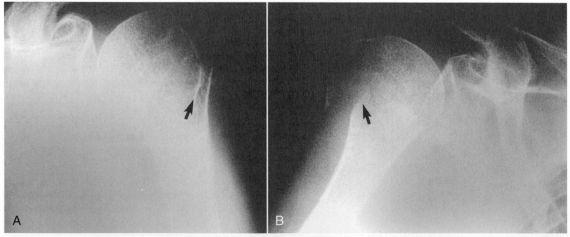

FIGURE 8-6 A, Slightly impacted fracture of the surgical neck is seen (*arrow*). **B,** A minimally distracted greater tuberosity fragment is also apparent (*arrow*). Although three fragments are involved, this is a Neer one-part fracture because no fragment is angulated more than 45 degrees or displaced more than 1 cm.

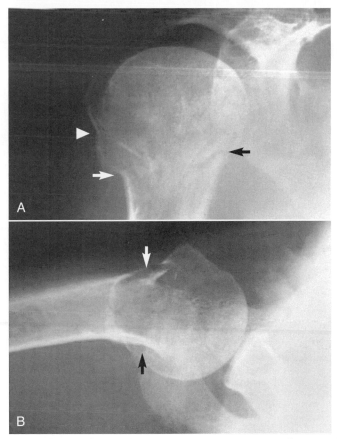

FIGURE 8-7 One-part surgical neck fracture (*arrows*). **A,** Anteroposterior view. **B,** Axillary view. (*From Browner BD, Jupiter JB, Levine AM, Trafton PG [eds]. Skeletal Trauma, vol 2. Philadelphia, WB Saunders, 1992.*)

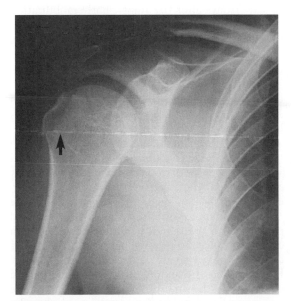

FIGURE 8-8 Nondisplaced avulsion fracture of the greater tuberosity (Neer one-part fracture) (*arrow*). If the avulsed fragment had been displaced more than 1 cm, this would have been classified as a two-part fracture.

Immobilization can be achieved with either a standard shoulder sling or a collar and cuff sling (Figure 8-9). Casting is not required for these fractures. The collar and cuff sling is superior for angulated fractures because the unsupported weight of the elbow may improve the degree of angulation via downward traction. A sling is preferred when disimpaction of the fragments would be undesirable such as in fractures with minimal angulation and minimal displacement. Ice and narcotic analgesics are usually required for pain relief. Patients may be more comfortable sleeping in a semi-recumbent position with adequate support under the arm.

For a patient being referred to an orthopedist, a sling and swath or shoulder immobilizer can be used to stabilize the shoulder until the patient can receive definitive care.

Follow-up Care

Impacted proximal humerus fractures with minimal angulation and displacement are generally very stable, and conservative treatment yields good

Table 8-1	*Management Guidelines for Proximal Humerus Fractures*
	INITIAL TREATMENT
Splint type and position	If referring, sling and swath (only for a limited time)
	Standard sling if there is minimal angulation or displacement
	Collar and cuff sling if >20 degrees of angulation is present
Initial follow-up visit	3 to 7 days to assess symptoms and begin ROM
Patient instruction	Wrist and finger ROM
	FOLLOW-UP CARE
Cast or splint type and position	If referring, sling and swath (only for a limited time)
	Standard sling if there is minimal angulation or displacement
	Collar and cuff sling if >20 degrees of angulation is present
Length of immobilization	2 to 4 weeks
	After 2 weeks, remove sling for part of the day
Healing time	6 to 8 weeks
Follow-up visit interval	Every 2 weeks until satisfactory function is regained
Repeat radiography interval	Consider at 1 to 2 weeks if the patient is unable to initiate ROM exercises (to rule out a change in fragment position)
	At 4 to 6 weeks to assess healing
Patient instruction	ROM exercises are crucial to regaining function
	Shoulder ROM as soon as tolerated
	Elbow ROM whenever the sling is removed
	After the sling is discontinued, aggressive ROM and strengthening exercises
Indications for orthopedic consult	Displaced Neer types (two-, three-, and four-part fractures)
	Neurovascular injury or open fracture
	Significant distortion of bicipital groove
	Fracture dislocation

ROM, range of motion.

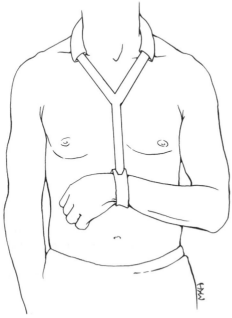

FIGURE 8-9 Collar and cuff sling. Note that the elbow is unsupported, producing some downward traction on the proximal humerus.

outcomes.[8,13] Healing is usually rapid owing to the large areas of impacted cancellous bone. The goal of treatment is to restore as much function as possible; thus, mobilization is begun as early as pain allows. In most patients, this can be done as early as 5 to 7 days after the injury. Early mobilization is associated with improved pain and mobility in the early phases and achieves results in the long term similar to those with treatment that includes longer periods of immobilization.[14,15]

The patient should return for follow-up within the first week after injury. After assessment of symptoms, the importance and safety of early mobilization should be discussed. During the follow-up visit, pendulum exercises performed with the sling in place (Figure 8-10) should be demonstrated and the patient encouraged to gently attempt them. Capable patients should be encouraged to begin home exercises, which can produce results similar to physical therapy in selected patients who are carefully instructed. Pendulum exercises should be repeated two or three times a day with progressively larger arm circles made. Patients who are unable to perform pendulum exercises at the first follow-up visit should be encouraged to initiate them at home during the upcoming week and then be evaluated again in 4 to 7 days. An inability to perform the exercises at that time should prompt reassessment of the injury

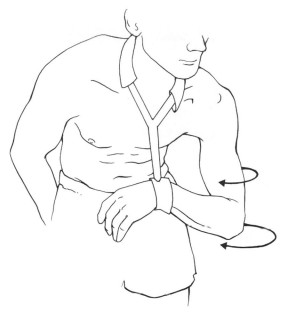

FIGURE 8-10 Pendulum exercises. The patient should bend forward at the waist and draw circles with the elbow, starting with small circles and progressing to larger circles. Circles should be drawn in both clockwise and counterclockwise directions.

and consideration of repeat radiography. If an associated injury or significant displacement or angulation is suspected, orthopedic consultation is desirable. Otherwise, referral to a physical therapist is probably necessary to assist the patient in regaining adequate function of the shoulder and arm.

Patients able to initiate home exercises can be reevaluated approximately 2 weeks after injury. At that point, the patient should be encouraged to go without the sling for most of the day and to begin elbow range of motion (ROM) exercises. Shoulder rehabilitation to restore mobility and strength should be done two or three times per day. Whenever possible, the patient should use the injured arm for activities of daily living. The sling should be discontinued completely 2 to 4 weeks after the injury. The rehabilitation progresses from pendulum exercises in the first 2 weeks to light functional exercises without resistance in weeks 2 to 6 (e.g., placing the hand on the wall in a seated position, lying on the side and externally rotating the arm) and then active strengthening with resistance bands and weights thereafter. Go to Expert Consult for the electronic version of a patient instruction handout for shoulder rehabilitation after a fracture.

A 2-week interval between subsequent follow-up visits allows the physician to monitor the patient's progress closely. Radiographs generally demonstrate abundant callus by 4 to 6 weeks. Functional measures of the patient's progress include an ability to touch the lumbar spine, touch the back of the neck, and fully abduct the arm over the head. After 6 to 8 weeks, follow-up visits can be scheduled at 3- to 4-week intervals, provided ROM and function are progressing well. In the event that little progress is made or an unacceptable plateau is reached, referral to a physical therapist is strongly advised. Rehabilitation and follow-up visits should ideally be continued until both the clinician and the patient are satisfied with the functional results.

Complications

The most significant complications of proximal humerus fractures are neurovascular injury, AVN of the humerus head, and adhesive capsulitis (frozen shoulder). Fortunately, neurovascular injury and AVN are rare unless the fracture involves the anatomic neck or is severely displaced or angulated. A frozen shoulder can occur after any proximal humerus fracture. This complication can be prevented in most cases by paying careful attention to ROM and promptly referring the patient to a physical therapist whenever recovery of arm function lags behind what is expected.

Proximal humerus fractures with associated rotator cuff tars or avulsed fragment can cause loss of motion or instability. Nonunion is rare unless significant displacement has occurred and soft tissue interposition is present.

Return to Work or Sports

Patients with proximal humerus fractures can often return to work within 1 week of the injury. The sling (or collar and cuff) allows use of the hand for many tasks. These tasks may actually help the patient maintain ROM of the wrist, hand, and fingers. However, jobs or duties that demand full use of both arms will not be possible until callus is present and adequate ROM and strength are achieved to permit safe performance of the activity. This generally takes 6 to 10 weeks but may take longer. Similar criteria should be met before return to most if not all sports. Athletes and other patients who wish to maintain aerobic fitness during the healing period may find this difficult. Walking or use of a stationary bike is likely to be the safest and most comfortable approach.

PROXIMAL HUMERUS FRACTURES (PEDIATRIC)

Fractures of the proximal humerus are relatively uncommon in children. They occur most often in adolescents and are usually Salter-Harris type II fractures. In younger children, the fracture usually involves the metaphysis. Rapid growth during adolescence weakens the physis, predisposing it to fracture. Figures 8-11 and 8-12 demonstrate fracture patterns commonly seen in this age group.

Mechanism of Injury

As in adults, proximal humerus fractures in children are generally caused by a fall on an outstretched arm or a direct blow to the lateral shoulder. Repetitive throwing stress on the physis can lead to a widening of the physis known as Little League shoulder.[16] A mechanism inconsistent with a fracture in an otherwise healthy child younger than 3 years of age should raise concern for child abuse.[17] Metaphyseal corner fractures at the proximal humeral physis may occur when the extremity is pulled or twisted forcibly.

Clinical Presentation

The child with a proximal humeral fracture typically presents with a history of trauma and marked pain on arm movement. The physical findings may be minimal for nondisplaced fractures. For displaced fractures, significant anterior swelling and altered shoulder appearance is often present (arm is usually shortened and held in extension).

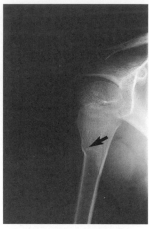

FIGURE 8-12 Buckle or torus fracture of the proximal humerus with minimal angulation (*arrow*). (*From Thornton A, Gyll C. Children's Fractures: A Radiological Guide to Safe Practice. Philadelphia, WB Saunders, 1999.*)

Imaging

Routine AP and axillary lateral views of the humerus are generally sufficient to make the diagnosis. A three-view shoulder trauma series should be obtained if clinical suspicion is high for other shoulder injuries. Proximal humerus fractures in children often have some displacement. Comparison views of the uninjured side may be helpful to determine if the physis is widened. Undulations in the physis of the proximal humerus are normal and should not be confused with a fracture.

It is difficult to make definitive statements about how much displacement to accept. In general, greater angulation and displacement can be accepted in younger children, and fractures in those younger than 11 years of age have good outcomes regardless of displacement.[18] As with adults, the extreme mobility of the shoulder means that some angulation can be well tolerated. Considerable remodeling of the area will also occur in younger children because most humerus growth occurs at the proximal physis. An acceptable position for fractures in children older than age 11 years of age is less than 50% displacement and less than 20% angulation.[18]

Indications for Orthopedic Referral

Consultation or referral is recommended if the physician is unsure about the acceptability of the fracture position. If displacement exceeds the previously mentioned range, referral is recommended because closed reduction or operative treatment may be needed. Patients with fractures that are intraarticular (Salter Harris type IV), associated with a shoulder dislocation, have an accompanying neurovascular injury or involve the physis should also be referred to an orthopedic surgeon.

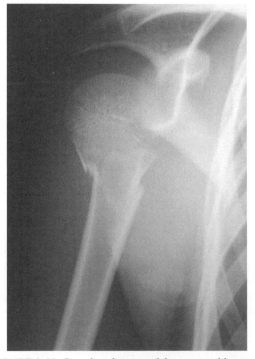

FIGURE 8-11 Complete fracture of the proximal humerus (metaphysis) in a 10-year-old child with approximately 20 degrees of apex medial angulation and 85% apposition. This position is well within the acceptable range for proximal humerus fractures in a patient of this age. If desired , a collar and cuff sling (see Figure 8-9) could be used to achieve ongoing gentle traction, which might restore a more anatomic position.

Treatment

Nondisplaced or minimally displaced fractures may be treated with a sling and swath or a shoulder immobilizer appropriate for the child's age. This usually provides adequate pain relief and prevents further displacement of the fracture. Healing is typically more rapid than in adults, and callus is usually evident in 2 to 3 weeks. If fracture stability is a concern, the first follow-up radiographs should be obtained much sooner (3 to 5 days) to detect a change in position while the fragments can still be manipulated. The sling or immobilizer can be completely discontinued when callus is present. Children generally regain ROM rapidly after this brief immobilization, especially if they are encouraged to swim or participate in other typical childhood activities. Most patients will have close to normal or normal function 2 months after the injury.[17]

Complications

Complications are rare after fractures of the proximal humerus. Arm function is usually very good even if some angulation persists. Abnormal growth may result if the physis was injured. In general, this leads only to one arm being slightly shorter than the other. This is generally well tolerated, although the patient may need to shorten a sleeve on any long-sleeved shirt or jacket. Nonetheless, patients and parents should be advised that future growth problems could occur whenever the physis has been injured.

MIDSHAFT FRACTURES OF THE HUMERUS

Mechanism of Injury

Midshaft humeral fractures generally result from a direct blow or a bending force applied to the middle humerus. They may also be caused by a fall onto an outstretched arm or elbow or by violent muscle contraction such as in weight lifting. Torsional forces produce long spiral fractures. Physical abuse should be suspected with these types of injuries in children. Stress fractures of the humerus are an uncommon but do occur in overhead athletes (e.g., baseball, tennis, gymnastics).

Clinical Presentation

Patients usually seek treatment for considerable swelling and pain of the mid-upper arm. The fracture site is tender. When significant displacement is present, shortening of the upper arm is apparent. In many cases, even gentle palpation produces painful crepitance. If report of the injury is delayed 1 to 2 days, the swelling and ecchymosis settle downward and are most prominent well below the fracture site. In such patients, initial inspection suggests that the elbow, rather than the midshaft, is fractured. Most midshaft fractures are readily suspected after initial clinical examination. A large hematoma caused by soft tissue injury may have a similar appearance.

A careful neurovascular examination is important. At a minimum, the clinician should assess the strength of the radial pulse and sensation in the territories supplied by the radial nerve (dorsum of the hand), median nerve (palmar aspect of thumb, index and middle fingers), and ulnar nerve (palmar aspect of little finger). Motor function can be assessed by tests of the strength of wrist dorsiflexion (radial nerve), finger abduction (ulnar nerve), and thumb opposition (median nerve).

Imaging

AP and lateral views of the humerus are usually adequate to detect a fracture and determine displacement and angulation. Transverse, spiral, oblique, and comminuted fractures may occur. The actions of muscles attached to the humerus cause characteristic angulation patterns in shaft fractures (Figure 8-13). Proximal fractures usually assume apex medial angulation. The proximal fragment is pulled medially by the pectoralis major muscle, and the distal fragment is pulled laterally by the deltoid muscle. A midshaft fracture usually assumes apex lateral angulation. In this type of fracture, the proximal fragment is pulled laterally by the deltoid, and the distal fragment is pulled medially by the biceps and triceps. The strong forces exerted across the fracture site by the biceps and triceps may also produce overriding of the fragments and shortening across the fracture site (Figure 8-14).

Many midshaft fractures are associated with injuries of either the shoulder or the elbow. If such injuries cannot be confidently excluded by physical examination, obtaining radiographs of these areas is advisable.

Indications for Orthopedic Referral

Emergent Referral (Within 30 to 60 Minutes)

Emergency referral of any patient with a neurovascular deficit is indicated because surgical exploration may be necessary. Similarly, patients with open fractures of the midshaft require emergent referral for operative debridement.

Nonemergent Referral (Within a Few Days)

Most midshaft fractures are treated nonsurgically with either functional bracing or traction with a hanging arm cast. Primary care providers who are not comfortable with the use of these approaches should refer patients with midshaft fractures. Ironically, transverse fractures, which often have the

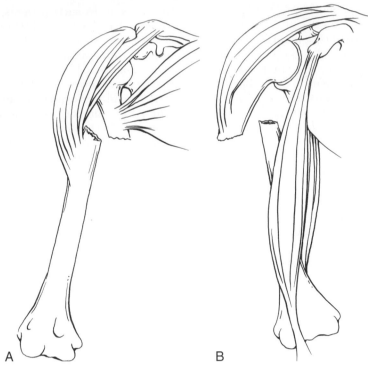

FIGURE 8-13 Displacement of humerus shaft fractures as a result of muscle action. **A,** Proximal fracture with apex medial angulation. **B,** Midshaft fracture with apex lateral angulation.

most "benign" radiographic appearance, may be more difficult to manage than displaced spiral fractures. They are prone to nonunion, especially if displaced or treated with too much traction. Transverse fractures also require close monitoring. Depending on their expertise, primary care providers probably should refer most patients with transverse fractures. Other indications for operative treatment include nonunion, pathologic fractures, fractures associated elbow injuries, extensive local associated injuries, and inadequate reduction with closed methods (uncommon except with segmental fractures).[19]

Initial Treatment

Table 8-2 summarizes management guidelines for midshaft humerus fractures.

Complete immobilization of the humerus is neither feasible nor desirable. Initial treatment is aimed at reducing movement at the fracture site and correcting any displacement. The neurovascular examination, as described above under Clinical Presentation, should be repeated after any manipulation of the fracture site, including splint or cast application. Typically, the displaced fragments of these fractures are so mobile that even these actions may occasionally cause a neurovascular injury.

Some degree of traction is needed for proper positioning of these fractures. In an acute care setting, a coaptation splint (Figure 8-15) can be used to initially stabilize the fracture and protect against further displacement. It is important to note that the unsupported splint tends to slide downward. This can be minimized by applying cast padding to wet benzoin on the skin, avoiding excess padding, and contouring the splint over the shoulder. The plaster slab should nestle comfortably in the axilla, wrap around the elbow, and extend over the deltoid. After application of the coaptation splint, the patient should be placed in a collar and cuff sling (Figure 8-9). The weight of the unsupported elbow provides some traction. In fractures with minimal shortening or patients with little muscle mass, this is often all that is needed to correct the shortening. A coaptation splint and collar and cuff sling is recommended if referral is planned.

If the amount of swelling is minimal, a hanging arm cast (described below) can be applied as the initial treatment provided the patient can be trusted to detect and respond appropriately to the early signs of an iatrogenic compartment syndrome. Alternatively, a coaptation splint can be applied and a hanging arm cast applied when swelling subsides. Proper use of a hanging arm cast requires essentially continuous traction by the cast. Therefore the patient must sleep upright and avoid supporting the elbow at all times.

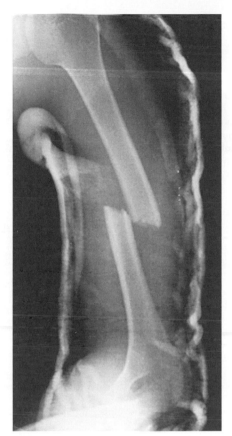

FIGURE 8-14 Midshaft fracture with overriding and shortening of the fragments. *(From Browner BD, Jupiter JB, Levine AM, Trafton PG [eds]. Skeletal Trauma: Fractures, Dislocations, Ligamentous Injuries. Philadelphia, WB Saunders, 1992.)*

The humerus is the most easily reduced long bone, and for most spiral or oblique fractures of the shaft, a reduction that exceeds the goals stated is not difficult to obtain. After adjustment of the cast, the signs and symptoms of compartment syndrome should be discussed and the patient encouraged to begin shoulder pendulum exercises as soon as possible (no later than 1 week).

Follow-up Care

The choices for nonoperative treatment of humeral shaft fractures are functional bracing and a hanging arm cast. The theory behind functional bracing, which does not immobilize the fracture, is that in most patients, gravity results in adequate alignment of the fracture fragments and motion at the fracture site induces bone healing. Varus angulation is common after treatment with a brace but this rarely leads to cosmetic or functional problems, and the incidence of nonunion is low.[19] Some clinicians favor bracing for all midshaft fractures without significant shortening or displacement.[20,21]

Compared with the hanging arm cast, bracing minimizes elbow stiffness, and some patients favor the brace because it is less bulky.

Functional Bracing

Functional bracing is the preferred definitive treatment for transverse fractures. Muscle movement around the fracture is encouraged. Compression by the contracting muscles helps restore the fragments to proper position and is thought to stimulate the development of callus. When swelling subsides and less mobility is present at the fracture site (usually 1 to 2 weeks after injury), the coaptation splint can be removed and the patient fitted for a humerus brace (Figure 8-16). Commercially made braces of various sizes (e.g., the Sarmiento brace) are available. The brace should be tight and should extend above and below the fracture site. The patient should continue to use the collar and cuff sling during recumbency until clinical union has been achieved. With this treatment, early directed ROM of the shoulder, elbow, and hand is stated as soon as symptoms allow.

Hanging Arm Cast

A hanging arm cast is shown in Figure 8-17. The cast should include the wrist and extend above the fracture site by at least 2 cm. The elbow is

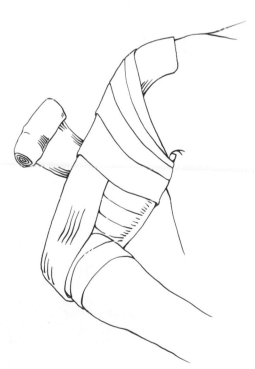

FIGURE 8-15 Coaptation or sugar-tong splint. Note that the plaster extends from the axilla around the elbow and up over the deltoid.

Table 8-2	*Management Guidelines for Midshaft Humerus Fractures*
INITIAL TREATMENT	
Splint type and position referral planned	Coaptation splint with collar and cuff sling if little traction is needed or if bracing or a hanging arm cast when traction is needed
	Coaptation splint and standard sling for transverse fractures
Initial follow-up visit	1 to 2 weeks
	1 to 2 days if cast is applied acutely
Patient instruction	Initiate shoulder, hand, and finger ROM as soon as tolerated
	If cast is applied acutely, carefully discuss symptoms of compartment syndrome
	If hanging arm is cast applied, patient must not support elbow and must sleep upright
FOLLOW-UP CARE	
Cast or splint type and position	Functional brace or hanging arm cast
Length of immobilization	10 to 12 weeks (continue until callus is present and the fracture site is nontender and stable to manual stress)
Healing time	10 to 12 weeks
	If not healed by 12 weeks, refer for surgical treatment for nonunion
Follow-up visit interval	Weekly for 4 to 6 weeks; then every 2 weeks
Repeat radiography interval	Weekly for 4 to 6 weeks; then every 2 weeks
Patient instruction	Continued shoulder, hand, and finger ROM is emphasized
	Directed elbow ROM if brace is used
	When cast or brace is removed, increased ROM and strengthening exercises with special emphasis on the elbow
Indications for orthopedic consult	Neurovascular injury or open fracture
	Transverse fractures
	Provider unfamiliar with use of hanging arm cast and functional bracing
	Suspected nonunion
	Miscellaneous: pathologic fracture, associated elbow injury, multiple injuries, adequate closed reduction

ROM, range of motion.

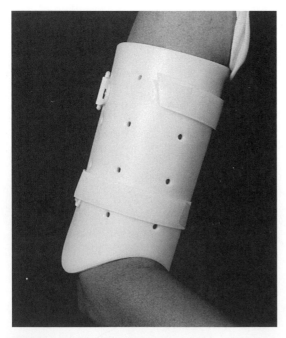

FIGURE 8-16 Functional humerus brace (Sarmiento humeral fracture brace). (*Courtesy of United States Manufacturing Company, Pasadena, CA.*)

immobilized at 90 degrees of flexion, and the forearm is in neutral position. The cast should hang free of the body to provide a traction force. It is important that the cast not be too heavy because this overly distracts the fragments and favors the development of nonunion. The weight of the cast should rarely exceed 2 lb (a maximum of three 4-inch rolls and one 3-inch roll of plaster or slightly more if fiberglass is used). The position of the cast must be adjusted to correct angulation, shortening, or distraction. This can be done by changing the length of the stockinette around the neck, changing the place where the stockinette is attached to the cast, or both. If a plate with multiple attachment points is not available, plaster or wire loops can be incorporated into the cast at the distal forearm in dorsal, neutral, and volar positions. After the cast has hardened, the stockinette should be attached and radiographs taken with the arm hanging dependently. The stockinette should be adjusted if needed and radiographs repeated until an acceptable position is obtained. An acceptable position is less than 20 degrees of AP angulation, less than 30 degrees of mediolateral angulation, and displacement of less than half the width of the humerus. This amount of angulation

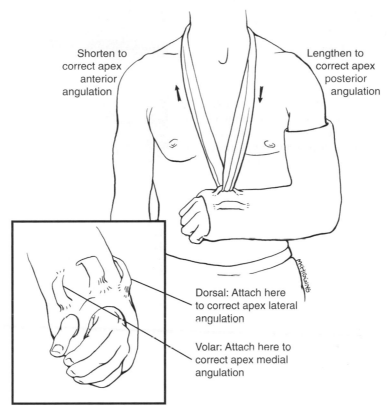

Shorten to correct apex anterior angulation

Lengthen to correct apex posterior angulation

Dorsal: Attach here to correct apex lateral angulation

Volar: Attach here to correct apex medial angulation

FIGURE 8-17 Adjustments to the hanging arm cast used to correct length and angulation.

and displacement is well tolerated both cosmetically and functionally. Radiographs should also be examined to be sure that the fracture fragments have not been distracted by too much traction. Pendulum exercises are started early to prevent stiffness.

Rehabilitation

Patients treated in a functional brace or hanging arm cast continue treatment until callus is detected and the fracture site is nontender and stable to manual stress. This frequently takes up to 12 weeks. Active abduction and elevation of the shoulder is avoided while the patient is in the cast or brace because this may lead to angular deformities. During the first 4 to 6 weeks, weekly radiographs are advisable until it is clear that the fragments are not moving appreciably. After stability of the fracture is established, the patient can be seen every 2 weeks. After the brace or cast is removed, elbow ROM and arm strengthening become paramount. The patient is followed up every 1 to 2 weeks until both the patient and physician are satisfied with the functional result. Many patients require referral to a physical therapist in order to obtain an optimal result. Go to Expert Consult for the electronic version of a patient instruction handout for shoulder rehabilitation after a fracture.

Complications

The most common complications associated with midshaft fractures are neurovascular injuries and nonunion. Radial nerve injury causes complications in 10% to 15% of midshaft fractures. Injuries to the brachial artery and other nerves may also occur. Fortunately, most nerve injuries associated with midshaft fractures are temporary neurapraxias. These injuries are best managed by orthopedists. Nerve injuries associated with distal shaft or open fractures and injuries resulting in complete loss of nerve function usually require operative exploration.

Transverse fractures, which have less surface area of bone contact, are more prone to nonunion. Nonunion is considered to be present if there is no radiographic healing by 12 weeks. At this point, conservative therapy is unlikely to produce healing and likely to produce further atrophy and joint stiffness. After nonunion is diagnosed, operative repair is indicated.

Because the humerus functions well even when it heals with some degree of shortening or angulation, clinically significant malunion is unlikely. Occasionally, a patient finds the cosmetic result suboptimal.

Return to Work or Sports

A hanging arm cast limits the use of the affected arm and hand, precluding many job tasks. Vigorous or quick movements may produce movement of the bone edges, causing a sensation some patients find unpleasant. This may also limit the activity, particularly during the first few weeks after injury. After 1 week, many patients will have adjusted to the cast well enough to return to work, although certain job tasks will still be impossible. A humerus brace allows greater arm use and typically interferes less with activities. Walking or a stationary bike can be used to maintain cardiovascular fitness. Patients should not return to contact sports or jobs that require significant arm strength until callus is present, the bone is stable to manual stress, and ROM of the shoulder and elbow is sufficient.

Pediatric Considerations

Midshaft humerus fractures make up about 2% of fractures in children. Spiral fractures predominate. Until approximately age 3 years, child abuse (usually a twisting injury) is the most common cause.[17] After this age, the usual cause is direct trauma, such as a blow to the arm or a fall onto an object. Pathologic fractures of the humerus may occur from minor trauma and occur because of the common occurrence of bone cysts or benign lesions of the humerus in children (Figure 8-18). The underlying lesion is often subtle and may be missed if the examiner focuses only on the fracture line. Neonates may sustain a humeral fracture from birth trauma.

After a midshaft fracture, the child will have mid-arm pain and swelling, and a visible deformity is uncommon. AP and lateral radiographs should suffice for diagnosis. The midshaft remodels much less than the metaphysis. Little remodeling of the shaft can be expected after age 6 years. As with proximal humerus fractures, authorities disagree on how much angulation is acceptable. A conservative goal for children younger than 7 years of age is less than 20 degrees of AP angulation, less than 30 degrees of mediolateral angulation, less than 15 degrees of rotation, approximately 50% apposition, and shortening of less than 2.5 cm. For older children and adolescents, the goal is somewhat less deformity than this. However, as in adults, even this degree of deformity is usually well tolerated.

Referral is indicated for patients with pathologic fractures, nerve injuries, open fractures, comminuted fractures, and multiple injuries. Referral is also indicated if the physician is not comfortable

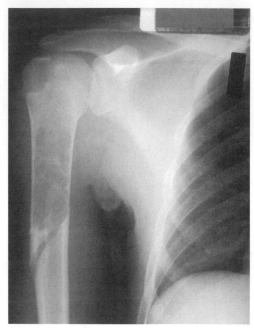

FIGURE 8-18 Spiral fracture of the midshaft of the humerus. The patient reported merely bumping his arm against the door frame while walking through a door. This suspicious cause of injury raised concerns about child abuse. However, the radiograph demonstrates that this is a pathologic fracture caused by an underlying benign bone tumor. Note the lucency and thinning of the cortex above the fracture site.

assessing the degree of displacement and using the following treatment methods.

After children reach adolescence, humerus shaft fractures should be treated as already described for adults. Children younger than 12 years of age can be treated with a sling and swath or shoulder immobilizer if little or no displacement is evident. If mild displacement is present, a collar and cuff sling (see Figure 8-9) may be used to help correct it. If displacement is unacceptable but little shortening is present, acute treatment may entail either a hanging arm cast or reduction followed by application of a coaptation splint (Figure 8-17) with a sling and swath. If unacceptable shortening is apparent, a hanging arm cast (Figure 8-18) should be used because this method best restores the humerus to an acceptable length. The hanging arm cast must not be too heavy because excessive traction could distract the bone ends and lead to nonunion. A pediatric humerus brace could be substituted for the coaptation splint or hanging arm cast if the right size is available. With children younger than 3 years of age, healing generally takes only 3 weeks. For older children, 4 to 6 weeks may be necessary.

Complications are relatively unusual. The radial nerve is occasionally injured, but this is less common than in adults. Nonunion is extremely rare. Some angulation usually persists at the fracture site, but it is generally well tolerated if it is not excessive. Mild shortening or overgrowth of the humerus may occur. This usually does not interfere with function. Rarely, paralysis of a nerve (usually radial) appears for the first time during healing. This suggests that the nerve is being compromised by the callus, and it is an indication for immediate referral and prompt surgical exploration.

SHOULDER (GLENOHUMERAL) DISLOCATIONS

The shoulder is an inherently unstable joint because only a small portion of the humeral head articulates with the glenoid, akin to a golf ball on a tee. This is the primary reason that the shoulder is the most frequently dislocated joint. This injury occurs most often in young adults but is not uncommon in elderly patients. It is rare in children. Patients report shoulder pain and are reluctant to move the shoulder. The differential diagnosis includes AC joint injury; rotator cuff tears; and fractures of the humerus, clavicle, or scapula. Shoulder dislocations can be divided into three categories: anterior, posterior, and inferior (luxatio erecta) dislocations.

Anterior Dislocations

Mechanism of Injury

The vast majority of shoulder dislocations (>90%) are anterior. The usual cause of injury is a combination of abduction and external arm rotation in addition to a force that drives the humeral head anteriorly. After losing contact with the glenoid fossa, the humeral head slips anterior and inferior, resulting in the characteristic positions shown in Figures 8-3, A Figure 8-19, A.

Clinical Presentation

Patients typically seek treatment with the arm held firmly in slight abduction and slight external rotation. The patient avoids joint movement because it is painful. Rotation is particularly resisted. A depression may be seen or palpated below the acromion, and there is a loss of the normal rounded contour of the shoulder. The head of the humerus may be felt below the coracoid. Special attention should be paid to the neurovascular examination. The brachial plexus, axillary nerve, or both may be injured. Axillary nerve injury can be detected by checking for loss of sensation in the area over the lateral deltoid. Loss of deltoid muscle function most likely has also occurred if sensation is absent or significantly diminished. Resistance to

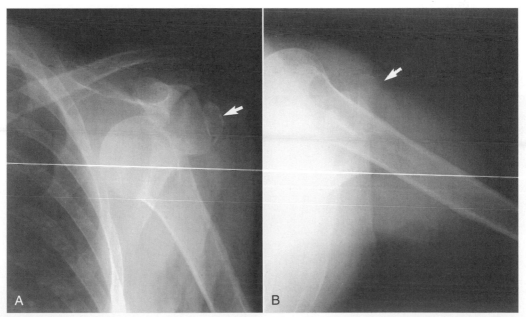

FIGURE 8-19 A, Anteroposterior view demonstrating anterior dislocation of the humeral head with avulsion fracture of the greater tuberosity. Note the typical position of the humeral head (inferior and medial to the glenoid), the fracture fragment lateral to the glenoid fossa (*arrow*), and the corresponding defect on the humeral head. **B,** Axillary view confirms that the humeral head has lost contact with the glenoid fossa and lies anterior. The fracture fragment can be seen at the edge of the acromion (*arrow*).

movement because of pain makes this difficult to confirm or refute during examination. The axillary artery may also be injured, especially in elderly patients. Some axillary nerve dysfunction is common after an anterior dislocation, but this is temporary in most patients.[22]

Imaging

In cases of anterior dislocation, a single AP view of the shoulder usually demonstrates the abnormal position of the humeral head, often in a subcoracoid position. Another view at roughly 90 degrees is necessary, however, to adequately search for associated fractures and to rule out posterior dislocations. A transcapular or "Y" view (Figures 8-3, B and 8-4, B) is recommended. Normally, the humeral head is in the center of the "Y" but will be medial to the "Y" with an anterior dislocation. An axillary view (Figures 8-4, C and 8-19, B) is another option, but getting the patient to move the arm into the necessary position is often very difficult.

Clinically important fractures occur with approximately one quarter of shoulder dislocations. Risk factors for fractures along with the dislocation include age older than 40 years, first-time dislocation, and traumatic mechanism.[23] When these three factors are absent, fracture is highly unlikely, and prereduction radiographs are unnecessary if none of these risks are apparent and the clinician feels certain of the diagnosis of an anterior shoulder dislocation.[24] Associated fractures include an avulsion of the greater tuberosity (Figure 8-19), a Hill-Sachs lesion (cortical depression of the posterolateral humeral head caused by

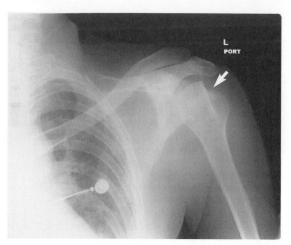

FIGURE 8-20 Hill-Sachs lesion. Note the cortical depression of the posterosuperior humeral head caused by impaction with the glenoid rim (*arrow*). (*Photo courtesy of Michael L. Richardson, MD.*)

impaction with the glenoid rim) (Figure 8-20), or a Bankart lesion (a fracture of the inferior aspect of the glenoid fossa) (Figure 8-21). The latter two fractures may predispose the patient to future dislocations.

Indications for Orthopedic Referral

Immediate orthopedic assistance should be obtained for patients with neurologic or vascular compromise. Patients with coexistent fractures should generally be referred as well, although the fracture fragments will often return to an acceptable position after reduction of the dislocation. If the associated fracture is an avulsion, it would be

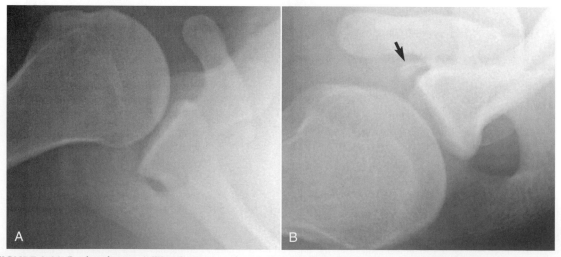

FIGURE 8-21 Bankart lesion. A West Point view shows a fracture of the inferior aspect of the glenoid fossa (*arrow*). (*From Pope T, Bloem H, Beltran J, Morrison WB, Wilson D. Imaging of the Musculoskeletal System. Philadelphia, WB Saunders, 2008.*)

reasonable to attempt reduction if orthopedic assistance is not available within a few hours. Failed reduction despite several attempts is also an indication for referral, consultation, or both. Dislocations that are more than a few days old are more difficult to reduce and are likely to require referral of the patient as well. The reduction is commonly performed under general anesthesia. Occasionally, interposition of soft tissue or fracture fragments necessitates operative reduction.

Initial Treatment

Most patients with uncomplicated anterior dislocations can be treated by primary care providers. Reduction is usually successful even without analgesia in dislocations that are recent, recurrent, or relatively atraumatic. Thus, many primary care attempt reduction at the scene of the injury (e.g., on the sidelines of a football game) before radiographs can be taken. The benefits of an easier, less traumatic reduction often outweigh the benefits of prereduction radiographs. On-the-scene reduction is even safer for recurrent dislocations in which a fracture is much less likely. After the first 30 to 60 minutes, progressive muscle spasm and edema make reduction more difficult. Prolonged dislocation (>24 hours) usually requires reduction under general anesthesia, and before reduction is attempted, obtaining radiographs is preferable to confirm the diagnosis and rule out a fracture.

Reduction is greatly facilitated by procedural sedation to relieve pain and reduce rotator cuff muscle spasm, although this may not be necessary if reduction is attempted soon after injury. A number of parenteral medications are available, including fentanyl and midazolam, ketamine, etomidate, and propofol. Another option is instillation of 10 to 20 mL of 2% lidocaine into the joint, which is less costly and provides pain relief while avoiding complications from intravenous sedatives.[25] A lateral approach is preferable when the humeral head is displaced anteriorly. If parenteral agents are used, it is highly recommended that oxygen saturation and vital signs be closely monitored, especially after the reduction. At this point, the patient typically becomes more comfortable and more susceptible to respiratory depression. The risk of respiratory depression is especially high in elderly patients and those with coexistent medical conditions.

Reduction Technique

Go to Expert Consult for a video on how to perform a reduction maneuver for a shoulder dislocation. No one method of reducing an anterior should dislocation has been shown to be superior, so the method used depends mostly on clinician preference.[26] An anterior dislocation can be reduced using one of several techniques. Successful reduction is characterized by a feeling of a "clunk" as the humeral head relocates and the return of the normal appearance of the shoulder. This is not always felt, especially with more gradual relocation techniques (e.g., external rotation). The ability of the patient to place the hand of the affected extremity on the opposite shoulder is another method of confirming the reduction.

Scapular Manipulation. Scapular manipulation is quick, easy, and well tolerated by the patient and therefore is a good first maneuver. Success rates exceed 80%.[27] The upright technique is preferred. The examination table or gurney is placed at 90 degrees, and the patient rests the unaffected shoulder against the upright portion of the bed while dangling the legs over the end. The patient is encouraged to relax the shoulder muscles against the upright portion. The clinician stands behind the patient, locates the scapula, and then simultaneously pushes the tip medially and the acromion inferiorly using the thumbs, thereby rotating the scapula. At the same time, an assistant provides gentle downward traction on the arm by grabbing the patient's wrist with one hand and the already flexed elbow with the other hand and pushes down on the elbow while holding the wrist in place.

Stimson's Technique. The patient is placed face down on the examining table with the affected arm hanging down toward the floor. A pillow is placed under the clavicle, and approximately 5 lb of weight is attached to the patient's wrist. Over time, the traction gradually overcomes the muscle forces, and the humeral head slips back into place. Reduction may take 15 to 20 minutes to occur.

Traction Countertraction. This technique involves laying the patient on his or her back and wrapping a sheet under the axilla and around the torso with the ends extending above the patient's head. An assistant applies countertraction by pulling on the two ends of the sheet while standing behind the top of the patient's head. Reduction is facilitated if a third assistant applies outward traction to a sheet wrapped around the proximal humerus (double-sheet method). The clinician grasps the wrist firmly and applies steady traction. The patient's arm should be held in a slightly abducted position with traction directed toward the patient's feet and slightly above horizontal. When the muscle spasm relaxes and the muscles lengthen, the patient's palm should be rotated upward (external rotation) to facilitate reduction. The maneuver is completed by internal rotation and relaxation of traction. When the head slips back into place, a clunk is generally felt. It may be necessary to apply steady traction for some time before the muscle forces are overcome. If no assistant is available, the clinician's foot can be placed against the side of the patient's chest just below the axilla while traction is applied (the Hippocratic method).

Follow-up Care

After reduction, the neurovascular examination should be repeated. Arterial injury may occur during relocation, especially in elderly patients with long-standing dislocations. Radiographs should be obtained after reduction to confirm that reduction has been achieved and to rule out fractures that may have been caused by the reduction. If this is the first time the shoulder has been dislocated, the patient should be immobilized in a sling and swath or shoulder immobilizer. Arthroscopic repair within 10 days is recommended in young people with first-time dislocations who engage in highly demanding physical activities because surgery reduces the high rate of subsequent redislocation in this group.[28] In patients older than 40 years old, the rate of redislocation is lower, and early mobilization should be started after 1 week to limit joint stiffness. Gentle pendular motion exercises are performed during the immobilization period to reduce the risk of frozen shoulder.

For recurrent dislocations, immobilization is less crucial. After the third dislocation, immobilization can stop as soon as the patient's symptoms allow, which is usually in a few days. After immobilization ends, ROM exercises should be begun and use of the sling quickly weaned. ROM exercises and strengthening can be approached as previously described for proximal humerus fractures, with the patient referred to physical therapy if progress is slow. Patients should not return to sports until arm strength and ROM are adequate. This may take 2 to 4 months. Because a complete tear of a rotator cuff tendon or muscle may accompany a dislocation, the function of the four rotator cuff muscles should be assessed during the rehabilitation process.

Recurrent Dislocations

Recurrent dislocations are very common in patients younger than 20 years of (occurring in 50% to 90% of patients), less common in those older than 40 years of age, and quite unusual in elderly people. Much less force is typically required to cause a recurrent dislocation than was necessary for the initial injury. Even trivial forces such as lifting a suitcase can cause a recurrent dislocation. Patients with these repeated injuries should be advised that surgery can dramatically reduce the risk of future dislocations and be referred to an orthopedic surgeon if they are interested in pursuing this level of treatment.

Posterior Dislocations

Posterior dislocations make up only 2% to 3% of shoulder dislocations. They are usually caused by a blow to the front of the shoulder or a fall onto an internally rotated, adducted, and outstretched arm. Unlike anterior dislocations, the abnormal position may be subtle on the AP view (Figure 8-22). As a result, it is not unusual for the diagnosis to be missed initially in up to 50% of cases.[29] Remaining alert for this condition and paying careful attention to the physical examination and radiographs can help prevent this. Typically, the patient holds the arm in internal rotation and slight abduction. A depression will usually be felt below the acromion anteriorly, and the bulge of the humeral head may be felt posteriorly. Shoulder motion, especially rotation, will be resisted. Although the AP view may seem unremarkable on first glance, lack of congruence between the curvature of the humeral head and that of the glenoid fossa is often present (compare Figures 8-22, C and 8-4, C). The posterior position of the head can be confirmed with an axillary view. Radiographs should also be scrutinized for concurrent fractures, which are often present. A CT scan should be obtained if plain radiographs are indeterminate.

For a number of reasons, posterior dislocations are more complicated to manage than anterior dislocations. General anesthesia may be required to achieve reduction, and coexistent fractures are often present. The reduction may not be stable, and special techniques may be required to maintain the reduction. Hence, most patients with these injuries should probably be referred to an orthopedic surgeon for prompt reduction. If referral is not feasible or the physician is more experienced with musculoskeletal injuries, reduction can often be achieved after procedural sedation. With the patient laying on his or her back, the elbow is bent to 90 degrees and the arm abducted to 90 degrees (i.e., arm sticking straight out to the side with fingers and hand pointing toward feet). Manual traction is then applied, pulling the arm straight outward. The arm is then externally rotated so the hand and fingers rotate upward toward the ceiling, completing the reduction.

The arm is then lowered to the patient's side and immobilized in a sling and swath. Postreduction radiographs should be carefully examined to be sure that the reduction was maintained after the arm was lowered to the patient's side and placed in the sling. If the reduction is maintained, immobilization should continue for 4 weeks and be followed by ROM and strengthening exercises. Consideration should be given to follow-up radiographs approximately 1 week after reduction to ensure that reduction has been maintained.

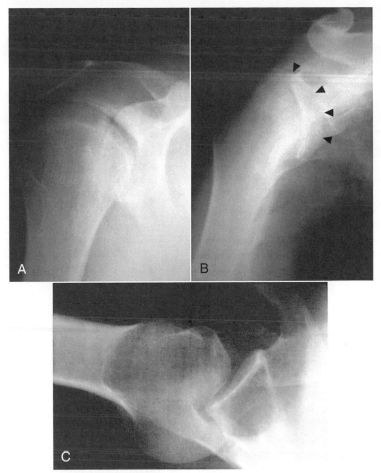

FIGURE 8-22 Anteroposterior radiographs. A, Sagittal plane of the body (missed posterior dislocation). B, Overlap of the head and glenoid indicates a dislocation in the sagittal plane of the scapula ("rim sign"). C, Optimally, axillary or computed tomography views are used to diagnose a posterior dislocation or fracture-dislocation. *(From Browner BD, Jupiter JB, Levine AM, Trafton PG [eds]. Skeletal Trauma, vol 2. Philadelphia, WB Saunders, 1992.)*

Inferior Dislocations (Luxatio Erecta)

The mechanism of injury of this relatively rare dislocation is an axial load with the arm abducted. It may occur when the patient falls and tries to grasp an object above the head, causing hyperabduction of the arm. The patient seeks treatment with the arm held straight outward at approximately 100 degrees of abduction and is unable to adduct the arm. Radiographs will reveal that the humeral head has slipped inferiorly and lies in the axilla below the glenoid. Neurovascular compromise, especially axillary nerve injury, is relatively common. Greater tuberosity fractures or rotator cuff tears are present in the majority of cases. Reduction is reportedly easy to achieve and should be accomplished promptly. Traction is applied directly along the existing axis of the arm, and the arm is then swung down to the patient's side. The arm is then immobilized in a sling and swath or shoulder immobilizer, and postreduction films are

obtained. Postreduction management is similar to that of anterior dislocations. Vascular compromise that persists after reduction requires emergency referral of the patient. Patients with persistent neurologic deficits are unlikely to need emergency intervention, but prompt orthopedic evaluation is still recommended.

REFERENCES

1. Visser CP, Coene LN, Brand R, Tavy DL. Nerve lesions in proximal humeral fractures. *J Shoulder Elbow Surg.* 2001;10:421-427.
2. Gallo RA, Sciulli R, Daffner RH, et al. Defining the relationship between rotator cuff injury and proximal humerus fractures. *Clin Orthop Relat Res.* 2007;458: 70-77.
3. Court-Brown CM, Garg A, McQueen MM. The epidemiology of proximal humeral fractures. *Acta Orthop Scand.* 2001;72:365-371.
4. Palvanen M, Kannus P, Niemi S, et al. Update in the epidemiology of proximal humeral fractures. *Clin Orthop Relat Res.* 2006;442:87-92.

5. Chu SP, Kelsey JL, Keegan TH, et al. Risk factors for proximal humerus fracture. *Am J Epidemiol*. 2004;160: 360-367.

6. Neer CS. Displaced proximal humeral fractures. I. Classification and evaluation. *J Bone Joint Surg Am*. 1970;52: 1077-1089.

7. Sidor ML, Zuckerman JD, Lyon T, et al. The Neer classification system for proximal humeral fractures: an assessment of interobserver reliability and intraobserver reproducibility. *J Bone Joint Surg Am*. 1993;75:1745-1750.

8. Gaebler C, McQueen, MM, Court-Brown CM. Minimally displaced proximal humeral fractures: epidemiology and outcome in 507 cases. *Acta Orthop Scand*. 2003;74: 580-585.

9. Koval KJ, Gallagher MA, Marsicano JG, et al. Functional outcome after minimally displaced fractures of the proximal part of the humerus. *J Bone Joint Surg*. 1997; 79:203-207.

10. Handoll HHG, Madhok R. Interventions for treating proximal humeral fractures in adults. *Cochrane Database Syst Rev*. 2003;(4):CD000434.

11. Lanting B, MacDermid J, Drosdowech D, et al. Proximal humeral fractures: a systematic review of treatment modalities. *J Shoulder Elbow Surg*. 2008;17:42-54.

12. Robinson CM. Proximal humerus fractures. In: Beaty JH, Kasser JR, eds. Rockwood & Wilkins Fractures in Adults. 7th ed. Philadelphia: Lippincott, Williams & Wilkins; 2010:1067-1068.

13. Tejwani NC, Liporace F, Walsh M, et al. Functional outcome following one-part proximal humeral fractures: a prospective study. *J Shoulder Elbow Surg*. 2008;17: 216-219.

14. Kristiansen B, Angermann P, Larsen TK. Functional results following fractures of the proximal humerus: a controlled trial comparing two periods of immobilization. *Arch Orthop Trauma Surg*. 1989;108:339-341.

15. Lefevre-Colau MM, Babinet A, Fayad F, et al. Immediate mobilization compared with conventional immobilization for the impacted nonoperatively treated proximal humeral fracture. A randomized controlled trial. *J Bone Joint Surg Am*. 2007;89:2582-2590.

16. Benjamin HJ, Hang BT. Common acute upper extremity injuries in sports. *Clin Pediatr Emerg Med*. 2007;8:15-30.

17. Shrader MW. Proximal humerus and humeral shaft fractures in children. *Hand Clin*. 2007;23:431-435.

18. Sarwark JF, King EC, Janicki JA. Proximal humerus, scapula and clavicle. In: Beaty JH, Kasser JR, eds. Rockwood & Wilkins Fractures in Adults. 7th ed. Philadelphia: Lippincott, Williams & Wilkins; 2010:649-655.

19. Sarmiento A, Waddell JP, Latta LL. Diaphyseal humeral fractures: treatment options. *Instr Course Lect*. 2002;51: 257-269.

20. Wallny T, Westermann K, Sagebiel C, et al. Functional treatment of humeral shaft fractures: indications and results. *J Orthop Trauma*. 1997;11:283-287.

21. Sarmiento A, Zagorski JB, Zych GA, et al. Functional bracing for the treatment of fractures of the humeral diaphysis. *J Bone Joint Surg Am*. 2000;82:478-486.

22. Visser CP, Coene LN, Brand R, Tavy DL. The incidence of nerve injury in anterior dislocation of the shoulder and its influence on functional recovery. A prospective clinical and EMG study. *J Bone Joint Surg Br*. 1999;81: 679-685.

23. Emond M, Le Sage N, Lavoie A, Rochette L. Clinical factors predicting fractures associated with an anterior shoulder dislocation. *Acad Emerg Med*. 2004;11:853-858.

24. Hendey GW, Chally MK, Stewart VB. Selective radiography in 100 patients with suspected shoulder dislocation. *J Emerg Med*. 2006;31:23-28.

25. Fitch RW, Kuhn JE. Intraarticular lidocaine versus intravenous procedural sedation with narcotics and benzodiazepines for reduction of the dislocated shoulder: a systematic review. *Acad Emerg Med*. 2008;15:703-708.

26. Kuhn JE. Treating the initial anterior shoulder dislocation—an evidence-based medicine approach. *Sports Med Arthrosc*. 2006;14:192-198.

27. Baykal B, Sener S, Turkan H. Scapular manipulation technique for reduction of traumatic anterior shoulder dislocations: experiences of an academic emergency department. *Emerg Med J*. 2005;22:336-338.

28. Handoll HHG, Al-Maiyah MA. Surgical versus nonsurgical treatment for acute anterior shoulder dislocation. *Cochrane Database Syst Rev*. 2004;(1):CD004325.

29. Gor DM. The trough line sign. *Radiology*. 2002;224: 485-486.

CLAVICLE AND SCAPULA FRACTURES

Clavicle fractures are common injuries, occurring most often in children and young adults. Treatment is determined largely by the location of the fracture and the degree of displacement. Many clavicle fractures lend themselves to management by primary care physicians. However, it is important to note that recently published studies have led to significant changes in treatment recommendations. Fractures of the scapula occur infrequently, accounting for fewer than 1% of all fractures. This low incidence may be attributable to the protective effects of the surrounding shoulder girdle muscles as well as the scapula's thickened edges and great mobility.

CLAVICLE FRACTURES

Clavicle fractures account for approximately 2% of all fractures and 5% of fractures seen by family physicians.[1,2] Most clavicle fractures (69%) occur in the middle third of the bone, 28% involve the distal third, and 3% involve the proximal third.[3] Diagnostic and treatment considerations vary depending on which third is fractured. Hence, discussions of clavicle fractures are typically divided into middle third, distal third, and proximal third fractures.

Anatomic Considerations

The clavicle is the only bony connection between the shoulder girdle and trunk. It acts to maintain width between the shoulders and provides some protection for the brachial plexus and great vessels. The clavicle forms an S-shaped curve—convex anterior in the proximal half and concave anterior in the distal half. The junction between these two curves is the thinnest portion of the bone and is untethered to ligamentous structures, which may explain why fractures are more common in this location. The acromioclavicular (AC) and coracoclavicular ligaments bind the clavicle to the scapula and contribute to the stability of the shoulder joint. The sternoclavicular ligaments firmly attach the clavicle to the chest. The sternocleidomastoid muscle attaches to the proximal segment of the clavicle and causes upward displacement of this portion of the bone when it is fractured. The soft tissues overlying the clavicle are quite thin. As a result, fracture hematomas and displacement are often easily seen on inspection. Open fractures of the clavicle are uncommon. However, because of the short distance between bone and skin, displaced fractures may cause tenting of the skin (taught stretching over a displaced bone end). Tenting should be addressed at the time of diagnosis to prevent skin necrosis and conversion to an open fracture.

Mechanism of Injury

Most clavicle fractures (87%) are caused by a fall onto the shoulder. Other causes include a direct blow to the clavicle (7%) and indirect trauma from falls onto an outstretched hand (6%).[4] There is no correlation between the mechanism of injury and the site of fracture (i.e., which third is involved).[4]

Fractures of the Middle Third of the Clavicle

Clinical Presentation

The patient with a fracture of the middle third of the clavicle usually complains of pain with any movement of the shoulder and holds the arm against the chest to protect against motion. The diagnosis of fracture is generally straightforward. A bulge is often visible at the fracture site either because of fracture hematoma or bone displacement. If displacement and shortening are present, downward and inward deformity of the shoulder is usually obvious. During examination, point tenderness over the fracture site is apparent. Crepitus or palpable motion of the fracture fragments is common given the subcutaneous position of the clavicle. Ecchymosis over the fracture or tenting of the skin may occur if the fragments are displaced.

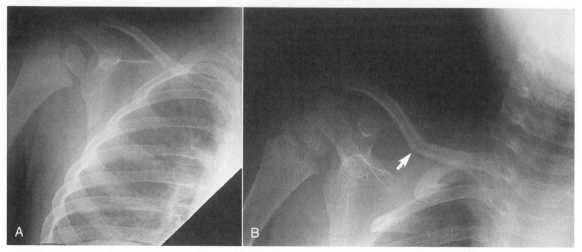

FIGURE 9-1 A, Fracture of the middle third of the clavicle. **B,** Note that the fracture is visible only in the 45-degree cephalic tilt view (*arrow*).

Pneumothorax, hemothorax, and neurovascular injury associated with clavicle fractures have been reported. These injuries are uncommon and are more likely to occur with fractures resulting from high-energy forces.

Imaging

An anteroposterior (AP) view is usually the only radiograph required to accurately diagnose a midshaft fracture. If the diagnosis is in question, a 45-degree cephalic tilt view can uncover the fracture (Figure 9-1). In displaced fractures, the strong pull of the sternocleidomastoid muscle results in upward displacement of the medial portion of the clavicle. The lateral fragment is usually displaced downward by the weight of the arm. These features are demonstrated radiographically and schematically in Figures 9-2 and 9-3. Comminution is frequently seen in middle third fractures (Figure 9-2).

Indications for Orthopedic Referral

Emergent Referral (Within 30 to 60 Minutes)

Neurovascular compromise, open fracture, and tenting of the skin are indications for emergent referral.

Nonemergent Referral (Within A Few Days of Injury)

Until recently, it was widely believed that these fractures almost always healed well, even if displaced. However, recent studies have shown that when complete displacement is present (i.e., displacement greater than one bone width; see Figure 9-2), conservative treatment produces unsatisfactory outcomes in more than 30 % of patients.[5,6] In a randomized trial of sling immobilization versus operative fixation, surgery produced faster healing, less nonunion, and fewer symptomatic malunions.[7]

Referral should therefore be considered for all patients with complete displacement, especially if there is comminution or significant shortening (>18 mm in men or >14 mm in women) because these factors are associated with even worse outcomes.[8,9] Surgery may also be more appealing if the patient is an athlete or is concerned about the prospect of a permanent visible lump at the fracture site, which is a common outcome. Surgery carries a risk of complications, including wound infections and hardware failure, and the benefits of

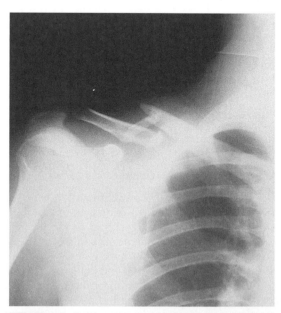

FIGURE 9-2 Anteroposterior view of the clavicle showing a comminuted fracture of the midshaft with upward displacement of the proximal fragment. Displacement is approximately 1.5 times the width of the clavicle with shortening of approximately 3 cm.

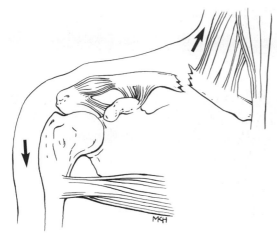

FIGURE 9-3 Deforming forces on a midshaft clavicle fracture. The pull of the sternocleidomastoid muscle causes upward displacement of the proximal fragment. The weight of the arm causes downward displacement of the distal fragment. The fracture is not completely displaced because displacement is only half of the bone width.

nonunion do not require treatment. If a glenoid neck fracture is present on the same side as the clavicle fracture ("floating shoulder"), referral is also indicated. This is an unstable injury and surgery appears to be the best treatment option.[10,11]

Initial Treatment

Table 9-1 summarizes management guidelines for middle third clavicle fractures.

The goal of conservative treatment for midshaft fractures is reduction of motion at the fracture site. The fracture site is best stabilized by restricting shoulder motion to less than 30 degrees of abduction, forward flexion, or extension. This can be achieved with a sling or a figure-of-eight bandage that keeps the shoulders back ("position of attention") (Figure 9-4). Treatment outcomes are nearly identical for the figure-of-eight bandage and sling support.[12] Figure-of-eight treatment has the advantage of leaving the elbow and hand free for daily activities, but it is more uncomfortable than a sling. It is not a good choice for patients who live alone because the bandage must be tightened regularly to maintain tension, and this requires assistance. Figure-of-eight treatment has the potential to minimize displacement and may be the preferred option for nonoperative treatment of completely displaced fractures. An arm sling can be used with a figure-of-eight bandage for additional comfort and support.

surgery must be weighed against these risks. For patients who are poor operative risks or prefer to avoid surgery, conservative treatment (described below) is a very reasonable alternative. Referral is also indicated for malunion and nonunion that is symptomatic. Asymptomatic malunion and

Table 9-1	Management Guidelines for Middle Third Clavicle Fractures	
	INITIAL TREATMENT	
Splint type and position	Figure-of-eight clavicle strap with shoulders in "position of attention" or arm sling	
	Sling preferable for nondisplaced fractures or plastic bowing in children	
Initial follow-up visit	1 to 2 weeks to assess pain level and healing	
Patient instruction	If using figure-of-eight, keep strap tight to hold shoulders in position	
	FOLLOW-UP CARE	
Cast or splint type and position	Figure-of-eight clavicle strap or arm sling	
Length of immobilization	4 to 8 weeks or until fracture site is nontender	
	3 to 6 weeks in children	
Healing time	6 to 12 weeks in adults	
	3 to 6 weeks in children	
Follow-up visit interval	Every 2 to 3 weeks	
Repeat radiography interval	At 6 weeks to assess callus and when clinical healing achieved	
Patient instruction	Use of the arm as pain permits	
	Avoid contact sports or activities with potential for falling for 1 to 2 months after clinical and radiographic healing	
	Bony deformity possible	
Indications for orthopedic consult	Tenting of skin	
	Open fracture	
	Consider referral for all patients with displacement greater than one bone width, especially if comminution or significant shortening is present or if the patient is concerned about cosmetic result	
	Symptomatic malunion and nonunion (after 12 weeks)	

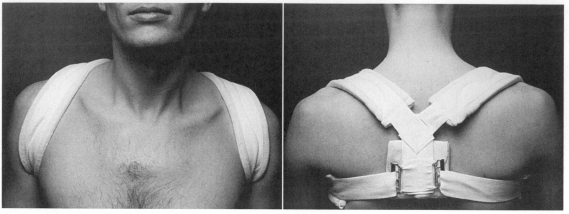

FIGURE 9-4 Figure-of-eight bandage with the shoulders held in a "position of attention."

Follow-up Care

Immobilization in the figure-of-eight bandage or arm sling should be continued until crepitus resolves and tenderness at the fracture site is minimal or absent. Follow-up visits should occur 1 to 2 weeks after injury to assess clinical symptoms and then every 2 to 3 weeks until the patient is asymptomatic. Clinical union has occurred when the fracture site is painless and the patient can move the arm fully without discomfort. Radiographic union progresses more slowly than clinical union and may not be present for 12 weeks. The usual healing time for this fracture is 3 to 6 weeks in children and 6 to 12 weeks in adults. Repeat radiographs of these fractures are not necessary at each return visit, but a final radiograph when clinical union is achieved is helpful to assess callus formation. During the period of immobilization, the patient may use the extremity as symptoms allow, but strenuous activities should be avoided. Patients who have sling immobilization should be instructed to perform elbow range of motion (ROM) exercises to maintain normal function. After immobilization, shoulder ROM and strengthening exercises speed recovery. Within several weeks, a visible "bump" (healing callus) may occur at the fracture site. This usually completely remodels and disappears in children but persists to some extent in adults because of relatively less remodeling. In adults, a permanent visible prominence over the fracture site is common, and they should be apprised of this likely outcome.

Return to Work or Sports

Return to work or sport activity can progress steadily as permitted by the patient's comfort level. Most patients are back to pre-injury levels of activity within 6 to 8 weeks. Those with occupations requiring heavy lifting, pushing or pulling, or overhead activity may need an additional 2 to 3 weeks to regain adequate strength for these tasks. Patients should refrain from contact sports or activities that put them at risk of falling for 8 to 10 weeks after the injury.

Complications

Serious complications resulting from fractures of the middle third of the clavicle, such as pulmonary, arterial, or nerve injury, are rare. Malunion resulting in angulation, shortening, and a poor cosmetic result is the most common complication. Malunion may lead to ongoing tenderness and reduction in shoulder function. Nonunion occurs less frequently. Predisposing factors include marked displacement, severe trauma, fracture comminution, and inadequate immobilization. A late complication associated with nonunion is brachial plexus compression neuropathy resulting from hypertrophic callus formation. The onset of symptoms of this condition may be early or quite late. Ulnar or median nerve symptoms are the most common.

Pediatric Considerations

Middle third clavicle fractures in children and adolescents are treated the same as in the adult patient. In the younger child, plastic bowing of the clavicle may occur, and these injuries should be treated just like other fractures to prevent an overt fracture. The healing time is much shorter than in adults, with most children back to full activity within 4 weeks after injury. Protection from contact or collision sports is advisable for an additional 2 to 3 weeks after adequate clinical and radiographic healing.

Birth Injuries

The clavicle may be fractured during childbirth trauma. These fractures usually involve the midshaft. Clavicle fractures in the newborn period are easily detected if the physician has a heightened awareness of the possibility of this lesion after difficult deliveries, especially those complicated by shoulder dystocia. Palpation of the clavicles should be part of every newborn examination. An infant with a clavicle fracture has decreased use of the arm on the injured side and reacts with pain to movement of the arm. Manipulation of the clavicle usually produces crepitus or palpable motion at the fracture site. Little treatment is needed for clavicle fractures in newborns because they almost always heal well within 2 weeks. Avoiding pressure on the clavicle and minimizing movement of the affected arm during feeding, dressing, and handling ensure greater comfort for the infant. Pinning the sleeve of the affected side to the chest with the elbow at 90 degrees is another treatment option. After symptoms resolve, the infant will begin to use the arm normally.

Fractures of the Distal Third of the Clavicle

Clinical Presentation

Fractures of the distal clavicle often produce no deformity and can easily be overlooked. These fractures can be difficult to distinguish from an AC separation. During examination, tenderness is apparent over the AC joint and in surrounding tissues. Pain increases with adduction of the arm across the chest. Ecchymosis and swelling over the AC joint may occur.

Imaging

Fractures of the distal third of the clavicle are classified into three types (Figure 9-5). In type I fractures, which are the most common, the supporting ligaments remain intact, and no significant displacement of the fracture fragments occurs (Figure 9-6). In type II distal fractures, a tear of the coracoclavicular ligament results in upward displacement of the proximal fragment (Figure 9-7). Type II fractures are particularly difficult to diagnose on standard clavicle views. Anterior and posterior 45-degree oblique views or a stress view of both shoulders with a 10-lb weight strapped to each wrist more clearly demonstrates the extent of separation of the fracture fragments. Type III fractures are intraarticular fractures through the AC joint. These fractures may be subtle and overlooked initially because there is often no displacement.

Indications for Orthopedic Referral.

Emergent Referral (Within 30 to 60 Minutes)

As with other clavicle fractures, neurovascular compromise, open fracture, and tenting of the skin are indications for emergent referral.

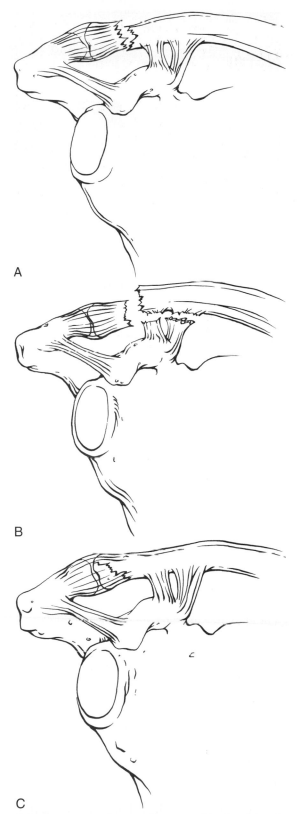

A

B

C

FIGURE 9-5 Classification of fractures of the distal clavicle. **A,** Type I: nondisplaced, intact ligaments. **B,** Type II: displaced coracoclavicular ligament tear. **C,** Type III: nondisplaced, intraarticular through the acromioclavicular joint.

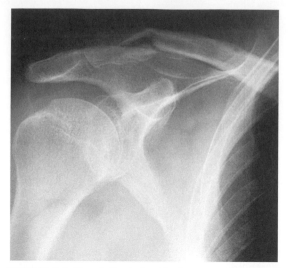

FIGURE 9-6 Type I distal clavicle fracture with minimal displacement.

Nonemergent Referral (Within A Few Days of Injury)

Types I and III distal clavicle fractures usually heal with symptomatic treatment only.[13] However, because type III fractures may lead to future degenerative changes of the AC joint, some primary care providers refer these intraarticular fractures for orthopedic management. Type II fractures are difficult to treat nonoperatively. Closed treatment is problematic because the fragments are distracted by muscle action, and the proximal fragment is unstable because it has no ligamentous attachment. Patients with type II fractures should be referred for possible open reduction and internal fixation.

Initial Treatment

Table 9-2 summarizes management guidelines for distal third clavicle fractures.

Type I and type III distal clavicle fractures are treated similarly with sling immobilization for comfort. These fractures are usually minimally displaced and heal well with conservative therapy. ROM exercises should begin when symptoms allow.[14] This may begin with pendulum exercises with the arm in the sling followed by progressive increase in use of the extremity as tolerated. Patients with type II fractures should have the fracture immobilized in a sling and swath while awaiting orthopedic consultation.

Follow-Up Care

Sling immobilization of types I and III fractures can usually be discontinued within 3 to 6 weeks as symptoms disappear. Clinical union occurs within 6 weeks in most cases. Patients should be reevaluated every 2 to 3 weeks to assess clinical healing. Avoidance of strenuous activities or contact sports

for an additional month after clinical union is advisable.

Return to Work or Sports

Guidelines for return to work or sport activity are similar to those described for fractures of the middle third except that the return to preinjury levels of activity is usually shorter (4 to 6 weeks) for distal third fractures.

Complications

Delayed union or nonunion occurs as a complication of type II fractures, particularly those treated nonoperatively. Overall, distal clavicle fractures are more prone to nonunion than shaft fractures. Symptomatic degeneration of the AC joint is a possible late complication of intraarticular (type III) fractures. The individual with this complication may report pain at the AC joint or show signs of shoulder impingement from osteophyte formation. Radiographic findings may include cystic changes, resorption of the distal clavicle, joint space narrowing, or spur formation. Occasionally, computed tomography (CT) scanning is necessary to diagnose this condition. If the patient's symptoms are not relieved with conservative therapy such as nonsteroidal medications or local steroid injections, orthopedic consultation is indicated for consideration of resection of the distal clavicle.

Pediatric Considerations

The classification of injuries to the distal clavicle in children is similar to the adult classification.

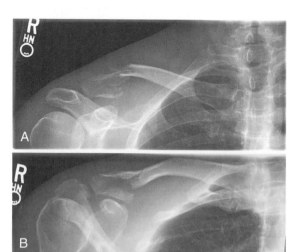

FIGURE 9-7 Anteroposterior (**A**) and oblique (**B**) views demonstrate a type II distal clavicle fracture with normal acromioclavicular and coracoclavicular distances but with upward displacement of the proximal fracture fragment. *(Reprinted with permission from Nett MH, Richardson ML. Open reduction and internal fixation of a distal clavicle fracture using a clavicle hook plate. Radiology Case Rep 2009;4:325.)*

Table 9-2	Management Guidelines for Distal Third Clavicle Fractures
INITIAL TREATMENT	
Splint type and position	Type I and III: arm sling
	Type II: do not use figure-of-eight; sling and swath until seen by orthopedist
Initial follow-up visit	1 to 2 weeks to assess pain level and healing
Patient instruction	Wear sling continuously until follow-up visit
FOLLOW-UP CARE	
Cast or splint type and position	Type I and III: arm sling
	Type II: sling and swath postoperatively
Length of immobilization	Type I and III: 3 to 6 weeks or until pain subsides
	Type II: 6 to 8 weeks
Healing time	Type I and III: 6 to 8 weeks
	Type II: 8 to 12 weeks
Follow-up visit interval	Every 2 to 3 weeks
Repeat radiography interval	After clinical healing or for late symptoms
Patient instruction	Type I and III: gradual increased activity as symptoms allow
	Avoid contact sports or activities with potential for falling for 1 to 2 months after clinical and radiographic healing
	Type II: persistent and painful arthritis of acromioclavicular joint possible
Indications for orthopedic consult	Type II fractures
	If type III fracture remains symptomatic despite conservative therapy, resection of the distal clavicle may be necessary

However, type II injuries in children are usually much more stable than the same fractures in an adult because the periosteal sleeve and the coracoclavicular ligament typically remain intact in children. Type I, II, and III distal clavicle fractures heal well with sling immobilization for comfort with early ROM exercises as soon as pain permits. Most fractures are healed within 4 to 6 weeks.

Fractures of the Proximal Third of the Clavicle

Clinical Presentation

Proximal clavicle fractures are usually caused by motor vehicle accidents and other severe trauma.[15] Hence, when evaluating patients with proximal clavicle fractures, one should consider the possibility of other potentially life-threatening injuries. The patient with a fracture of the proximal third of the clavicle usually complains of pain, tenderness, and swelling over the sternoclavicular area. Pain is exacerbated by any movement of the shoulder. There may be ecchymosis over the fracture site, especially if significant ligamentous injury has occurred with displacement of the fracture fragments. A sitting position with support of the arm on the injured side is usually more comfortable than a supine position. An associated anterior sternoclavicular dislocation results in visible displacement of the medial end of the clavicle. The usually prominent medial end of the clavicle is not palpable in a posterior sternoclavicular dislocation.

Chronic pain over the sternoclavicular area may indicate a stress fracture. Proximal clavicle stress fractures have been reported in rowers, gymnasts, and others who repetitively stress this area.

Imaging

Proximal clavicle fractures can be difficult to diagnose radiographically because of bony overlap in the standard AP view. The 45-degree cephalic tilt view more clearly demonstrates this fracture (Figure 9-8). Plain radiographs miss approximately 20% of proximal fractures.[15] A CT scan is able to detect these fractures and help exclude more serious intrathoracic injuries. Sternal fractures and sternoclavicular dislocations may also accompany these fractures.

Indications for Orthopedic Referral

Emergent Referral (Within 30 to 60 Minutes)

Emergency operative treatment is indicated if significant intrathoracic or neurovascular injury results from posterior displacement of fracture fragments. Even if posterior displacement is not present, other potentially life-threatening injuries may be present and should be considered during evaluation.

Nonemergent Referral (Within A Few Days from Injury)

Orthopedic referral is indicated for any patient with a proximal clavicle fracture with significant displacement or an associated sternoclavicular dislocation.

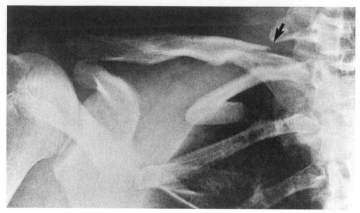

FIGURE 9-8 Fracture of the proximal clavicle seen on a 45-degree cephalic tilt view (*arrow*).

Initial Treatment

Table 9-3 summarizes management guidelines for proximal third clavicle fractures.

Analgesics, ice, and a sling for support constitute the acute treatment of nondisplaced proximal clavicle fractures.[16] After an initial period of rest, functional use of the arm is allowed as symptoms permit.

Follow-up Care

Most proximal clavicle fractures are successfully treated with sling immobilization. Healing generally occurs within 6 to 8 weeks. Definitive treatment of this fracture is similar to the treatment of types I and III distal fractures. Nonunion and posttraumatic arthritis are the most likely complications.

Pediatric Considerations

Fractures of the medial end of the clavicle in children are extremely uncommon, accounting for fewer than 1% of all clavicle fractures in the pediatric age group. Nondisplaced fractures are often discovered well after the acute injury because of the lack of deformity and symptoms. The child may be brought for treatment at a later date because of concern about a mass that represents callus formation around the healing fracture site. Nondisplaced medial fractures, whether they involve the physis or not, can be treated with a sling for comfort. Progressive motion and strengthening are allowed as pain permits.

Fractures that are displaced anteriorly can be treated without reduction because the displacement is usually well tolerated by the patient, and

Table 9-3	Management Guidelines for Proximal Third Clavicle Fractures
INITIAL TREATMENT	
Splint type and position	Arm sling
Initial follow-up visit	1 to 2 weeks to assess pain level and healing
Patient instruction	Wear sling continuously until follow-up visit
FOLLOW-UP CARE	
Cast or splint type and position	Arm sling for comfort
Length of immobilization	3 to 6 weeks or until fracture site is nontender
Healing time	6 to 8 weeks
Follow-up visit interval	Every 2 to 3 weeks
Repeat radiography interval	After clinical healing or for late symptoms
Patient instruction	Use of the arm as pain permits
	Avoid contact sports or activities with potential for falling for 1 to 2 months after clinical and radiographic healing
Indications for orthopedic consult	Neurovascular injury
	Symptomatic nonunion
	Posttraumatic arthritis

tremendous potential for remodeling exists. Patients having fractures with posterior displacement should be referred promptly for emergency reduction if neurovascular compromise occurs.

SCAPULA FRACTURES

Anatomic Considerations

The anatomic parts of the scapula include the body, spine, glenoid neck, glenoid fossa, acromion, and coracoid process (Figure 9-9). The scapula assists the arm in forward elevation and stabilizes the arm against the thorax. It is protected by thick muscles that cover its surface almost entirely. The anterior surface is covered by the subscapularis and serratus anterior muscles. Posteriorly, the supraspinatus muscle covers the surface above the scapular spine, and the infraspinatus muscle covers that below the spine. Some of the many inserting muscles may cause scapular fractures if they undergo violent contraction or cause displacement of fracture fragments. The triceps muscle attaches to the inferior glenoid rim. The pectoralis minor, coracobrachialis, and the short head of the biceps all insert on the coracoid process.

Mechanism of Injury

Significant force is required to fracture the scapular body or spine. Direct trauma from a blow or fall is the most common cause of injury. The scapular neck may be fractured indirectly from a fall on an

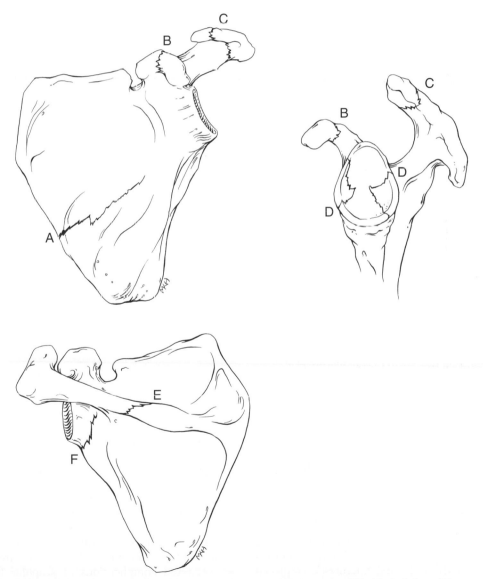

FIGURE 9-9 Fractures of the scapula: body (**A**), coracoid process (**B**), acromion (**C**), glenoid fossa (**E**), spine (**F**), and glenoid neck (**F**).

outstretched hand or a fall on the point of the shoulder. Glenoid fractures may result from a fall on the lateral shoulder or on a flexed elbow and may be associated with a shoulder dislocation, a fractured clavicle, or AC separation. Acromion fractures result from a direct downward blow to the shoulder. A direct blow to the point of the shoulder or a violent contraction of one of the attached muscles may result in a fracture of the coracoid process. Motor vehicle accidents are the cause of injury in more than half of cases of scapular fractures.

Scapular fractures are frequently associated with other traumatic injuries. The high incidence of other serious injuries reflects the degree of force necessary to fracture the scapula. Pneumothorax, fractured ribs, pulmonary contusion, clavicle fractures, and brachial plexus injury occur with sufficient frequency to warrant consideration and evaluation in any patient with a scapular fracture. Body fractures have the highest incidence of associated injury (Figure 9-10).

Clinical Presentation

After a fracture of the scapula, the patient typically holds the arm in adduction and resists any motion of the shoulder, especially abduction. Localized tenderness, pain, and swelling are present. Bruising is variable and often minimal. Deep swelling after a fracture of the body may mimic a rotator cuff tear. The shoulder may appear flattened after a displaced glenoid neck or acromion fracture.

Imaging

A true AP view of the shoulder, axillary view, and true scapular lateral view demonstrate most fractures of the scapular neck, glenoid, body, and acromion. The neck and body are the most commonly fractured areas of the scapula (10% to 15% and 50% to 80%, respectively). The cephalic tilt view is helpful in the evaluation of coracoid fractures. A CT scan is often needed in the evaluation of glenoid fractures to accurately assess the position of the humeral head and determine the size and amount of displacement of the fracture fragments.

An os acromiale, formed from a failed fusion of the ossification center of the acromion, can be confused with an acute fracture. The majority of patients with this finding are affected bilaterally, so a radiograph of the uninjured side may be beneficial.

Indications for Orthopedic Referral

Most scapular fractures heal well without operative treatment.[17,18] Orthopedic referral of the patient is indicated for the following fractures: a displaced glenoid neck fracture that is associated with a clavicle fracture or exceeds 1 cm displacement or

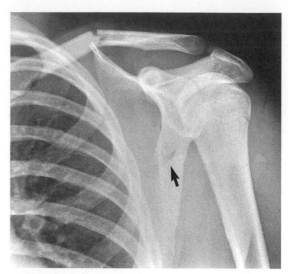

FIGURE 9-10 Fracture of the body of the scapula with an associated midshaft clavicle fracture.

20 degrees of inferior angulation (especially in a younger patient); glenoid fractures that involve more than 25% of the articular surface, have more than a 5 mm stepoff on the articular surface or are associated with a subluxed humeral head; significantly displaced coracoid fractures, especially if combined with complete AC separation; and displaced acromion fractures.[19,20] Body fractures with more than 1 cm of separation at the spine or lateral border may also require surgery.[20] Certain scapula fractures may widen during conservative treatment. If this occurs, surgery may be required.[21]

Initial Treatment

Table 9-4 summarizes management guidelines for scapular fractures. The acute management of fractures of the scapula entails symptomatic local care with ice, analgesics, and a sling for comfort. Some patients feel more comfortable with a sling and swath. The treatment of other associated traumatic injuries may take precedence.

Follow-up Care

General Considerations

Repeat radiographs should be obtained for all types of scapular fractures within 2 to 4 weeks after the initial injury. If progressive widening of the fracture occurs, referral is recommended for possible surgery. Evidence of radiographic healing should be present before resistance exercises for the shoulder are initiated. Patients should be seen every 2 to 4 weeks to ensure adequate progress in their rehabilitation program. The most frequently encountered complications of scapular fractures are posttraumatic arthritis and decreased shoulder mobility. Nonunion of scapular fractures is rare.

Table 9-4	*Management Guidelines for Scapular Fractures*
INITIAL TREATMENT	
Splint type and position	Arm sling for comfort
Initial follow-up visit	Within 1 to 2 weeks of injury
Patient instruction	Icing in the first 48 to 72 hours
	Early ROM exercises as pain permits within the first week
FOLLOW-UP CARE	
Cast or splint type and position	Body, spine, coracoid: none
	Glenoid neck: sling for comfort
	Acromion: sling for 2 to 3 weeks
Healing time	4 to 6 weeks
Follow-up visit interval	Every 2 to 4 weeks to assess progress with shoulder rehabilitation
Repeat radiography interval	Within 2 to 4 weeks of injury
	Must see radiographic healing before starting resistance exercises (usually within 2 to 4 weeks)
Patient instruction	Pendulum exercises followed by progressive ROM, including extension and abduction
	Resistance exercises especially for rotator cuff muscles
Indications for orthopedic consult	Displaced glenoid neck fractures with clavicle fracture or with more than 1 cm displacement or 20 degrees inferior angulation
	Glenoid fracture with more than 25% articular involvement, >5 mm stepoff, or displaced humeral head
	Displaced coracoid and acromion fractures

ROM, range of motion.

Specific Considerations

Body and Spine

Symptomatic treatment alone should suffice for these fractures. Early ROM exercises as tolerated are encouraged within 1 week of the injury. Within 2 to 4 weeks, the patient should begin progressive resistance exercises for the rotator cuff and deltoid muscles. Normal anatomic alignment is not necessary for good function in a healed scapular body fracture.

Glenoid Neck

Reduction of a displaced scapular neck fracture is generally not necessary to achieve a good clinical outcome, although surgical fixation may be considered in young patients and patients with more than 1 cm displacement or 20 degrees of inferior angulation.[19,20] Sling immobilization for comfort followed by early mobilization allows for adequate fracture healing in most cases. Shoulder muscle strengthening exercises should be started after pain-free motion is restored and evidence of radiographic healing exists. Neck fractures combined with a displaced clavicle fracture (Figure 9-11) or coracoclavicular ligament tear result in an unstable segment and require operative stabilization.

Glenoid

Nonsurgical treatment is indicated for a glenoid fracture in which the humeral head is centered on the glenoid, there is less than 5 mm stepoff on the joint surface, and less than 25% of the articular surface is involved. Pendulum exercises should be started as soon as the patient's comfort level allows. Progressive resistance exercises should be started after fracture union.

Acromion

Nondisplaced acromion fractures heal well with sling immobilization for 2 to 3 weeks followed by shoulder rehabilitation. Passive ROM exercises should be started within the first week. Active progressive resistance exercises for the rotator cuff and deltoid muscles should begin after fracture union occurs. Displaced acromion fractures often require internal fixation.

Coracoid

Isolated coracoid fractures heal adequately with symptomatic treatment, as outlined in the treatment of scapular body and spine fractures. A displaced fracture with an associated complete AC separation requires surgical repair of both injuries.

Return to Work or Sports

Patients should be advised that it may take several months of rehabilitation before they regain full function after a scapular fracture. Progressive return to occupational activities is appropriate. Contact or strenuous activities of the shoulder should be avoided for 8 to 10 weeks after injury.

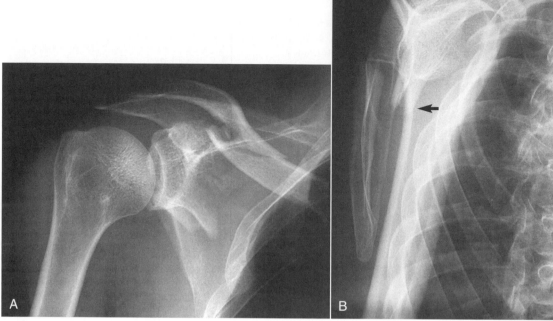

FIGURE 9-11 A, Anteroposterior view demonstrates the fracture of the glenoid neck and a midshaft clavicle fracture. **B,** Transscapular view reveals no apposition of the fracture fragments with lateral displacement and shortening of the body of the scapula. This is an unstable fracture because of the associated clavicle fracture.

REFERENCES

1. Postacchini F, Gumina S, De Santis P, Albo F. Epidemiology of clavicle fractures. *J Shoulder Elbow Surg.* 2002;11:452-456.
2. Hatch RL, Rosenbaum CI. Fracture care by family physicians: a review of 295 cases. *J Fam Pract.* 1994;38:238-244.
3. Robinson CM. Fractures of the clavicle in the adult. Epidemiology and classification. *J Bone Joint Surg Br.* 1998;80:476-484.
4. Stanley D, Trowbridge EA, Norris SH. The mechanism of clavicular fracture. A clinical and biomechanical analysis. *J Bone Joint Surg Br.* 1988;70:461-464.
5. Hill JM, McGuire MH, Crosby LA. Closed treatment of displaced middle-third fractures of the clavicle gives poor results. *J Bone Joint Surg Br.* 1997;79:537-539.
6. Nowak J, Holgersson M, Larsson S. Sequelae from clavicular fractures are common: a prospective study of 222 patients. *Acta Orthop.* 2005;76:496-502.
7. Canadian Orthopedic Trauma Society. Nonoperative treatment compared with plate fixation of displaced midshaft clavicular fractures. A multicenter, randomized clinical trial. *J Bone Joint Surg Am.* 2007;89:1-10.
8. Zlowodzki M, Zelle BA, Cole PA, et al. Treatment of acute midshaft clavicle fractures: systematic review of 2144 fractures: on behalf of the Evidence-Based Orthopaedic Trauma Working Group. *J Orthop Trauma.* 2005;19:504-507.
9. Lazarides S, Zafiropoulos G. Conservative treatment of fractures at the middle third of the clavicle: the relevance of shortening and clinical outcome. *J Shoulder Elbow Surg.* 2006;15:191-194.
10. Edwards SG, Whittle AP, Wood GW. Nonoperative treatment of ipsilateral fractures of the scapula and clavicle. *J Bone Joint Surg Am.* 2000;82:774-780.
11. Leung KS, Lam TP. Open reduction and internal fixation of ipsilateral fractures of the scapular neck and clavicle. *J Bone Joint Surg Am.* 1993;75:1015-1018.
12. Anderson K, Jensen PO, Lauritzen J. Treatment of clavicular fractures. Figure-of-eight bandage versus a simple sling. *Acta Orthop Scand.* 1987;58:71-74.
13. Nordqvist A, Petersson C, Fedlund-Johnell I. The natural course of lateral clavicle fracture. 15 (11-21) year follow-up of 110 cases. *Acta Orthop Scan.* 1993;64(1):87-91.
14. Anderson K. Evaluation and treatment of distal clavicle fractures. *Clin Sports Med.* 2003;22:319-326.
15. Throckmorton T, Kuhn JE. Fractures of the medial end of the clavicle. *J Shoulder Elbow Surg.* 2007;16:49-54.
16. Ring D, Jupiter JB, Miller ME, Ada JR. Part II, fractures of the clavicle. In: Browner BD, Jupiter JB, Levine AL, Trafton PG, eds. Skeletal Trauma: Fractures, Dislocations, Ligamentous Injuries, vol II. Philadelphia: WB Saunders; 1998:1670.
17. Schofer MD, Sehrt AC, Timmesfeld N, et al. Fractures of the scapula: long-term results after conservative treatment. *Arch Orthop Trauma Surg.* 2009;129:1511-1519.
18. Gosens T, Speigner B, Ninekus J. Fracture of the scapular body: functional outcome after conservative treatment. *J Shoulder Elbow Surg.* 2009;18:443-448.
19. Bahk MS, Kuhn JE, Galatz LM, et al. Acromioclavicular and sternoclavicular injuries and clavicular, glenoid, and scapular factures. *J Bone Joint Surg Am.* 2009;91:2492-2510.
20. Lapner PC, Uhtoff HK, Papp S. Scapula fractures. *Orthop Clin North Am.* 2008;39:459-474.
21. Anavian J, Khanna G, Plocher EK, Wijdicks CA, Cole PA. Progressive displacement of scapula fractures. *J Trauma.* 2010;69:156-161.

SPINE FRACTURES

Orthopedic surgeons or neurosurgeons manage most acute fractures of the spine. Knowledge of the signs of fracture instability is the key to appropriate selection of fractures that can be managed safely by primary care providers. Cervical spine fractures are nearly always the result of significant trauma and are frequently unstable. Cervical spine injuries are common in children, and the inherent ligamentous laxity allows the child's spine to absorb and dissipate forces, leading to fewer serious spinal injuries. Thoracolumbar spine fractures are more common than fractures of the cervical spine. Younger patients fracture their thoracolumbar spine after a high-energy force, but fractures in elderly patients may occur secondary to minimal or no trauma because of underlying osteoporosis. Osteoporotic compression fractures are probably the most common type of spine fracture encountered in the office setting.

CERVICAL SPINE FRACTURES (ADULT)

Anatomic Considerations

The cervical spine is composed of seven vertebrae (Figure 10-1). The bony ring of the first cervical vertebra (C1) does not contain a vertebral body or a distinct spinous process but is composed of anterior and posterior arches and lateral masses. Its articulation with C2 is circular and flat. The odontoid process of C2 is an extension of the vertebral body and is tightly bound to C1 by the dense fibers of the transverse ligament. The transverse ligament prevents forward subluxation of C1 relative to C2 during flexion. In the lower cervical vertebrae (C3-C7), the laminae arise from the pedicles on the posterior aspect of the vertebral body and join posteriorly to form the spinous processes. With the exception of C8, the cervical nerve roots exit superior to the pedicle at each level (e.g., the C5 nerve root passes between C4 and C5; the C8 nerve root passes between C7 and T1).

The three-column model is a useful way to evaluate spine fractures (Figure 10-2). The anterior column is composed of the anterior half of the vertebral body and the anterior ligamentous complex (anterior portion of the annulus fibrosus and the anterior longitudinal ligament). The middle column is composed of the posterior half of the vertebral body, the posterior portion of the annulus fibrosus, and the posterior longitudinal ligament. The posterior column is composed of the facet joints, the laminae, the spinous processes, and the posterior ligamentous complex (the facet capsules and the interspinous ligaments). Simple wedge compression fractures are caused by failure of the anterior column while the middle column remains intact. These fractures are usually stable. Burst fractures result in failure of the anterior and middle columns and are usually unstable as a result of retropulsion of bony fragments into the spinal canal. Fracture dislocations of the spine, resulting from flexion rotation forces, disrupt all three columns and are highly unstable fractures.

Mechanism of Injury

Cervical spine fractures occur in a bimodal age distribution: most injuries occur among subjects 15 to 24 years old, but a second smaller peak occurs among subjects older than 55 years old. Whereas patients younger than 30 years of age most commonly injure their cervical spine during motor vehicle accidents (MVAs) or sports (mostly diving), cervical spine fractures in patients older than 35 years are more likely caused by falls or gunshot wounds. The cause of injury is highly correlated with the anatomic site of injury. MVAs most commonly cause injuries at C1 followed by C5, C6, and C7. Falls and sports-related injuries cause fractures at C5, C6, or C7. Gunshot wounds are randomly distributed.

Clinical Presentation

The first step in recognition of cervical spine fractures is to be especially alert to their possible occurrence. A significant number of patients with an acute cervical spine injury suffer from a delayed or missed diagnosis. Factors that contribute to a delayed diagnosis include head injury, altered consciousness (resulting from head injury or alcohol or other drugs), multiple traumatic injuries, and poor-quality radiographs.

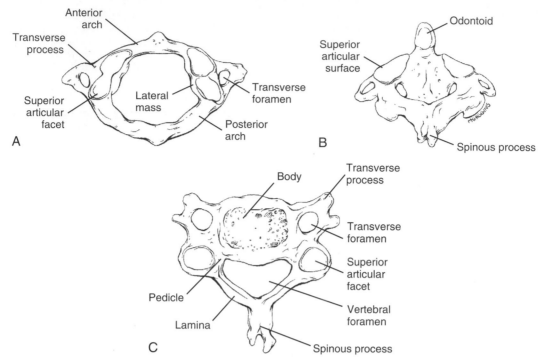

FIGURE 10-1 Anatomy of the cervical vertebrae. **A,** Superior view of C1 (atlas). **B,** Posterior view of C2 (axis). **C,** Superior view of C4.

The conscious patient may complain of neck pain, pain with motion of the neck, or loss of motor strength to one or more extremities. Complaints of sensory loss, numbness, or tingling are variable. Pain or tenderness of the neck should be elicited by palpation only, not by movement of the neck or spine. Motor function is tested by having the patient move the extremities on command. Sensation to light touch is tested to help assess the level of injury. The unconscious patient with a head injury must be presumed to have a neck injury until proven otherwise.

After a traumatic primary injury to the spinal cord, several metabolic abnormalities can cause secondary injury to the cord. This secondary injury includes loss of local vascular control, neurogenic shock, hypoperfusion of the cord, edema, and inflammation.

Imaging

Immobilization of the cervical spine should be maintained until imaging can rule out an unstable injury. Even with less severe trauma, imaging of the cervical spine must be performed in the presence

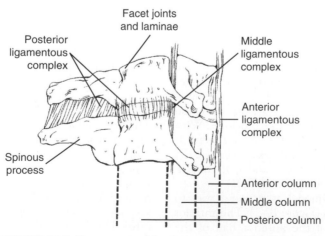

FIGURE 10-2 Components of the three-column model of the spine.

of an abnormal mental status, neurologic deficit, disproportionate midline neck pain, intoxication, or painful distracting injury. Either plain radiographs or a computed tomography (CT) scan may be used to evaluate the cervical spine in low-risk patients. If CT imaging is being performed to assess for other traumatic internal injuries of the head or chest, then plain radiographs are unnecessary.

Imaging Decision Rules

Well-validated and sensitive clinical decision rules have been developed to determine the need for cervical spine imaging. The NEXUS Low-risk Criteria (NLC) was prospectively validated in a large, multicenter, observational study.[1] The NLC has been shown to have a sensitivity of 99.6% and a specificity of 12.9%. The NLC decision rule

stipulates that imaging is *unnecessary* if patients satisfy *all* five of the following low-risk criteria:

1. Absence of posterior midline cervical tenderness
2. Normal level of alertness
3. No evidence of intoxication
4. No abnormal neurologic findings
5. No painful distracting injuries (e.g., long bone fractures, large lacerations, burns)

Plain Radiographs

Routine radiographs to assess the cervical spine include cross-table lateral, anteroposterior (AP), and open-mouth odontoid views (Figure 10-3). The lateral view detects the majority of cervical spine fractures, but a technically adequate three-view series increases the diagnostic yield.[2] The

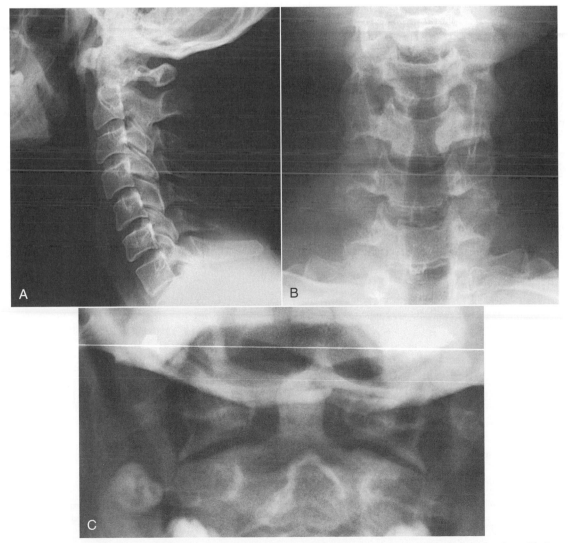

FIGURE 10-3 Routine cervical spine series. **A,** Lateral view. **B,** Anteroposterior view. **C,** Open-mouth odontoid view.

normal odontoid view shows the dens projecting from the body of C2, symmetrically flanked by the lateral masses of C1. A systematic review of plain radiographs of the cervical spine is essential if serious injuries are to be recognized. Examining the radiographs in a stepwise fashion helps ensure that cervical spine instability or fracture is not missed. Table 10-1 lists the steps to follow in reviewing cervical spine films.

All vertebrae on the Lateral View

All seven cervical vertebrae must be clearly visible on the lateral view, or repeat films must be taken. If the C7 vertebra is obscured by soft tissue, an attempt should be made to lower the shoulders by pulling the arms toward the feet with slow traction. If this is unsuccessful, the swimmer's view may be necessary to demonstrate C7 adequately. For this view, one of the patient's arms is abducted 180 degrees while traction is applied to the other arm, and the beam is directed at 15 to 20 degrees caudal. If the lower cervical vertebrae still cannot be seen on this view, CT evaluation is required.

Presence of Lordosis

The presence or absence of the normal cervical lordosis should be observed. Straightening of the cervical spine or loss of the normal cervical lordosis may be attributable to a simple muscle spasm or

may be a clue to a more serious injury (Figure 10-4).

Vertebral Alignment

The anterior and posterior aspects of the vertebral bodies should be well aligned, forming smooth continuous curves (Figure 10-5). Signs of instability include angulation between adjacent vertebral bodies of more than 11 degrees, anterior or posterior displacement of the vertebral body of more than 3.5 mm, increased distance between the spinous processes, and facet joint widening. A stepoff of up to 3.5 mm may be a normal variant along the posterior vertebral bodies. In the context of trauma to the cervical spine, further radiologic testing with dynamic flexion-extension views or CT scanning is required to determine whether the stepoff is abnormal or a normal variant. If the amount of stepoff increases in flexion or extension, the spine is unstable.

Spinolaminal Line

The spinolaminal line is behind the posterior vertebral line (see Figure 10-5). On the lateral radiograph, the junction of the lamina and the base of the spinous process appears as a bright radiodensity posterior to the vertebral bodies. The line connecting these junctions should form a smooth lordotic curve.

Table 10-1	*Systematic Review of Cervical Spine Radiographs*
	LATERAL VIEW
All vertebrae on the lateral	If all seven cervical vertebrae are not easily seen on the lateral view, repeat radiographs should be taken.
Presence of lordosis	Straightening of the cervical spine or loss of the normal cervical lordosis may be caused by simple muscle spasm or indicate a more serious injury.
Vertebral alignment	Anterior and posterior aspects of the vertebral bodies should form smooth continuous curves. Signs of instability include angulation of more than 11 degrees between adjacent vertebral bodies, more than 3.5 mm anterior or posterior displacement of the vertebral body, increased distance between the spinous processes, and facet joint widening.
Spinolaminal line	The spinolaminal line should form a smooth lordotic curve behind the posterior vertebral lines. This line connects the bases of the spinous processes and appears as a bright radiodensity posterior to the vertebral bodies.
Spinous processes	Examine the tips of the spinous processes for evidence of displacement or increased space between the spinous processes. The size and shape of the spinous processes vary, so a line connecting the tips is of limited use.
Soft tissue examination	Measure the soft tissues anterior to the upper cervical vertebrae. The soft tissue anterior to C1 through C3 should be no more than 7 mm wide.
	AP VIEW
Spinous processes	The spinous processes should be well aligned vertically. Any lateral displacement usually indicates a fracture.
	ODONTOID VIEW
C1–C2 articulation	The spaces between the lateral edges of the odontoid and the medial borders of the lateral masses should be approximately equal. The lateral masses should line up directly over the body of C2 without overlapping.

AP, anteroposterior.

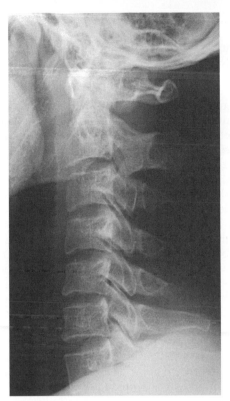

FIGURE 10-4 Lateral view of the cervical spine demonstrating loss of normal lordosis.

Spinous Processes

On the lateral view, the tips of the spinous processes are examined for evidence of displacement or increased space between the spinous processes. The size and shape of the spinous processes are variable, so a line connecting the tips is of limited use. On the AP view, the spinous processes should be well aligned vertically. Any lateral displacement usually indicates a fracture.

Odontoid View

The position of the odontoid in relation to the lateral articulating masses of C1 should be examined. The spaces between the lateral edges of the odontoid and the medial borders of the lateral masses should be approximately equal. The lateral masses should line up directly over the body of C2 without overlap.

Soft Tissue Examination

The soft tissues anterior to the upper cervical vertebrae should be measured. The soft tissue anterior to the body of C2 should be no more than 7 mm wide. More soft tissue swelling may indicate an occult cervical spine fracture. The thickness of the soft tissue anterior to C4 through C7 varies from 14 to 22 mm wide; thus, measurements are of limited diagnostic value at this level.

Flexion-Extension Radiographs

The utility of these views is uncertain. Dynamic flexion-extension cervical spine radiographs should only be considered in alert cooperative patients and may demonstrate previously undetected ligamentous disruption. They are indicated if initial radiographs show a stable cervical spine but a small possibility of instability remains.[3] The patient must be able to actively flex and extend the neck at least 30 degrees in each direction and have no neurologic deficit. Neither the radiology technician nor the attending physician should manipulate the neck to obtain these radiographs. The patient should slowly flex and extend the neck actively as far as possible, stopping for pain or paresthesias. Signs of instability on these dynamic views include more than 3.5 mm of horizontal displacement between adjacent disks, displaced apophyseal joints, widened disk spaces, loss of more than 30% of disk height, or prevertebral hematoma.

Computed Tomography

CT is useful in demonstrating bony lesions, particularly when a cervical spine fracture is suspected but not confirmed on plain radiographs. Based on a systematic review, in patients with blunt trauma, CT is superior to plain radiographs in the detecting

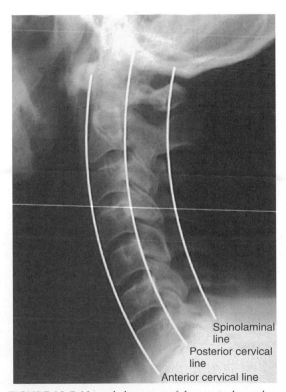

Spinolaminal line
Posterior cervical line
Anterior cervical line

FIGURE 10-5 Normal alignment of the cervical vertebrae on the lateral view.

a cervical spinal injury.[4] If a fracture or subluxation is detected on plain films, a CT scan should always be obtained to better visualize the fracture and determine whether any displacement has occurred. Plain radiographs are still adequate as the initial screen in patients at low risk for cervical spine injury.

Magnetic Resonance Imaging

Magnetic resonance imaging (MRI) is useful for visualization of soft tissues, including ligamentous structures and clear definition of canal compromise. It is useful in diagnosing nerve root avulsion, hematoma, and other vascular injury of the neck.

Fracture Patterns

C1 Fractures

Fractures of C1 may be caused by axial loads or extension forces. The most common fracture is a bilateral burst fracture (Jefferson fracture) through the posterior arch and lateral masses. Fortunately, this fracture does not typically result in neurologic injury. Posterior arch fractures are usually caused by hyperextension. The transverse ligament is disrupted, and the fracture is unstable if the lateral masses extend laterally beyond those of the axis on the open-mouth odontoid view (Figure 10-6). CT scanning is required in the complete evaluation of C1 fractures.

C2 fractures

Fractures of C2 usually occur at the arch or the odontoid. Fractures of the arch are caused by hyperextension. The unstable hangman's fracture occurs when breaks occur through both arches. In this type of C2 fracture, C2 is subluxated anteriorly relative to C3, and the posterior elements of C2 may be displaced posteriorly. CT scanning may be needed to detect a nondisplaced hangman's fracture. Fractures of the odontoid most commonly occur at the junction of the odontoid process and the body as a result of a forced flexion or extension of the head (e.g., a fall forward onto the forehead). These fractures often require surgical treatment. Avulsion fractures of the tip of the odontoid are usually horizontal and are stable, requiring only simple collar immobilization.

Facet Dislocations

Unilateral or bilateral facet dislocations cause subluxation of one vertebra relative to another. Signs

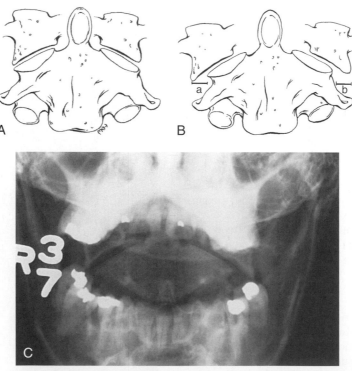

FIGURE 10-6 A, Normal alignment of the lateral masses of C1 on C2. **B,** Displacement of the lateral masses caused by of the transverse ligament. The sum of the left and right displacement is used to measure instability (a + b >7 mm). **C,** Open-mouth odontoid view of a Jefferson fracture of C1 with displacement of the lateral masses. Compare the position of the lateral masses on this view with the normal odontoid view in Figure 10-3, C.

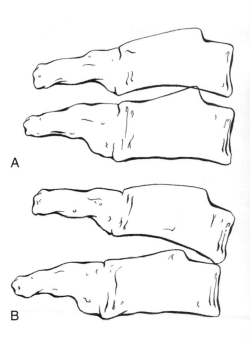

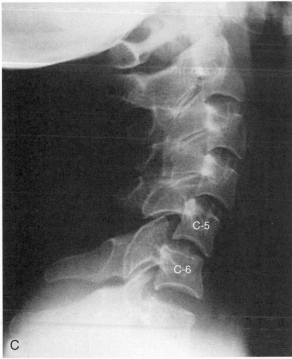

FIGURE 10-7 A, Normal alignment of the cervical vertebrae in the lateral view. **B,** Subluxated position with narrowing of the intervertebral disk, anterior angulation, and widening of the space between the spinous processes. **C,** C5–C6 subluxation. Note the widened space between the spinous processes.

of subluxation include narrowing of the intervertebral disk space, anterior angulation, and increased distance between the spinous processes (Figure 10-7). Unilateral facet dislocation, caused by axial loading with flexion and rotation, results in partial anterior subluxation of less than 50% of the vertebral body width. This is usually a stable injury. Bilateral facet dislocation is caused by severe flexion forces and disrupts both the middle and posterior columns. This unstable injury results in significant subluxation with the vertebra displaced more than 50% of the width of the body relative to the adjacent vertebra (Figure 10-8).

Wedge Fractures

Simple wedge (compression) fractures of the cervical spine can occur with even minor flexion loading forces. On the lateral radiograph, the anterior vertebral body end plate is compressed, usually in the absence of any subluxation or displacement of the vertebra (Figure 10-9). In stable simple wedge fractures, the height of the posterior vertebral cortex is maintained. These fractures must be further evaluated with dynamic flexion-extension views of the cervical spine to detect any subluxation. Fractures causing loss of more than 25% of the vertebral body height may be associated with disruption of the posterior ligamentous complex (two-column fracture).

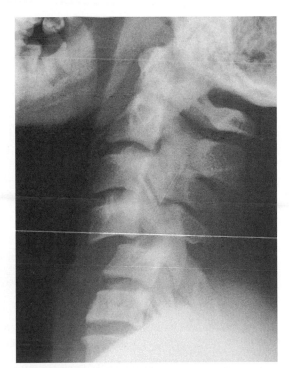

FIGURE 10-8 Bilateral facet dislocation with significant C4–C5 subluxation.

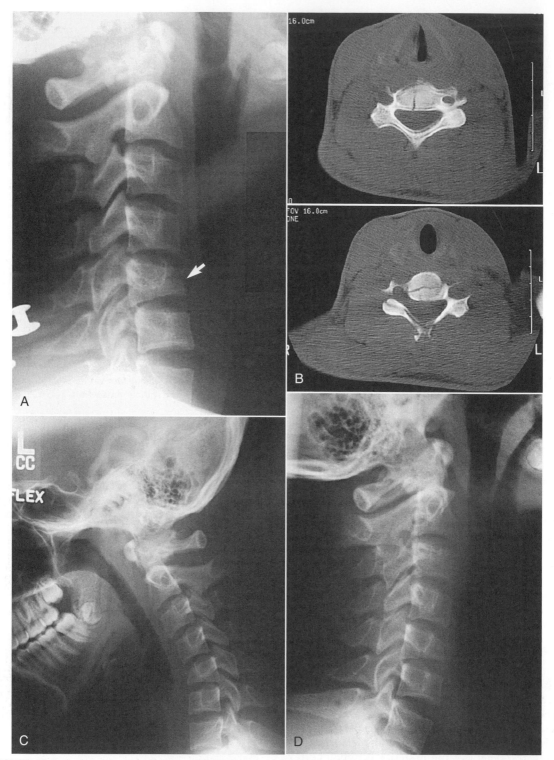

FIGURE 10-9 **A,** Anterior wedge fracture of C5 with normal alignment of the cervical spine (*arrow*). **B,** Computed tomography scan reveals fracture lines in two planes, which could indicate fracture instability. The fracture is not significantly displaced, and no protrusion of fragments into the spinal canal is apparent. **C,** Flexion and, **D,** extension views show no subluxation, indicating that this is a stable fracture. The patient was successfully treated with a rigid cervical collar.

Flexion Teardrop Fractures

This injury, caused by combined flexion and compression forces, is actually a fracture dislocation and is among the most unstable of all cervical spine fractures. A small anteroinferior teardrop fragment is present with subluxation of the vertebral body or facets or angulation of the spine (Figure 10-10). The teardrop fragment typically remains aligned with the inferior vertebra, and the posterior fragment remains aligned with the vertebra superior to the level of injury. These fractures must be distinguished from a small anteroinferior avulsion fracture that has no signs of subluxation, comminution, or angulation.

Burst Fractures

These fractures, caused by compression and flexion forces (e.g., diving injury), are comminuted and disrupt both the anterior and middle columns. Severe spinal cord injury occurs if the fracture fragments displace anteriorly and posteriorly. The middle and lower cervical vertebrae are most frequently involved.

Spinous Process Fractures

Fractures of the spinous processes occur as a result of direct trauma to the process, sudden deceleration and resultant neck flexion after high velocity trauma, or avulsion forces from severe muscular

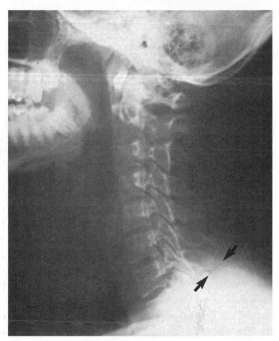

FIGURE 10-11 Avulsion fracture of the spinous process of C7, the so-called clay shoveler's fracture (*arrows*). (*From Mettler FA Jr. Essentials of Radiology. Philadelphia, WB Saunders, 1996.*)

contraction. An avulsed tip of the spinous process of C6 or C7 is known as the "clay shoveler's fracture" (Figure 10-11) because historically the strong pull of neck and shoulder muscles during heavy physical work could result in an avulsion fracture. On the AP radiograph, the affected spinous process may be seen displaced laterally from the midline. Fractures of the tip of the spinous process are stable and must be distinguished from fractures at the base of the process that may disrupt the posterior ligamentous complex. Dynamic flexion-extension radiographs of the cervical spine should be checked to ensure that the anterior and posterior columns remain aligned. A nonfused apophysis of a spinous process can be confused with an acute fracture.

Indications for Referral

Most cervical spine fractures are unstable and require definitive care by a specialist. Even minor fractures noted on plain radiographs may be associated with significant ligamentous injuries that render the cervical spine unstable. Although stable fractures such as a simple anterior wedge fracture or a spinous process fracture can be managed by the primary care provider, consultation with a spine orthopedist or neurosurgeon and review of the radiographs are helpful in the management of these patients.

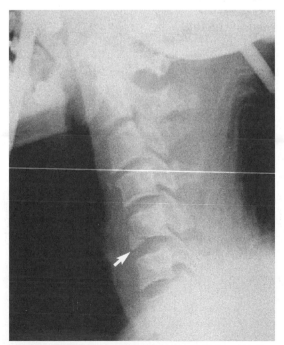

FIGURE 10-10 Flexion teardrop fracture of C5. Note that the teardrop fragment is aligned with C6, and the posterior fragment remains aligned with C4 (*arrow*).

Initial Treatment

Prehospital Care

Before transport, the patient with a suspected cervical spine fracture should be placed in the neutral supine position on a backboard. A scoop-type stretcher should be used if available. The neck should then be stabilized with a firm, preferably two-piece, cervical collar to minimize neck motion. The head and neck should then be stabilized with sandbags and the chest and extremities securely strapped to the backboard. During transport to an appropriate facility, the patient should be kept in slight Trendelenburg position to minimize the effects of neurogenic shock.

Emergent Care

On the patient's arrival at a well-staffed facility, Advanced Trauma Life Support (ATLS) protocols should be followed. Hemodynamically unstable patients typically are taken to the operating room rather than delaying further with any imaging because they are presumed to have an unstable cervical spine injury in this circumstance. The cervical spine and paraspinous musculature should be palpated for tenderness or deformity followed by a complete neurologic survey.

Follow-up Care

Stabilization of the cervical spine with early mobilization and rehabilitation is the key to treating cervical spine fractures and may be accomplished by either nonoperative or operative means. Stabilization in more severe and unstable cervical spine fractures is usually achieved by using a halo and vest or through operative stabilizing procedures.

Stable fractures such as nondisplaced anterior wedge fractures or isolated spinous process fractures with intact ligamentous support may be treated with a rigid cervical orthosis (e.g., Philadelphia collar) and analgesics for 4 to 8 weeks. The patient should wear this orthosis until the neck is nontender and then begin gentle range of motion (ROM) exercises under the guidance of a physical therapist. Some patients may benefit from the use of muscle relaxants during the rehabilitation period. Neck muscle strengthening exercises can be started after full painless ROM is achieved. Normal activities should be resumed gradually, and vigorous physical activity is best avoided until normal motion and strength are restored. Patients with anterior wedge fractures should have repeat radiographs taken at weekly intervals to document healing and check for any further loss of vertebral height. A follow-up radiograph of a spinous process fracture is advised after the neck is nontender to document evidence of radiographic healing.

Return to Work or Sports

Patients with simple wedge compression fractures or spinous process fractures may return to nonstrenuous occupations after the tenderness is gone and they have regained normal or near-normal ROM of the cervical spine. Decisions about returning to work must be individualized for patients who have sustained an unstable fracture, flexion teardrop fracture, fracture dislocation, or burst fracture. Close consultation with a neurosurgeon is recommended.

CERVICAL SPINE FRACTURES (PEDIATRIC)

Anatomic Considerations

Cervical spine injuries among children are fundamentally different from adults' injuries because of anatomic differences and dissimilar causes of injury. Cervical spine injuries are relatively uncommon among children: fewer than 1% of all cervical spine injuries occur among children younger than 15 years of age. Typically, the child's cervical spine does not take on an adult-like appearance until 8 years of age. In children younger than 8 years of age, anatomic differences specific to children include the greater relative mass of the head, underdeveloped neck muscles, greater ligamentous laxity, horizontally oriented posterior facets, and incomplete ossification of the vertebral bodies. Ligamentous laxity allows the child's cervical spine to absorb and dissipate traumatic forces without injury to the vertebra or the spinal cord. However, these anatomic differences predispose children to wedge-shaped anterior vertebral fractures and anterior sliding injuries, especially in the upper cervical region (C1 to C4). The most common sites for fractures in children younger than 8 years of age are the upper cervical vertebrae C1 to C3.[5] In children older than 8 years of age, fractures of C6 and C7 are the most common.

Mechanism of Injury

The cause of injury varies with the patient's age. Infants may sustain neck injuries during birth or because of child abuse. Injuries in this age group involve the occiput, C1, or C2 and are usually of a spinal cord injury without radiographic abnormality (SCIWORA). Young children usually sustain cervical spine injuries from falls or MVAs. Older children and adolescents' neck injuries may be sports related or caused by bicycle, motor vehicle–pedestrian, or all-terrain vehicle accidents.

Cervical spine injury can occur through various mechanisms, and the type of deforming forces may predict the type of injury and radiologic findings.

Hyperflexion injuries are the most common and may cause wedge fractures of the anterior vertebral body along with injury of the posterior elements. Hyperextension injuries may cause compression of the posterior elements and a tear of the anterior longitudinal ligament. Axial loading may cause burst or comminuted fractures of the arches of the upper cervical spine or compression fractures of the lower cervical vertebra. Rotational injuries may cause a fracture or dislocation of the facets.

Clinical Presentation

The most common symptoms are localized neck pain, decreased ROM, and muscle spasm. The patient may also report transient paresthesias or weakness. The history should include symptoms present at any time after the injury even if they are transient. Transient symptoms may be the only indication of SCIWORA, and it is important to have a high index of suspicion and to ask specifically about transient symptoms in any patient whose mechanism of injury is consistent with cervical spine injury. Patients who have sustained serious trauma, multiple injuries, or both are particularly at risk for unrecognized neck injuries. Physical examination should include assessment of vital signs, a neck examination, and a neurologic examination. Midline cervical tenderness is more common than paraspinous muscular spasm or tenderness in the presence of a cervical spine injury. The neurologic assessment should include evaluation of tone, strength, sensation, and reflexes. Up to half of children with cervical spine trauma also have neurologic deficits.[6] Children who have findings suggestive of spinal injury should have immobilization maintained and undergo immediate radiologic evaluation.

Imaging

Although by 8 to 10 years of age the child's spine is similar to that of an adult, interpretation of cervical spine radiographs in children is difficult. Normal variants at various ages must be distinguished from pathologic findings. The tip of the odontoid process shows a cartilage line until the 12 years of age, and the vertebral ring apophyses do not fuse until 25 years of age. In the open-mouthed AP view, the odontoid process appears sandwiched between the neural arches. Between 3 and 6 years of age, the odontoid fuses with the neural arches and the body of C2. Therefore, no physis should be seen at the odontoid of a child 6 years of age or older. Vertebrae C3 through C7 arise from three ossification centers: one for the anterior vertebral body and one each for the neural arches. Between 3 and 6 years of age, the neural arches fuse with the anterior segment. On the lateral view, the child's vertebral bodies appear wedge shaped until the age of 7 years, at which time they develop the more "squared-off" appearance.

Criteria have been developed to identify those with low probability of cervical spine injury to determine when radiographic evaluation is not necessary.[7] In children older than 8 years of age, if they meet all five of these criteria, radiographs can safely be avoided: no midline cervical tenderness, no focal neurologic deficit; normal alertness; no intoxication; and no painful, distracting injury. If radiographs are indicated, three views of the cervical spine are recommended: cross-table lateral, AP, and open-mouth odontoid. The cross-table lateral identifies the majority of fractures, subluxations, and dislocations.[8] The most common cause of an overlooked vertebral fracture is an inadequate film series so obtaining appropriate views is essential. Flexion-extension views may identify cervical instability and may be useful when the three views are negative despite the presence of cervical pain, tenderness, or spasm. They do require that the patient is alert and cooperative. MRI is the imaging procedure of choice in any patient with neurologic signs or symptoms and normal plain radiographs.

The lateral view should be systematically evaluated looking for bony integrity, alignment of the three cervical spine contour lines (Figure 10-5), and soft tissue spaces. Absence of cervical lordosis may be attributable to muscle spasm and may be normally absent in children up to age 15 years. The examiner should be aware that the spinolaminal line is not as easily seen in children as in adults. Some children demonstrate significant anterior subluxation of C2 on C3 often accentuated by neck flexion (Figure 10-12). This is because of the increased mobility of the child's cervical spine and to the horizontal orientation of the facet joints. If the patient has no history of neck injury or neck pain and has normal neck ROM, "pseudosubluxation" can be presumed. The posterior cervical (Swischuk) line between the anterior aspects of the C1 and C3 spinous processes is used to distinguish pseudosubluxation from true subluxation. True subluxation should be suspected if the posterior cervical line misses the anterior aspect of the C2 spinous process by 2 mm or more.

Widening of the predental and prevertebral soft tissue space is caused by hemorrhage or edema, which may indicate dislocation or fracture of a cervical vertebra. The predental space is between the posterior surface of the anterior arch of C1 and the anterior surface of odontoid process of C2. In children younger than 8 years of age, the predental space should be no more than 4 to 5 mm. The prevertebral space at the level of C3 and C4 should be no more than one third the AP diameter of the vertebral body. The amount of adenoid tissue,

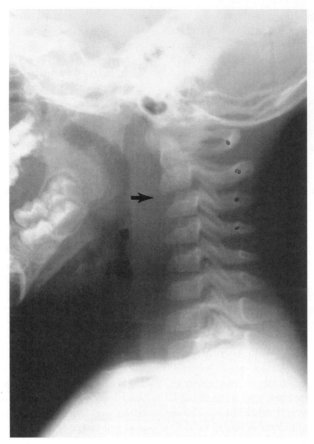

FIGURE 10-12 Pseudosubluxation. The arrow points to an apparent subluxation of C2 on C3, which in reality is normal. A line drawn between the anterior aspects of the C1 and C3 processes would course within 2 mm of the anterior aspect of the C2 spinous process. *(From Green NE, Swiontkowski MF [eds]. Skeletal Trauma in Children, 2nd ed. Philadelphia, WB Saunders, 1998.)*

position changes, and crying may give the false impression of a widened prevertebral soft tissue space. These soft tissues are fairly uniform in adults but vary more widely in children, making them more difficult to evaluate.

The AP view should be examined for the presence of lateral mass fractures. The odontoid process should be examined for any longitudinal or transverse fractures. The lateral aspects of C1 should be symmetric, and they should have equal amounts of space on both sides of the odontoid.

The incidence of multilevel injury is high for children with cervical spine injury, approaching 25%; therefore, the presence of one cervical abnormality should prompt close evaluation for other associated injuries.

Fracture Patterns

Spinal Cord Injury without Radiographic Abnormality

SCIWORA is defined as objective signs of myelopathy resulting from trauma in the absence of findings on imaging studies. MRI has decreased the true incidence of this condition since it was originally described in 1982.[9] SCIWORA is unique to children and occurs because of the higher mobility of the child's cervical spine, relative ligamentous laxity, and immature vascularization of the child's spinal cord. Acceleration–deceleration or rotation are the usual mechanisms of injury. Transient neurologic symptoms may be the only indication that the cervical spine has been injured. Children younger than 8 years of age are especially at risk of SCIWORA.

Odontoid Fracture

Fracture of the odontoid process is the most common cervical spine fracture among children. The average age at occurrence is 4 years. Fractures usually occur at the base of the odontoid process and are in reality "physeal" injuries through the synchondrosis between the odontoid process and the body of C2. The patient reports facial or head trauma, usually after a fall or MVA, although this injury may also occur after relatively minor trauma.

The patient complains of neck pain and may be unwilling to extend the neck. The AP view may only show the normal synchondritic line, with typical anterior displacement of the odontoid process apparent only on the lateral view (Figure 10-13). CT is preferable for distinguishing a fracture from a normal synchondrosis and detecting displacement. Acute injuries must also be distinguished from os odontoideum, which represents an odontoid nonunion or a developmental anomaly (Figure 10-14). Os odontoideum can lead to neck pain and neurologic symptoms or may be asymptomatic. Stable odontoid fractures are usually treated nonoperatively in a halo brace. After 6 to 10 weeks of immobilization, lateral flexion-extension views should be examined to confirm fracture union.

True C2 on C3 Subluxation

As previously discussed in the Imaging section, hypermobility of the child's cervical spine allows significant pseudosubluxation of C2 on C3. True subluxation can be suspected if the patient reports trauma sufficient to cause a neck injury, has neck pain and muscle spasm, and has decreased ROM and point tenderness when examined. Some patients report continued symptoms despite an appropriate course of conservative therapy; these patients may have a true subluxation. Radiographic findings suggestive of true subluxation include

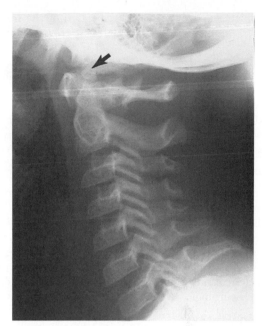

FIGURE 10-14 Os odontoideum (arrow). (From Thornton A, Gyll C. Children's Fractures: A Radiological Guide to Safe Practice. Philadelphia, WB Saunders, 1999.)

ossification of the posterior longitudinal ligament, avulsion fracture of the tips of the spinous processes, and compensatory lordosis.

Wedge Compression Fractures

Wedge compression fractures below the level of C3 are the most common cervical spine injury among children. The usual cause of injury is flexion with axial loading, leading to the wedge compression fracture. Radiographs may show associated injuries such as anterior teardrop fracture, laminar fracture, or spinous process fracture. The wedge compression fracture may go unrecognized because of the typical pediatric ossification pattern. Simple compression fractures (no displacement with intact posterior elements) are stable injuries and heal within 3 to 6 weeks. A cervical collar is worn for 2 to 4 weeks until the injury no longer is tender; then follow-up flexion-extension radiographs are obtained to confirm AP stability.

Indications for Referral

Cervical spine injuries in children are difficult to detect and pose potentially lethal complications. Children suspected of having such serious injuries should be stabilized on a backboard and referred to a neurosurgeon.

Initial Treatment

The patient should be placed in the supine position with the head and neck stabilized. The neck should be stabilized in a hard cervical collar,

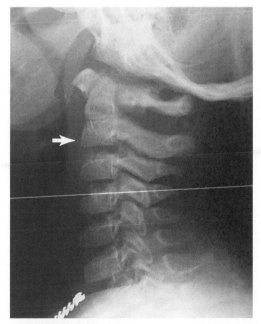

FIGURE 10-13 Synchondrosis at the base of the odontoid (arrow), simulating a fracture in a 3-year-old child. (From Thornton A, Gyll C. Children's Fractures: A Radiological Guide to Safe Practice. Philadelphia, WB Saunders, 1999.)

supplemented by further stabilization of the head (e.g., taping, sandbags, and foam head immobilizer). Because the child's head is relatively large compared with the body, the occiput should be placed 1 or 2 inches below the level of the supine child's back to obtain better supine cervical alignment. This can be accomplished by use of a backboard with a cutout to recess the occiput or a backboard with padding to raise the chest relative to the neck.

Follow-up Care

Definitive treatment is individualized. Patients with instability usually require immobilization in a Minerva body jacket or halo vest. Occasionally, a patient requires posterior fusion of the involved cervical spine. Close follow-up for years after the injury is needed for early detection of common late complications such as spinal deformity or progressive neurologic deficit.

Complications

Associated injuries are common. Among children with cervical spine injuries caused by MVAs, approximately 50% have an associated head injury, 24% an associated orthopedic injury, and 25% an abdominal injury. Mortality is closely related to the presence of head injury.

A common complication is development of late spinal deformity. The younger the patient and the higher the cervical lesion, the greater the likelihood of late spinal deformity. Deformities include scoliosis, kyphosis, and hyperlordosis. Another late complication is development of intramedullary spinal cord cysts caused by spinal cord trauma. These can be detected by MRI and may require surgical drainage. Children who undergo posterior spinal fusion because of cervical spine injury are likely to have chronic neck pain and stiffness.

Return to Sports

Allowing return to sports after cervical spine injury is controversial. No return to sports is possible until all spinal instability is corrected or resolved. Patients who have undergone spinal fusion have decreased cervical spine mobility and should avoid contact and collision sports and be directed toward noncontact sports. MRI that documents a cerebrospinal fluid (CSF) "reserve" around the spinal cord should be obtained before return to sports is allowed.

THORACOLUMBAR SPINE FRACTURES (ADULT)

The thoracolumbar spine is the predominant site of vertebral fractures. Most of these fractures (75%) occur among patients 15 to 64 years of age, but a significant percentage occur among older patients. These fractures are caused by high-energy trauma in younger patients and minimal or no trauma in older patients with osteoporosis. Traumatic fractures include compression fractures, spinous process and transverse process fractures, and burst fractures. Nontraumatic fractures may occur as a result of osteoporosis, tumors, or vertebral osteomyelitis (VO).

Anatomic Considerations

The 12 thoracic vertebrae are intermediate in size between the smaller cervical and larger lumbar vertebrae (Figure 10-15). The thoracic spine maintains a slight kyphosis, and each vertebral body articulates with the rib cage. The rib cage and sternum stabilize the upper part of the thoracic spine (T1–T9). The thoracolumbar junction is particularly susceptible to injury and instability because the spinal column progresses from the stable thoracic spine to the more mobile lumbar spine at this level. Fractures in the lower lumbar area (L2–L5) tend to be stable owing to the large vertebral bodies, the surrounding musculature, and the lordosis, which places the vertebral bodies anterior to the center of gravity. Fractures at L5 and S1 tend to be unstable as a result of the

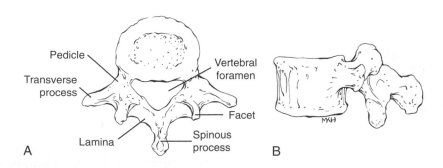

FIGURE 10-15 Anatomy of the thoracic and lumbar vertebrae. **A,** Superior view. **B,** Lateral view.

high-energy forces required to cause injury at this level.

Compression Fractures

Mechanism of Injury

Acute compression fractures are caused by an axial load combined with flexion or lateral bending of the spine. Flexion forces account for 89% of compression fractures; lateral bending leads to another 11%. Significant trauma, such as a fall or an MVA, is the usual cause of spine fractures in young to middle-aged adults. A compression fracture with a history of minimal or no trauma in an adult without osteoporosis should raise suspicion of a metastatic or primary malignant process.

Clinical Presentation

Patients report acute onset of pain sharply localized to the midline of the spine. The area of maximal point tenderness should be noted and the midline carefully palpated for a stepoff deformity over the vertebral body. Testing of motor and sensory function is essential. Injuries to the thoracolumbar spine can have a variety of neurologic deficits arising from injuries to the thoracolumbar nerve roots, terminal spinal cord, cauda equina, or conus medullaris.

Pulmonary, vascular, and visceral injuries are often associated with thoracolumbar spine fractures. Patients with thoracic spine fractures may have a hemopneumothorax, aortic tear, or ruptured diaphragm. Patients with lumbar fractures may have abdominal trauma, including injuries to the bowel, liver, spleen, and genitourinary tract.

Imaging

Initial radiographs should include AP, lateral, and oblique views of the entire thoracolumbar spine because many patients have fractures at more than one level. Most compression fractures occur at the level of T11 to L2, and a fracture of the superior end plate is the most common pattern.[10] Radiographs should be examined in a systematic way to avoid missing subtle signs of a fracture. A wedge-type deformity of the anterior aspect of the vertebral body is common (Figure 10-16). The anterior and posterior vertebral body heights should be compared because loss of more than 50% of the original height is indicative of instability. The Cobb angle is the most accurate and reproducible measure of local kyphosis.[11] This angle is calculated from the intersection of a line drawn perpendicular to the superior end plate of the vertebra above the fracture and a line perpendicular to the inferior end plate of the vertebra below the fracture. The superior and inferior vertebral body end plates should be examined for fracture and the

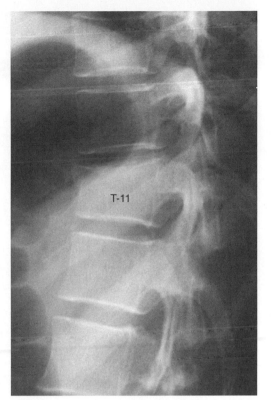

FIGURE 10-16 Traumatic compression fracture of T11. This is a stable fracture because the loss of anterior vertebral body height is not more than 50% compared with the posterior vertebral height. The posterior height has been preserved.

integrity of the anterior cortex of the vertebral body assessed. On the lateral view, the spinous processes are examined with particular attention paid to the space between adjacent processes.

On the AP view, the width of each vertebral body is examined, with particular attention to the interpedicular distance. The pedicles are seen end on in the AP view and appear as ringlike structures on either side of the vertebral body. Compared with adjacent vertebrae, a widening of the space between pedicles of more than 3 mm is an important indication of a fracture of the vertebral body (Figure 10-17). Alignment of the superior and inferior facets should be noted when the facet joints on the oblique views are examined. The facet joints should be tightly apposed, symmetric, and paired.

CT scanning should follow plain radiographs and is particularly useful in detecting occult fractures or bony impingement on the spinal canal and is helpful in determining fracture stability.[12] MRI is recommended in the presence of a neurologic deficit to evaluate soft tissue injuries such as spinal cord compression, cord edema or contusion,

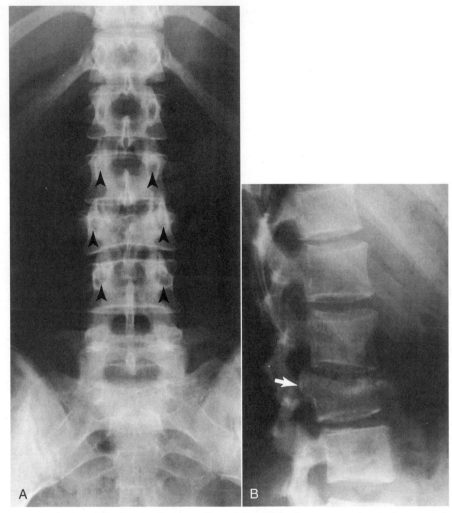

FIGURE 10-17 A, Widening of the distance between the pedicles of L3 when compared with the interpedicle distance of the adjacent vertebrae. **B,** Lateral view of the same patient showing a wedge fracture of L3. This is an unstable fracture because of the posterior displacement of bone fragments into the spinal canal. *(From Raby N, Berman L, DeLong G. Accident and Emergency Radiology: A Survival Guide. Philadelphia, WB Saunders, 1995.)*

epidural hematoma, ligamentous disruption, or nerve root involvement.

Indications for Referral

Patients with unstable fractures or stable fractures with any sign of neurologic injury should be referred for neurosurgical evaluation. Radiographic findings that suggest instability and the need for further evaluation include loss of more than 50% of vertebral body height, presence of more than 20 degrees of angulation, an increased space between the spinous processes, and disruption of the posterior column. Unstable compression fractures may be managed operatively or nonoperatively, and treatment is individualized and best left to the specialist to determine the appropriate course of therapy.

Initial Treatment

Table 10-2 summarizes management guidelines for compression fractures of the thoracolumbar spine.

Nonsurgical treatment achieves good functional results for stable anterior and lateral compression fractures of the thoracic spine at the thoracolumbar junction.[13] Patients should be prescribed 24 to 48 hours of bed rest. Because serial neurologic reevaluation is important in the monitoring of these patients, bed rest is best accomplished during a hospital stay. Patients with an acute spine fracture often have an associated ileus; oral intake should be restricted until this resolves, usually within 2 to 3 days.

Management of pain after an acute fracture may require narcotic analgesics for 2 to 3 days.

Table 10-2	*Management Guidelines for Thoracolumbar Compression Fractures*
	INITIAL TREATMENT
Splint type and position	Bed rest and serial neurologic monitoring for 24 to 48 hours
	Narcotic analgesics
	Observe for signs of ileus
Initial follow-up visit	Within 7 to 10 days
Patient instruction	Ambulate with assistance (cane) after 48 hours
	FOLLOW-UP CARE
Cast or splint type and position	TLSO (usually not necessary with minimal compression)
Length of immobilization	4 to 6 weeks (if TLSO used)
Healing time	8 to 12 weeks
Follow-up visit interval	Every 2 to 4 weeks until healed
Repeat radiography interval	At 3, 6, and 12 weeks to look for kyphotic deformity
Patient instruction	Isometric back extension exercises followed by back strengthening exercises and aerobic conditioning when pain is minimal and no progressive deformity is apparent
Indications for orthopedic consult	>50% loss of vertebral height
	>20 degrees of angulation
	Increased space between spinous processes
	Disruption of facet joints
	Neurologic deficit
	Progressive kyphotic deformity during healing

TLSO, thoracolumbosacral orthosis.

Nonsteroidal antiinflammatory drugs (NSAIDs) are also useful in controlling pain and inflammation. Physical measures such as gentle massage, moist heat, or ice packs can be used to relieve pain. Bed rest in the supine position on a firm mattress helps ease pain, particularly if the patient uses a thin pillow under the head and a fuller pillow under the knees. The lateral decubitus position with a pillow between the knees and the hip and knee in slight flexion may be more comfortable for some patients. Sitting is allowed as soon as pain begins to lessen, usually within 2 to 5 days. Ambulation with assistance is encouraged as early as possible, and use of a cane in the hand opposite to the painful side reduces the pain of weight bearing.

Follow-up Care

After a brief period of bed rest, stable compression fractures may be treated with early ambulation, with or without a thoracolumbosacral orthosis (TLSO), and regular radiographic follow-up. A recent review found no evidence for improved outcomes using a brace, although high-quality studies are lacking.[14] Radiographs are obtained at 3, 6, and 12 weeks to rule out a progressive kyphotic deformity. If pain is minimal and no progressive deformity is detected, patients may be advanced to isometric back extension exercises followed by back-strengthening exercises and aerobic conditioning.

Return to Work or Sports

Patients with a simple wedge compression fracture or spinous process fracture may return to nonstrenuous occupations after they have no pain and have regained normal or near-normal ROM. Return to work decisions must be individualized for patients who have sustained an unstable fracture, fracture dislocation, or burst fracture. Close consultation with a neurosurgeon is recommended.

Spinous Process and Transverse Process Fractures

Fractures of either the spinous process or transverse process of the thoracolumbar spine are generally benign injuries and do not result in neurologic deficits or spine instability. However, because significant force is usually required to cause these injuries, the clinician must be alert to signs of concomitant intraabdominal organ injuries.[15] The cause of injury of a transverse process fracture is a lateral bending force with a subsequent avulsion of the process on the convex side. The usual site for these fractures is L2, L3, or L4, and multiple contiguous fractures are common. Spinous process fractures are caused by hyperflexion or direct blows.

After these injuries, the patient has point tenderness over the fracture site, and the surrounding paraspinous muscles may be in spasm. An accompanying ileus is common. A urinalysis should be obtained because renal contusion may be associated with these fractures. The AP view can demonstrates transverse process fractures, and this view should be examined for a lateral compression fracture on the side opposite the fractured process. Because transverse process fractures can be missed on plain films, CT should be obtained to rule out this injury in patients with blunt trauma. Spinous process fractures can be detected on the lateral view.

Treatment of these fractures includes bed rest as needed for the first few days and adequate analgesics. The patient can resume normal activity gradually as tolerated. Patients may be symptomatic for 4 to 6 weeks. Healing may result in a nonunion, but this is usually not of functional consequence. Patients with persistent pain after a nonunion should be referred for consideration of surgical excision of the avulsed fragment.

Burst Fractures

Axial loading forces, usually from a fall, cause burst fractures of the thoracolumbar spine that result in failure of both the anterior and middle columns of the spine. Fractures of the middle column (i.e., posterior vertebral body) often result in displacement of bony fragments posteriorly and spinal cord injury. The radiographic appearance of burst fractures includes loss of vertebral body height and retropulsion of bony fragments on the lateral view. On the AP view, the interpedicular distance is increased. CT scanning is recommended to adequately evaluate impingement of bony fragments on the spinal cord.

By definition, most burst fractures are unstable with a high risk for spinal cord injury, so patients should be referred for definitive care. Emergency care includes stabilization and resuscitation with transport of the patient to an appropriate trauma center as needed. In patients without a neurologic deficit, nonoperative and operative treatment have similar outcomes.[16] Nonoperative treatment includes bed rest and immobilization with a brace. Operative therapy involves anterior or posterior stabilization and removal of bone fragments extruded into the spinal canal.

THORACOLUMBAR SPINE FRACTURES (PEDIATRIC)

Fractures involving the thoracic or lumbar spine among children are rare. Most fractures occur in the adolescent age group and are caused by recreational or sports activities, MVAs, or falls from a significant height. In infants, these fractures may indicate nonaccidental trauma. More than one vertebra is fractured in 50% to 75% of thoracolumbar fractures.

Anatomic Considerations

By the time a child has reached the age of 10 years, the spine is quite similar to an adult's. The pediatric vertebral column is more malleable to deforming forces than the adult spine and has a higher cartilage component. In children, the intervertebral disk is firm, and compression of the spine usually results in failure of the vertebral end plate. Moreover, these elastic disks transmit forces through several segments, resulting in multiple compression fractures that usually occur in the midthoracic and midlumbar sections of the spine. The vertebral end plate is particularly susceptible to shear forces because the vertebral apophysis (analogous to the epiphysis of long bones) is separated from the end plate by a narrow cartilaginous physis.

Mechanism of Injury

The most common type of thoracolumbar fracture in children is a vertebral body compression fracture caused by axial loading or a hyperflexion injury. A fracture pattern seen from a seatbelt injury is the Chance fracture, in which forward flexion causes compression of the anterior column of the vertebral spine and simultaneous tension along the posterior column of the spine. Burst fractures occur in patterns similar to those seen in adults and occur mainly at the thoracolumbar junction. Compression forces and activities such as weightlifting, gymnastics, or shoveling may cause slipping of the vertebral apophysis. This injury usually affects adolescents, most commonly at the L4 level.

Clinical Presentation

The patient typically reports involvement in an MVA, sports activity, or significant fall. During physical examination, the patient may have midline tenderness of the involved spinal segment, muscle spasm, inability to walk, or a combination of these symptoms. The patient may also have obvious ecchymosis, significant soft tissue swelling, and marked tenderness in the posterior spinal area. Acute slipping of the vertebral apophysis may cause symptoms similar to those of acute disk herniation in an adult, including muscle weakness, altered deep tendon reflexes, or positive results on a straight-leg raising test.

Intraabdominal injury commonly accompanies traumatic thoracolumbar fracture, especially seatbelt fractures. Up to 20% of patients with fractures of the thoracic or lumbar spinous processes have intraabdominal injuries that include the liver, spleen, pelvis, or urinary tract.

Imaging

Suspected thoracic or lumbar spine injury indicates a need for AP and lateral views. The radiographic findings of compression fractures vary. Minor injuries may show some flattening of the normal slightly convex appearance of the thoracic vertebrae and angulation less than 30 degrees. More severe injuries cause anterior wedging of the body or loss of the posterior border concavity. Fracture at more than one level is common. Adolescents may show a more typical adult pattern of fracture such as fracture dislocation. Fractures of the posterior arch may require CT scanning for adequate visualization. In cases of slipped vertebral apophysis, the CT scan may show a small bony fragment within the spinal canal. MRI is used to delineate injury to the spinal cord or cauda equina. MRI may demonstrate spinal cord edema, contusion, or hemorrhage.

Chance fractures most typically affect the upper lumbar vertebrae (L1 to L3) and are best seen on the lateral view. A bilateral facet dislocation or lamina fracture will cause splaying of the posterior elements (Figure 10-18). The fracture usually extends through the vertebral body, but this is often invisible on plain films.

Indications for Orthopedic Referral

All patients with a suspected spinal cord injury or multisystem trauma should be immobilized on a

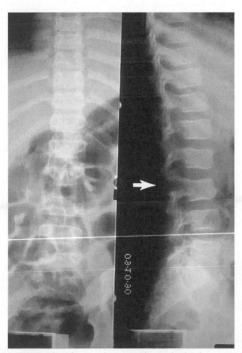

FIGURE 10-18 Chance fracture through the lamina of L3 (*arrow*). Splayed posterior elements on the lateral view are the clue to the diagnosis. The anteroposterior view appears normal. (*From Thornton A, Gyll C. Children's Fractures: A Radiological Guide to Safe Practice. Philadelphia, WB Saunders, 1999.*)

backboard and referred for definitive care. Patients with an unstable fracture, a Chance fracture, vertebral apophysis avulsion, or fracture dislocation must be referred to a specialist. Selected patients who have no radiographic abnormality but have significant trauma and neurologic complaints, findings, or both should also be referred to rule out the possibility of SCIWORA. Some burst fractures can be managed nonoperatively, but all should be referred to a specialist to make the treatment decisions.

Treatment

Stable fractures, including most compression fractures, spinous process fractures, and transverse process fractures, respond well to conservative treatment. The patient may be immobilized in a TLSO or simply prescribed bed rest for a few days. The patient should be seen again within 1 week. Repeat radiographs should be obtained to confirm that the fracture is indeed stable. Many patients do well with simple restriction of activity; more symptomatic patients may require continued use of the TLSO. Most patients are asymptomatic within 10 to 14 days.

Complications

Growth arrest is relatively uncommon after a compression fracture or Chance fracture. Bony remodeling is expected for children 10 years of age and younger; children older than 10 years of age show less potential for remodeling. Injury to the vertebral end plate seldom results in significant scoliosis.

Spinal deformity is a late complication, especially if neurologic deficit (e.g., paraplegia) is present. Scoliosis, kyphosis, or hyperlordosis may develop. The younger the patient and the more proximal the lesion, the greater the likelihood of spinal deformity.

Return to Sports

After simple compression fracture, the patient can return to sports activity after pain is resolved and flexibility is normal, usually 8 to 12 weeks after injury. The decision to resume sports activities after a Chance fracture, burst fracture, or vertebral apophysis avulsion must be individualized and managed in consultation with an orthopedic surgeon or neurosurgeon.

SPONDYLOLYSIS

Mechanism of Injury

Spondylolysis is a defect of the pars interarticularis (usually lumbar), the narrow portion of bone between the superior and inferior articular facets.

The defect can result from congenital, degenerative, traumatic, or stress-related causes. Approximately 10% of the adult white population has a pars defect on radiographs.[17] Spondylolysis is more common in adolescents than adults and can occur in those involved in repetitive mechanical loading of the back, especially with hyperextension and the performance of heavy physical work. Three types of sporting activities are implicated in pars stress injuries from repetitive motion: weight-loading sports (weightlifting), rotation-associated sports (tennis, baseball, golf), and back-arching sports (gymnastics, swimming, diving, football [especially linemen], and volleyball).[18]

Clinical Presentation

Spondylolysis should be suspected in an adolescent with unilateral low back pain of 2 to 3 weeks' duration. Typically, the patient reports unilateral low back pain without radiation at the level of the belt. The pain worsens with extension and rotation, and symptoms may begin after the intensity of usual activities has been increased. During physical examination, the patient is usually able to localize the pain with "one-finger" accuracy, and most of the time the pain is at the L5 level. The patient usually has full ROM, but the pain is accentuated with the single-leg extension test, also know as the "stork test": the patient balances on the leg on whichever side of the body has the lumbar pain and then hyperextends the back. Unfortunately, this test has low sensitivity ad specificity for spondylolysis.[19] Hamstring tightness is a common finding. Sensory and motor functions are normal.

Imaging

Oblique radiographs, which eliminate bony overlap, are necessary to detect a fracture of the pars. The classic finding is a defect (lucent line) appearing at the neck of the "Scottie dog" (Figure 10-19). Most pars defects are at the L5 level. Bilateral pars fractures result in spondylolisthesis or slippage of the affected vertebra anterior to the vertebra below it (Figure 10-20).

Oblique plain radiograph results may be negative in acute cases because the stress fracture is not yet complete. If spondylolysis is clinically suspected, a bone scan may help confirm the diagnosis. The combination of plain films and a bone scan can theoretically determine whether the bone-healing process is active or completed. A positive plain radiography result and a negative bone scan

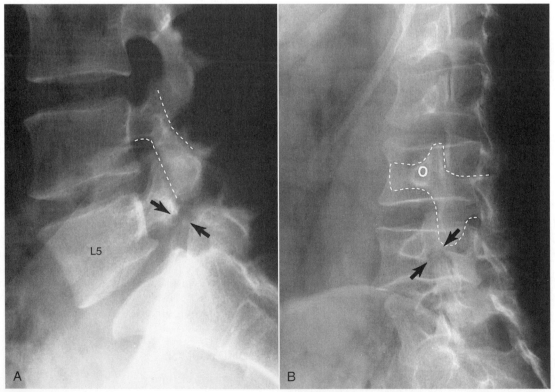

FIGURE 10-19 Spondylolysis. **A,** On the lateral view, a fracture of the posterior elements of L5 is apparent (*arrows*). The normal contour of the posterior elements is outlined by the *white dotted lines.* **B,** On the oblique view, a fracture line through the neck of the "Scottie dog" is shown (*arrows*). (*From Mercier L. Practical Orthopedics, St. Louis, Mosby, 2000.*)

result indicate the absence of bony activity at the fracture site, presumably secondary to a fibrous union of an old pars injury. In contrast, a positive or negative plain radiography result and a positive bone scan result indicate an acute fracture with healing activity at the fracture site, suggesting a good prognosis for bony union.[20]

The optimal imaging modality to evaluate spondylolysis is controversial. Plain oblique radiographs are the least expensive but have a low sensitivity, result in a fairly high radiation dose, and are not "physiologic" (i.e., do not determine healing activity). A routine bone scan is more sensitive than plain radiography, but it is not as sensitive as other modalities and does not show detailed anatomy. A single-photon emission computed tomography scan has greater accuracy for diagnosing pars injuries than conventional bone scan or plain radiography and is the preferred imaging modality for this condition (Figure 10-21).[21] A thin-section CT scan (3-mm cuts) is sensitive and shows anatomic detail, but the examiner must know which level to image first, and getting images of the pars injury is technically more challenging.

Indications for Orthopedic Referral

Consultation with an orthopedic surgeon, particularly someone with more expertise in treating

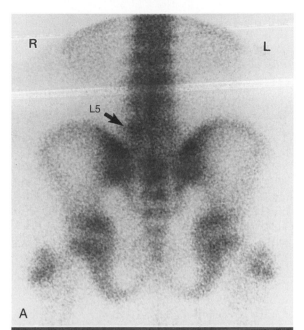

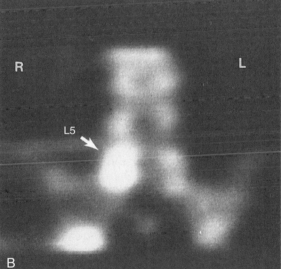

FIGURE 10-21 Occult spondylolysis. In this teenage athlete with back pain, plain radiography findings were normal. **A,** A regular nuclear medicine bone scan was obtained with images over the lower lumbar spine and pelvis. A very minimal increase in activity may possibly be seen on the right side of L5. **B,** An additional tomographic or coronal single photon emission computed tomography image was obtained. It shows markedly increased activity on the right side of L5 resulting from a traumatic fracture of the pars interarticularis on that side. (*From Mercier L.* Practical Orthopedics. *St. Louis, Mosby, 2000.*)

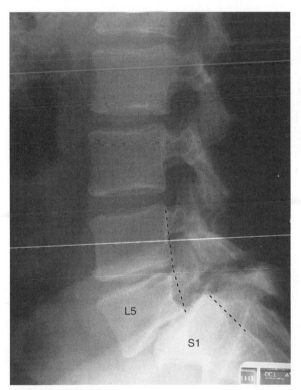

FIGURE 10-20 Spondylolisthesis. A bilateral pars defect at L5 has allowed it to slip forward on S1. (*From Mercier L.* Practical Orthopedics. *St. Louis, Mosby, 2000.*)

patients with this injury, should be considered to help establish a treatment regimen and a plan for monitoring healing and activity level. Patients with persistent pain beyond 6 months despite conservative treatment and proper rehabilitation should be referred to an orthopedic surgeon.

Treatment

The majority of patients with spondylolysis respond favorably to nonoperative treatment. Common features of most treatment plans include stopping the offending activities, stretching the hamstring and gluteal muscles, and strengthening the abdominal and back extensor muscles. The use of a lumbar support brace to decrease lordosis is controversial, and no clear evidence exists that it leads to improved outcomes. No value is apparent in bracing patients who have negative bone scan and positive radiography findings because the fracture is likely to be old.

The optimal length of treatment and activity restriction is unknown but varies between 6 weeks and 6 months. Patients with positive bone scan findings should be completely asymptomatic for 3 to 4 weeks before active rehabilitation exercises are started. Activity should be resumed slowly. Rehabilitation can begin earlier if the patient is asymptomatic and no bony activity is apparent (negative bone scan findings).

Observation of fracture healing is probably best accomplished with plain oblique radiography every 4 weeks and the addition of a CT scan if healing is questionable. The bone scan may show positive results up to 1 year after the injury and is not a reliable indicator of healing. Patients with bilateral spondylolysis are at risk of spondylolisthesis. Lateral radiographs of the lumbar spine should be obtained every 2 to 4 weeks, and the patient should be monitored closely. If significant spondylolisthesis (>50% slip) has occurred, the patient should be referred to a back surgeon for consideration of a surgical stabilization procedure.

Complications

Nonunion is a common complication, although the long-term prognosis is quite good even with continuation of sports. Bilateral nonunion can sometimes lead to slippage of the vertebra (spondylolisthesis). In patients older than 13 years of age, it is unusual for the initial slip to progress. Only rarely does spondylolisthesis become severe enough to impinge on the cauda equina and cause neurologic symptoms.

Return to Sports

Patients recovering from acute pars stress fracture or stress reaction can return to sports after they are pain free after a period of restricted activity with or without bracing followed by gradual resumption of spine-loading activities.[22] For most patients, this process takes 2 to 6 months. For patients with an established nonunion after presumed spondylolysis, return to sports can be directed by symptoms: after an initial period of restricted or modified activity and a brief period of rehabilitation, the asymptomatic athlete can return to sports under close supervision.

NONTRAUMATIC THORACOLUMBAR FRACTURES

Osteoporotic Fractures

Osteoporosis is a disease characterized by low bone mass, altered bone architecture, increased bone fragility, and increased risk of fracture. Of 9 million fractures linked each year to osteoporosis, 1.4 million are vertebral fractures.[23] Vertebral osteoporotic fractures are associated with an increased mortality rate, loss of independence, and impaired quality of life. The majority of osteoporotic vertebral fractures occur in the absence of specific trauma, begin at an earlier age than osteoporotic hip fractures, and affect many more women than men.

Fracture risk increases as bone mineral density (BMD) decreases.[24] BMD is classified according to the standard deviation (SD) difference between a patient's BMD and that of a young-adult reference population.[25] This value is called the "T-score." A T-score that is equal to or less than -2.5 is consistent with a diagnosis of osteoporosis, a T-score between -1.0 and -2.5 is classified as low bone mass (osteopenia), and a T-score of -1.0 or higher is normal. There is an approximate twofold increased risk of osteoporotic fractures for each SD decrease in BMD. Individuals with T-scores below -2.5 have the highest risk of fracture. Non-BMD factors that contribute to fracture risk include older age, female gender, prior osteoporotic fracture, low body weight, smoking, chronic heavy alcohol consumption, vitamin D deficiency, chronic glucocorticoid use, rheumatoid arthritis, and secondary osteoporosis (chronic liver disease, inflammatory bowel disease, premature menopause).

Fracture Risk Assessment

In 2008, the World Health Organization introduced a Fracture Risk Assessment Tool (FRAX), which estimates the 10-year probability of major osteoporotic fracture (hip, clinical spine, proximal humerus, or forearm) for untreated patients between age 40 to 90 years using clinical risk factors for fracture and femoral neck BMD using dual-energy x-ray absorptiometry (DEXA).[26] This tool is based on data collected from large prospective observational studies of men and women from different parts of the world and has been validated in numerous independent cohorts.[27] The tool is available online at http://www.shef.ac.uk/FRAX.

Mechanism of Injury

Most vertebral fractures caused by osteoporosis occur related to low level trauma such as a fall from standing height. There may be a history of seemingly harmless trauma such as driving over a speed bump.[28]

Clinical Presentation

Many osteoporotic vertebral fractures are asymptomatic and are diagnosed incidentally by radiographs taken for other purposes. Patients may report a sudden onset of sharp localized back pain with a history of minimal trauma or no trauma or even after coughing. Pain often radiates to the flank, the anterior chest, or the abdomen but rarely to the legs. Physical examination reveals midline back tenderness and an intact neurologic system. Kyphosis or height loss may indicate previous osteoporotic fractures.

Osteoporotic vertebral fractures are not usually associated with neurologic symptoms or spinal cord compression. If such symptoms are present or arise during therapy, other causes of the fracture must be considered, including congenital abnormalities, degenerative changes, infection, or tumor.

Imaging

Osteoporotic vertebral fractures are typically defined by changes in vertebral body heights or ratios of heights, but this can lead to many false-positive assessments. Height loss itself can be caused by other processes and is therefore a nonspecific finding. Comparison with old spine radiographs, if available, is sometimes helpful in distinguishing a new from an old fracture. New vertebral body fractures usually result in substantial loss of vertebral body height (Figure 10-22). The anterior, midbody, and posterior vertebral body measurements must be compared with adjacent vertebrae or a "standard" vertebra such as T4 or T5. Fractures occur most commonly at two levels: at the thoracolumbar junction (T12 to L1) or midthoracic (T7 to T9). This bimodal distribution is probably related to vertebral body shape and load distribution. Findings suggestive of an osteoporotic compression fracture include accentuation of the vertical trabeculation, biconcavity of the vertebral body end plates, and anterior wedging of the vertebral body. If a fracture is suspected and plain radiographs are equivocal, CT is useful in resolving the diagnosis and distinguishing between old and new fractures. CT is also helpful in determining

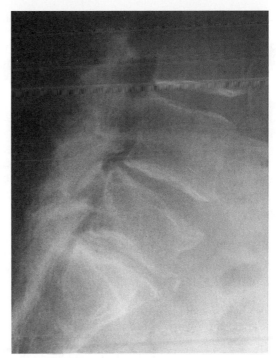

FIGURE 10-22 Compression fracture of L5 in a 65-year-old woman with osteoporosis.

fracture stability. Neurologic findings should prompt an urgent CT or MRI to assess for fracture fragments in the spinal canal.

Indications for Orthopedic Referral

Patients with unstable osteoporotic compression fractures as described in the Compression Fractures section should be referred to an orthopedic surgeon.

Initial Treatment

The acute treatment of osteoporotic compression fractures is the same as described earlier for traumatic compression fractures. Early ambulation is even more important for elderly patients to prevent complications from prolonged immobility, such as skin breakdown and thromboembolic disorders.

Follow-up Care

The definitive treatment of osteoporotic compression fractures should address three major areas: pain relief, prevention of further injury, and increasing bone mass. Both narcotic and NSAID analgesics can have bothersome side effects in older adults, and the lowest possible dose that achieves adequate pain control should be used. A TLSO is usually not necessary and may impair return to function in older adults. Back extension exercises should be done as early as possible when pain has diminished, preferably under the supervision of a physical therapist. Flexion exercises should be avoided because they may increase the risk of compression fractures. Follow-up radiographs are indicated if the patient is not gradually improving or shows signs of any neurologic deficit.

Prevention of further injury includes adequate physical therapy to strengthen weight-bearing muscles and improve balance, use of assistive devices for ambulation, proper footgear, appropriate lighting, and fall prevention in the home.

A thorough discussion of the medical treatment of osteoporosis is beyond the scope of this book, and readers are directed to recent reviews on the subject.[29,30]

Complications

Patients with one osteoporotic vertebral fracture are at approximately twofold greater risk for a second fracture.[31] This may be because of inherent abnormalities of bone formation or because of abnormal loads placed on other vertebrae after the initial fracture. Chronic back pain may affect some patients, particularly those with multiple osteoporotic fractures, loss of height, kyphosis, or kyphoscoliosis. These patients may benefit from a multidisciplinary approach involving the primary care provider, pain management specialist, and physical therapist.

TUMORS

Metastatic and primary bony tumors occur in all age groups and at all levels of the spinal column. Metastatic lesions are most common among patients with breast, lung, or prostate primary malignancies. Tumors of the spinal column may remain asymptomatic for years. Symptoms usually develop as a consequence of tumor expansion, vertebral body fracture, compression or invasion of adjacent nerve roots, spinal instability, or spinal cord compression. The most common presenting complaint is progressive and unrelenting pain. The pain, which occurs at night, is usually poorly localized, not clearly related to activity, and not relieved by rest or the recumbent position. Initial plain radiography findings may be negative because 30% to 50% of trabecular bone must be destroyed before radiographic changes are evident. The contour and size of the vertebra are usually preserved unless a compression fracture has occurred. Sites of involvement that are visible early in the course of metastatic disease are the anterior margins of the vertebral body (lateral view) and unilateral involvement of the pedicle, seen as "loss" of a pedicle on the AP view (Figure 10-23).

Treatment of patients with bony tumors of the spine must be individualized and done in concert with both medical and surgical oncologists. Supportive therapy, pain management, and palliative

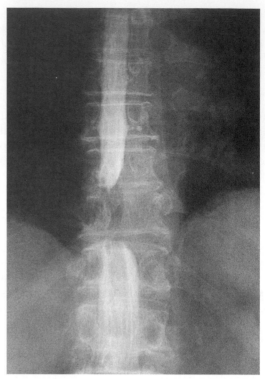

FIGURE 10-23 Myelogram of the spine in a patient with metastatic colon cancer. Note the interruption of contrast and "loss" of the pedicle on the left at T11 compared with the ringlike end-on appearance of the pedicles at other vertebral levels.

use of radiation therapy are appropriate for patients with a rapidly progressive and fatal lesion. For patients whose survival may be expected to exceed 6 months or even years, prompt treatment of symptomatic spinal lesions may further prolong survival or prevent the catastrophic consequences of spinal cord compression. Surgery is recommended to treat isolated primary or metastatic lesions or to correct spinal cord compression after pathologic fracture.

Pediatric Considerations

Tumors of the spine are rare among children but should be suspected in children with unrelenting back pain. The most common tumor causing back pain in children is an osteoid osteoma, a benign tumor. Dense sclerotic areas on plain radiographs are indicative of this tumor.[32] Extramedullary intradural tumors are usually benign and arise from neural crest tissue (e.g., neurofibroma, ganglioneuroma, or meningioma). Extramedullary extradural tumors are usually metastatic and include neuroblastoma, sarcoma, and lymphoma. Patients usually have some combination of gait disturbance, scoliosis, and back pain. Back pain at night or at rest should suggest this diagnosis. If an extramedullary extradural tumor causes acute blockage of CSF, the patient may have a flaccid paraplegia, urinary retention, and loss of anal sphincter tone. Radiographs may show widening of the interpedicular distance on the AP view or destruction or sclerosis of the vertebral body on the lateral view. MRI is the diagnostic test of choice to delineate spinal tumors among children. Early diagnosis is important to prevent irreversible damage to the spinal cord. Modern surgical techniques allow total resection for most patients. Use of radiation therapy, chemotherapy, or both depends on the primary tumor type.

VERTEBRAL OSTEOMYELITIS

VO occurs from three sources: hematogenous spread from a distant site (most common), direct inoculation from trauma or spine surgery, and contiguous spread from soft tissue infection. Sources of hematogenous infection include genitourinary tract, respiratory tract, infected intravenous catheter sites, endocarditis, and dental infection. Although *Staphylococcus aureus* is the most common organism, accounting for more than 50% of cases, a significant number of cases are caused by gram-negative organisms, especially after genitourinary manipulation. Methicillin-resistant strains (MRSA) are also on the rise.[33] Other pathogens include *Pseudomonas aeruginosa* and *Candida* spp., hemolytic streptococci (especially in people with diabetes), and tuberculous organisms. Hematogenous VO is usually a monomicrobial disease. Polymicrobial disease usually results from spread of a contiguous infection, most commonly sacral decubitus ulcers. Factors associated with higher rates of VO include age 50 years or older, male gender, intravenous drug use, and diabetes mellitus.

Clinical Presentation and Laboratory Studies

Back or neck pain is the most commonly reported symptom of VO, occurring in 90% of patients. The pain is well localized, continuous, and unrelated to movement or position. It can be mild or excruciating and is often accompanied by stiffness. Tenderness with spine percussion is often present. The majority of patients have an elevated erythrocyte sedimentation rate (ESR) and C-reactive protein, and these laboratory markers can be used to follow treatment efficacy.[34] Blood culture results are positive in the majority of patients but may require multiple blood cultures. CT-guided needle biopsy for culture is recommended, especially for patients with negative blood culture results.

Imaging

Plain radiograph findings are often normal when obtained in the early phases of infection and bone destruction may not be apparent for 2 to 4 weeks. Typical findings on AP and lateral plain radiographs are erosive irregularities at contiguous vertebral end plates with collapse of the intervening disc space (Figure 10-24). MRI is the most sensitive modality to detect VO, and abnormalities consistent with osteomyelitis can be seen before plain radiography findings become abnormal. If clinical suspicion is high for VO and plain radiography findings are negative, an MRI scan should be obtained to further evaluate the possibility of osteomyelitis.

Treatment

VO is a serious and complicated disease with the potential for abscess formation or catastrophic vertebral collapse leading to spinal cord compression. Early consultation with infectious disease specialists and orthopedic surgeons or neurosurgeons is recommended. Parenteral antimicrobial therapy directed at the isolated pathogen leads to good outcomes in most cases. The optimal duration of treatment is unknown, but most experts recommend 6 to 12 weeks. Most patent require parenteral therapy throughout the duration of treatment, but a suitable oral drug with proven susceptibility can be considered if the patient is responding well

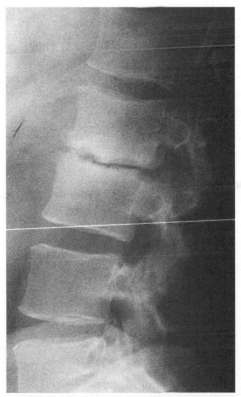

FIGURE 10-24 Erosions of the end plates of L2 and L3 in a patient with vertebral osteomyelitis.

to parenteral therapy after several weeks. Early rest and adequate pain control are helpful adjuncts. Surgery is indicated if antimicrobial therapy fails, if neurologic deficits develop, if previous neurologic deficits progress, or for marked instability of the spine or an epidural abscess.

Pediatric Considerations

VO is uncommon among children, accounting for only 1% to 2% of cases of pediatric osteomyelitis, but it can be devastating if left untreated. Diagnosis is made more difficult because symptoms are similar to those reported among children with discitis. Most children with VO are older than 8 years of age. Whereas symptoms are usually age related: children younger than 3 years of age may limp or refuse to walk, older children with verbal skills report back pain. The course may be indolent with several weeks of low-grade fever and mild symptoms.[35] The lumbar spine is involved in about two thirds of cases, and one third of cases involve thoracic spine involvement. During physical examination, patients appear to be ill, and approximately 80% have a fever. Point tenderness during back examination is usually present. Both the white blood cell count and the ESR are usually elevated, but these changes are nonspecific. A single set of blood cultures yields positive identification of the pathogen in slightly more than 50% of cases. Needle or open biopsy may be required for definitive identification.

Early in the course of disease, radiographs show rarefaction of the involved vertebral body; later, bony destruction is apparent, usually in the anterior portion of the vertebral body. Osteophytic bridging between vertebral bodies may also be a late finding. However, diagnostic abnormalities are present in only 50% of cases. MRI is the diagnostic study of choice for children with suspected VO.

Treatment requires intravenous antimicrobial therapy, usually a semisynthetic penicillin. In cases of MRSA, intravenous vancomycin can be used. The duration of therapy must be individualized and depends on the site and severity of infection and the causative organism.

REFERENCES

1. Hoffman JR, Mower WR, Wolfson AB, Todd KH, Zucker MI. Validity of a set of clinical criteria to rule out injury to the cervical spine in patients with blunt trauma. National Emergency X-Radiography Utilization Study Group. N Engl J Med. 2000;343:94-99.
2. Mower WR, Hoffman JR, Pollack CV Jr, et al. Use of plain radiographs to screen for cervical spine injuries. Ann Emerg Med. 2001;38:1-7.
3. Lewis LM, Docherty M, Ruoff BE, et al. Flexion-extension views in the evaluation of cervical-spine injuries. Ann Emerg Med. 1991;20:117-121.
4. Holmes, JF, Akkinepalli, R. Computed tomography versus plain radiography to screen for cervical spine injury: a meta-analysis. J Trauma. 2005;58:902-905.
5. Patel JC, Tepas JJ, Mollitt DL, Pieper P. Pediatric cervical spine injuries: defining the disease. J Pediatr Surg. 2001; 36:373-376.
6. Finch GD, Barnes MJ. Major cervical spine injuries in children and adolescents. J Pediatr Orthop. 1998;18: 811-814.
7. Viccellio P, Simon H, Pressman BD, et al. A prospective multicenter study of cervical spine injury in children. Pediatrics. 2001;108(2):E20.
8. Jacobs LM, Schwartz R. Prospective analysis of acute cervical spine injury: a methodology to predict injury. Ann Emerg Med. 1986;15:44-49.
9. Felsberg GJ, Tien RD, Osumi AK, Cardenas CA. Utility of MR imaging in pediatric spinal cord injury. Pediatr Radiol. 1995;25:131-135.
10. Vaccaro AR, Kim DH, Brodke DS, et al. Diagnosis and management of thoracolumbar spine fractures. J Bone Joint Surg Am. 2003;85:2456-2470.
11. Keynan O, Fisher CG, Vaccaro A, et al. Radiographic measurement parameters in thoracolumbar fractures: a systematic review and consensus statement of the spine trauma study group. Spine. 2006;31:E156-E165.
12. Campbell SE, Phillips CD, Dubovsky E, et al. The value of CT in determining potential instability of simple wedge compression fractures of the lumbar spine. AJNR Am J Neuroradiol. 1995;16:1385-1392.
13. Weninger P, Schultz A, Hertz H. Conservative management of thoracolumbar and lumbar spine compression and burst fractures: functional and radiographic outcomes in 136 cases treated by closed reduction and casting. Arch Orthop Trauma Surg. 2009;129:207-219.
14. Giele BM, Wiertsema SH, Beelen A, et al. No evidence for the effectiveness of bracing in patients with thoracolumbar fractures. Acta Orthop. 2009;80:226-232.
15. Miller CD, Blyth P, Civil ID. Lumbar transverse process fractures—a sentinel marker for abdominal organ injuries. Injury. 2000;31:773-776.
16. Yi L, Jingping B, Gele J, Baoleri X, Taixiang W. Operative versus non-operative treatment for thoracolumbar burst fractures without neurological deficit. Cochrane Database Syst Rev. 2006;(4):CD005079.
17. Tsirikos AI, Garrido EG. Spondylolysis and spondylolisthesis in children and adolescents. J Bone Joint Surg Br. 2010;92:751-759.
18. Baker RJ, Patel D. Lower back pain in the athlete: common conditions and treatment. Prim Care. 2005;32:201-229.
19. Masci L, Pike J, Malara F, et al. Use of the one-legged hyperextension test and magnetic resonance imaging in the diagnosis of active spondylolysis. Br J Sports Med. 2006;40:940-946.
20. Sairyo K, Sakai T, Yasui N. Conservative treatment of lumbar spondylolysis in childhood and adolescence: the radiological signs which predict healing. J Bone Joint Surg Br. 2009;91:206-209.
21. Takemitsu M, El Rassi G, Woratanarat P, Shah SA. Low back pain in pediatric athletes with unilateral tracer uptake at the pars interarticularis on single photon emission computed tomography. Spine. 2006;31:909-914.
22. Bono CM. Low back pain in athletes. J Bone Joint Surg Am. 2004;86:382-396.
23. Johnell O, Kanis JA. An estimate of the worldwide prevalence and disability associated with osteoporotic fractures. Osteoporos Int. 2006;17:1726-1733.
24. Leslie WD, Tsang JF, Caetano PA, Lix LM. Effectiveness of bone density measurement for predicting osteoporotic fractures in clinical practice. J Clin Endocrinol Metab. 2007;92:77-81.

25. World Health Organization: WHO Study Group on Assessment of Fracture Risk and its Application to Screening for Postmenopausal Osteoporosis. Geneva: World Health Organization; 1994.
26. Kanis JA, Johnell O, Oden A, et al. FRAX and the assessment of fracture probability in men and women from the UK. *Osteoporos Int.* 2008;19:385-397.
27. Kanis JA, Oden A, Johnell O, et al. The use of clinical risk factors enhances the performance of BMD in the prediction of hip and osteoporotic fractures in men and women. *Osteoporos Int.* 2007;18:1033-1046.
28. Aslan S, Karcioglu O, Katirci Y, et al. Speed bump-induced spinal column injury. *Am J Emerg Med.* 2005;23:563-564.
29. MacLean C, Newberry S, Maglione M, et al. Systematic review: comparative effectiveness of treatments to prevent fractures in men and women with low bone density or osteoporosis. *Ann Intern Med.* 2008;148:197-213.
30. National Osteoporosis Foundation. NOF's New Clinician's Guide to Prevention and Treatment of Osteoporosis. Accessed September 19, 2010, at http://www.nof.org/professionals/Clinicians_Guide.htm.
31. Kanis JA. A meta-analysis of previous fracture and subsequent fracture risk. *Bone.* 2004;35:375-382.
32. Khoury NJ, Hourani MH, Arabi MM, et al. Imaging of back pain in children and adolescents. *Curr Probl Diagn Radiol.* 2006;35:224-244.
33. Lew DP, Waldvogel FA. Osteomyelitis. *Lancet.* 2004;364:369-379.
34. An HS, Seldomridge JA. Spinal infections: diagnostic tests and imaging studies. *Clin Orthop Relat Res.* 2006;444:27-33.
35. Fernandez M, Carrol CL, Baker CJ. Diskitis and vertebral osteomyelitis in children: an 18-year review. *Pediatrics.* 2000;105(6):1299-1304.

11

FEMUR AND PELVIS FRACTURES

Fractures of the proximal femur are common in elderly individuals, who have decreased bone mass and a higher frequency of falls. Women are more likely than men to sustain femoral neck or intertrochanteric fractures because of their higher incidence of osteoporosis. The vast majority of patients with hip fractures require operative treatment, and the primary care provider's knowledge of the patient's medical condition and preinjury functional level is essential in making decisions regarding surgery.

Fractures of the femoral shaft and distal femur are relatively uncommon and are usually the result of significant trauma from automobile accidents in younger patients and falls in elderly people. Pelvic fractures are a leading cause of traumatic morbidity and mortality. The primary care provider involved in trauma care plays an important role in the recognition and stabilization of patients with pelvic fractures.

Femoral Neck Fractures

As the population ages, the number of hip fractures will increase substantially. Current estimates are 500,000 hip fractures at a cost of $8 billion per year in the United States.[1] Risk factors in the elderly population include falls and altered bone density.

Anatomic Considerations

The femoral neck lies within the hip joint capsule, and fractures of the femoral neck are considered intracapsular. The hip capsule, composed of supporting ligaments, arises from the acetabular ring and attaches to the intertrochanteric crest anteriorly and the midportion of the neck posteriorly.

The most significant anatomic feature of the femoral neck is its precarious vascular supply. Circumflex branches of the profunda femoris artery form an extracapsular ring at the base of the neck (Figure 11-1). Ascending branches, also known as the retinacular arteries, traverse the superficial surface of the neck. The close proximity of these vessels to the bone makes them vulnerable to injury in any fracture of the femoral neck. The greater the displacement, the more likely that a

fracture will result in compromise of the blood supply to the femoral head. The incidence of avascular necrosis (AVN) of the femoral head and nonunion is increased because of the potentially tenuous blood supply after a femoral neck fracture.

Several proposed classification schemes are based either on fracture location or on the amount of displacement of the fracture fragments. The Garden classification based on radiographic appearance is most commonly used.[2] Stage I involves an incomplete or impacted fracture; stage II involves a complete fracture without displacement; stage III involves a complete fracture with partial displacement; and stage IV involves a complete fracture with total displacement.

Mechanism of Injury

The majority of femoral neck fractures occur in elderly patients, especially those with osteoporosis. In these patients, the usual cause of injury is minor or indirect trauma. A stress fracture that may develop in the osteoporotic femoral neck combines with a torsion injury to cause a more significant fracture. This event may actually precipitate the fall that patients associate with the fracture. The fall then often causes further displacement or comminution of the fracture. In younger patients, femoral neck fractures result from major trauma caused by incidents such as motor vehicle accidents (MVAs).

Clinical Presentation

Patients with nondisplaced or minimally impacted femoral neck fractures may be ambulatory with only diffuse groin or thigh pain. Typically, a patient with a displaced fracture complains of significant hip pain, and the leg may appear slightly shortened and externally rotated. Pain is increased with any movement of the hip. Because neck fractures are intracapsular, ecchymosis is not usually present. The neurovascular status of the distal extremity is nearly always intact, so any evidence of nerve or arterial damage warrants a search for other injuries. The clinician should look for any conditions that may have precipitated a fall in the elderly patient

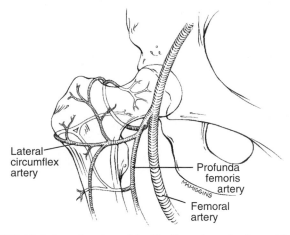

FIGURE 11-1 Anterior view of the blood supply to the femoral head and neck.

with a hip fracture. In those with a stress fracture or impacted fracture, the clinical signs may be less pronounced. These patients may be ambulatory; have groin, medial thigh, or knee pain; and have no clear history of trauma. The leg is not shortened or rotated.

Imaging

A true anteroposterior (AP) view with the hip in as much internal rotation as possible and a lateral view are usually adequate to diagnose a femoral neck fracture (Figure 11-2). The radiographs should be examined for disruption of the trabecular pattern, cortical defects, and shortening of the femoral neck. Comparison views of the other hip may aid in the diagnosis of more subtle fractures.

The normal neck shaft angle is 45 degrees on the AP view. The normal angle of the trabecular lines from the medial femur to the head on the AP view is 160 to 170 degrees (Figure 11-3). Any increase or decrease in these angles may indicate a fracture.

The proximal femur is at risk for occult fracture because of the high percentage of trabecular bone, in which disruption is more difficult to detect than in cortical bone. Occult fractures about the hip can lead to significant morbidity and mortality if left undetected; therefore, determining which patients are at risk and performing additional imaging studies in the event of negative plain radiograph findings is imperative in high-risk patients. High-risk characteristics include (1) new inability to bear weight; (2) pain with hip range of motion (ROM); (3) low-energy trauma, such as a fall from standing height; and (4) conditions leading to osteoporosis. A limited magnetic resonance imaging (MRI) scan of the hip can be used in the first 24 hours to confirm the diagnosis and is the preferred form of examination[3] (Figure 11-4). It is

quick, noninvasive, and just as accurate as bone scanning. If MRI is not available, a bone scan is a useful diagnostic tool. The disadvantage of using bone scanning is that it may take up to 72 hours after the injury to get optimal results, especially in an elderly patient with osteopenia, and it has lower specificity. This delay in the diagnosis of a hip fracture may result in a longer hospital stay for the patient.

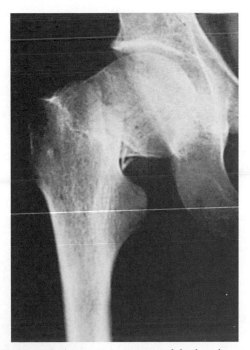

FIGURE 11-2 Anteroposterior view of the hip showing a displaced and impacted femoral neck fracture. (*From Browner BD, Jupiter JB, Levine AM, Trafton PG [eds]. Skeletal Trauma: Fractures, Dislocations, Ligamentous Injuries. Philadelphia, WB Saunders, 1992.*)

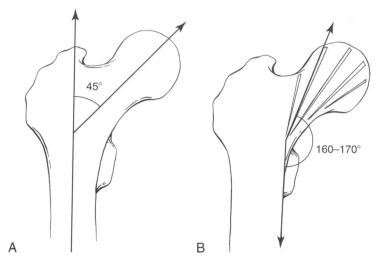

FIGURE 11-3 A, Normal angle of the femoral shaft and neck. **B,** Normal angle of trabecular lines from the shaft to the femoral head.

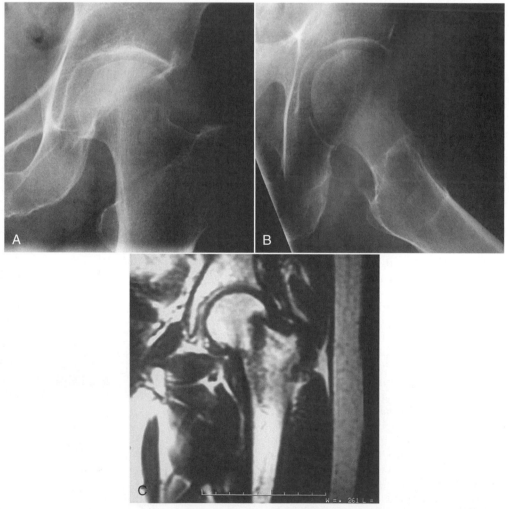

FIGURE 11-4 A, Normal anteroposterior view of the hip of an 80-year-old woman who sustained a fall. **B,** Lateral view demonstrating a very faint lucency crossing the femoral neck. **C,** Magnetic resonance image obtained on the same day reveals edema and fracture of the femoral neck.

Indications for Orthopedic Referral

Although impacted or nondisplaced fractures may appear benign, they are at risk of displacement, especially with conservative treatment (Figure 11-5). Nondisplaced fractures are rarely treated nonoperatively because the risk of disability, complications, and mortality is increased with conservative management. Therefore, all patients with femoral neck fractures should be referred to an orthopedic surgeon.

Especially in elderly patients, the primary care provider should coordinate the timing of surgery with the orthopedist based on the patient's medical condition and the need for stabilization of other medical problems. In general, surgery should proceed when the patient's condition is optimized, but the decision needs to be individualized. Patients with medical comorbidities have a significantly higher overall mortality regardless of the timing of surgery, and priority should be given to improving their medical status preoperatively at the expense of surgical delay.[4] In young healthy patients, current best evidence shows no association between the time to surgery and the risk of AVN or nonunion, although surgery is usually performed in the first 24 hours.[4]

Initial Treatment

The acute management of femoral neck fractures includes analgesia, assessment and stabilization of the patient's medical condition, and prompt orthopedic consultation. Patients should receive prophylaxis against deep venous thrombosis and wound infection. The use of traction before surgery has not been shown to provide any benefit in reducing pain or improving fracture reduction.[5]

Follow-up Care

In elderly independent patients with proximal femur fractures, total hip arthroplasty (prosthetic replacement of femoral head and acetabulum) is the preferred treatment based on current best evidence showing improved functional outcomes.[4] Hemiarthroplasty (replacement of the femoral head only) is reserved for patients with cognitive dysfunction. In younger patients, achieving anatomic reduction and a stable fixation is the goal, and which technique is used and surgical timing are determined by the orthopedic surgeon. Patients with osteoporosis should receive therapy to increase bone mass and thus prevent future osteoporotic fractures.

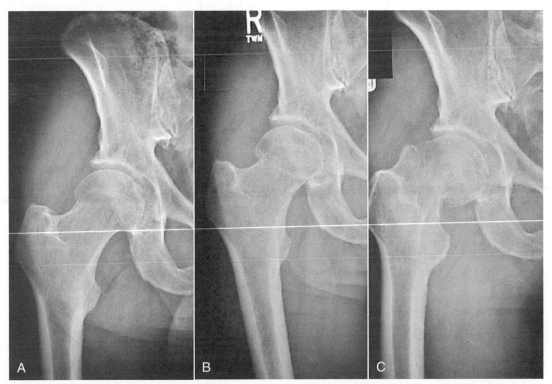

FIGURE 11-5 A, Initial anteroposterior view demonstrating a nondisplaced fracture of the femoral neck that was missed initially. **B,** A follow-up radiograph 2 weeks later shows impaction and displacement of the femoral head. **C,** At 5 weeks, the fracture became significantly displaced after a minor foot twist.

Complications

The long-term complications of nonunion and AVN are related to the risk of injury to the blood supply of the femoral head and neck after a fracture. These complications occur more frequently in displaced fractures and in fractures in younger patients, which involve greater injury violence than does the usual fracture in an older patient. Radiographs should be obtained periodically for up to 3 years after injury to screen for AVN. Complications after surgical repair include failure of the fixation device, chronic pain, infection, dislocation, and posttraumatic arthritis.

INTERTROCHANTERIC FRACTURES

Anatomic Considerations

By definition, an intertrochanteric fracture is extracapsular and occurs along a line between the greater and lesser trochanters (Figure 11-6). Muscle attachments on the femur may cause displacement after an intertrochanteric fracture because the internal rotators remain attached to the distal fragment, and the external rotators stay attached to the proximal head and neck fragment. The vascular supply to the intertrochanteric area is usually adequate for healing because of the surrounding muscles and periosteum.

Mechanism of Injury

Intertrochanteric fractures account for almost half of all fractures of the proximal femur and occur primarily in elderly individuals. This fracture usually results from a fall involving both direct and indirect forces. Direct forces act along the axis of the femur or over the greater trochanter. Indirect forces from the pull of the iliopsoas muscle on the lesser trochanter or the pull of the abductor muscles on the greater trochanter may also cause a fracture.

Clinical Presentation

Patients report hip pain, swelling, and ecchymosis. The injured leg may be noticeably shortened and externally rotated if the fracture is displaced. Any movement of the hip is painful. Distal pulses and nerve function are usually intact.

Elderly patients who have fallen and fractured a hip are at risk of dehydration if help has been delayed and they have been unable to drink fluids. Intertrochanteric fractures can cause a loss of up to 3 units of blood, which leads to intravascular volume depletion, especially when combined with dehydration. Skin breakdown is possible in the acute setting if the patient has been unable to get up from the fall for a prolonged period. After a fall, patients with osteoporosis may also have associated fractures of the distal radius, proximal humerus, ribs, or spine.

Imaging

A true AP view in internal rotation and a lateral view should be obtained for a patient with a suspected hip fracture. The AP view should be examined for bone quality (trabecular architecture) and fracture displacement. The lateral radiograph is useful in determining the size, location, and comminution of the fracture fragments.

Patients with negative radiographic results and a clinical examination that suggests an intertrochanteric fracture should undergo additional diagnostic studies to confirm the diagnosis. MRI can be used if a diagnosis is imperative in the first 24 hours. A bone scan can be used to detect an occult fracture 24 to 72 hours after injury.

A number of classification systems exist for intertrochanteric fractures, but these can be simplified by distinguishing a stable from an unstable fracture. This distinction determines the possibility of obtaining an anatomic fracture reduction, as well as the risk of loss of fracture reduction after internal fixation. Stable fractures have no displacement of the lesser trochanter and no comminution, and the medial cortices of the proximal and distal fragments are aligned (i.e., no displacement between the femoral shaft and neck) (Figure 11-7). Unstable fractures are comminuted, have multiple fracture lines, or are displaced, with medial displacement of the shaft occurring most frequently (Figure 11-8).

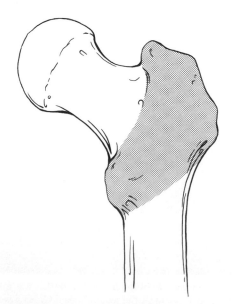

FIGURE 11-6 Intertrochanteric fracture zone.

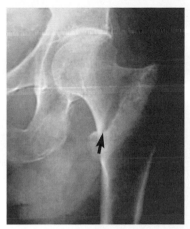

FIGURE 11-7 Nondisplaced stable intertrochanteric fracture (arrow). (From Browner BD, Jupiter JB, Levine AM, Trafton PG [eds]. Skeletal Trauma: Fractures, Dislocations, Ligamentous Injuries. Philadelphia, WB Saunders, 1992.)

Indications for Orthopedic Referral

All patients with intertrochanteric fractures should be referred to an orthopedic surgeon because the vast majority of them need operative treatment. Nonoperative management can be considered for nonambulatory or patients with dementia. The primary care provider plays an important role by informing the orthopedic surgeon of the patient's functional status before the fracture so that an appropriate decision regarding surgery can be made.

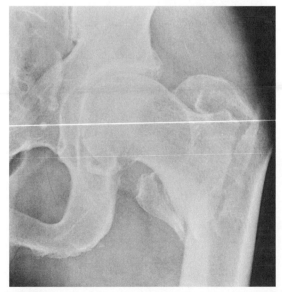

FIGURE 11-8 Displaced comminuted intertrochanteric fracture.

Initial Treatment

As is the case for patients with femoral neck fractures, in the acute period, the patient's medical condition—particularly the fluid status—must be assessed and stabilized. Analgesia and prompt orthopedic consultation are next. Although surgery can be performed within 24 to 48 hours after hospital admission, the decision regarding operative versus nonoperative treatment should be made in the acute setting.

Follow-up Care

The goal of treatment for intertrochanteric fractures is restoring the patient to his or her preinjury level of function and activity as soon as possible. A systematic review found insufficient evidence to recommend arthroplasty over internal fixation.[6] Nonoperative treatment may be a safer and less expensive option for patients who have little or no chance to walk based on their preinjury functional level. In nonambulatory patients, the fracture itself is ignored, and the resultant deformity of shortening and external rotation is accepted. The patient is given pain medication as needed and mobilized to a sitting position within 2 to 3 days. When the pain has subsided, the patient can resume a preinjury level of care and activity. Medical therapy to increase bone mass and thus prevent future fractures should be considered for any patient with osteoporosis.

Complications

Patients with intertrochanteric fractures have an increased mortality rate in the first year after fracture. Survival is most closely related to the patient's age and medical condition at the time of the fracture, not the method of treatment used. Complications from intertrochanteric fractures are similar to those occurring after femoral neck fractures and include infection, fixation failure, AVN, and nonunion. The incidence of nonunion and AVN is significantly lower than the incidence of these complications in femoral neck fractures because of the better blood supply in these extracapsular fractures.

Pediatric Considerations

Proximal femur fractures in children are rare compared with fractures in adults. They represent fewer than 1% of pediatric fractures and fewer than 1% of all hip fractures. Most orthopedic surgeons may treat only four or five of these injuries in a lifetime. When they do occur, they are usually the result of severe trauma. A hip fracture that occurs with minor trauma should arouse suspicion of a pathologic fracture or child abuse (Figure 11-9). Because of the weak proximal femoral epiphysis, a

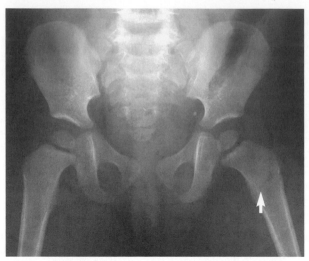

FIGURE 11-9 Intertrochanteric fracture of the left hip, 1.5-year-old girl, suggestive of nonaccidental injury (*arrow*). (*From Thornton A, Gyll C. Children's Fractures: A Radiological Guide to Safe Practice. Philadelphia, WB Saunders, 1999.*)

transepiphyseal separation may occur after significant trauma. Nearly all hip fractures in children require surgical intervention. Complications include AVN, malunion, nonunion, and premature physeal closure.

TROCHANTERIC FRACTURES

Trochanteric fractures are usually avulsion injuries in adolescents. Fractures of the lesser trochanter are caused by avulsion of the attachment of the iliopsoas muscle when the muscle contracts forcefully in an extended leg. Greater trochanter fractures may result from avulsion of the abductor muscles (gluteus medius and minimus) or direct trauma from a fall onto the hip. An isolated fracture of the lesser trochanter in the older adult should raise suspicion of underlying metastatic disease.

Examination of the patient with a lesser trochanter fracture reveals tenderness in the femoral triangle and pain that is increased with hip flexion and rotation. Patients with a greater trochanter fracture have localized tenderness that is exacerbated by hip abduction. AP and lateral views of the hip are usually adequate to diagnose these fractures (Figure 11-10). Standard radiographs should be examined to determine the amount of displacement, but internal and external rotation views may be necessary to assess this accurately. Patients with decreased bone density are at risk of extension of a trochanteric fracture into the intertrochanteric zone or femoral neck and should undergo additional imaging with an MRI to rule out this possibility.

Patients with displaced fractures (>1 cm) should be referred to an orthopedic surgeon for consideration of open reduction and internal fixation

(ORIF). Nondisplaced fractures of the trochanters heal well with conservative treatment that includes bed rest until pain subsides followed by gradual ambulation with crutches. Partial weight bearing should be continued for 3 to 4 weeks or until the patient has pain-free ROM. Physical therapy should be considered to help guide the patient through a progressive exercise program. Most

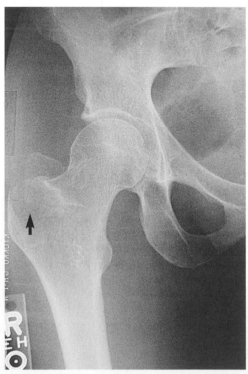

FIGURE 11-10 Fracture of the greater trochanter with superior displacement of the avulsed fragment (*arrow*).

patients resume normal physical activity within 2 to 3 months. Repeat radiographs should be taken at 4 weeks to document evidence of callus formation. Complications from isolated trochanteric fractures are rare.

FEMORAL SHAFT FRACTURES

The overall annual incidence of fractures of the femoral shaft is approximately 10 per 100,000 person-years.[7] There is a bimodal distribution of femoral shaft fractures in both genders, with the first peak in children younger than 10 years of age and the second peak in very old individuals (older than 90 years of age). Up to approximately 50 years of age, femoral shaft fractures are more common in males than females but this difference reverses in those older than 60 years of age. The majority of femoral shaft fractures occur in the proximal third of the bone.

Anatomic Considerations

Femoral shaft fractures can be subdivided into proximal third (subtrochanteric), middle third (midshaft), and distal third (supracondylar, intercondylar, condylar). The pull of the numerous muscles surrounding the femoral shaft results in displacement and angulation of the fracture fragments. The excellent blood supply to the femoral shaft, mostly from the profunda femoral artery, leads to good fracture healing, but it also accounts for significant volume loss after an acute fracture, 1000 to 1500 mL on average.[8] The popliteal artery and vein and the tibial and common peroneal nerves are in close proximity to the distal femur and may be injured when a fracture occurs in this location.

Mechanism of Injury

Approximately 25% of fractures of the femoral shaft are the result of MVA or falls from a significant height, particularly in the younger population. More than half of femoral shaft fractures result from low-energy trauma such as a fall on the same level in older adults. Transverse fractures result from bending forces or direct trauma. Spiral fractures result from torsional force—the greater the force, the greater the degree of comminution and displacement. Pathologic fractures of the femur after minor trauma are associated with metastatic disease or, in rare cases, primary tumors such as osteogenic sarcoma (Figure 11-11).

Clinical Presentation

The clinical presentation of a patient with a femoral shaft fracture is not subtle. The patient has a history of violent trauma or a fall, significant pain, and swelling and bruising of the thigh. The injured extremity may appear shortened or rotated. If high-energy trauma is involved, stabilization of

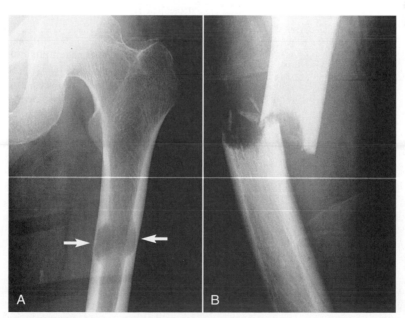

FIGURE 11-11 A, A view of the femur in this patient with known lung carcinoma shows a destructive lesion expanding from the marrow space and thinning the cortex (*arrows*). This lesion has no clear margin or white rim to distinguish it from normal bone. Lesions such as this in weight-bearing bones are important to find so therapy can be undertaken to prevent pathologic fracture. **B,** A view of the femur in the same patient, who returned 2 weeks later with a pathologic fracture. (*From Mettler FA. Essentials of Radiology. Philadelphia, WB Saunders, 1996.*)

the patient's airway, breathing, and circulation takes priority. Once the patient is stabilized, the pelvic ring, hip and knee should be inspected for tenderness, swelling, and ecchymosis, which may indicate associated injuries such as pelvic disruption, hip fracture, or soft tissue injuries of the knee. The patient's vital signs should be closely monitored because significant hemorrhage can occur after a femoral shaft fracture.

The patient should be examined carefully for signs of compartment syndrome because of the risk of massive bleeding into the soft tissues around the femur. If a distal femur fracture is suspected, the popliteal space should be examined for signs of an expanding hematoma indicating a popliteal artery injury. Neurovascular injury is rare with closed femoral shaft fractures, but nerve function and distal pulses must be well documented.

Imaging

Radiographs (AP and lateral views) should be obtained only after the patient is hemodynamically stable and has been placed in a splint or traction device. Fractures of the femoral shaft may be transverse, oblique, spiral, or comminuted. They are usually noticeably displaced and display signs of overriding, angulation, or rotation. Examples of femoral shaft fractures are shown in Figures 11-12 and 11-13.

Several classification schemes exist for subtrochanteric, midshaft, and supracondylar femur

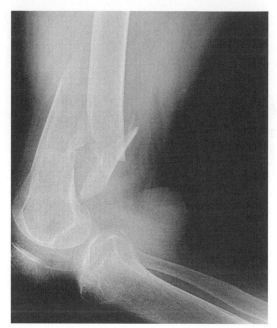

FIGURE 11-13 Obvious displaced, comminuted supracondylar femur fracture.

fractures. Because these schemes are designed to assist the orthopedic surgeon in making decisions regarding operative treatment and long-term outcome, a working knowledge of them is not essential for the primary care provider. The degree of comminution is an important factor in the prognosis for healing.

Initial Treatment

Essential initial management consists of stabilization of the patient's hemodynamic status, evaluating the patient for associated injuries and treating them as appropriate, providing analgesia, and immobilizing the injured extremity. Patients with open fractures should receive antibiotics and tetanus prophylaxis.

A traction splint such as a Hare or Sager splint is used to reduce patient pain, secure the leg in an appropriate position and restore length to the femur (Figure 11-14). Relative contraindications to the use of traction splints include hip dislocation, fracture-dislocation of the knee, and concomitant ankle injury.

Follow-up Care

All patients with a femoral shaft fracture, regardless of its location or degree of displacement, should be referred promptly to an orthopedic surgeon for early operative treatment. Intramedullary nailing is the most widely used technique for midshaft fractures and achieves excellent results. Subtrochanteric and supracondylar

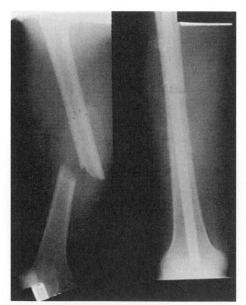

FIGURE 11-12 A displaced midshaft femur fracture fixed with intramedullary nailing. *(From Browner BD, Jupiter JB, Levine AM, Trafton PG [eds].* Skeletal Trauma: Fractures, Dislocations, Ligamentous Injuries. *Philadelphia, WB Saunders, 1992.)*

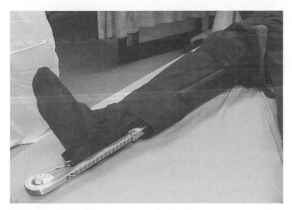

FIGURE 11-14 Positioning of the Sager traction splint used in the acute management of femoral shaft fractures.

fractures usually require a combination of fixation devices to achieve adequate healing. Long-term traction was used in the treatment of femoral shaft fractures in the past, but it is rarely used in adults today, except in those unable to undergo surgery or in remote locations without surgical capability.

Management of femur fractures requires careful balancing of the need for anatomic alignment and the need for early functional rehabilitation. If fixation has been successful, the patient can be ambulating on crutches with toe touch within a few days of surgery. Most patients with an isolated femoral shaft fracture treated with early operative fixation have a good prognosis. Soft tissue damage, infection, and inadequate fracture stabilization may delay healing. Patients usually have good ambulation within 1 month and can expect to return to normal activity within 3 to 6 months in younger patients and up to 12 months in elderly patients. Physical therapy is an essential part of rehabilitation to restore lower extremity muscle strength after the fracture has healed.

Complications

Disability, including post traumatic arthritis and a limp when walking, can result from fracture malalignment, fracture shortening, or prolonged immobilization. Other complications include breakage of nails and plates, postsurgical wound infection, and refracture. Peroneal nerve palsy from compression can complicate skeletal traction.

Pediatric Considerations

Although femoral shaft fractures in children are usually dramatic injuries, most heal rapidly without significant complications. A bimodal distribution occurs, with the first peak in early childhood and the second in mid-adolescence. The femur is relatively weak in early childhood and can fracture under loads typical of normal play. The specific

mechanism of injury is most often related to the patient's age.[9] In infants and toddlers, falls and abuse are the typical causes of femoral shaft fractures. Falls are the most common mechanism in children from toddler age to school age, and high-velocity trauma from MVAs or sports-related injuries account for most of the fractures in adolescents. Pathologic femoral fractures can occur after minor injury in those with predisposing conditions such as osteogenesis imperfecta, osteopenia, or neoplasms.

An unusual femoral fracture occurs in infants when the parent falls on a child who is straddling the parent's hip. This results in a greenstick fracture of the medial distal femoral metaphysis and is caused by bending of the femur. Because fractures with this cause of injury can occur at an age when abuse is the most common cause of femoral fracture, it is important to distinguish greenstick fractures from those caused by abuse.

Children and adolescents with femoral shaft fractures will be in considerable pain and unable to walk. Swelling, instability, and crepitance are usually present. Initial radiographs of the entire femur, including the hip and knee joints, should be obtained with the leg in the presenting position. The leg is then rotated to obtain a view at right angles to the first view. When resulting from high-energy trauma, a femur fracture is frequently associated with other serious concomitant injuries and warrants a comprehensive assessment for traumatic injuries.

For children with an isolated femoral shaft fracture without other serious injuries, initial therapy consists of pain management and immobilization consisting of a lateral slab from the iliac crest to the ankle. All patients should be referred to an orthopedic surgeon for definitive management. The diagnosis of a femoral shaft fracture with a questionable mechanism of injury, especially in a nonambulatory infant, should prompt consultation with an experienced child protection team.

Of the many factors that affect the ultimate treatment plan, the age of the patient is a primary determinant. Whereas younger children are managed with a variety of nonoperative techniques, older children often require operative fixation. Femoral fractures in infants younger than 12 months of age are usually stable and can be successfully treated with a Pavlik harness (0 to 6 months of age), splinting, or spica casting if significant shortening (>3 cm) or angulation is apparent. Children between the ages of 12 months and 6 years are most often treated in a hip spica cast. A brief period of traction may be required for fractures with greater degrees of shortening or those with considerable instability. Spica cast care can be quite daunting for families, so children placed in spica casts are best served by an initial hospital admission for cast care and parental education. Beyond age 6 years, it is more appropriate to avoid a hip spica cast because they are much more difficult to manage in larger children, and older children are more capable of walking with crutches or a walker. Closed reduction and flexible intramedullary rod fixation are the treatments of choice in children 6 to 10 years of age. After age 11 years, the diameter of the femur will allow intramedullary fixation with a rigid rod, which is then the preferred treatment.

Full weight bearing is typical by 6 weeks after initiation of treatment. Most patients are able to gradually progress to normal activity by 3 months and get back to full function by 6 months.

Complication after femoral shaft fractures in pediatric patients are uncommon. Early complications include neurovascular injury, compartment syndrome, and infection and are more often associated with higher energy trauma. Late complications such as shortening, overgrowth, leg length discrepancy, malunion (angular and rotational), and nonunion are unusual and infrequently require intervention. In younger children, discrepancies in length, rotation, and angle often resolve spontaneously with growth.

STRESS FRACTURES OF THE FEMUR

Stress fractures of the femur account for approximately 7% to 10% of all stress fractures in athletes.[10] The femoral neck is the most common site of injury, accounting for approximately half of the femoral stress fractures, followed by the shaft. Prolonged or significant increase in physical activity as seen in distance runners or military recruits can cause excessive stress, leading to fracture.

Femoral Neck Stress Fractures

Two types of femoral neck stress fractures have been described: distraction or tension type and the compression type. Distraction fractures are more common in patients older than the age of 60 years and occur on the superior lateral border of the femoral neck. Compression fractures occur on the inferior medial border of the femoral neck and are more common in younger more athletic patients. Other risk factors include coxa vara, osteopenia, and the female athlete triad (amenorrhea, eating disorder, and osteoporosis).

Clinical Presentation

These fractures should be considered in athletes, especially distance runners, who present with insidious onset of hip, thigh, or inguinal pain. The pain is exacerbated by weight-bearing activity. Night pain may develop, especially if diagnosis is delayed. Findings on physical examination are usually nonspecific but may include discomfort at the extremes of hip motion, especially internal rotation.

Imaging

Radiographic changes usually do not become apparent until 2 to 4 weeks after symptoms begin. Early radiographic findings of a compression fracture are subtle endosteal lysis or sclerosis along the inferior cortex of the femoral neck (Figure 11-15, A). This may be followed by progressive sclerosis and a definite fracture line. The fracture line may extend across the femoral neck, but fracture displacement is rare. Distraction fractures are characterized radiographically by a cortical defect in the superior cortex or tension side of the femoral neck. Because this fracture develops perpendicular to the lines of stress, it is less stable and more prone to displacement with continued stress.

A bone scan or MRI can confirm the diagnosis if a stress fracture is suspected in a patient with progressive or nonresponding inguinal pain, limitation of hip motion, and no radiographic evidence of fracture (Figure 11-15, B). MRI, although more expensive, is superior to radionuclide imaging because it is noninvasive; lacks the radiation exposure of a bone scan; and has higher diagnostic sensitivity, especially in the early stages of bone injury.

Indications for Orthopedic Referral

Because distraction stress fractures are at increased risk of becoming displaced, patients with these injuries should be referred early for consideration of operative fixation to prevent potentially serious complications. Displaced compression fractures, those that progress to completion across the femoral neck, or those that fail to heal with non–weight-bearing ambulation should be referred to an orthopedist for possible internal fixation.

Treatment

Nondisplaced, incomplete compression fractures can be treated conservatively with rest until the patient is pain free and the hip regains full motion. Non–weight-bearing ambulation with crutches is continued until radiographic evidence of healing is seen (usually 6 weeks). The patient can resume non–weight-bearing conditioning such as swimming or cycling during this initial healing period. To detect any progression of the stress fracture, the physician should obtain serial radiographs every 1 to 2 weeks or at any time the patient stops improving. In general, 2 to 3 months are required to return to pre-injury levels of activity after a compression-type femoral neck stress fracture. Patients can resume full activity when they have achieved

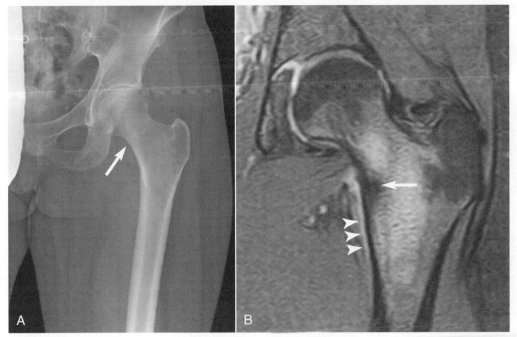

FIGURE 11-15 A, Frontal radiograph shows a subtle linear area of sclerosis at the medial femoral neck, representing a small, nondisplaced fracture (*arrow*). (*From Ouellette HA. The Teaching Files: Musculoskeletal. Philadelphia, WB Saunders, 2009.*) **B,** STIR (short tau inversion recovery) magnetic resonance image shows a focus of hypointensity at medial cortex of femoral neck (*arrow*) along with periosteal thickening (*arrowheads*) and regional bone marrow edema indicative of a stress fracture. (*From Pope T, Bloem H, Beltran J, Morrison WB, Wilson D. Imaging of the Musculoskeletal System. Philadelphia, WB Saunders, 2008.*)

asymptomatic full weight bearing and pain-free passive ROM of the hip and radiographs show signs of a healed fracture.[11]

Femoral Shaft Stress Fractures

Femoral shaft stress fractures may occur anywhere along the shaft, but the medial side of the femur at the junction of the proximal and middle thirds is the most common location. This is the site of the origin of the vastus medialis and the insertion of the adductor brevis. These muscle attachments have been implicated as causal factors in the development of stress fractures from overuse activity.[12] Risk factors include a sudden and abrupt change in training regimen, poor nutrition, and abnormal menstrual cycles.[13]

Clinical Presentation

The combination of vague thigh pain, diffuse tenderness, and no history of trauma should raise suspicion of a femoral shaft stress fracture, especially in a recreational or competitive runner. Patients often initially think they have strained a quadriceps muscle, but continued or worsening symptoms lead them to seek evaluation. Diffuse tenderness is more characteristic of a stress fracture; quadriceps muscle strain usually has a definitive traumatic etiology, and localized swelling and tenderness are

usually present. The location of the pain does not necessarily correlate with the location of the fracture. Hopping may reproduce the pain, and the patient may have a positive fulcrum test result. This test is performed by placing an arm under the symptomatic thigh of the seated patient on the examination table. The examiner's arm is used as a fulcrum and is moved from distal to proximal as gentle pressure is applied to the dorsum of the knee. At the point of the stress fracture, the patient experiences a sharper and more localized pain.

Imaging

Because the majority of patients delay seeking medical attention for at least 4 to 6 weeks from the onset of symptoms, a femoral shaft stress fracture may be apparent on initial radiographs (Figure 11-16, A). If periosteal callus or an overt fracture line is not present on plain radiographs, a bone scan or MRI should be obtained to confirm the diagnosis (Figure 11-16, B). Both MRI and a bone scan are sensitive in detecting early stress changes. If the primary goal is to exclude a stress fracture by the most cost-effective means, a bone scan is the best initial test. However, MRI is more specific. MRI evaluates a narrower field than bone scanning, it does not expose the patient to radiation, and the surrounding soft tissues can also be assessed.

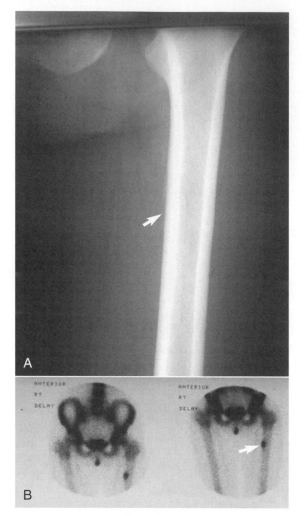

FIGURE 11-16 A, Radiograph of the left femur demonstrates periosteal reaction in the proximal medial cortex (*arrow*) consistent with a stress fracture. **B,** Bone scan reveals intense uptake in the medial cortex of the left proximal femur consistent with a stress fracture. (*Photos courtesy of Karl B. Fields, MD.*)

Treatment

Most femoral shaft stress fractures do not progress to complete fracture or displacement, but these injuries are possible if the patient continues vigorous training despite symptoms. Patients with these conditions should be referred to an orthopedic surgeon. Provided there is no evidence of a full cortical break, the patient is allowed protected weight bearing with crutches until pain-free ambulation is achieved. A cross-training program consisting of non–weight-bearing activity such as swimming or bicycling can be started during this healing period. Impact-loading activity should be avoided for 6 to 8 weeks. Patients typically return to full activity within 8 to 12 weeks. Return-to-play decisions should be guided by the absence

of clinical symptoms. Follow-up radiographs are useful at 6 to 8 weeks to document radiographic healing. Training errors and other risk factors should be evaluated to prevent recurrence. Delayed union or nonunion is rare.

HIP DISLOCATIONS

Go to Expert Consult for a video on how to perform a reduction maneuver for a hip dislocation. Hip dislocations are orthopedic emergencies. They are difficult to manage, are prone to complications, and generally require reduction under procedural sedation or anesthesia. Essentially all hip dislocations should be managed by orthopedists. However, primary care physicians may be called upon to recognize the injury and assess and stabilize the patient.

High-energy forces are usually necessary to dislocate the hip. Most hip dislocations are caused by automobile accidents. Dislocation is a complication of prosthetic hip joints, and the force required to dislocate in this circumstance is far less. These are extremely painful injuries, and patients are usually in agony unless their sensorium is clouded by intoxicants or a head injury. Posterior dislocation is the most common type of hip dislocation. It is often caused by the knee hitting the dashboard. Characteristically, the hip in patients with a posterior dislocation is flexed, adducted, and internally rotated (Figure 11-17). An anterior dislocation is most commonly caused by a hyperextension force against an abducted leg. Patients with this injury present with the hip typically flexed, abducted, and externally rotated (Figure 11-18). It is important to note, however, that a concomitant fracture of the femur may obscure these characteristic deformities and disguise a hip dislocation. The third type of hip dislocation, a central dislocation, occurs when the femoral head is driven through the acetabulum, fracturing the acetabulum in the process.

When a hip dislocation is suspected, initial management should focus on stabilizing the patient, carefully surveying the patient for other injuries (which may be much more serious than the hip dislocation), and making a neurovascular assessment of the affected extremity. A single AP view of the pelvis will usually show the dislocation. A 15-degree oblique lateral view could be used to differentiate anterior from posterior dislocations. Computed tomography (CT) accurately delineates the type of dislocation and identifies any associated acetabular fractures and the small intraarticular bone and cartilage fragments that are often present. If such fragments remain in the joint, severe degenerative changes are likely to develop in the future.

Various techniques have been described to reduce a posterior dislocation with no evidence

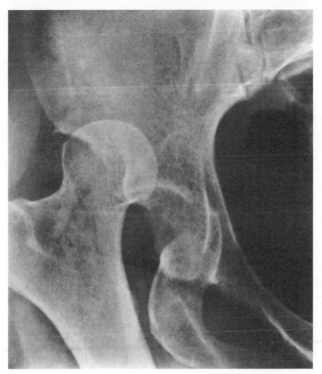

FIGURE 11-17 Posterior dislocation with classic position of leg in adduction and internal rotation. (*From Browner BD, Jupiter JB, Levine AM, Trafton PG [eds]. Skeletal Trauma, vol 2. Philadelphia, WB Saunders, 1992.*)

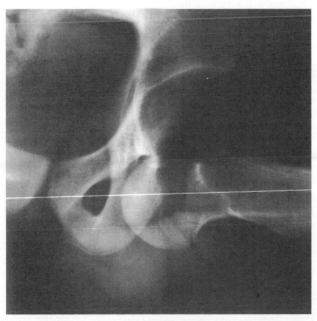

FIGURE 11-18 Anterior dislocation with classic position of leg in abduction and external rotation. (*From Browner BD, Jupiter JB, Levine AM, Trafton PG [eds]. Skeletal Trauma, vol 2. Philadelphia, WB Saunders, 1992.*)

that one technique is preferable. The choice of technique depends on the patient's condition and physician experience. Conscious sedation is used before the reduction maneuver. In the Allis maneuver, the patient is supine, and an assistant applies downward pressure on the pelvis by pushing down on both anterior superior iliac spines. With the hip flexed to 90 degrees and adducted, the physician applies axial traction to the femur while the physician applies longitudinal traction. Reduction is confirmed with feeling a click and restoration of normal leg position and ROM. Postreduction AP and lateral radiographs of the hip should be obtained to confirm normal anatomic alignment.

Hip dislocations are fraught with complications. Sciatic nerve injury occurs in up to 10% of cases, and associated fractures of the acetabulum, femur, or patella are common. Arterial injury may also occur. The femoral head has a precarious blood supply, which may be compromised by the dislocation. This can lead to AVN of the femoral head, especially if reduction was delayed. Degenerative joint disease is also common after hip dislocations, and reduction maneuvers may cause additional injuries.

PELVIC FRACTURES

Pelvic fractures vary from benign to life threatening injuries. Distinguishing stable from unstable pelvic fractures helps the primary care provider with management decisions. Stable fractures, those with only one break in the pelvic ring or fractures external to the ring, can usually be treated

Table 11-1	*Stable Pelvic Fractures*
EXTERNAL TO PELVIC RING	
Avulsion	
Single pubic or ischial ramus	
Iliac wing	
Isolated sacrum	
Coccyx	
PELVIC RING	
Two ipsilateral rami	
Near or subluxation of symphysis pubis	
Near or subluxation of sacroiliac joint	

symptomatically with rest followed by progressive activity (Figure 11-19). Stable pelvic fractures are listed in Table 11-1. Fractures involving two breaks in the ring require more aggressive treatment and are more commonly associated with visceral injury. Conditions that increase the risk of pelvic fractures include smoking, low bone mass, older age and propensity to fall.[14]

Anatomic Considerations

The pelvis is made up of three bones that unite to form a ring: the sacrum and two innominate bones composed of the ischium, ilium, and pubis (Figure 11-20). The two rigid half-rings are joined at the sacroiliac (SI) joints and the symphysis pubis. The SI joint is supported by strong ligamentous attachments and has little motion. The interpubic ligament joins the two pubic bones. These joints are the primary yield points when traumatic force is applied to the pelvis. For a pelvic fracture to be

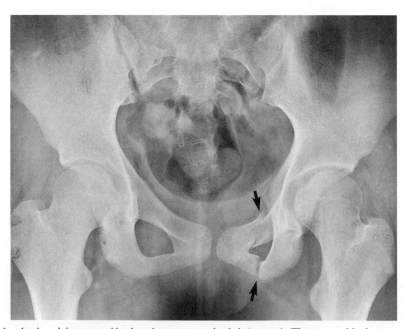

FIGURE 11-19 Nondisplaced fracture of both pubic rami on the left (*arrows*). This is a stable fracture of the pelvic ring.

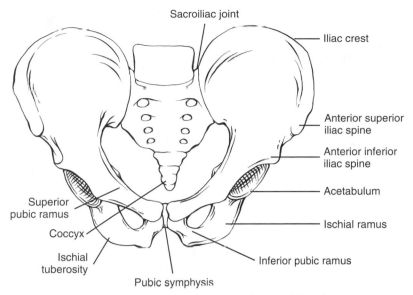

Sacroiliac joint

Iliac crest

Anterior superior
iliac spine

Anterior inferior
iliac spine

Acetabulum

Ischial ramus

Superior
pubic ramus

Coccyx

Ischial
tuberosity

Inferior pubic ramus

Pubic symphysis

FIGURE 11-20 Anterior view of the bones of the pelvis.

unstable, two breaks must occur in the pelvic ring, either from two fractures or from a fracture plus a joint dislocation (usually the SI joint).

Several muscles attach to the pelvis, serving to support the body when standing and provide motion to the legs. The muscles that may lead to avulsion fractures when forcefully contracted include the sartorius (inserts on the anterior superior iliac spine), the rectus femoris (inserts on the anterior inferior iliac spine), and the hamstring muscles (insert on the ischial tuberosity) (Figure 11-21).

Pelvic fractures can be associated with massive hemorrhage because of the extensive blood supply to the area. The internal iliac artery, a branch of the common iliac artery, provides the major vascular supply to the pelvic muscles and viscera. A rich venous plexus surrounds the pelvic organs and the pelvic walls. Because of the close relationship of the arterial and venous supply to the SI joint, fractures of the posterior pelvis are usually associated with more extensive bleeding than anterior fractures.

The bladder, rectum, and anus are contained within the bony pelvis and are the most commonly injured viscera associated with pelvic fractures. Anterior pelvic fractures may cause urethral or external genitalia injury, especially in men. Urinary tract injury is the most frequent visceral injury, and the clinician evaluating a patient with pelvic trauma must assume that a bladder or urethral injury exists until proven otherwise.

The spinal nerves exit the lumbar vertebrae and sacrum and course along the posterior aspect of the pelvis. Fractures involving the posterior half of the

pelvic ring may cause damage to these peripheral nerves.

Mechanism of Injury

Most pelvic fractures are the result of violent trauma from impact during an MVA or a fall from a considerable height. The primary types of force are lateral compression, AP compression, vertical

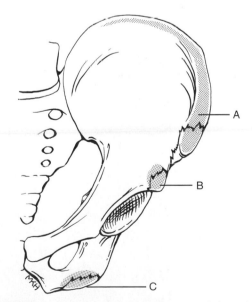

FIGURE 11-21 Sites of avulsion fractures of the pelvis. **A,** The sartorius muscle inserts on the anterior superior iliac spine. **B,** The rectus femoris muscle inserts on the anterior inferior iliac spine. **C,** The hamstring muscles insert on the ischial tuberosity.

shear, and a combination of these forces. In elderly individuals, a less significant fall may cause a pelvic fracture in osteoporotic bone. A fall that lands a person in the sitting position may result in an ischial body, sacral, or coccygeal fracture. Iliac wing fractures are usually the result of a medially directed force. Stress fractures of the pubic rami occur in long-distance runners and military recruits. Avulsion fractures occur in skeletally immature individuals as the result of sudden forceful contraction of attached muscles.

Clinical Presentation

The patient with a pelvic fracture usually is the victim of violent trauma. If the patient is conscious, he or she may complain of generalized pelvic or groin pain or pain localized to the area of the fracture, depending on injury location. Swelling and ecchymosis may be present in the pelvis, groin, scrotum, or perineum. Palpation and pressure (pushing the iliac spines together and apart) usually exacerbate pain, and the examiner may detect motion if the pelvis is unstable. Applying pressure to detect instability should be done gently and only in a hemodynamically stable patient because this maneuver may exacerbate hemorrhage.

Gross hematuria or blood in the urethral meatus, rectum, or vagina indicates visceral injury. Genital injuries in female patients may be overlooked initially, and the clinician must perform a thorough examination of the vagina to detect lacerations. A high-riding, boggy prostate is indicative of injury to the membranous urethra. Decreased anal

sphincter tone may accompany a sacral fracture. A careful examination of neurologic function and pulses in the lower extremities is also part of a complete evaluation of patients with pelvic fractures. Because patients with pelvic fractures often have incurred multiple trauma, a systematic evaluation to exclude life-threatening injuries of the head, chest, and abdomen must be performed.

Imaging

It is generally recommended that a portable AP pelvis radiograph be obtained in unstable trauma patients suspected of having a pelvic injury, although clinical examination may be at least as good as the portable radiograph in detecting fractures.[15] Obvious fractures are usually readily apparent on the AP view (Figure 11-22). The role of bedside ultrasound examination in the assessment of pelvic trauma is not yet clearly defined.[16] Hemodynamically stable patients should undergo CT to delineate the exact extent of injury and help guide surgical decisions. Inlet, outlet, and oblique views can help further define pelvic fractures.

A retrograde urethrogram must be performed if any suspicion of urethral injury exists. If this test is normal, a Foley catheter can be placed into the bladder and retrograde cystography performed to detect bladder injury.

Indications for Orthopedic Referral

The presence of life-threatening injuries such as hemorrhage and visceral organ damage requires emergency referral to a trauma care team after patient stabilization. Patients with unstable

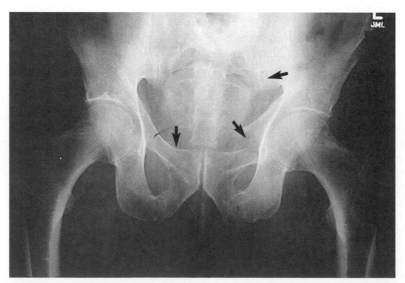

FIGURE 11-22 Anteroposterior view of the pelvis demonstrating an unstable pelvic fracture with multiple breaks in the ring. Fractures are present in the right superior pubic ramus, the left superior and inferior pubic rami, and the inferior left sacroiliac joint (*arrows*).

fractures of the pelvis should be referred promptly to an orthopedic surgeon.

Initial Treatment

Emergent Treatment

The primary care provider's top priority in the acute management of a patient with a pelvic fracture is stabilization of the patient's airway, breathing, and circulation. Hemorrhagic shock is the major cause of death in patients with pelvic fractures, so volume resuscitation is of paramount importance. If the patient has sustained significant pelvic trauma or remains unstable after a pelvic fracture, the pelvis should be "wrapped" to reduce volume and stabilize the fracture fragments. This can be accomplished by wrapping a sheet around the greater trochanters with towel clamps for fixation or using commercial pelvic binder devices. Care should be taken to not overreduce the fracture by making sure the patient's legs, greater trochanters, and patellae lie in an anatomically neutral position.

After the patient is stable, the diagnosis and management of associated injuries such as the genitourinary or gastrointestinal system injury take priority over treatment of the pelvic fracture itself. Patients with stable pelvic fractures without associated visceral injury can be treated symptomatically in the acute period with analgesics and bed rest. Hospital admission should be considered for patients without adequate home care resources and for those with sacral fractures because of the risk of sacral nerve injury and subsequent bowel or bladder difficulties.

Follow-up Care

Unstable Fractures

Patients with unstable fractures of the pelvic ring are treated with internal fixation, skeletal traction, or both. External fixation is sometimes used in combination with traction and internal fixation.

Stable Fractures

Patients with stable pelvic fractures can be treated symptomatically with bed rest, analgesics, and progressive mobilization, depending on pain tolerance. The length of bed rest needed usually varies from 2 to 4 weeks. The patient may sit as much as is manageable. Gentle ROM exercises of the lower extremity should be performed during the period of bed rest, especially in elderly people. Protected weight bearing (with a cane or crutch used on the injured side) is allowed after pain subsides. Repeat radiographs should be obtained when the patient is mobile to ensure that no displacement has occurred with weight bearing. A donut-ring cushion, sitz baths, and stool softeners used to avoid straining are beneficial adjuncts in the management of patients with coccygeal fractures.

Complications

The mortality rate from pelvic fractures is substantial, ranging from 10% to 15%. Long-term pain and disability relate to the amount of residual deformity of the pelvic ring after treatment. Complications include infection, thromboembolism, malunion, posttraumatic arthritis, and complications associated with visceral organ damage.

Pediatric Considerations

Avulsion Fractures

Avulsion fractures commonly occur in young athletes at apophyseal sites (see Figure 11-21). The ischial tuberosity is the most commonly injured apophysis and occurs typically after forceful contraction of the hamstrings in sports such as football, track, and gymnastics. With the hip in extension, the sartorius is fully stretched and is susceptible to strain that results in an avulsion fracture of the anterior superior iliac spine. An avulsion of the anterior inferior iliac spine can be caused by excessive force on the rectus femoris muscle when the hip is hyperextended and the knee is flexed. This injury usually occurs in sports that involve kicking and is much less common than avulsion of the anterior superior iliac spine. The anterior inferior iliac spine apophysis fuses earlier than the anterior superior iliac spine, which may explain the less frequent occurrence of avulsion fractures of the anterior inferior iliac spine.

Symptoms include tenderness and localized swelling around the avulsion site. Passive stretch of the attached muscle will exacerbate the pain, and the muscle may be weak compared with the uninjured side. If the avulsion is attributable to chronic repetitive traction, pain and loss of motion worsen. An AP radiograph of the pelvis should be adequate to diagnose common avulsion injuries. Avulsion fractures of the anterior inferior or superior iliac spine are usually minimally displaced (Figure 11-23). Avulsion of the hamstring attachment to the ischial tuberosity may result in a large displaced fragment. Because these avulsion fractures occur primarily through secondary ossification centers in adolescents, comparison views of the contralateral apophysis may be necessary to distinguish a true fracture from an anatomic variant. A CT scan should be obtained if the injury is suspected but plain radiographs are inconclusive.

Conservative treatment consisting of a brief period of rest with the hip positioned to lessen stretch on the affected muscle followed by

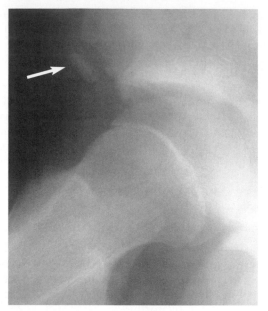

FIGURE 11-23 Minimally displaced avulsion fracture of the anterior inferior iliac spine (*arrow*).

crutch-assisted ambulation for 2 to 3 weeks leads to good outcomes in most cases. Progressive rehabilitation to regain motion and full strength is necessary before the individual can return to athletic activities. Return to full function may take 8 to 12 weeks. Surgery is reserved for those with symptomatic nonunions and fractures with significant displacement (>2-3 cm). Excessive callus formation, especially after ischial tuberosity avulsions, may cause prolonged symptoms and impair function.

ACETABULAR FRACTURES

Fractures of the acetabulum pose a great challenge to orthopedic surgeons for several reasons: they are frequently comminuted; surgical exposure is difficult; they are intraarticular, which requires near-anatomic reduction; and they often occur in patients with multiple trauma. The primary care provider plays an important role in identifying these fractures and any associated injuries and in stabilizing the patient before orthopedic care.

Acetabular fractures are the result of high-energy forces. Force applied directly to the greater trochanter or directed up the femoral shaft, as occurs when the knee strikes the dashboard in a MVA, is a common cause of injury. Elderly patients with osteopenia may fracture the acetabulum during a minor fall. Associated musculoskeletal injuries include hip dislocation, femur fractures, and knee injuries. Sciatic nerve injury may occur after posterior acetabular fractures, and injury to the femoral artery may complicate anterior fractures.

Three views are required in the evaluation of acetabular fractures: the AP view, the obturator oblique view (45 degrees of internal rotation), and the iliac oblique view (45 degrees of external rotation). CT is routinely used to delineate the degree of comminution, the size of fracture fragments, the presence of intraarticular fragments, and associated femoral head fractures (Figure 11-24).

Patients with acetabular fractures should be managed by orthopedic surgeons. Nondisplaced fractures of the acetabulum in which the congruity and stability of the hip joint are maintained are usually treated with traction and close monitoring

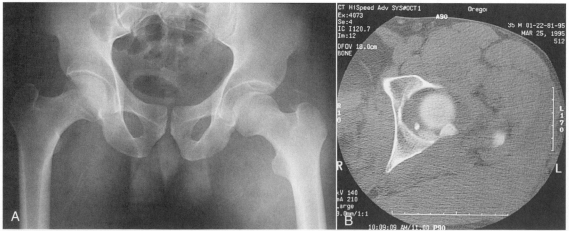

FIGURE 11-24 A, Anteroposterior of the pelvis showing a widened joint space of the left hip. This finding can be a clue to the presence of an acetabular fracture. **B,** Computed tomography scan of the left hip demonstrating intraarticular bone fragments from an acetabular fracture.

to ensure that the fracture stays well aligned. Displaced and unstable fractures are treated with either closed reduction and skeletal traction or ORIF. Surgical decision making and technique are complex. Common complications after acetabular fractures include sciatic nerve injury, AVN, traumatic arthritis, and heterotopic ossification.

REFERENCES

1. Cummings SR, Rubin SM, Black D. The future of hip fractures in the United States. Numbers, costs, and potential effects of postmenopausal estrogen. *Clin Orthop Relat Res.* 1990;Mar:163-166.
2. Garden RS. Low-angle fixation in fractures of the femoral neck. *J Bone Joint Surg.* 1961;43B:647.
3. Cannon J, Silvestri S, Munro M. Imaging choices in occult hip fracture. *J Emerg Med.* 2009;37(2):144-152.
4. Lowe JA, Crist BD, Bhandari M, Ferguson TA. Optimal treatment of femoral neck fractures according to patient's physiologic age: an evidence-based review. *Orthop Clin North Am.* 2010;41:157-166.
5. Parker MJ, Handoll HH. Pre-operative traction for fractures of the proximal femur in adults. *Cochrane Database Syst Rev.* 2006;(3):CD000168.
6. Parker MJ, Handoll HH. Replacement arthroplasty versus internal fixation for extracapsular hip fractures in adults. *Cochrane Database Syst Rev.* 2006;(2):CD000086.
7. Weiss RJ, Montgomery SM, Al Dabbagh Z, Jansson KA. National data of 6409 Swedish inpatients with femoral shaft fractures: stable incidence between 1998 and 2004. *Injury.* 2009;40:304-308.
8. Lee C, Porter KM. Prehospital management of lower limb fractures. *Emerg Med J.* 2005;22:660-663.
9. Loder RT, O'Donnell PW, Feinberg JR. Epidemiology and mechanisms of femur fractures in children. *J Pediatr Orthop.* 2006;26:561-566.
10. Matheson GO, Clement DB, McKenzie DC, et al. Stress fractures in athletes: a study of 320 cases. *Am J Sports Med.* 1987;15:46-58.
11. DeFranco MJ, Recht M, Schils J, et al. Stress fractures of the femur in athletes. *Clin Sports Med.* 2006;25:89-103.
12. Boden BP, Speer KP. Femoral stress fractures. *Clin Sports Med.* 1997;16:307-317.
13. Kang L, Belcher D, Hulstyn MJ. Stress fractures of the femoral shaft in women's college lacrosse: a report of seven cases and a review of the literature. *Br J Sports Med.* 2005;39:902-906.
14. Kelsey JL, Prill MM, Keegan TH. Risk factors for pelvis fractures in older persons. *Am J Epidemiol.* 2005;162:879-886.
15. Duane TM, Dechert T, Wolfe LG. Clinical examination is superior to plain films to diagnose pelvic fractures compared to CT. *Am Surg.* 2008;74:476-479.
16. Tayal VS, Neilsen A, Jones AE, et al. Accuracy of trauma ultrasound in major pelvic injury. *J Trauma.* 2006;61:1453-1457.

12

PATELLAR, TIBIAL, AND FIBULAR FRACTURES

Fractures of the patella are uncommon and occur primarily in patients between 20 and 50 years of age. Determining the integrity of the quadriceps extensor mechanism is crucial in the diagnosis of these fractures. Patients with nondisplaced fractures and intact knee extension heal well with immobilization and rehabilitation. Most patellar fractures in children are avulsion or osteochondral fractures

The tibia is the most frequently fractured long bone. Near-anatomic alignment is important in minimizing the risk of nonunion or malunion in these fractures. Even minimal displacement in tibial fractures necessitates referral to an orthopedist. Primary care providers must stay alert to the signs of an acute compartment syndrome when evaluating fractures of the tibia. Tibial fractures in children can result from relatively minor injuring forces. The accidental toddler's fracture is common and must be distinguished from a fracture caused by child abuse.

Recognition of neurovascular and ligamentous injuries or compartment syndromes that may accompany fibular fractures is essential in distinguishing uncomplicated from complicated fractures. Truly isolated fractures of the fibula shaft are treated symptomatically and heal well with minimal treatment.

See Appendix for stepwise instructions for short- and long-leg casts and splints used in the treatment of patellar, tibial, and fibular fractures.

PATELLAR FRACTURES AND DISLOCATIONS

Anatomic Considerations

The patella is the largest sesamoid bone in the body and serves to increase the leverage and efficiency of the quadriceps muscle. The patella is generally triangular, with the apex pointing distally. The rectus femoris and vastus muscles (lateralis, medialis, intermedius) all insert on the proximal pole. The patellar ligament attaches to the distal pole of the patella and inserts on the tibial tuberosity. The medial patellofemoral ligament is the primary restraint to lateral subluxation of the patella, particularly in early flexion.[1] Other medial stabilizers include the medial retinaculum, the medial patellotibial ligament, and the vastus medialis obliquus muscle. A thin layer of quadriceps tendon passes over the patella and joins the patellar ligament distally. The medial and lateral retinacula, which are extensions of the quadriceps muscle, bypass the patella and insert directly on the tibia. If the retinacula are intact after a patellar fracture, the patient is able to extend the knee actively. The primary blood supply of the patella enters the central portion and the distal pole. Fractures through the midportion of the patella compromise the vascular supply to the proximal pole and leave it at risk for avascular necrosis (AVN).

Fractures of the patella are broadly classified as transverse, stellate or comminuted, vertical, and osteochondral. Any of these fracture types can be displaced or nondisplaced. Transverse fractures are the most common type followed by stellate fractures. The majority of transverse fractures are in the lower third of the patella. Vertical fractures usually occur along the margins of the patella. An osteochondral fracture involving the medial patellar facet can occur after a patellar dislocation or subluxation.

Mechanism of Injury

Patellar fractures result from either direct or indirect forces. Most fractures are due to direct forces such as a fall on the anterior aspect of the knee or striking the knee on the dashboard in a motor vehicle accident (MVA). Indirect injuries occur when patients stumble and attempt to prevent themselves from falling. The quadriceps muscle contracts forcefully, exceeding the intrinsic strength of the patella. The patella actually fractures before the patient strikes the ground. Continued quadriceps muscle contraction tears the medial and lateral retinacula, which results in

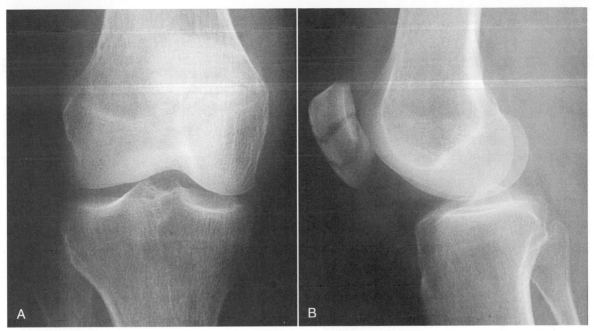

FIGURE 12-1 Anteroposterior (**A**) and lateral (**B**) views of a nondisplaced transverse fracture of the patella.

fracture displacement. Fractures caused by direct trauma are usually stellate and nondisplaced; fractures caused by indirect forces are usually transverse and displaced.

Clinical Presentation

The patient has tenderness and swelling over the anterior knee. When the fracture is displaced, a defect or separation is usually palpable if swelling is not excessive. The most important aspect of the examination is to check for the patient's ability to actively extend the knee against gravity. If this capability is absent, the quadriceps mechanism is disrupted. Local anesthetic can be injected into the knee joint to relieve pain before testing extensor function.

Imaging

Anteroposterior (AP), lateral, and sunrise views of the knee should be adequate for diagnosing most patellar fractures (Figure 12-1). The lateral view is the most useful view in delineating fracture lines and determining displacement (Figure 12-2). A separation of more than 3 mm between fragments or an articular stepoff of more than 2 mm constitutes a displaced fracture. Marginal vertical fractures are best visualized on the sunrise view. A bipartite patella may be mistaken for an acute fracture. This variation of ossification is best seen on the AP view and can be distinguished from an acute fracture by the well-defined zone of separation usually in the superolateral aspect of the patella (Figure 12-3). A radiograph of the opposite knee can confirm this diagnosis because bipartite patella is usually a bilateral finding. Another common finding on lateral radiographs of the knee is a small sesamoid bone in the tendons posterior to the knee joint (Figure 12-4). This normal variant is called the fabella and is of no clinical significance.

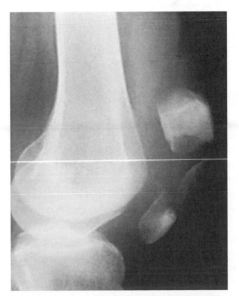

FIGURE 12-2 Lateral view of the knee demonstrating a markedly displaced transverse fracture of the patella. (*From Browner BD, Jupiter JB, Levine AM, Trafton PG [eds]. Skeletal Trauma: Fractures, Dislocations, Ligamentous Injuries. Philadelphia, WB Saunders, 1992.*)

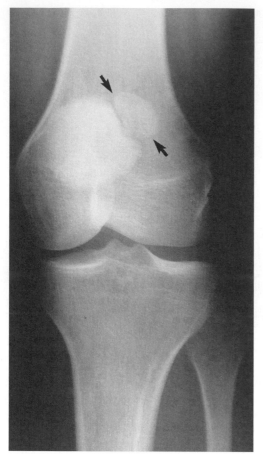

FIGURE 12-3 Anteroposterior view showing a bipartite patella with the characteristic finding of a well-demarcated lucent zone in the superolateral aspect of the patella (*arrows*). (*From Mettler FA. Essentials of Radiology. Philadelphia, WB Saunders, 1996.*)

Indications for Orthopedic Referral

Displaced patellar fractures require operative fixation and referral to an orthopedic surgeon. Patients with severely comminuted fractures should also be referred for consideration of partial or complete patellectomy. Quadriceps tendon repair and preservation of as much of the patella as possible are important in restoring knee extension. Total patellectomy is indicated only for highly displaced, severely comminuted fractures in which no large fragments remain. The timing of the surgery depends somewhat on the integrity of the overlying skin, which is often abraded during the injury. If the abrasions are clean and the wound is less than 8 hours old, the operative risk of infection is low. Extensive abrasions or a contaminated wound may necessitate delaying surgery until the skin heals.

Initial Treatment

Table 12-1 summarizes management guidelines for nondisplaced patellar fractures.

Aspiration of the knee joint hemarthrosis with use of aseptic technique should be considered to reduce pain and swelling, especially if a tense effusion is present. The knee should be wrapped with a compressive elastic bandage and the patient placed in a knee immobilizer with the knee in full extension. Icing and elevation of the knee are important in keeping the swelling to a minimum. The patient should remain non–weight bearing until examined again 5 to 7 days later.

Follow-up Care

Patients who have nondisplaced patellar fractures that have a smooth articular surface and an intact quadriceps mechanism and who are capable of extending the knee against gravity can be treated effectively nonoperatively. A cylinder cast from the groin (not the midthigh) to just above the ankle malleoli with the knee in extension (not

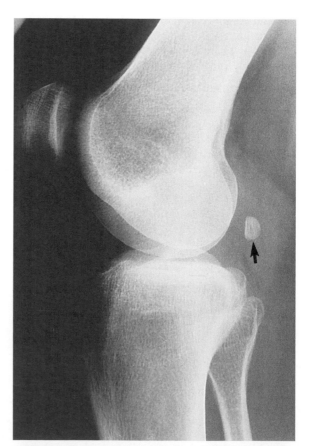

FIGURE 12-4 Fabella. A lateral view shows a normal variant, a small sesamoid bone in the tendons posterior to the knee joint (*arrow*). (*From Mettler FA. Essentials of Radiology. Philadelphia, WB Saunders, 1996.*)

Table 12-1	*Management Guidelines for Nondisplaced Patellar Fractures*
	INITIAL TREATMENT
Splint type and position	Knee immobilizer Knee in full extension
Initial follow-up visit	5 to 7 days
Patient instruction	Icing and elevation of the knee Non–weight bearing until follow-up visit
	FOLLOW-UP CARE
Cast or splint type and position	Cylinder cast above ankle to groin Knee in full extension, not hyperextension Knee immobilizer brace for reliable patients
Length of immobilization	4 to 6 weeks
Healing time	8 to 10 weeks
Follow-up visit interval	Every 3 to 4 weeks
Repeat radiography interval	At 2 weeks to check position At 4 to 6 weeks to document union
Patient instruction	Weight bearing as tolerated and straight-leg raises while in cast or brace Knee ROM and strengthening exercises after the cast or brace is removed Physical therapy referral is usually required to restore knee function
Indications for orthopedic consult	>3 mm of separation of fragments or >2 mm of articular stepoff Severely comminuted fractures

ROM, range of motion.

hyperextension) is the most reliable form of immobilization. Selected compliant patients can be treated with a removable hinged knee brace locked in extension for walking provided they wear the brace at all times except for bathing. Weight-bearing and straight-leg-raising exercises should be started in the cast or brace. The hinged brace is lighter than a cast and is an especially good choice for an elderly patient so early motion can be started to minimize loss of function.

A follow-up radiograph should be taken after 2 weeks to confirm that the fracture remains nondisplaced. Any displacement beyond the aforementioned limits warrants referral to an orthopedic surgeon. Immobilization should continue until radiographic evidence of union is apparent, which usually occurs in 4 to 6 weeks. Once the cast or brace is discontinued, the patient should be instructed in knee range of motion (ROM) exercises and quadriceps-strengthening exercises. A physical therapy referral is usually necessary to help the patient regain normal strength and motion.

Nondisplaced marginal vertical fractures do not have to be immobilized and can be treated with reduced activity for 3 to 6 weeks and progressive ROM and strengthening exercises.

Return to Work or Sports

The level of activity required by the patient's job should be considered when deciding how soon a patient may return to work. Patients with relatively sedentary jobs could return to work after several days of elevating and icing the knee if their symptoms allow, but it may be best to wait until after the first follow-up visit (5 to 7 days after injury). Patients whose jobs involve squatting, climbing stairs, or other activities requiring knee flexion should not return until the cast or brace is discontinued and knee ROM has progressed to the point at which they can perform these activities with reasonable comfort. This level of recovery is likely to take a minimum of 6 to 8 weeks. Athletes may begin activities that require little knee flexion (e.g., walking or freestyle swimming with gentle turns) soon after immobilization ends. Patients may begin gentle running when they are able to walk with little or no discomfort and knee ROM permits. This activity can be advanced as symptoms permit, with jumping and cutting activities added last. Patients can return to active jobs or sports more quickly by performing regular weight bearing, straight-leg raises, and ankle ROM while the knee is immobilized and by working diligently on regaining leg ROM and strength after immobilization ends. Referral to a physical therapist can greatly facilitate this process.

Complications

Complications after treatment of nondisplaced patellar fractures are rare, although patellofemoral pain and post traumatic osteoarthritis may occur.[2] Persistent patellofemoral pain after a patellar fracture should be managed with nonsteroidal antiinflammatory drugs (NSAIDs) and physical therapy. Prolonged immobilization may result in significant weakness in the extremity and loss of knee motion, and patients should work with physical therapists to restore function. Fracture fragment separation and dehiscence of fracture repair, infection, and AVN may complicate operative repair of patellar fractures.

Pediatric Considerations

The patella ossifies in early childhood, first becoming visible on plain radiographs between the ages of 3 and 6 years. Up to six separate ossification centers may be present, simulating the presence of a fracture. Palpation for tenderness and a comparison view of the normal knee may be used to distinguish a fracture from a growth plate.

Unlike injuries in adults, a knee effusion in a child is rarely caused by ligament injury. Patellar dislocation or fracture is far more likely. If a child has a traumatic knee effusion, a patellar dislocation that has spontaneously become reduced should be suspected. In a child with a traumatic knee effusion that was not caused by a patellar dislocation, an occult fracture is probably present. Such patients should either be referred or undergo aspiration of the joint. In the presence of normal radiographs, fat in the aspirate would indicate an occult fracture. Because the fracture may primarily involve cartilage, magnetic resonance imaging (MRI) is often required for adequate evaluation.

Most patella fractures in children are either osteochondral fractures or avulsion fractures. Osteochondral fractures occur in approximately 40% of childhood patellar dislocations.[3] Patients with osteochondral fractures should be referred to an orthopedic surgeon.

In children, patellar avulsion fractures may appear deceptively small on radiographs. However, the fragment typically includes a portion of unossified patella, making the fracture much larger than it appears. In patellar sleeve fractures, for instance, much or all of the articular surface of the patella is avulsed along with a small fragment of bone from the inferior pole of the patella. This injury is characterized by a high-riding patella (Figure 12-5), tenderness over the inferior pole, and an extensor lag when leg extension is tested. Patients with sleeve fractures should be referred, as should patients with avulsion fractures that are displaced or complicated by an inability to fully extend the knee. Nondisplaced fractures may be managed as previously described for adults. Healing is likely to be more rapid, allowing earlier discontinuation of the cast.

Transverse fractures of the patella are rare in children. They may be managed as described for adults, with special emphasis on assessing the patient's ability to actively extend the knee. If the patient is unable to fully extend the knee, referral is indicated.

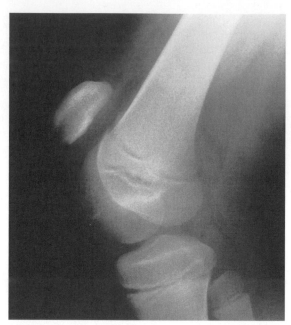

FIGURE 12-5 Sleeve fracture of the patella. On the lateral view, the patella is high riding, and a defect is noted on the inferior border of the patella, which represents the avulsed inferior pole. The fractured inferior portion of the patella overlies the femoral condyle and is not easily seen. *(From Green NE, Swiontkowski MF [eds]. Skeletal Trauma in Children, 2nd ed. Philadelphia, WB Saunders, 1998.)*

Patellar Dislocation

Dislocation of the patella usually occurs in patients with underlying patellofemoral malalignment. Predisposing factors that put the patient at risk of subluxation or dislocation include a shallow femoral groove, hypoplasia of the lateral femoral condyle, ligament hyperlaxity, a small or high-riding patella, genu valgum, external tibial torsion, and atrophy of the vastus medialis muscle. Nearly all patellar dislocations are lateral.

Mechanism of Injury

The usual cause of injury is an external pivotal motion on a partially flexed knee followed by a forceful contraction of the quadriceps that pulls the patella laterally. A direct blow to the medial patella, forcing it laterally, may also result in a dislocation.

Clinical Presentation

If the patient reports that the knee went out of place and slipped back after extension of the knee, the patella has spontaneously become reduced. If the patella remains dislocated, the knee is obviously deformed, and a hemarthrosis may occur. Findings related to injury to the medial stabilizers include hemarthrosis, tenderness along the medial patella edge, or tenderness proximal to the medial femoral condyle. A larger hemarthrosis volume (~50 mL) suggests a more major injury to the medial stabilizers or osteochondral injury and is actually associated with a lower recurrence rate because this larger volume usually represents a more traumatic dislocation. This is in contrast to the patient with a lower energy mechanism who may have one or more predisposing risk factors and a less traumatic injury and thus a minimal hemarthrosis. The presence of fat in the knee aspirate is indicative of an osteochondral fracture.

Reduction Maneuver

See Expert Consult for a video on how to perform a reduction maneuver for an a patellar dislocation. Reduction of the dislocation can be preformed safely before obtaining radiographs. To reduce a laterally dislocated patella, the clinician places the patient in the supine position and flexes the hip to 90 degrees to relax the quadriceps muscle. The clinician then gradually extends the knee while gently pushing the patella medially. If moderate swelling and muscle spasm prevent relocation, aspiration of the hemarthrosis and instillation of a local anesthetic usually provide enough pain relief to accomplish the reduction. A benzodiazepine can also be used to relax the patient.

Imaging

Radiographs should be obtained to rule out an accompanying fracture even if the dislocation spontaneously became reduced. The AP, lateral, and sunrise views should be examined, particularly for an osteochondral fracture of the patella, which occurs in up to 25% of cases.[4] Unfortunately, these fractures are often missed on initial radiographs.[5] All patients with a first-time traumatic dislocation should be considered to have an osteochondral injury until otherwise proven, and MRI is indicated to look for this injury as well as injury to the medial stabilizers.[3] Postreduction radiographs are necessary to check patellar position.

Indications for Orthopedic Referral

If an osteochondral fracture is associated with the dislocation, the patient should be referred to an orthopedic surgeon. Other indications for operative treatment include significant injury to the medial patellar stabilizers, a persistently laterally subluxed patella, or a second dislocation.

Initial Treatment

Initial treatment includes limitation of knee flexion with a knee immobilizer, icing, and elevation of the knee. The patient should remain non–weight bearing for 2 to 3 days. The patient should remain in the knee immobilizer for the first 2 to 3 weeks for comfort.

Follow-up Care

Weight-bearing and return to work duties are allowed as soon as the patient is able. After 2 to 3 weeks, functional rehabilitation and progressive knee flexion are allowed over the next 3 weeks. Commercially available patellofemoral braces provide needed protection during this time because quadriceps strength is inadequate for full independent function. Physical therapy referral is indicated in most cases to help the patient restore strength and motion gradually. Guidelines for return to work or sports are the same as outlined previously for patellar fractures.

Complications

Redislocation is common, with those who are younger and female being at greater risk. There are some reports of higher redislocation rates with closed treatment versus operative treatment for first-time dislocators, but a well- designed, randomized, prospective trial with an adequate length of follow-up has failed to show a significant difference in rates based on initial treatment choice.[3,6] Other complications after a patellar dislocation include patellar instability and patellofemoral arthritis.

Pediatric Considerations

The evaluation, indications for referral, and treatment of patellar dislocations in children are similar to those in adults. In children, if the patella remains dislocated when the child seeks treatment and prereduction radiographs do not reveal a fracture, reduction should be performed as previously described for adults. Films should be repeated after reduction because fracture fragments are often visible only on postreduction views.

TIBIAL FRACTURES

Anatomic Considerations

The tibia and fibula are bound together proximally by the tibiofibular articulation, a synovial joint reinforced with strong anterior and posterior ligaments. Distally, the tibia and fibula are connected by the tibiofibular syndesmosis, which is composed of the anterior and posterior tibiofibular ligaments and the interosseous membrane. The bones and muscles of the leg are surrounded by the crural fascia. The interosseous membrane and fibrous extensions of the crural fascia separate the leg into four distinct compartments (Figure 12-6).

The popliteal artery divides to form the anterior and posterior tibial arteries after it exits the popliteal fossa. The anterior tibial artery enters the anterior compartment just below the level of the fibular head and descends along the interosseous

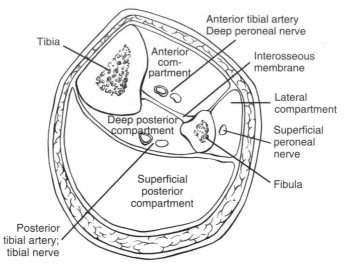

FIGURE 12-6 Cross section of the lower leg demonstrating the four compartments.

membrane. It is vulnerable to direct injury in proximal tibial fractures.

The medial and lateral tibial plateaus are the articular surfaces of the medial and lateral tibial condyles. The two plateaus are separated by the intercondylar eminence, which serves as the attachment for the anterior cruciate ligament (ACL). The outer aspect of each plateau is covered by the cartilaginous meniscus. The medial plateau and condyle are larger and stronger than on the lateral side, and fractures of the relatively weaker lateral plateau are more common.

Tibial Plateau Fractures

Mechanism of Injury

Many tibial plateau fractures occur as a result of a car–pedestrian accident in which the bumper strikes the outside of the leg with a force directed medially (valgus). This results in a depressed or split fracture of the lateral tibial plateau as the femoral condyle is driven into it. Because of the greater strength of the medial plateau, fractures on this side of the joint usually suggest a much higher energy injuring force (varus). Axial compression caused by a fall from height can also fracture the proximal tibia. Elderly patients with osteoporosis are more likely to sustain a fracture of the tibial plateau than a ligamentous or meniscal tear after a twisting injury to the knee. The intercondylar eminence can be fractured in association with an ACL tear as a result of hyperextension or rotatory forces.

Clinical Presentation

Patients with a tibial plateau fracture have a painful swollen knee and are unable to bear weight. During examination, they have tenderness over the proximal tibia and limited flexion and extension of the knee. The clinician should determine whether the cause of injury was a low- or high-energy force because associated neurovascular and ligamentous injuries and compartment syndromes are much more common after high-energy injuries. Distal pulses and peroneal nerve function should be documented. The skin should be carefully examined for any evidence of abrasions or lacerations that may indicate an open fracture. Presence of an effusion suggests an osteochondral fracture or a ligament or meniscal injury.

Assessment of knee stability is an important element in the evaluation of tibial plateau injuries. Aspiration of the knee hemarthrosis and instillation of a local anesthetic may be necessary to get an accurate examination. Compared with the uninjured side, a stable knee should not have more than 10 degrees of joint widening on varus or valgus stressing at any point in the arc of motion from full extension to 90 degrees of flexion. The integrity of the ACL should be assessed by means of the Lachman test.

Tibial plateau fractures are frequently associated with soft tissue injuries around the knee.[7] Medial collateral ligament and lateral meniscal tears often accompany lateral plateau fractures. Medial plateau fractures are associated with lateral collateral ligament and medial meniscus tears. The ACL can be injured in fractures of either plateau. Tibial plateau fractures, especially those with extension of the fracture into the tibial shaft, can lead to an acute compartment syndrome resulting from hemorrhage and edema (see discussion of acute compartment syndrome in the section on Clinical Presentation for tibial shaft fractures).

Imaging

AP, lateral, and internal and external oblique views of the knee should be obtained in the evaluation of a suspected proximal tibial fracture. A tunnel (notch) view is useful in visualizing the intercondylar eminence. The tibial plateau normally slopes from anterosuperior to posteroinferior. Findings on the AP view may be subtle and fail to define fracture depression because this view does not demonstrate the normal plateau slope (Figure 12-7). An area of increased bone density from fracture depression may be the only finding on the AP view (Figure 12-8). Split fractures of the tibial plateau are more common in younger patients with dense cancellous bone. Depressed fractures or split fractures with depression are more common in older patients with decreased bone density. Fractures can also occur in both plateaus simultaneously.

Additional imaging with computed tomography (CT) scanning is useful in delineating the extent of articular involvement and the degree of fracture depression. MRI has replaced CT scanning in many centers because of its superior ability to detect associated ligamentous and meniscal injuries.

Indications for Orthopedic Referral

A tibial plateau fracture in association with a vascular injury or compartment syndrome requires emergent orthopedic referral and treatment. Displaced or depressed tibial plateau fractures and fractures with associated ligamentous or meniscal injuries should be referred within 24 to 48 hours. The goal in treating these fractures is to achieve a stable knee with a congruous healthy articular surface. Decisions regarding operative versus nonoperative treatment of displaced or depressed fractures must take into account the patient's age, current and expected level of activity, presence of associated injuries, and current medical conditions.

Initial Treatment

Table 12-2 summarizes the management guidelines for nondisplaced tibial plateau fractures.

The patient should be immobilized in a long-leg splint or compressive dressing such as a Jones dressing (see Figure 13-22) from the thigh to the metatarsals with the knee in full extension and the ankle at 90 degrees. The patient should remain non–weight bearing. Icing and strict elevation of the leg are important to minimize swelling and the risk of

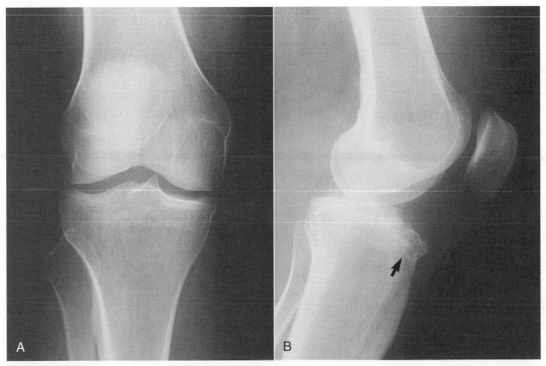

FIGURE 12-7 A, Anteroposterior view of the knee, showing subtle irregularity of the superior edge of the lateral tibial condyle. **B,** Lateral view clearly demonstrates a depressed fracture of the anterior aspect of the lateral plateau (*arrow*).

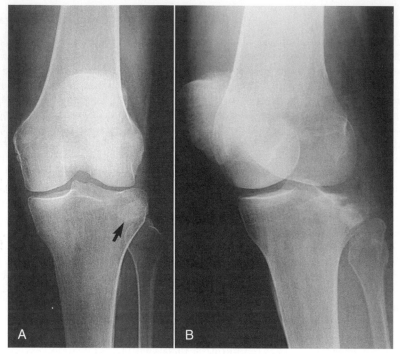

FIGURE 12-8 A, Anteroposterior view of the knee showing minimal findings of increased bone density of the lateral tibial condyle (*arrow*). **B,** The oblique view more clearly demonstrates a depressed, displaced fracture of the lateral plateau.

Table 12-2	*Management Guidelines for Nondisplaced Tibial Plateau Fractures*
INITIAL TREATMENT	
Splint type and position	Long-leg splint or compressive dressing
	Knee in full extension; ankle at 90 degrees
Initial follow-up visit	Within 3 to 5 days
Patient instruction	Icing and strict elevation of the leg
	Non–weight bearing
FOLLOW-UP CARE	
Cast or splint type and position	Hinged brace initially in full extension
	Gradual flexion in brace after 10 to 14 days
	Flexion to 90 degrees within 3 to 4 weeks
Length of immobilization	8 to 12 weeks until evidence of radiographic union
Healing time	12 to 20 weeks until full function restored
Follow-up visit interval	Every 2 to 3 weeks while in brace; then monthly until full function is restored
Repeat radiography interval	At first follow-up visit; then weekly for 3 weeks to check position
	Every 2 to 3 weeks
Patient instruction	Non–weight bearing for 4 to 6 weeks; then partial weight bearing with crutch assistance until solid fracture union
	Active knee flexion while in brace
	Quadriceps strengthening after brace is removed
Indications for orthopedic consult	Vascular injury or compartment syndrome
	Displaced or depressed fractures
	Associated ligamentous or meniscal injury

compartment syndrome. Patients with displaced fractures should be referred promptly to an orthopedic surgeon. Patients with nondisplaced fractures should be seen within 3 to 5 days for definitive care.

Follow-up Care

The patient is placed in a hinged brace initially in full extension. After 10 to 14 days, the brace is adjusted to allow gradual flexion so the patient is flexing the knee to 90 degrees in 3 to 4 weeks. The brace should be continued for 8 to 12 weeks until radiographic evidence of union is seen. Repeat radiographs should be obtained at the first follow-up visit and weekly thereafter for at least 3 weeks to ensure no loss of position. If position is lost, the patient should be referred promptly, because correction becomes more difficult with each passing day. Radiographic healing can be assessed every 2 to 3 weeks after fracture stability is documented. The patient should remain non–weight bearing for 4 to 6 weeks until radiographic evidence of some healing is evident. After that point, partial weight bearing with crutch assistance is used until solid union of the fracture has occurred. Patients should continue active ROM exercises during the entire healing period, and those who fail to achieve 90 degrees of knee flexion by 4 weeks after injury should be referred for physical therapy. More aggressive rehabilitation, especially quadriceps-strengthening exercises, is started after fracture union is apparent. Physical therapy supervision of the rehabilitation is warranted. Return to full function typically takes 4 to 5 months.

Return to Work or Sports

For the first few weeks, patients will be unable either to bear weight or to bend the knee, making it impossible for many to get to work and perform even sedentary jobs. As knee flexion increases and the patient begins partial weight bearing, sedentary jobs should become quite manageable. Jobs requiring standing or walking may be gradually resumed after a solid union is present and full weight bearing is well tolerated. Patients should not return to jobs that place greater demands on the knee until ROM and strength allow the patient to perform the tasks comfortably and safely. A physical therapist can speed recovery and provide useful guidance about advancing activity levels. Athletes should be able to safely resume non–weight-bearing aerobic activities such as swimming or biking after full weight bearing is started. It may be wise to limit prolonged or stressful weight bearing activities for many months until healing is nearly complete.

Complications

Loss of knee motion is a common complication after tibial plateau fractures. This outcome may be caused by the fracture itself or the prolonged immobilization necessary for treatment. Post-traumatic arthritis may develop, especially if joint instability and articular incongruity accompanied the fracture. Infection may complicate surgical treatment of these fractures, particularly if a breakdown of overlying contused skin occurred.

Pediatric Considerations (Proximal Tibia)

Two important growth centers lie in the proximal tibia: a physis that allows longitudinal growth of the tibia and an apophysis lying beneath the tibial tubercle. The latter allows growth at the patellar tendon insertion site. Injuries that would produce knee dislocations or tibial plateau fractures in adults are likely to produce fractures through the physis in children. Fractures through this physis are more common in young adolescents and are usually caused by high-velocity trauma. A metaphyseal corner or bucket handle fracture is associated with intentional trauma when pulling or rotational forces are forcibly applied to the leg and should warrant further evaluation for child abuse.

The child with a proximal physeal facture will be unable to bear weight and have a hemarthrosis. In rare circumstances, these fractures are complicated by injuries to the popliteal artery, especially if there is a large joint effusion or posterior displacement of the fracture. A careful distal vascular examination is warranted. The young toddler with a metaphyseal corner fracture typically presents with a limp or inability to bear weight, but swelling and deformity are lacking.

All fractures involving the proximal tibial physis should be referred to an orthopedic surgeon because of the risk of growth disturbance and valgus angular deformity. Emergent referral must be obtained if there is any evidence of vascular compromise. The leg should be immobilized in a long-leg posterior splint from the metatarsal heads to the proximal thigh with the knee in extension and with adequate padding over bony prominences until the patient is seen by the specialist. Patients with displaced fractures should be seen within a few hours for closed or open reduction, and those with nondisplaced fractures can be seen within 1 week.

Tibial Tubercle

The tibial tubercle apophysis is susceptible to avulsion injuries, especially in adolescents. In evaluating a teenager with tibial tubercle pain, the physician must distinguish between Osgood-Schlatter disease and an acute avulsion. Osgood-Schlatter disease, a painful inflammation of the tubercle, is thought to result from repetitive microfractures in the cartilaginous portion of the tendon insertion site. Typically, patients report progressive tubercle pain that began gradually and was not associated with an acute injury. The pain generally interferes with certain activities and may produce a limp. During examination, point tenderness of the tubercle is apparent. The tubercle may also be somewhat enlarged. Radiographs usually reveal an irregular ossification center (Figure 12-9, A). Radiographs are not necessary when the history and examination strongly suggest Osgood-Schlatter disease but should be performed if the physician suspects an acute avulsion injury superimposed on a background of preexisting Osgood-Schlatter disease. Patients with Osgood-Schlatter disease usually respond well to activity limitation. Icing and NSAIDs may also help patients who are very symptomatic.

With acute avulsions, tubercle pain typically occurs after a discrete jumping incident. The symptoms may mimic those of Osgood-Schlatter disease except that knee extension may be limited or impossible, especially if displacement is present (Figure 12-9, B). A joint effusion is seldom present. Patellar sleeve fractures, previously discussed, have a similar presentation and should be considered in the differential diagnosis. Nondisplaced fractures can be treated initially with a knee immobilizer until swelling has decreased to allow for casting with a long-leg cast for 4 to 6 weeks. Displaced avulsions require referral. Rehabilitation with a focus on quadriceps strengthening occurs after immobilization has been discontinued. The patient should avoid jumping or strenuous sport activity until quadriceps strength has returned to near normal.

Tibial Spine

In general, bone or the physis will fail before ligaments in children. A cause of injury that would produce an ACL tear in an adult will instead produce a fracture through the anterior tibial spine in a child (Figure 12-10). This injury occurs during late childhood to mid-adolescence and is often associated with bicycling. Hyperextension of the knee during abruptly braking while biking causes the fracture through the tibial spine. Children with this injury will have a hemarthrosis and decreased knee motion. Patients with nondisplaced fractures may be managed initially in a knee immobilizer and kept non–weight bearing for the first few days followed by a long-leg cast with 5*10 degrees of flexion for 5*6 weeks. Patients with displaced tibial spine fractures should be referred to an orthopedic surgeon.

Tibial Shaft Fractures

Mechanism of Injury

Tibial shaft fractures occur as a result of low-energy forces such as a fall with a twisting motion on a fixed foot or high-energy forces such as MVAs or

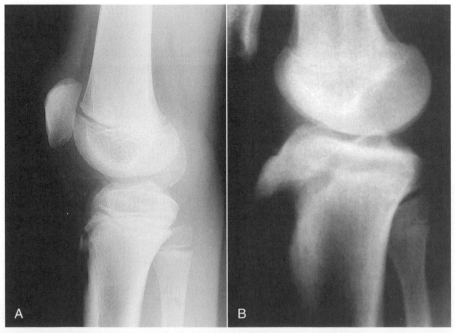

FIGURE 12-9 A, Irregular ossification of the tibial tubercle characteristic of Osgood-Schlatter disease. *(From Thornton A, Gyll C. Children's Fractures: A Radiological Guide to Safe Practice. Philadelphia, WB Saunders, 1999.)* **B,** Lateral view of the knee demonstrating a displaced avulsion fracture of the tibial tubercle.*(From Green NE, Swiontkowski MF [eds].Skeletal Trauma in Children, 2nd ed. Philadelphia, WB Saunders, 1998.)*

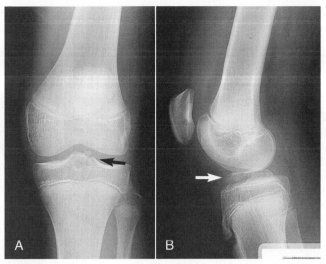

FIGURE 12-10 Avulsion of the anterior tibial spine after a fall in a 15-year-old (*arrows*). (*From Thornton A, Gyll C. Children's Fractures: A Radiological Guide to Safe Practice. Philadelphia, WB Saunders, 1999.*)

falls from a significant height. Proximal fractures are more often high-energy injuries, and distal fractures are more often low-energy injuries. Direct trauma tends to cause transverse and comminuted fractures, and indirect forces cause oblique or spiral fractures. Usually, the amount of comminution is proportional to the amount of energy that caused the fracture. The relatively superficial position of the anteromedial aspect of the tibia puts this area at higher risk for fracture from a direct blow.

Clinical Presentation

Patients with tibial shaft fractures report an inability to bear weight and significant pain and swelling over the fracture site. Open fractures are common, and the skin should be examined thoroughly for evidence of small lacerations caused by sharp underlying fracture fragments puncturing the skin from the inside. Direct injury to major blood vessels is unlikely with closed tibial fractures except for proximal fractures, which may injure the anterior tibial artery. A thorough neurovascular examination, including the dorsalis pedis and posterior tibial pulses and lower extremity motor and sensory function, must be documented.

Compartment Syndrome

Fractures of the tibia, especially those in the diaphysis and in younger patients, are associated with acute compartment syndromes, and prompt recognition of this complication is essential in the management of patients with these fractures.[8] Any one of the four compartments of the lower leg may be affected (see Figure 12-6). A compartment syndrome results from increased pressure within a defined space that interferes with capillary blood flow within that space. This leads to ischemia with resultant loss of nerve and muscle function. Hemorrhage into the lower leg after a tibial fracture can significantly raise intracompartmental pressure.

The symptoms and signs of compartment syndrome change over time, so serial examination is important.[9] Pain is the most reliable early symptom, but it is not present in all cases. Typically, pain caused by compartment syndrome is disproportionate, deep, and poorly localized (analogous to the pain of cardiac ischemia). The presence of such pain after a tibial shaft fracture strongly suggests a compartment syndrome. Other symptoms of acute compartment syndrome include tense swelling in one or more compartments, increased pain with passive motion or stretching of the muscles in the involved compartment, and paresthesias. Any of these symptoms may or may not be present in a given case. Diminished or absent pulses are late findings. Anterior compartment syndrome symptoms are pain on passive ankle or toe plantarflexion and numbness of the web space between the first and second toes (deep peroneal nerve). Symptoms that suggest a lateral compartment syndrome are pain with passive inversion of the foot and numbness along the lateral dorsum of the foot, excluding the first web space (superficial peroneal nerve). Patients with a deep posterior compartment syndrome have pain on dorsiflexion of the toes and paresthesias along the sole of the foot (tibial nerve). Superficial posterior compartment syndrome symptoms are pain with passive ankle dorsiflexion and numbness of the lateral aspect of the heel (sural nerve). After paralysis and pulselessness are present, permanent damage, loss of the limb, or both are likely.

To detect compartment syndrome early, the clinician must remain extremely alert to its potential occurrence, be aware of the early symptoms, and pursue further evaluation with compartment pressure measurement and orthopedic consultation in suspected cases. Interpreting the results of compartment pressure measurements can be complex because accuracy depends on proper calibration of the device and needle placement, and the pressure necessary to cause injury varies depending on the clinical scenario. Serial or continuous pressure measurements are usually more helpful than a single measurement.[10] Although there is no agreed upon compartment pressure threshold above which fasciotomy is indicated, this surgical procedure to decompress the affected compartments is the definitive treatment in the vast majority of cases.

Imaging

Before radiographs are obtained, the leg should be immobilized with a radiolucent splint to prevent further movement of the fracture fragments and subsequent soft tissue injury. AP and lateral views of the entire tibia, including the knee and ankle joints, should be obtained.

Several classification schemes have been developed for tibial shaft fractures.[11] No one scheme is preferred. The following features are important to note in the description of a tibial shaft fracture:

1. Open versus closed injury
2. Anatomic location (proximal, middle, distal)
3. Pattern(s) of fracture lines (transverse, oblique, spiral, segmental, comminuted)
4. Amount of displacement in the AP and mediolateral planes measured in millimeters
5. Degree of angulation in the AP and mediolateral planes
6. Amount of shortening measured in millimeters
7. Degree of rotation (detected as a discrepancy in the transverse widths of the proximal and distal fragments)
8. Presence or absence of an associated fibular fracture
9. Extent of soft tissue damage

A fracture is considered nondisplaced if it meets the following criteria: less than 5 mm of displacement and less than 10 degrees of angulation in both the AP and mediolateral planes and less than 10 degrees of rotation (Figure 12-11).

Indications for Orthopedic Referral

Emergent Referral

Emergent orthopedic referral is required for open tibial shaft fractures, fractures with evidence of

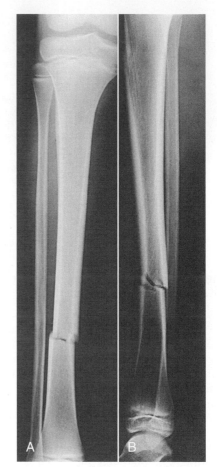

FIGURE 12-11 Anteroposterior (**A**) and lateral (**B**) views of a nondisplaced tibial shaft fracture. This fracture is considered nondisplaced if it meets the following criteria: less than 5 mm of displacement in both the anteroposterior and mediolateral planes, less than 10 degrees of angulation in either plane, and less than 10 degrees of rotation.

neurovascular injury or compartment syndrome, and fractures associated with dislocation of the knee or ankle (which must be reduced immediately). A delay of longer than 6 hours to operative intervention for open tibial fractures increases the risk of infection.[12]

Referral Within 1 to 2 days

Optimal management of displaced fractures is controversial, so early evaluation by an orthopedic surgeon is needed to determine the treatment strategy and when intermedullary nailing is indicated.[13,14] Patients with comminuted and segmental fractures should also be referred to an orthopedic even if displacement is minimal. Before being seen by the orthopedist, the patient should be immobilized in a long-leg splint as described below.

Initial Treatment

Table 12-3 summarizes the management guidelines for nondisplaced tibial shaft fractures.

The leg should be immobilized in a long-leg posterior splint from the metatarsals to the midthigh, with the knee in 10 to 15 degrees of flexion and the ankle at 90 degrees. The leg should be well padded before the application of the splint to allow for swelling. The patient must remain non–weight bearing. Hospitalization is often needed for 2 to 3 days to achieve adequate elevation and pain control and to monitor for a compartment syndrome. For selected reliable patients who can perform strict elevation and icing and who will return at the first sign of a compartment syndrome, home care in the acute treatment phase is appropriate. Patients sent home should receive telephone follow-up in 24 hours to assess their symptoms and be seen within 48 hours.

Follow-up Care

Only nondisplaced, noncomminuted tibial shaft fractures in which acceptable position can be maintained with long-leg cast immobilization should be managed by a primary care provider provided he or she is comfortable with long-leg cast application and management. A circumferential cast should not be applied until the amount of swelling has stabilized or is decreasing and minimal risk of compartment syndrome exists (usually 3 to 5 days). If the fracture is potentially unstable, a long-leg cast may be applied acutely to better maintain position, provided it is bivalved to accommodate any swelling and the patient is reliable and compliant with follow-up. A stepwise description of how to apply a long-leg cast is included in the Appendix. Plaster is easier to mold and is the preferred material for the initial cast.

Radiographs should be obtained after casting to ascertain that the fracture has not lost position. A change from acceptable to unacceptable position usually necessitates referral. Patients are kept non–weight bearing weight for the first 1 to 2 weeks. The cast will most likely need to be changed in 2 to 3 weeks because of loosening as swelling decreases. Fiberglass can be used at the first cast change because it is lighter and more durable. The long-leg cast is continued for 4 to 6 weeks. When there is radiographic evidence of adequate healing, the patient may be converted to a short-leg walking cast or preferably a walking cast boot. This treatment is continued until clinical and radiographic evidence of fracture union is observed. The majority of nondisplaced fractures heal within 10 to 14 weeks. Signs of clinical healing are minimal tenderness over the fracture site and no motion or pain accompanying bending stress in any direction.

Table 12-3	*Management Guidelines for Nondisplaced Tibial Shaft Fractures*
INITIAL TREATMENT	
Splint type and position	Long-leg posterior splint, well padded
	Knee in 10 to 15 degrees of flexion; ankle at 90 degrees
Initial follow-up visit	24 to 48 hours if patient sent home
	Consider admission for elevation, pain control, and neurovascular monitoring
Patient instruction	Strict elevation
	Non–weight bearing
	Explain signs of compartment syndrome
FOLLOW-UP CARE	
Cast or splint type and position	Long-leg cast when swelling stabilized
	Knee at 0 to 5 degrees of flexion; ankle at 90 degrees
	Use plaster cast initially
Length of immobilization	Long-leg cast for 4 to 6 weeks
	Short-leg walking castor boot casting until clinical and radiographic union (10 to 14 weeks)
Healing time	6 to 9 months until full function restored
Follow-up visit interval	Weekly for 3 to 4 weeks; then every 2 to 4 weeks until brace is removed; then every 1 to 2 months until full function is restored
Repeat radiography interval	Weekly for 3 to 4 weeks to ensure alignment; then every 2 to 4 weeks
Patient instruction	Weight bearing as soon as possible
	Crutch assistance with ambulation
Indications for orthopedic consult	Displaced: >5 mm displaced >10 degrees of angulation in any plane >10 degrees of rotation
	Open fracture
	Comminuted fracture

Signs of radiographic union are new bone formation (callus) that bridges the fracture defect on all four views (AP, lateral, right and left oblique).

Weekly radiographs (AP and lateral) for 3 to 4 weeks are required to document that fracture alignment is maintained. When fracture stability is evident (callus is present and the position is unchanged), radiographs can be obtained every 2 to 4 weeks until fracture union is confirmed. If displacement, angulation, or shortening increases at any time during healing, the patient should be referred to an orthopedist.

After immobilization is discontinued, the patient should use crutches to assist with ambulation until balance and strength are restored. Because patients have significant muscle atrophy and weakness after immobilization, physical therapy supervision during the rehabilitation period is advisable. The patient should begin with ankle and knee ROM and muscle-stretching exercises followed by progressive strengthening and endurance training. It may take as long as 6 to 9 months from the time of injury for the patient to resume a preinjury level of activity. Any type of contact sport, skiing, or jumping activity should be avoided until the patient has sufficient strength to jump in place and do a full squat and radiographs show that the tibial intramedullary canal has remodeled.

Return to Work or Sports

The guidelines for return to work or sports after tibial shaft fractures are the same as outlined previously for tibial plateau fractures.

Complications

Although they mend more slowly than most other fractures, nondisplaced fractures of the tibial shaft generally heal without complication as long as normal alignment is maintained. Some patients experience prolonged symptoms lasting longer than 1 year from the injury, and all patients should be advised that this is a possibility regardless of treatment.[15] A fracture that has shown no evidence of progress toward radiographic healing after 12 weeks is considered a nonunion. Nonunion and delayed union are more common in severely displaced or comminuted fractures. Malunion can occur, but as long as the patient has good function of the leg, operative correction is not needed. Varus angulation is the most common deformity. Other complications include joint stiffness caused by prolonged immobilization, infection (open fractures or postoperative), refracture, and complex regional pain syndrome.

Pediatric Considerations

Tibial shaft fractures are common in children, and concurrent fractures of both the tibia and fibula

occur in up to 30% of cases.[16] Because the management of both bone fractures is much more complicated and usually requires referral to an orthopedic surgeon, the physician must carefully scrutinize the entire length of the fibula for a coexisting fracture. The fibula fracture may be of the plastic deformity type, which can easily be missed (Figure 12-12).

Pediatric tibia fractures may be of the torus or buckle type (Figure 12-13), the greenstick type (Figure 12-14), or complete (Figure 12-15). The most frequent pattern is a short oblique or transverse fracture in the middle or distal third of the bone. Compared with fractures of both the tibia and fibula, isolated fractures of the tibia may be caused by relatively mild forces in younger children. Falls and twisting injuries of the foot are common causes of injury. The periosteum generally remains intact. The combination of low force, an intact periosteum, and support from the intact fibula prevents significant displacement in most cases.

Patients with open fractures, pathologic fractures, displaced fractures (>10 degrees anterior angulation, >5 degrees of varus or valgus angulation, >1 cm of shortening), and both-bone fractures should be referred. Bowing or torus fractures are quite stable and usually heal completely with 3 to 4 weeks of immobilization in a short-leg

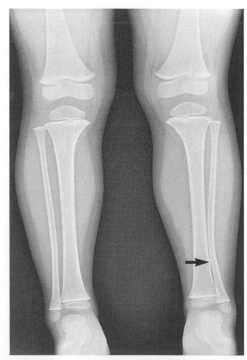

FIGURE 12-12 Anteroposterior view of both legs demonstrating plastic deformation of the left fibula. A torus fracture of the distal tibia is also apparent.

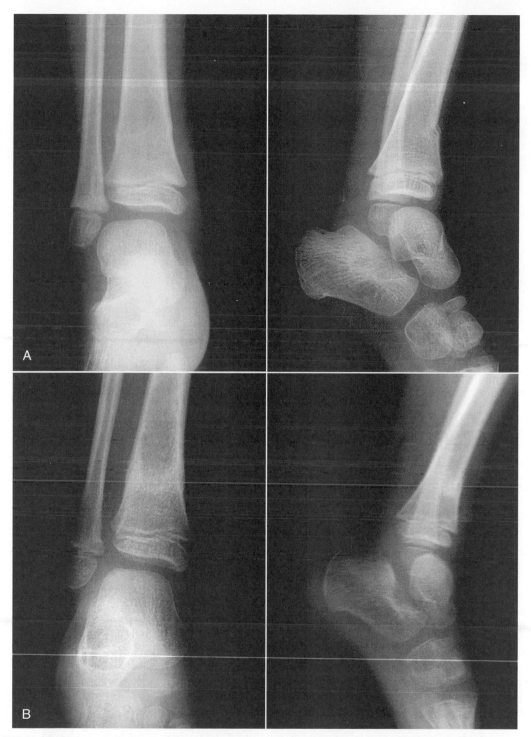

FIGURE 12-13 A, Anteroposterior and lateral views of an acute buckle fracture of the distal tibia in a 3-year-old child, demonstrating minimal angulation (<10 degrees) in the anteroposterior plane. The fibula appears normal. **B,** Follow-up radiograph 5 weeks later demonstrating good healing without change in position. Lack of callus in the fibula confirms that the fibula was not fractured.

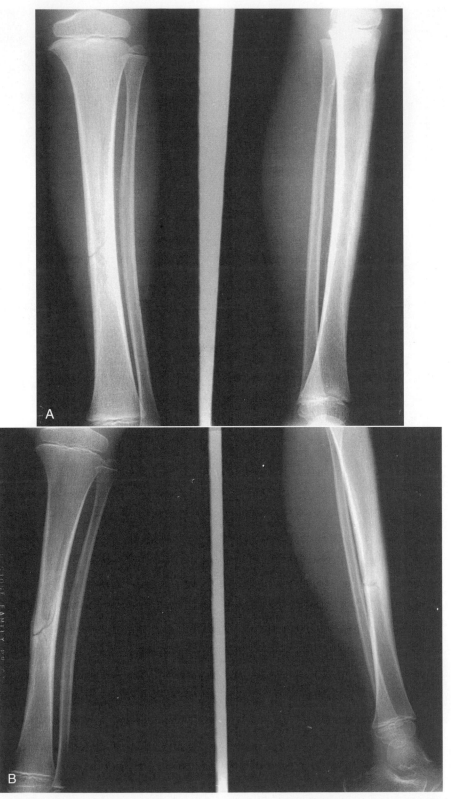

FIGURE 12-14 A, Subtle fracture of the midtibia in a 4-year-old child. The medial cortex is broken, but the lateral cortex is intact, which is consistent with a greenstick fracture. **B,** Follow-up radiograph 3 weeks later. The fracture line is now much more obvious, callus is present, and varus angulation has increased minimally if at all.

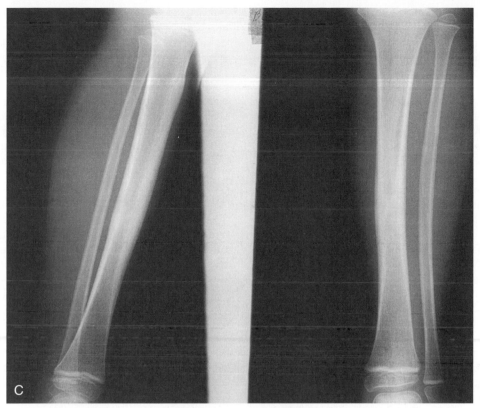

FIGURE 12-14, cont'd C, Eight weeks after injury, the fracture is healing well, and the cast may be discontinued. Varus angulation has increased slightly but is less than 10 degrees and should remodel easily.

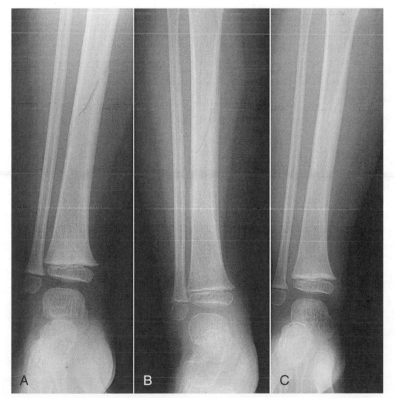

FIGURE 12-15 A, Anteroposterior view of the tibia demonstrating a nondisplaced spiral fracture of the midtibial shaft, the so-called toddler's fracture. B, Follow-up radiograph 1 month later shows fracture healing. C, Follow-up radiograph 2 months after original injury shows complete healing.

walking cast. Patients with nondisplaced tibial shaft fractures are managed with a bent knee long-leg cast for 4 to 6 weeks. As with adults, radiographs should be repeated weekly and the patient referred at the first sign of increasing angulation. After some callus is present and position maintained, the cast is changed to a short-leg walking cast for an additional 4 to 6 weeks with progressive weight bearing as tolerated. Healing is more rapid than in adults, usually occurring by 6 to 10 weeks. Mild varus deformity is common. It should remodel well if it is less than 10 degrees. Compartment syndrome is much less common in children than adults with tibial shaft fractures.[17]

Toddler's Fracture

This is a distinct subtype of tibia fracture seen in young children. In children from 9 months to 3 years of age, a torsional force applied to the foot may result in a spiral fracture of the middle or distal tibia. Toddler's fractures occur most commonly in children younger than 2 years of age who are learning to walk. Frequently, no definite history of a traumatic event exists, and the child is brought to the office for evaluation because of reluctance to bear weight on the leg. A thorough physical examination may be limited by the child's degree of cooperation, but maximal tenderness over the fracture site and pain elicited by grasping the knee and ankle and gently twisting in opposite directions are common findings. The hip, thigh, and knee should be examined first to rule out other causes of the limping.

AP and lateral views of the entire tibia and fibula should be obtained if a toddler's fracture is suspected. Additional oblique views may be necessary to define the fracture. The typical findings are a nondisplaced spiral fracture of the tibia and no fibular fracture (see Figure 12-15). It is common for findings of initial radiographs to be normal and the diagnosis of this fracture to be made several days after the injury when follow-up radiographs show a lucent line or periosteal reaction.

Distinguishing a toddler's fracture from a fracture caused by child abuse may be somewhat difficult because often no witnessed trauma occurs, and the spiral fracture suggests a twisting force. The child should be examined carefully for signs of soft tissue trauma such as bruises on the buttocks and the back of the legs, head, or neck. Bruises over the shins, knees, elbows, and forehead are typical in a toddler and are not signs of abuse. The clinician should suspect abuse more strongly if the caregivers are vague or evasive, a significant delay from the time of initial symptoms (limping) to obtaining treatment has occurred, the reported mechanism does not match the degree of injury, or current evidence or a history of other suspicious

injuries exists. Transverse fractures of the midshaft and both-bone fractures of the tibia and fibula are more often caused by abuse and should arouse greater suspicion.

A toddler's fracture should be immobilized in a bent knee long-leg cast for 3 weeks followed by 2 weeks in a short leg walking cast. Weight bearing is allowed as tolerated. If the fracture is discovered as a late finding ($\geq$2 weeks after the injury), immobilization may not be necessary unless the child is quite symptomatic. The fracture is usually completely healed within 6 to 8 weeks.

Stress Fractures of the Tibia

The tibia is one of the most common sites for stress fractures in young athletic individuals. Stress fractures can be caused by repetitive forces applied to the tibia during strenuous physical activity, which involves walking, running, or jumping. Possible risk factors include lower extremity malalignment, poor footwear, and training errors or excesses. Women are at increased risk of stress fractures perhaps because of higher rates of eating disorders leading to altered bone density, more malalignment issues, or other endocrine factors.[18] Tibial stress fractures are on the rise in older children and adolescents because of increases in the length and intensity of training regimens for young athletes.

Clinical Presentation

In most cases, the initial symptoms of a tibial stress fracture are indistinguishable from medial tibial stress syndrome, also known as "shin splints." Symptoms start insidiously with soreness over the shin that increases with physical activity. Eventually, pain increases to the point at which discontinuing the offending activity becomes necessary. The pain may become severe enough to persist for hours after activity or continue even at night. The patient may experience an abrupt change in pain at the site of milder chronic symptoms, indicating that the stressed area has been fractured. Findings suggestive of a stress fracture include localized point tenderness or swelling and pain that increases with the impact of running. An inability to hop on the affected leg for 10 repetitions (positive hop test result) is suggestive but not diagnostic of a stress fracture. Any of these findings should prompt further evaluation to confirm the presence of a stress fracture. Exertional compartment syndrome, posterior tibial tendinitis, and periostitis can also be confused with a tibial stress fracture.

Imaging

Radiographs frequently give no indication of fracture within the first 2 to 4 weeks after the onset of symptoms. Localized periosteal thickening, cortical sclerosis, or a true fracture line are positive findings of tibial shaft stress fractures (Figure 12-16). MRI has become the preferred imaging study to evaluate tibial stress fractures (Figure 12-17).[19] It is especially useful in distinguishing stress fractures from soft tissue injuries and shin splints. After a stress fracture has been diagnosed, follow-up imaging is not necessary to document healing unless the patient fails to improve with treatment. In this circumstance, imaging is done to determine if the fracture has extended or developed a nonunion, and CT is the best study to detect this.

Indications for Orthopedic Referral

The most difficult to manage tibial stress fracture is one involving the anterior tibial cortex. Stress fractures in this location appear as a linear lucency on plain radiographs, a finding commonly known as "the dreaded black line" (Figure 12-18). These fractures are very slow to heal, frequently go on to nonunion, and are at risk of recurrence. All of these factures should be referred for management by an orthopedic surgeon. Other indications for

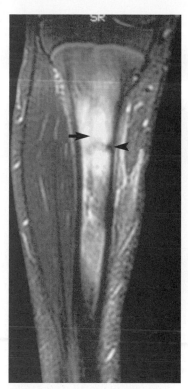

FIGURE 12-17 T2-weighted coronal magnetic resonance image reveals increased marrow signal intensity (*arrow*) representing marrow edema and focal low signal intensity indicative of a stress fracture (*arrowhead*) in the right proximal tibia. (*From Pope T, Bloem H, Beltran J, Morrison WB, Wilson D. Imaging of the Musculoskeletal System. Philadelphia, WB Saunders, 2008.*)

referral include intraarticular stress fractures and failure to improve with conservative treatment.

Initial Treatment

The initial treatment entails rest and immobilization in a long air splint or knee brace for 1 to 2 weeks. The patient should remain non–weight bearing during this time.

Follow-up Care

The rehabilitation of a patient with a tibial stress fracture should be customized based on the patient's symptoms, preinjury activity level, and the intended goals of treatment. Use of a long air splint may allow the patient to return to activity sooner than more standard treatment protocols.[20] A fairly aggressive rehabilitation regimen over the course of 12 weeks is appropriate for active individuals. Referral to a physical therapist is strongly advised to ensure proper progression of activity to allow the bone to heal with activity so weight-loading capacity continues to increase. Any persistent swelling or pain indicates that rest is needed before progressing to the next level of activity.

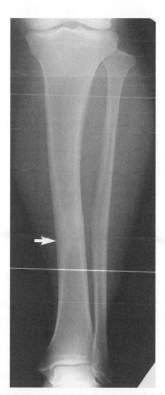

FIGURE 12-16 Anteroposterior radiograph of the left tibia demonstrates thickening of the left tibial cortex (*arrow*) extending approximately 4 cm in length over the distal shaft of the left tibia. These findings are indicative of a healing tibial stress fracture in this area. (*From Pope T, Bloem H, Beltran J, Morrison WB, Wilson D. Imaging of the Musculoskeletal System. Philadelphia, WB Saunders, 2008.*)

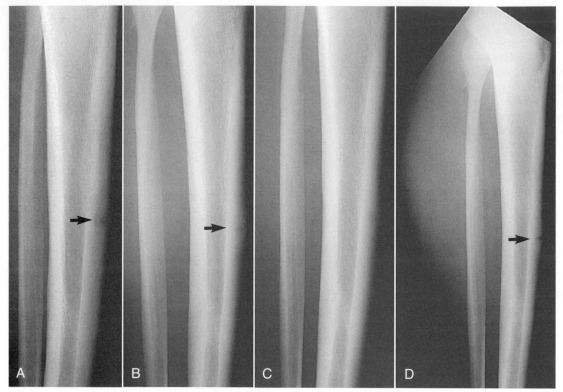

FIGURE 12-18 A, Stress fracture of the anterior midshaft of the tibia in a 16-year-old basketball player (*arrow*). **B,** After 3 months of rest, the fracture is only minimally healed (*arrow*). **C,** Six months after the original injury, the fracture is radiographically healed. **D,** Seven months after the original fracture had healed, another stress fracture developed at the same site.

Return to Work or Sports

Patients with fairly physically demanding jobs should return to full work when healing is nearly complete. Patients with less physically demanding jobs can often return to work with an air splint within a few weeks, and those with sedentary jobs may be able to return to work as soon as pain is controlled. Tibial stress fractures sometimes heal rapidly, and some athletes can begin vigorous training as early as 8 weeks after their injury. More commonly, most uncomplicated fractures are sufficiently healed by 12 weeks to allow athletes to return to their sports.

Fractures of the Shafts of the Tibia and Fibula

Both-bone fractures of the lower extremity are unstable injuries that result from high-energy direct impact forces or indirect rotatory forces. As with tibial shaft fractures, these fractures put patients at risk for acute compartment syndromes and neurovascular injuries. Nondisplaced fractures are rare. Emergency orthopedic referral is recommended in the management of these fractures. While the patient awaits orthopedic care, the leg should be splinted as described earlier for the acute treatment of tibial shaft fractures. Close monitoring for signs of compartment syndrome or neurovascular compromise is essential.

FIBULAR FRACTURES

Anatomic Considerations

The fibula is a non–weight-bearing bone. It helps anchor the lateral supports of the knee, and its distal end, the lateral malleolus, is a crucial lateral support of the ankle. The peroneus longus and brevis muscles originate from the proximal and middle fibular shaft and provide some protection from direct injury. The common peroneal nerve crosses the neck of the fibula just below the fibular head and may be contused or stretched in a proximal fibular fracture. The common peroneal nerve divides at the level of the proximal fibula into a superficial branch (ankle plantarflexion and eversion) and a deep branch (ankle and toe dorsiflexion). The lateral collateral ligament of the knee and the biceps femoris tendon attach to the fibular head.

Mechanism of Injury

Isolated fibular fractures are caused by a direct blow to the lateral leg. Proximal fibular fractures can also occur from a varus stress and result in avulsion of the lateral collateral ligament of the knee. Significant external rotational force at the ankle may cause a proximal fibular fracture, the Maisonneuve fracture (see Figure 13-8).

Clinical Presentation

The evaluation of a patient with a possible fibular fracture should be considered a diagnostic challenge. Most of these patients have other injuries requiring treatment that often takes precedence over management of the fibular fracture. The clinician must carefully assess the injured patient to exclude neurovascular injury, ligament tears, compartment syndrome, or tibial shaft fractures. Examination of the knee and ankle joint is essential to rule out associated ligamentous injuries. Distal pulses should be palpated, and the integrity of the peroneal nerves should be documented (ankle dorsiflexion and plantarflexion). Paresthesias over the lateral aspect of the middle to distal leg and dorsum of the foot may result from a neurapraxia of the superficial peroneal nerve.

Patients with isolated fibular fractures have pain and tenderness over the fracture site. Swelling is usually more diffuse because of the effects of gravity, and pain may radiate down the length of the fibula. Patients are able to ambulate, although walking may exacerbate the pain. Lateral compartment syndrome after an isolated fibular fracture is unusual, but it is more likely if a crush injury of the leg occurred.

Imaging

AP and lateral radiographs of the entire fibula are usually adequate to diagnose fractures. Significant fracture displacement or angulation is uncommon (Figure 12-19 and 12-20). If ankle pain or tenderness occurs, a complete ankle series should be obtained to detect evidence of fracture or ligamentous disruption.

Indications for Orthopedic Referral

Whereas isolated fractures of the fibula rarely need operative fixation, patients with a fibular fracture and a nerve injury, knee or ankle joint instability, compartment syndrome, or tibial shaft fracture must be promptly referred to an orthopedic surgeon. Orthopedic referral should also be considered for severely displaced or comminuted fractures, and patients with a painful nonunion after treatment should be referred for possible surgical correction.

Initial Treatment

Table 12-4 summarizes the management guidelines for nondisplaced fractures of the fibular shaft.

A patient with an isolated fibular fracture should be placed in a stirrup splint with the ankle

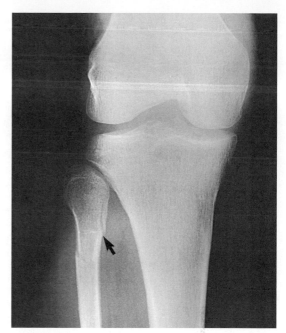

FIGURE 12-19 Nondisplaced isolated fracture of the proximal fibular shaft (*arrow*).

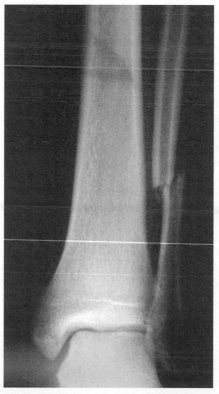

FIGURE 12-20 Transverse fracture of the fibular shaft with 50% apposition. This fracture will heal well with cast immobilization or crutch-assisted ambulation if the patient has only mild symptoms.

Table 12-4	*Management Guidelines for Isolated Fibular Shaft Fractures*
INITIAL TREATMENT	
Splint type and position	Stirrup splint
	Ankle at 90 degrees
Initial follow-up visit	3 to 5 days
Patient instruction	Icing and elevation of leg
	Non–weight bearing until follow-up visit
FOLLOW-UP CARE	
Cast or splint type and position	Short-leg walking cast or cast boot
	Prefabricated splint if symptoms are minimal
Length of immobilization	3 to 4 weeks
Healing time	6 to 8 weeks
Follow-up visit interval	Every 3 to 4 weeks to document union
Repeat radiography interval	At 6 to 8 weeks to document union
Patient instruction	Weight bearing as tolerated
	Gradual progression of activity as tolerated after cast or brace is removed
Indications for orthopedic consult	Significant displacement or comminution
	Associated neurovascular or ligament injury, compartment syndrome, tibial shaft fracture
	Painful nonunion

at 90 degrees. A prefabricated padded splint that applies compression and prevents ankle motion can be substituted for a more rigid splint in compliant patients. The patient should remain non–weight bearing until seen for definitive care in 3 to 5 days.

Follow-up Care

A short-leg walking cast or cast boot is indicated for relief of moderate to severe pain. The proximal fibula should be well padded, and care should be taken to avoid pressure indentations in this area to prevent an iatrogenic peroneal nerve injury. A period of 3 to 4 weeks of immobilization is sufficient. If the patient's symptoms are minimal, casting is not necessary, and a prefabricated splint and crutch assistance when walking provide adequate support and comfort. A follow-up radiograph at 3 to 4 weeks that documents radiographic healing (callus or some filling in of the fracture line) is an indication to move to as-needed splint use and begin progressive rehabilitation. The fracture is usually clinically healed within 6 to 8 weeks.

Return to Work or Sports

Patients with more sedentary jobs can return to work within the first week after their injury. Those with jobs that require a great deal of walking, standing, or climbing stairs may need to delay returning to work until the rigid immobilization is discontinued. Rehabilitation exercises to restore ankle ROM and calf muscle strength should be started after the period of immobilization. Most individuals will be able to return to a full preinjury

activity level within 6 to 8 weeks from the date of injury. Diligent effort during the rehabilitation period should enable patients to resume more physically demanding activities sooner. Athletes can return to high-level sports as soon as they have near-normal ankle motion and lower extremity strength.

Complications

Fibular fractures heal well without complication in the vast majority of cases. Occasionally, a nonunion that is symptomatic occurs, and patients with this outcome may respond to operative fixation and bone grafting.

Pediatric Considerations

Isolated fibular fractures are rare in children. As with adults, a direct blow is the most common cause of injury. Plastic bowing caused by axial loading and buckle fractures caused by compressive forces can also occur (see Figure 12-12). These fractures can be quite subtle, and comparison views may be needed to confirm the presence of a fracture. When evaluating an apparent isolated fibula fracture, the physician must carefully rule out a coexistent tibia fracture. Proximal fibular fractures in children may be associated with a fracture through the distal tibial physis. This injury, which is analogous to the adult Maisonneuve fracture, should be suspected if the physician detects tenderness of this physis in conjunction with a proximal fibular fracture. Patients with this injury and with nearly all fractures involving both the tibia and fibula should be referred. Isolated fibular fractures in children can be managed as outlined previously for adults, using a short-leg walking cast or stirrup splint for 3 to 4 weeks.

Stress Fractures of the Fibula

Stress fractures of the fibula occur primarily in runners and ballet dancers. Conditions placing athletes at greater risk of fibular stress fractures include hyperpronation, leg length discrepancy, and varus or valgus deformities of the knee. The most common location is in the lower third of the fibula approximately 4 to 7 cm proximal to the lateral malleolus. Symptoms are usually insidious and increase with activity. Pain and tenderness are localized to the fracture site. Radiographic changes often do not appear until 3 to 4 weeks after onset of symptoms of a stress fracture, so MRI is indicated if this injury is suspected and confirmation of the fracture is needed. Follow-up imaging to document healing is not necessary unless the patient fails to improve with treatment. Crutch-assisted ambulation can be used for comfort in the early stages if necessary. Immobilization is rarely needed, and weight bearing is allowed during the healing period. Stress fractures of the fibula usually heal within 6 to 8 weeks if the patient refrains from the offending activity and training progresses gradually to maintain fitness without impairing fracture healing. Pain should be used as a guide for when to decrease training intensity. Patients are usually able to resume some level of training within 3 weeks of the injury.

REFERENCES

1. Desio SM, Burks RT, Bachus KN. Soft tissue restraints to lateral patellar translation in the human knee. Am J Sports Med. 1998;26:59-65.
2. Nummi J. Fracture of the patella: a clinical study of 707 patellar fractures. Ann Chir Gyneacol Fenn Suppl. 1971, 179:1-85.
3. Nietosvaara Y, Aalto K, Kallio PE. Acute patellar dislocation in children: incidence and associated osteochondral fractures. J Pediatr Orthop. 1994;14:513-515.
4. Stefancin JJ, Parker RD. First-time traumatic patellar dislocation: a systematic review. Clin Orthop Relat Res. 2007;455:93-101.
5. Stanitski CL, Paletta GA Jr. Articular cartilage injury with acute patellar dislocation in adolescents: arthroscopic and radiographic correlation. Am J Sports Med. 1998;26:52-55.
6. Nikku R, Nietosvaara Y, Aalto K, Kallio PE. Operative treatment of primary patellar dislocation does not improve medium-term outcome: a 7-year followup report and risk analysis of 127 randomized patients. Acta Orthop. 2005;76:699-704.
7. Mustonen AO, Koivikko MP, Lindahl J, Koskinen SK. MRI of acute meniscal injury associated with tibial plateau fractures: prevalence, type, and location. AJR Am J Roentgenol. 2008;191:1002-1009.
8. Park S, Ahn J, Geo AO. Compartment syndrome in tibial fractures. J Orthop Trauma. 2009;23:514-518.
9. Shadgan B, Menon M, O'Brien PJ, Reid WD. Diagnostic techniques in acute compartment syndrome of the leg. J Orthop Trauma. 2008;22:581-587.
10. Harris IA, Kadir A, Donald G. Continuous compartment pressure monitoring for tibia fractures: does it influence outcome? J Trauma. 2006;60:1330-1335.
11. Schmidt AH, Finkemeier CG, Tornetta P 3rd. Treatment of closed tibial fractures. Instr Course Lect. 2003;52:607-622.
12. Khatod M, Botte MJ, Hoyt DB, et al. Outcomes in open tibia fractures: relationship between delay in treatment and infection. J Trauma. 2003;55:949-954.
13. Busse JW, Morton E, Lacchetti C, Guyatt GH, Bhandari M. Current management of tibial shaft fractures: a survey of 450 Canadian orthopedic trauma surgeons. Acta Orthop. 2008;79:689-694.
14. Coles CP, Gross M. Closed tibial shaft fractures: management and treatment complications. A review of the prospective literature. Can J Surg. 2000;43:256-262.
15. Ferguson M, Brand C, Lowe A, et al. Outcomes of isolated tibial shaft fractures treated at level 1 trauma centres. Injury. 2008;39:187-195.
16. Mashru RP, Herman MJ, Pizzutillo PD. Tibial shaft fractures in children and adolescents. J Am Acad Orthop Surg. 2005;13:345-352.
17. Bae DS, Kadiyala RK, Waters PM. Acute compartment syndrome in children: contemporary diagnosis, treatment, and outcome. J Pediatr Orthop. 2001;21:680-688.
18. Bennell KL, Brukner PD. Epidemiology and site specificity of stress fractures. Clin Sports Med. 1997;16:179-196.
19. Gaeta M, Minutoli F, Scribano E, et al. CT and MR imaging findings in athletes with early tibial stress injuries: comparison with bone scintigraphy findings and emphasis on cortical abnormalities. Radiology. 2005;235:553.
20. Rome K, Handoll HHG, Ashford RL. Interventions for preventing and treating stress fractures and stress reactions of bone of the lower limbs in young adults. Cochrane Database Syst Rev. 2005;(2):CD000450.

13

ANKLE FRACTURES

The key to successful management of ankle fractures is distinguishing between those that are stable and those that are unstable. In the evaluation of any traumatic or twisting injury to the ankle, a fracture of the distal fibula or tibia must be considered in the differential diagnosis. Isolated nondisplaced fractures of the lateral, medial, or posterior malleolus and nondisplaced fractures of the distal fibular shaft are stable and can be managed by primary care providers. Ankle fractures in children are usually epiphyseal injuries caused by the relative weakness of the physis.

See Appendix for stepwise instructions for weight bearing and non-weight bearing short leg casts and a lower extremity splint used in the treatment of ankle fractures.

Go to Expert Consult for the electronic version of a patient instruction sheet named "Broken Foot or Ankle," which covers the steps of care from pain relief to rehabilitation exercises. This can be copied to hand out to patients to assist them during the treatment period.

Ankle Fractures (Adult)

Most ankle fractures are malleolar fractures with the following distribution: 60% to 70% unimalleolar fractures, 15% to 20% bimalleolar fractures, and 7% to 12% trimalleolar fractures.[1,2] Men and women have similar rates overall, but men have a higher rate as young adults, and women have higher rates in older age groups.[1,2]

A high body mass index and cigarette smoking have been associated with ankle fractures.[3,4] In contrast to other fractures common among perimenopausal and postmenopausal women, bone density does not appear to be a major risk factor.[5]

Anatomic Considerations

Three bones make up the ankle joint: the distal tibia, the distal fibula, and the talus. They are bound together by a joint capsule and uniting ligaments that form a functional unit. The normal movement of the ankle mortise is dorsiflexion and plantarflexion. The perpendicular motions of inversion and eversion, which occur primarily at

the subtalar joint, are the most common injuring mechanisms of the ankle joint.

There is no single widely accepted definition of the margins of the lateral malleolus. For the purpose of managing ankle fractures in primary care, the lateral malleolus refers to the distal part of the fibula that is adjacent to the talus and tibia in the tibial grove (Figure 13-1). The lateral malleolus guards against excessive eversion of the ankle and foot. The most distal portion of the tibia where it articulates with the medial aspect of the talar dome constitutes the medial malleolus. The posterior aspect of the distal tibia is usually referred to as the *posterior malleolus*. It primarily includes the part of the tibia where the posterior tibiofibular ligament attaches.

The ligaments of the ankle include the medial deltoid ligament, three lateral ligaments (anterior talofibular, calcaneofibular, and posterior talofibular), and the distal tibiofibular ligaments (Figure 13-2). The deltoid ligament, a thick triangular band with superficial and deep fibers, originates from the medial malleolus and attaches to the navicular bone, calcaneus, and talus. The posterior tibial and flexor hallucis longus tendons cross it superficially. The lateral ligaments arise on the lateral malleolus and are in close proximity to the peroneal muscle tendons. The anterior talofibular ligament provides stability during plantarflexion. The calcaneofibular ligament stabilizes both the ankle and subtalar joints, especially during inversion. The posterior talofibular ligament protects against posterior displacement of the talus but is rarely torn unless the ankle becomes dislocated. The anterior and posterior tibiofibular ligaments, the transverse ligament, and the interosseous membrane bind the tibia and fibula together just above the joint line. Together these ligaments form the ankle syndesmosis.

The posterior tibial artery and tibial nerve course together posterior and lateral to the medial malleolus. The anterior tibial artery and deep peroneal nerve run together and cross the ankle joint anteriorly, approximately in the midline.

Several features of the bones of the ankle relate to ankle biomechanics and injury patterns. The

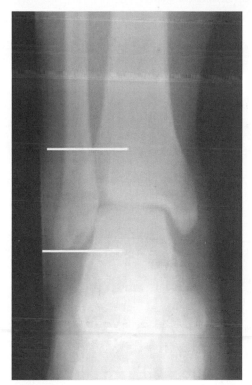

FIGURE 13-1 The anatomic margins of the lateral malleolus. The lateral malleolus lies between the distal tip of the fibula (*inferior line*) and the proximal portion of the fibula directly adjacent to the tibia in the tibial groove (*superior line*).

inferior surface of the distal tibia, articular and concave, is referred to as the *tibial plafond* or *ceiling*. The talus, covered largely by cartilage, is interposed between the tibia and calcaneus. The talus fits more snugly under the tibial plafond during ankle dorsiflexion. The plafond is broader anteriorly than posteriorly, which results in increased bony contact and stability in the dorsiflexed position. This anatomic relationship between the distal tibia and the talus explains why the plantarflexed ankle has the least amount of bony stability and is more vulnerable to injury in this position.

Classification

A number of classification systems exist for ankle fractures, which use the force applied and the position of the foot at the time of injury. The two most commonly used systems are the Lauge-Hansen and the Danis-Weber systems.[6] These classification schemes are complex and do not necessarily help the primary care provider distinguish stable from unstable fractures. Rather, knowledge of the typical patterns of ankle injury and the ligamentous injuries that accompany ankle fractures helps primary care providers accurately assess the stability of the

ankle joint. The bones and ligaments of the ankle essentially form a ring around the joint (Figure 13-3). If the ring has only one break, the ankle joint remains stable. For a talar shift and consequent instability to develop, a ligamentous injury or fracture on both the medial and lateral sides of the ring must occur. Truly isolated malleolar fractures in the absence of injury on the opposite side of the joint are stable fractures and do not lead to abnormal joint biomechanics.

Mechanism of Injury

The forces acting on the ankle that result in a fracture are typically combination motions. Patients often cannot accurately describe the cause of injury other than reporting a twisting motion. Lateral malleolus fractures result from inversion and adduction forces that cause medial displacement. Injury to the medial malleolus generally results from eversion and abduction forces that displace the joint laterally. Eversion, abduction, vertical loading, or a combination of these forces causes fractures of the posterior lip of the tibia (posterior malleolus). Axial compression of the ankle resulting from a fall from a great height or from some other high-energy injury may produce a severely comminuted fracture of the tibial plafond called a *pilon fracture*.

The direction of the injuring force and the position of the foot at the time of injury determine which structures are affected and the sequence in which they are injured. An inversion force first sprains the lateral ligament complex or avulses the distal lateral malleolus (Figure 13-4). If the force continues, the talus impacts the medial malleolus, causing an oblique fracture of the malleolus (Figure 13-5).

On the medial side of the ankle, an eversion force first sprains the deltoid ligament or avulses the distal medial malleolus (Figure 13-6). As the eversion force continues, an impaction (oblique) fracture of the lateral malleolus may occur or the syndesmosis may be ruptured (Figure 13-7). External rotation combined with eversion of the ankle may result in a proximal fibula fracture, the so-called Maisonneuve fracture (Figure 13-8). In this type of fracture, the medial side of the ankle is injured first followed by rupture of the anterior tibiofibular ligament, disruption of the syndesmosis, and finally a fracture through the proximal fibula.

Clinical Presentation

Identifying the area of maximal tenderness, other areas of tenderness, and localized swelling can aid in determining which ankle structures are injured. The degree of swelling present during examination is not a reliable indicator of injury severity or of

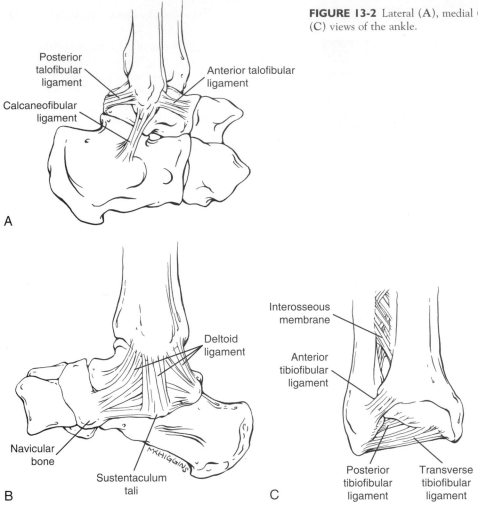

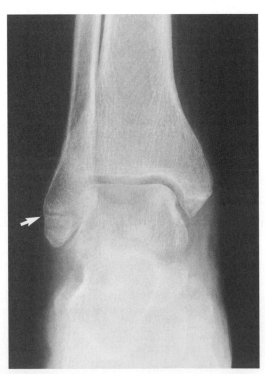

FIGURE 13-2 Lateral (A), medial (B), and anterior (C) views of the ankle.

Posterior talofibular ligament

Anterior talofibular ligament

Calcaneofibular ligament

A

Deltoid ligament

Navicular bone

Sustentaculum tali

B

Interosseous membrane

Anterior tibiofibular ligament

Posterior tibiofibular ligament

Transverse tibiofibular ligament

C

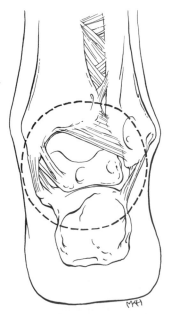

FIGURE 13-3 The ring of the ankle mortise.

FIGURE 13-4 Transverse avulsion fracture of the lateral malleolus resulting from an inversion force (*arrow*).

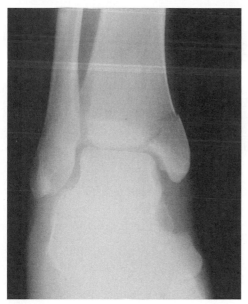

FIGURE 13-5 Oblique fracture of the medial malleolus resulting from an inversion force causing talar impact.

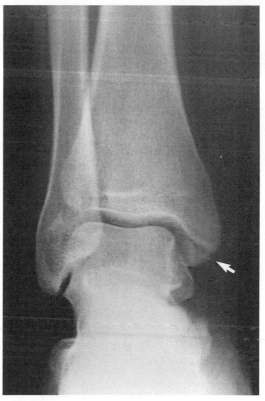

FIGURE 13-6 Avulsion fracture of the medial malleolus caused by an eversion force (*arrow*).

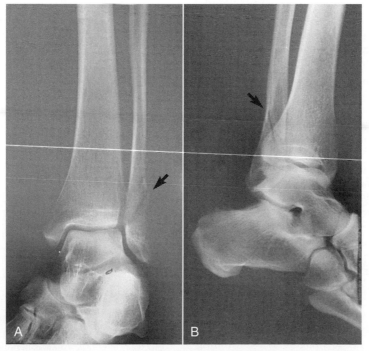

FIGURE 13-7 Nondisplaced oblique fracture of the lateral malleolus. **A,** Mortise view (*arrow*). **B,** Lateral view (*arrow*).

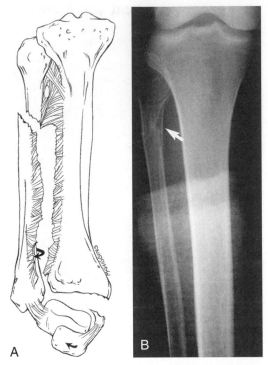

FIGURE 13-8 Maisonneuve fracture. **A,** External rotation causes a medial malleolus fracture and a fracture of the proximal fibula. **B,** Fracture of the proximal fibula seen on the anteroposterior view (*arrow*). Note the opaque line demarcating the top of the cast below the fibular fracture. This fracture was undetected initially, and only the ankle injury was treated.

the presence of a fracture because swelling is probably more related to the amount of time that elapsed between injury and presentation and the patient's actions after the injury. Although tenderness on the opposite side of the ankle may occur as a result of talar impact, an unstable ankle should be suspected when a patient has significant medial and lateral pain. Because of the possibility of associated proximal fractures, the full length of the fibula and tibia should be palpated on any patient with an acute ankle injury. Physical examination of the ankle joint to detect stability is often difficult in the acute setting because of swelling and voluntary guarding from pain and can be deferred until after radiographs are obtained. The skin and neurovascular integrity should be closely examined for signs of compromise or ischemia. Pulses of the dorsalis pedis and posterior tibialis arteries, distal capillary refill, and sensation and motor function should be assessed.

Imaging

Along with detecting a fracture after ankle injury, a primary goal of ankle imaging is determining joint stability. Typically, an ankle fracture is stable

if it includes *all* of these elements: not associated with a ligamentous injury, nondisplaced, and isolated to one malleolus.

The Ottawa Ankle Rules are well validated guidelines to aid in making decisions about the need for radiographs in a patient with an acute ankle injury (Table 13-1).[7] These standards perform well in ruling out a fracture (high sensitivity and high negative predictive value) but are poor in ruling in a fracture (low specificity and low positive predictive value). In other words, patients with negative findings based on the rules are highly unlikely to have a fractured ankle. The diagnosis for patients with positive findings based on the rules is much less certain, suggesting the need for radiography.

The standard ankle radiographic series consists of anteroposterior (AP), lateral, and mortise (AP with the foot in 15 degrees of adduction) views (Figure 13-9). In reviewing ankle radiographs for signs of instability, the clinician should look for any displacement of the talus in the mortise view (Figure 13-10), where the joint space between the talus and the lateral malleolus, distal tibia, and medial malleolus should be equidistant. A nondisplaced fracture of the ankle is commonly identified on only one view (Figure 13-11). The lateral view must be examined carefully, especially for oblique fractures of the distal fibula and fractures of the posterior malleolus.

In general, fractures resulting from avulsion forces are transverse, and fractures caused by talar impact against the malleoli are oblique. An oblique medial malleolus fracture after an inversion injury should raise suspicion of an associated lateral ligament sprain and a possibly unstable ankle (i.e., two breaks in the ring). An oblique fracture of the distal fibula 2 to 3 inches proximal to the ankle mortise may be associated with a medial joint injury and disruption of the tibiofibular ligaments (Figure 13-12). Displaced malleolar fractures are usually accompanied by a ligamentous injury on the opposite side of the ankle.

Table 13-1	*Ottawa Ankle Rules: Guidelines for Ordering an Ankle Radiography Series**

Patient has pain over the malleolus
and
Tenderness exists over the malleolus
or
Patient was unable to bear weight both immediately and at the time of the initial visit

*See Bachmann LM, Kolb E, Koller MT, Steurer J, ter Riet G. Accuracy of Ottawa Ankle Rules to exclude fractures of the ankle and mid-foot: systematic review. *BMJ* 2003;3:25.

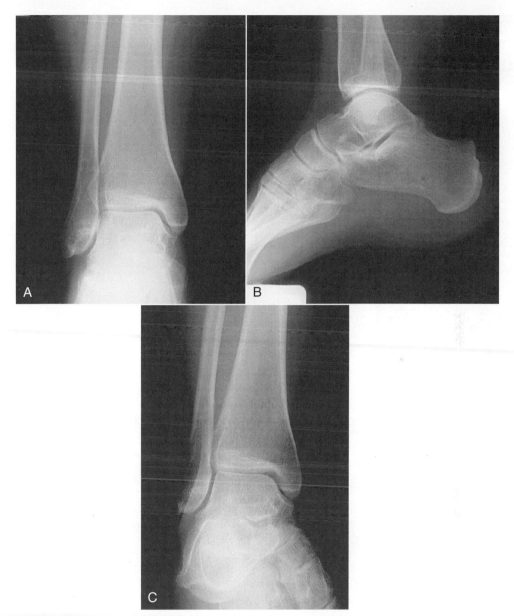

FIGURE 13-9 Standard ankle radiograph series. **A,** Anteroposterior view. **B,** Lateral view. **C,** Mortise view.

Indications for Orthopedic Referral

Emergent Referral (Within 30 to 60 Minutes)

Open fractures and injuries associated with vascular or neurologic compromise require immediate surgical referral. Fracture dislocations must be reduce immediately to prevent complications and should be referred immediately if orthopedic consultation is readily available. See description of how to reduce an ankle dislocation at the end of this chapter.

Nonemergent Referral (Within a Few Days from Injury)

Any patient with loss of joint congruity (intraarticular fracture) or an unstable ankle or in whom the stability of the ankle joint is in doubt should be referred to an orthopedic surgeon promptly for treatment. Examples of unstable ankle injuries are fractures of both medial and lateral malleoli (bimalleolar fracture) (Figure 13-13), a trimalleolar fracture (bimalleolar plus posterior malleolus fracture)

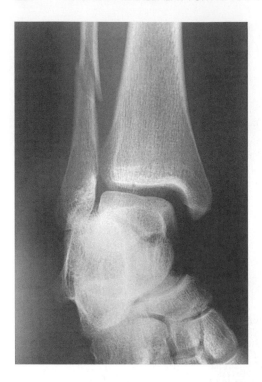

FIGURE 13-10 Mortise view demonstrating a talar shift. Note the widened space between the talus and medial malleolus. Instability was caused by a tear of the deltoid ligament and an oblique fibular shaft fracture.

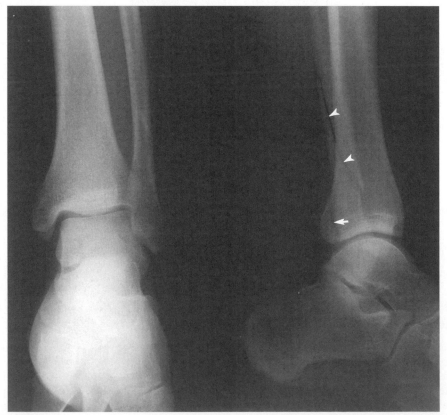

FIGURE 13-11 The mortise view of this injured ankle appears normal. The lateral view reveals a nondisplaced oblique fracture of the distal fibular shaft (*arrowheads*) and a posterior malleolus fracture (*arrow*). (*From Raby N, Berman l, Delong G. Accident and Emergency Radiology: A Survival Guide. Philadelphia, WB Saunders, 1995.*)

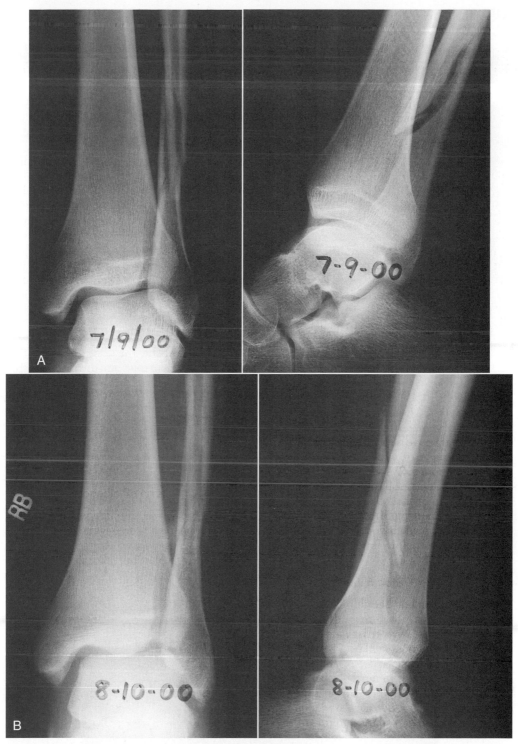

FIGURE 13-12 A, Anteroposterior and lateral views of a minimally displaced fracture of the distal fibular shaft. The medial aspect of the mortise appears slightly widened. **B,** Repeat radiographs 1 month later after immobilization in a short-leg walking cast reveal evidence of callus and a stable mortise.

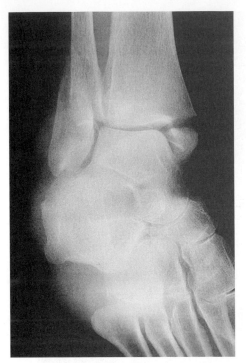

FIGURE 13-13 Bimalleolar fracture from an eversion force.

(Figure 13-14), or a malleolar fracture on one side with an associated ligament disruption on the opposite side. Injuries that lead to a distal fibular fracture above the tibiotalar joint line are frequently associated with a syndesmotic disruption and instability and should be referred for possible operative management (Figure 13-15). Operative treatment is recommended for posterior malleolar fractures involving more than 25% of the articular surface or displaced more than 2 mm.

Management of unstable fractures varies from closed reduction with immobilization to open reduction and internal fixation. The goal of treatment of displaced fractures is near-anatomic alignment with less than 1 mm of displacement on any view. Any displacement greater than this significantly reduces the area of contact force between the tibia and talus. This increases the degree of force on the talar articular surface, which predisposes the patient to posttraumatic arthritis in the ankle joint.

Initial Treatment

Swelling is probably the leading cause of pain after nondisplaced malleolar and distal fibular shaft fractures; therefore, measures to reduce swelling should be the primary objective of acute treatment of these fractures. External compression, applied early and used continuously, is an effective deterrent to

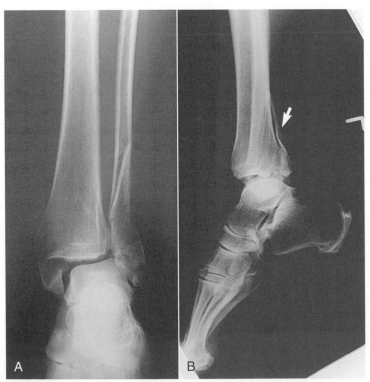

FIGURE 13-14 Trimalleolar fracture. **A,** Anteroposterior view shows displaced fractures of the medial and lateral malleoli. **B,** Lateral view shows a fracture of the posterior malleolus (*arrow*).

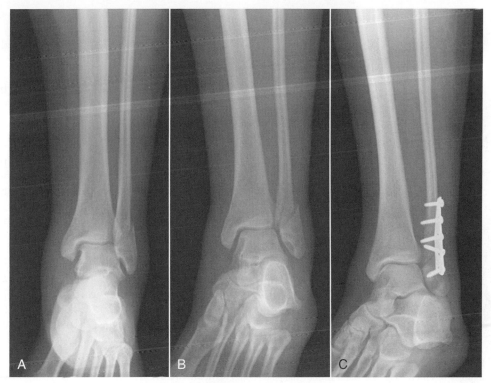

FIGURE 13-15 Unstable mildly displaced oblique distal fibular fracture. **A,** Anteroposterior view shows a fracture of the lateral malleolus just above the tibiotalar joint line. **B.** Mortise view shows some displacement. **C.** Postoperative view after surgical fixation.

swelling. The ankle should be splinted at 90 degrees (i.e., neutral position) and placed in a lower extremity splint. This form of compression combined with cryotherapy is very effective in the first 24 to 48 hours in reducing swelling. Draping an ice bag over the ankle for 20 to 30 minutes every 2 to 4 hours is recommended. Elevating the ankle higher than the knee and avoiding weight bearing also help minimize swelling in the first 24 to 48 hours.

Patients awaiting orthopedic consultation or surgery should remain non–weight bearing in a lower extremity splint, apply ice while keeping the splint dry, and use pain medication as needed. Warning signs to be given to the patient indicating possible vascular compromise or other complication include pain that is severe or increasing, skin discoloration distal to the splint, or numbness that is new or increasing. Before the first follow-up visit, the patients should be brought back in for reevaluation if he or she complains of excessive skin irritation, the splint has become subjectively too tight or too loose, or the splint has gotten wet.

Follow-up Care

Isolated Nondisplaced Lateral Malleolar Fractures

Isolated nondisplaced lateral malleolar fractures have a low risk of complications and have good clinical results regardless of treatment.[8,9] Small nondisplaced avulsion fractures of the tip of the lateral malleolus (Figure 13-4) are best treated with early mobilization similar to treatment of an ankle sprain. A functional stirrup splint that can be worn in a shoe works well during the healing process. Ankle rehabilitation exercises can be started as soon as symptoms allow.

Isolated oblique lateral malleolar fractures at or below the level of the ankle joint (Figure 13-7) should be immobilized in a commercially available walking fracture boot or short-leg walking cast for 4 to 6 weeks. Care should be taken to immobilize the ankle in a neutral position (90 degrees flexion) to minimize Achilles tendon shortening. Careful patient selection is required if use of a commercial fracture boot (Figure 13-16) is considered. Compliance with immobilization is essential to ensure adequate fracture healing, and patients may be tempted to alter treatment when using a removable fracture brace.

The patient should be seen in 10 to 14 days to check the condition of the cast or compliance with wearing the fracture boot and to ensure that alignment remains acceptable. At 4 weeks, if the fracture site is nontender and repeat radiographs show evidence of fracture union, the patient may begin gradual weight bearing and ankle rehabilitation. If

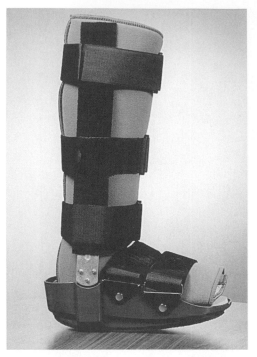

FIGURE 13-16 Walking boot fracture brace (BK Fracture Brace). *(Courtesy of United States Manufacturing Company, Pasadena, CA.)*

no radiographic evidence of healing is apparent in 4 weeks, the patient should remain immobilized for an additional 2 weeks and then return for repeat radiographs. If the patient is still not clinically healed (nontender over the fracture site and with some callus evident on the radiograph) at 6 weeks, a removable fracture boot should be used and daily range of motion (ROM) exercises started to minimize the stiffness and disuse muscle atrophy that can be caused by further immobilization. Radiographs are repeated and the patient reexamined at 8 weeks. If there is no evidence of callus on the radiograph, orthopedic consultation should be considered. An acceptable alternative is to continue rehabilitation exercises to restore function, use a functional stirrup splint as needed for support, and repeat the radiographs at 12 weeks after the injury. If there is still no radiographic healing, the patient should be referred to an orthopedist.

Isolated Nondisplaced Medial or Posterior Malleolar Fractures

These fractures often have associated injuries leading to instability, so the clinician should be on the look out for these so appropriate orthopedic referral can be accomplished. If the fractures are truly isolated injuries, they can be treated as described above for isolated oblique lateral malleolar fractures.

Distal Fibular Shaft Fractures

Nondisplaced fractures of the distal third of the fibular shaft can be treated in a short-leg walking cast or fracture boot as described previously for isolated malleolar fractures. Because these fractures can be associated with a medial ligament injury and thus are at risk of instability, follow-up radiographs must be examined closely for any evidence of talar shift. Repeat radiographs should be taken within 7 to 10 days to check fracture alignment and the position of the mortise. Most adults require 6 weeks of immobilization to achieve clinical healing. Occasionally, up to 8 weeks of immobilization is required before fracture union is apparent radiographically. It may take several months before complete resolution of the fracture line occurs on the radiographs, but some healing should be apparent in 8 weeks. As with malleolar fractures, immobilization past 6 weeks should be accompanied by daily ROM exercises and the use of a removable fracture boot.

Table 13-2 summarizes management guidelines for isolated malleolar and distal fibular shaft fractures.

Rehabilitation

The goal of rehabilitation after an ankle fracture is to restore loss of motion, strength, or proprioception that occurs as a result of the injury or disuse related to immobilization. There is no evidence to suggest that any specific rehabilitation program improves outcomes.[10] Some patients may return to their preinjury level of activity more quickly by following a stepwise rehabilitation that includes stretching, ROM exercises, strengthening, and balance exercises. Calf muscle stretching maintains muscle flexibility and restores ankle dorsiflexion. After the patient has achieved near-normal ROM, exercises to strengthen the muscles of the lower extremity should be started. Surgical tubing or some other elastic material can be used to provide resistance as the patient performs ROM exercises. Because the peroneal muscles are important in overall ankle function and stability, emphasis should be on strengthening these muscles through resistance of ankle eversion. Walking on the heels or toes is an additional way to strengthen the calf muscles. Patients should be seen within 2 weeks of discontinuing immobilization so their progress with these rehabilitation exercises and their return to function can be monitored.

Return to Work or Sports

Patients with more sedentary jobs can return to work within the first week after their injury. Those with jobs that require a great deal of walking, standing, or climbing stairs may need to delay returning to work or be put on light duty work

Table 13-2	*Management Guidelines for Isolated Malleolar and Distal Fibular Shaft Fractures**
ACUTE TREATMENT	
Splint type and position	Lower extremity splint with ankle in neutral position
Initial follow-up visit	3 to 5 days for definitive casting
Patient instruction	Non–weight bearing until definitive casting
	Icing and elevation to minimize swelling
DEFINITIVE TREATMENT	
Cast or splint type and position	Short-leg walking cast or walking cast fracture boot with the ankle in neutral position
Length of immobilization	Malleolar: 4 to 6 weeks
	Distal fibular: 6 to 8 weeks
	Immobilization continued up to 8 weeks if there is no evidence of radiographic healing
Healing time	6 to 8 weeks
	Possibly several months for complete radiographic healing
Follow-up visit interval	Malleolar: at 4 weeks to assess healing
	Distal fibular: every 2 to 4 weeks
	Every 2 weeks after immobilization to assess ankle rehabilitation
Repeat radiography interval	Malleolar: at 4 weeks to check for radiographic healing
	Distal fibular: at 7 to 10 days to check positioning
	Every 2 weeks if no healing at 4 weeks
Patient instruction	Ankle ROM exercises, calf stretching, and strengthening after immobilization
	Regaining full dorsiflexion and peroneal muscle strength emphasized
Indications for orthopedic consult	Unstable fractures
	Bimalleolar and trimalleolar fractures
	Posterior malleolar fractures with >25% articular involvement >2 mm displacement
	Symptomatic nonunion

*Excludes small nondisplaced avulsion fractures, which are best treated with early immobilization similar to treatment for an ankle sprain.
ROM, range of motion.

restriction until the rigid immobilization is discontinued. Rehabilitation exercises to restore ankle ROM and calf muscle strength should be started after the period of immobilization. Most individuals are able to return to a full preinjury activity level within 6 to 10 weeks from the date of injury. Diligent effort during the rehabilitation period could help patients resume more physically demanding activities sooner. Athletes can return to high-level sports as soon as they have near-normal ankle motion and calf muscle strength.

Complications

Complications after nonoperative treatment of isolated malleolar and distal fibular shaft fractures are uncommon. Most complications that do occur follow the treatment of unstable fractures. Avulsion fractures of the medial malleolus may go on to nonunion, but these are rarely symptomatic. Nonunion of the lateral or posterior malleolus is uncommon, but malunion may occur if the mortise is unstable or incongruity of the articular surface occurs during healing. Traumatic arthritis can result from altered joint biomechanics or damage to the articular cartilage after an ankle fracture. Degenerative changes may occur in up to 10% of adequately aligned fractures. Arthritis increases in incidence with the severity of the initial injury and is more common in older patients.

ANKLE FRACTURES (PEDIATRIC)

In contrast to adults, ligamentous injuries of the ankle are rare in children because the ligaments are stronger than growing bone. The joint itself is rarely disrupted in children because the physis is the weak point in the ankle joint. Injuries to the distal tibial and fibular physes are second in frequency only to fractures of the distal radius physis. Physeal ankle fractures are more common in boys than girls and occur mainly between the ages of 9 to 14 years. Fractures of the distal fibular physis are the most common types of pediatric ankle fractures and are at low risk for complications.[11] The goals of treatment for all pediatric ankle fractures are to achieve and maintain an acceptable reduction and to avoid growth arrest.

Classification

The widely accepted mechanism-of-injury classification of ankle fractures in children is that described by Dias and Tachdjian, who modified the adult Lauge-Hansen classification scheme. This classification is based on the position of the foot and the abnormal force applied to the ankle at the moment of injury. Because children are seldom able to recall this information, this system has limitations. As with adults, the primary care provider does not need a working knowledge of this classification system to distinguish between complicated and uncomplicated ankle fractures. However, knowledge of the Salter-Harris classification is useful because most ankle fractures in children involve the physis.

Distal Tibial Fractures

Anatomic Considerations

The distal tibial physis begins to close around age 12 years in girls and age 14 years in boys. The fusion of the physis is asymmetric, beginning in its midportion and progressing medially and then laterally before final fusion. This irregular fusion pattern and the resulting areas of relative strength and weakness are responsible for specific epiphyseal fracture patterns not seen in younger children. These fractures, specifically Tillaux and triplane fractures, are called "transitional" fractures because they occur during the transition from a skeletally immature ankle to one that is skeletally mature.

Mechanism of Injury

The Salter-Harris type I injury is rare and generally occurs in children younger than those with other types of fractures. The cause of injury varies. The typical type II fracture of the distal tibial epiphysis is an external rotation injury with the foot supinated, although other combinations of motions and foot positions can lead to this injury as well. In addition, the fibula is also often fractured. The cause of injury in type III and IV fractures is usually a supination–inversion force to the ankle that has driven the medial corner of the talus into the junction of the distal tibial articular surface and the medial malleolus. In the Tillaux fracture, the anteroinferior tibiofibular ligament avulses a fragment of the lateral epiphysis corresponding to the portion of the physis that is still open. Most juvenile Tillaux and triplane fractures are caused by inversion of the ankle with the foot pointed away from the midline (supination with external rotation).

Clinical Symptoms and Signs

The ankle is swollen, painful, and obviously deformed if the fracture is displaced. Patients with nondisplaced fractures may have minimal swelling, no deformity, and reasonably good ROM. The ankle should be examined systematically for areas of maximum tenderness, keeping in mind the physeal anatomy of the ankle. Subtle Tillaux fractures may present with tenderness isolated to the anterior joint line and swelling laterally over the distal fibula, while the medial malleolus is free of tenderness and swelling. ROM of the knee and hip and the ability to ambulate along with the status of the skin and neurovascular function should be assessed and recorded.

Radiographic Findings

A standard three-view ankle series should be used in evaluating pediatric ankle injuries. The Ottawa Ankle Rules, initially derived and validated in adults, appear to be a reliable tool to exclude fractures in children older than 5 years of age presenting with blunt trauma to the ankle and midfoot.[12,13] Clinicians can reassure patients and their families that this clinical decision rule has a low likelihood of missing a significant fracture and that conservative management and delayed radiographs for continued pain is a safe alternative.

Although obtaining views above and below the joint should be considered in the evaluation of pediatric fractures, centering the x-ray beam over the midtibia to include the ankle and knee joints is not recommended because it significantly decreases the quality of ankle views. Type I injuries may be difficult to detect radiographically and must be suspected in a child with marked soft tissue swelling and no visible fracture. A joint effusion will displace fat pads around the ankle joint and is a clue to the presence of an occult fracture (Figure 13-17). Stress views can be considered to document a type I fracture, but a child with clinical signs of this injury should be treated appropriately regardless of the stress view findings. Radiographs may show significant widening of the tibial physis if the fracture is accompanied by a transverse or oblique fracture of the fibular shaft (Figure 13-18).

Type II fractures are usually displaced laterally or posteriorly. The location of the Thurston-Holland

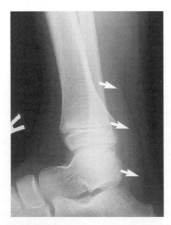

FIGURE 13-17 Large joint effusion (*arrows*) displaces the posterior fat pad. An occult fracture is likely. (*From Thornton A, Gylf C. Children's Fractures: A Radiological Guide to Safe Practice. Philadelphia, WB Saunders, 1999.*)

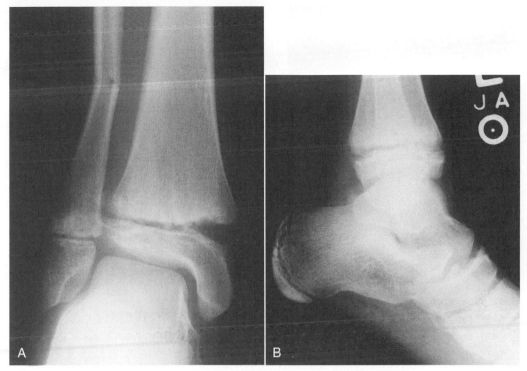

FIGURE 13-18 Salter-Harris type I fracture of the distal tibial physis with significant widening. A slightly angulated transverse fracture of the fibular shaft is also present. The irregular ossification and fragmentation of the calcaneal apophysis on the lateral view are normal. **A,** Mortise view. **B,** Lateral view.

fragment, the metaphyseal spike left attached to the epiphysis, is helpful in determining the mechanism of injury. A medial fragment indicates a supination–external rotation injury (Figure 13-19), and a lateral fragment indicates a pronation–eversion–external rotation injury.

Type III fractures typically involve less than one third of the medial lateral distance across the epiphysis (Figure 13-20). Determining the precise extent of displacement in type III fractures is crucial and may require computed tomography (CT) evaluation. Failure to reduce the interfragmentary gap to less than 2 mm has been associated with growth arrest and angular deformity.

The Tillaux fracture is a Salter-Harris type III fracture of the lateral part of the distal tibial epiphysis and results from an epiphyseal avulsion at the site of the attachment of the anterior inferior tibiofibular ligament (Figure 13-21). This is a relatively weaker section of the physis after fusion begins in the midportion. The triplane fracture, a Salter-Harris Type IV injury, is a combination fracture resulting in fractures in three planes: coronal, sagittal, and transverse. The fracture line crosses the articular surface through the epiphysis, physis, and finally the posterior tibial metaphysis. The fracture appears to be a type III injury on the AP view and a type II injury on the lateral view. CT

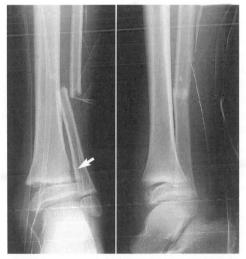

FIGURE 13-19 Type II fracture of the distal tibial physis. Note the triangular metaphyseal fragment (*arrow*) and the typical lateral displacement with associated fibular fracture. (*From Thornton A, Gyll C. Children's Fractures: A Radiological Guide to Safe Practice. Philadelphia, WB Saunders, 1999.*)

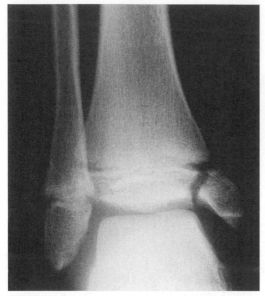

FIGURE 13-20 Type III fracture of the distal tibial epiphysis. The interfragmentary gap is greater than 2 mm and would require reduction.

is particularly useful in the evaluation of Tillaux and triplane fractures.

Indications for Orthopedic Referral

Most fractures of the ankle in children should be managed by an orthopedic surgeon because nearly all involve the growth plate, and clinical decisions regarding optimal management can be quite complicated. Only nondisplaced type I and II fractures should be managed by primary care providers. Indications for surgical management include an inability to obtain or maintain closed reduction, displaced intraarticular fracture, displaced physeal fracture, massive soft tissue injury, or neurovascular compromise.

Treatment

Displaced type I and II fractures and all type III, type IV, Tillaux, and triplane fractures should be managed by an orthopedic surgeon because most will require operative treatment. The child should be placed in a bulky compression dressing (Figure 13-22) and kept non–weight bearing until seen by an orthopedic surgeon.

Type I and II Fractures

Children with nondisplaced type I fractures are often treated initially for a sprain and return with continued pain and swelling. Immobilization in a short-leg walking cast for 4 weeks is usually sufficient treatment. A long-leg (above-knee) cast with 30 degrees of knee flexion is used in the treatment of a nondisplaced type II fracture. The patient initially is immobilized in the long-leg cast for 3

weeks followed by a short-leg walking cast for another 3 to 4 weeks.

Follow-up radiographs should be obtained every 6 months for 2 years or until Park-Harris growth arrest lines parallel to the physis appear (Figure 13-23). These lines represent transient calcification of physeal cartilage during injury repair and are parallel to the physis if growth is normal. If damage to the physis has occurred, the lines may appear tented or angulated.

Complications

The prognosis after a distal tibial physeal fracture depends on the skeletal maturity of the child, the fracture type, the severity of the injury, and the adequacy of the reduction. Delayed union and nonunion are rare. Deformity resulting from malunion and growth arrest are the most common complications and occur more often after displaced type II, III, or IV fractures.

Distal Fibular Fractures

The distal fibular physis begins to close approximately 1 to 2 years after closure of the distal tibial physis.

A Salter-Harris type I fracture of the distal fibula is the most common ankle fracture in children and

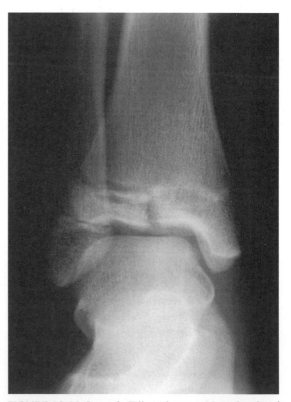

FIGURE 13-21 Juvenile Tillaux fracture. Note the closed physis from the midportion medially and the open physis laterally.

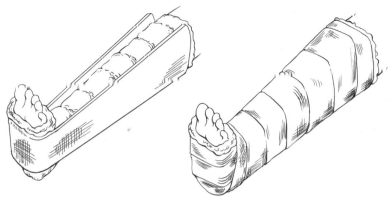

FIGURE 13-22 Jones dressing. The leg is wrapped with cotton batting and reinforced with a plaster stirrup slab. This dressing provides compression and immobilization while allowing for considerable swelling.

is typically caused by supination–inversion. During physical examination, the patient has localized tenderness and swelling over the lateral malleolus. Fracture displacement is usually minimal, making detection of the fracture on radiographs more difficult. A clue to the diagnosis is the presence of soft tissue swelling ("goose egg") over the lateral malleolus (Figure 13-24).

Patients with displaced or unstable fractures, which are usually associated with tibial physeal injuries, should be referred to an orthopedic surgeon. Internal fixation of the tibial fracture

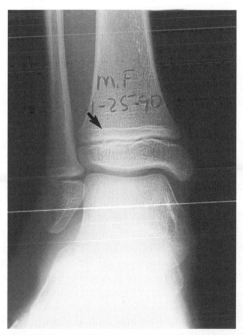

FIGURE 13-23 Park-Harris growth arrest line just superior to the tibial physis . The line should always be parallel to the physis when growth is normal. (*From Green NE, Swiontkowski MF [eds]. Skeletal Trauma in Children, 2nd ed. Philadelphia, WB Saunders, 1998.*)

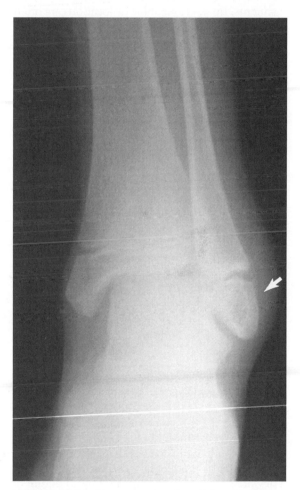

FIGURE 13-24 Anteroposterior view of the ankle with a "goose egg" soft tissue swelling over a nondisplaced type I fracture of the distal fibula. (*From Green NE, Swiontkowski MF [eds]. Skeletal Trauma in Children, 2nd ed. Philadelphia, WB Saunders, 1998.*)

generally results in adequate stability of the fibular fracture. Treatment with a removable ankle brace for 3 to 4 weeks for nondisplaced type I and II fractures of the distal fibula has been shown to have superior outcomes to casting.[11] Children with appropriate capability may be given crutches to remain non–weight bearing until pain subsides. Pain gradually resolves over 2 to 4 weeks and return to preinjury levels of activity typically occurs by 6 to 10 weeks. Complications are rare.

ANKLE DISLOCATION

Ankle dislocations without fractures are rare because of the mechanical stability of the mortise and the great amount of force required to tear the ligaments. In addition, ankle dislocations are often open because of the thin layer of tissue that lies over the malleoli. Individuals at increased risk for ankle dislocation injuries include those with a history of ankle fractures, ankle sprains, weakness of the peroneal muscles, or ligamentous laxity such as may occur with connective tissue disorders such as Ehlers-Danlos syndrome. The three types of dislocations are anterior, posterior, and lateral. The specific type is determined by the position of the talus in relation to the distal tibia, with posterior dislocations being the most common.

An ankle dislocation usually represents a high-force traumatic injury that often occurs in motor vehicle collisions or sports that involve jumping. The clinician must therefore be alert to the presence of other injuries and examine the patient thoroughly. Because subtalar dislocations may have presentations similar to those of dislocated ankles but are reduced with a different method, evaluation of the ankle injury must sufficiently demonstrate that the dislocation is of the ankle joint. The two injuries are clearly differentiated from each other radiographically.

Posterior Dislocation

Posterior dislocations are caused by a sudden excessive force applied to the joint, usually with inadequate muscle resistance while the foot is in a plantarflexed position. These injuries most often occur in young individuals and are associated with falls, vehicular accidents, or sporting activities. They are commonly accompanied by a fracture of one or both malleoli. When initially examined, the foot is plantarflexed and shortened.

Anterior Dislocation

Anterior dislocations are the least common type and are almost always accompanied by a fracture of the anterior lip of the tibia. The typical cause of injury is a force that produces posterior displacement of the tibia on the fixed foot similar to the position of the foot on the foot peg of a motorcycle. Anterior dislocations can also result from forceful dorsiflexion such as occurs from a fall from a significant height. A patient with this injury will have a dorsiflexed and elongated foot.

Lateral Dislocation

Lateral dislocations are always associated with a fracture of the lateral malleolus or of both malleoli. The usual cause is a forceful eversion with rotation. The ankle will be grossly deformed with the foot laterally displaced and the skin on the medial side very taut.

Treatment

Most important in the management of ankle dislocations is recognition of neurovascular compromise. If evidence of neurovascular injury exists and orthopedic consultation is not immediately available, closed reduction of a dislocated ankle must be attempted under intravenous sedation and analgesia by the primary care provider. In patients without neurovascular compromise, radiographs should be obtained before reduction to determine the presence of any fractures.

Reduction Maneuvers

Go to Expert Consult for a video on how to perform a reduction maneuver for an ankle dislocation. For all reductions, the knee should be flexed.

For a posterior dislocation, the foot and heel are grasped and pulled forward in a position of plantarflexion while an assistant grasps the tibia proximal to the dislocation and applies force on the distal leg in a posterior direction.

For an anterior dislocation, the foot is dorsiflexed slightly while downward traction is applied to disengage the talus; then the foot is pushed posteriorly.

For a lateral dislocation, longitudinal traction is applied on the plantarflexed foot while an assistant applies countertraction on the leg. This is followed with medial pressure over the talus to relocate it back into its normal position.

The neurovascular examination of the foot and ankle should be repeated after reduction. If reduction was successful but neurovascular compromise is apparent after reduction, emergent operative management is indicated. A bulky Jones dressing (Figure 13-22) should be applied to hold the ankle joint in a position of 90 degrees of flexion, maintain the reduction is maintained, and postreduction radiographs are obtained. Patients should remain non–weight bearing and remain in the splint at all times until seen in follow-up by an orthopedic surgeon. Many patients will require surgical repair.

REFERENCES

1. Daly PJ, Fitzgerald RH Jr, Melton LJ, Ilstrup DM. Epidemiology of ankle fractures in Rochester, Minnesota. *Acta Orthop Scand.* 1987;58:539.
2. Court-Brown CM, McBirnie J, Wilson G. Adult ankle fractures—an increasing problem? *Acta Orthop Scand.* 1998;69:43.
3. Valtola A, Honkanen R, Kroger H, et al. Lifestyle and other factors predict ankle fractures in perimenopausal women: a population-based prospective cohort study. *Bone.* 2002;30:238.
4. Honkanen R, Tuppurainen M, Kroger H, et al. Relationships between risk factors and fractures differ by type of fracture: a population-based study of 12,192 perimenopausal women. *Osteoporos Int.* 1998;8:25.
5. Seeley DG, Kelsey J, Jergas M, Nevitt MC. Predictors of ankle and foot fractures in older women. The Study of Osteoporotic Fractures Research Group. *J Bone Miner Res.* 1996;11:1347.
6. Carr JB. Malleolar fractures and soft tissue injuries of the ankle. In: Browner, BD, Jupiter, JB, Levine AM, Trafton PG, eds. Skeletal Trauma: Basic Science, Management and Reconstruction, 3rd ed. Philadelphia: Saunders; 2003:2326.
7. Bachmann LM, Kolb E, Koller MT, Steurer J, ter Riet G. Accuracy of Ottawa Ankle Rules to exclude fractures of the ankle and mid-foot: systematic review. *BMJ.* 2003; 3:25.
8. Ryd L, Bengtsson S: Isolated fracture of the lateral malleolus requires no treatment. *Acta Orthop Scand.* 1992;63: 443-446.
9. Port AM, McVie JL, Naylor G, Kreibich DN. Comparison of two conservative methods of treating an isolated fracture of the lateral malleolus. *J Bone Joint Surg (Br).* 1996;78(suppl B):568.
10. Lin CW, Moseley AM, Refshauge KM. Rehabilitation for ankle fractures in adults. *Cochrane Database Syst Rev.* 2008;(3):CD005595.
11. Boutis K, Willan AR, Babyn P, et al. A randomized controlled trial of a removable brace versus casting in children with low-risk ankle fractures. *Pediatrics.* 2007;119: e1256.
12. Dowling S, Spooner CH, Liang Y, et al. Accuracy of Ottawa ankle rules to exclude fractures of the ankle and midfoot in children: a meta-analysis. *Acad Emerg Med.* 2009;16:227.
13. Runyon MS. Can we safely apply the Ottawa Ankle Rules to children. *Acad Emerg Med.* 2009;16:352.

14

CALCANEUS AND OTHER TARSAL FRACTURES

Fractures of the tarsal bones are relatively uncommon. The calcaneus is the tarsal bone most often fractured, representing 60% of all tarsal fractures. The talus is the second most frequently fractured tarsal bone. Despite advances in the treatment of fractures over the years, the common calcaneal fractures still have a poor prognosis in regard to time lost from work and recreation. Isolated fractures of the tarsal bones of the midfoot—the navicular, cuboid, and cuneiform bones—are unusual. Typically, midfoot injuries involve multiple fractures or fracture dislocations. Calcaneus fractures in children are usually nondisplaced but are difficult to detect on plain radiographs.

See Appendix for stepwise instructions for weight-bearing and non–weight-bearing short-leg casts and a lower extremity splint used in the treatment of calcaneus and other tarsal fractures.

Go to Expert Consult for the electronic version of a patient instruction sheet named "Broken Foot or Ankle," which covers the steps of care from pain relief to rehabilitation exercises. This can be copied to hand out to patients to assist them during the treatment period.

CALCANEUS FRACTURES (ADULT)

Calcaneal fractures are generally subdivided into intraarticular and extraarticular fractures. Approximately one third are extraarticular, and compared with those with an intraarticular fracture, those who sustain an extraarticular fracture are typically younger, and the incidence of bilateral fractures is lower.[1] These differences relate to the different mechanisms of injury. Extraarticular fractures result from deforming forces, and intraarticular fractures result from high-energy accidents. Fractures of the anterior process and the tuberosity are the most common types of extraarticular fractures. Controversy exists in the treatment of calcaneal fractures in general but less so in the management of extraarticular fractures compared with the intraarticular type.

Anatomic Considerations

The foot is divided into the hindfoot (calcaneus and talus), midfoot (navicular, cuboid, and cuneiforms), and forefoot (metatarsals and phalanges) (Figure 14-1). The calcaneus is the largest of the tarsal bones. It provides support for the weight of the body and functions as a springboard for locomotion. The calcaneus has only a thin cortical shell, which makes it susceptible to fracture.

Figure 14-2 demonstrates the important anatomic relationships of the calcaneus. Superiorly, the calcaneus articulates with the talus through three facets that form the subtalar joint. Anteriorly, the calcaneus articulates with the cuboid bone. On the plantar surface are medial and lateral processes that serve as the insertion points for the plantar fascia and muscles. The medial surface has a projection known as the sustentaculum tali. The Achilles tendon inserts into the superior aspect of the calcaneal tuberosity, the hindmost portion of the bone.

The bifurcate ligament connects the anterior process of the calcaneus to both the cuboid and navicular bones. This ligament is stretched with inversion stress similar to a lateral ankle sprain mechanism.

Imaging

The initial radiographic series obtained for any patient who complains of hindfoot pain after an injury consists of three views: lateral, axial, and dorsoplantar (Figure 14-3). Most calcaneal fractures can be seen on at least one of these views. The axial view is obtained by directing the beam obliquely through the heel from the plantar surface while the ankle is held fully dorsiflexed. Because calcaneal fractures can be bilateral, obtaining radiographs of both feet should be strongly considered. Even if no fracture has occurred on the other side, comparison views are especially helpful in the measurement of normal anatomic angles. Views of the lumbar spine and ipsilateral ankle should be obtained when a patient has a calcaneus fracture

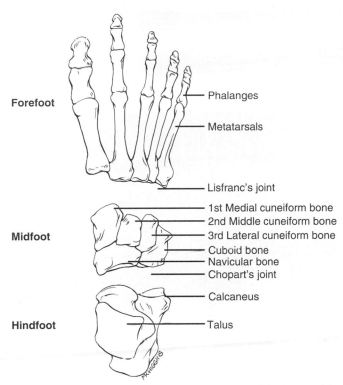

FIGURE 14-1 Hindfoot, midfoot, and forefoot divisions of the bones of the foot.

because of the likelihood of associated fractures in these areas.

The normal alignment of the calcaneus in relation to the talus can be assessed on a lateral view by looking for the preservation of two angles

(Figure 14-4). Bohler's angle is measured by drawing a line from the highest point of the posterior aspect of the calcaneus to its highest midpoint. A second line is drawn from this point to the highest point of the anterior process. This

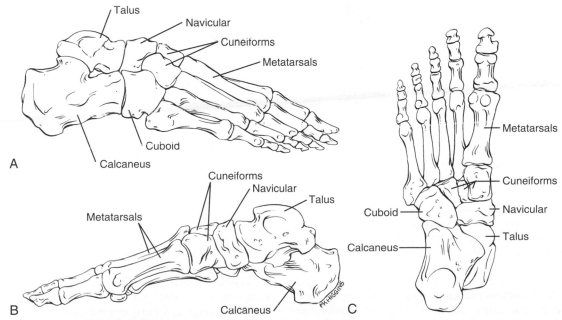

FIGURE 14-2 Lateral (**A**), medial (**B**), and plantar (**C**) views of the bones of the foot.

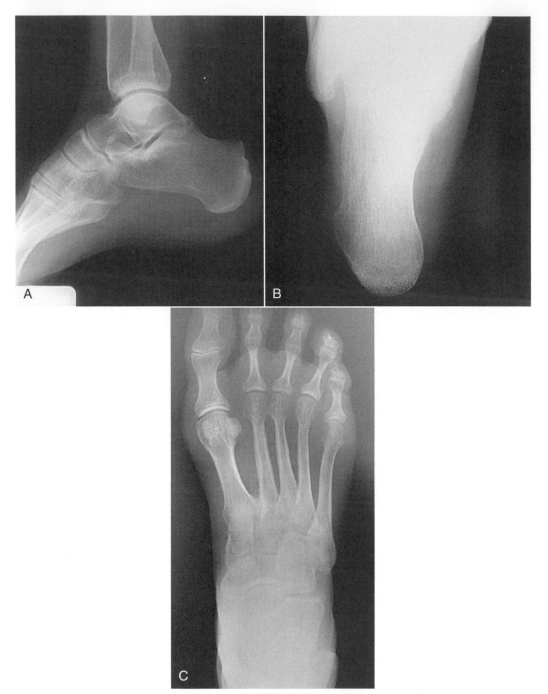

FIGURE 14-3 Standard calcaneus radiographic series. **A,** Lateral view. **B,** Axial view. **C,** Dorsoplantar view.

angle normally measures between 20 and 40 degrees and is usually similar in the two calcanei of one individual. If the angle is less than 20 degrees, a depressed fracture is present. The apex of the lateral process of the talus (LPT) points directly at the crucial angle, also known as the crucial angle of Gissane. Driven by compressive forces, the talus acts as a wedge to disrupt the subtalar joint and distort the crucial angle.

Classification

The primary function of a classification scheme for calcaneal fractures is to distinguish those with a good prognosis (the extraarticular fractures outside the subtalar joint) from those that require more aggressive treatment and do poorly (the intraarticular fractures involving the subtalar joint). The extraarticular fractures include fractures of the

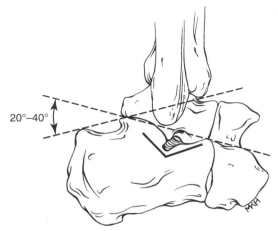

FIGURE 14-4 Lateral view of the calcaneus demonstrating Bohler's angle and the crucial angle of Gissane. The normal Bohler's angle is 20 to 40 degrees.

anterior process, the medial or lateral process, the tuberosity, the sustentaculum tali, and the body not involving the subtalar joint. The intraarticular fractures are more common and are difficult to subclassify because of the wide variety of patterns with varying degrees of displacement that can be present. Patients with intraarticular fractures should be referred to an orthopedic surgeon early because the specialist's knowledge and experience with these basic patterns are essential in developing a reasonable treatment program.

Extraarticular Fracture: Anterior Process

Mechanism of Injury

The anteriormost portion of the calcaneus may be fractured in two ways. An *avulsion* fracture caused by adduction and plantarflexion of the foot resulting in a pull-off of the attached bifurcate ligament is the most common type. A *compression* fracture of the anterior calcaneal articular surface occurs infrequently and is caused by forceful abduction of the forefoot with compression of the calcaneocuboid joint with the heel fixed to the ground. Treatment of these two anterior process fractures varies, so distinguishing them is important.

Clinical Presentation

Patients with an anterior process fracture usually report a twisting injury of the foot and complain of pain and swelling just distal to the lateral malleolus. Noting the point of maximal tenderness, which is typically over the calcanealcuboid joint (~1 cm inferior and 3 to 4 cm anterior to the lateral malleolus), can help the clinician distinguish an anterior avulsion fracture from a lateral ankle sprain.[2] This point can be best located by placing a thumb on the lateral malleolus and the third digit on the base of the fifth metatarsal with the index finger pointing out the tender area.

Imaging

The lateral oblique view of the calcaneus is the best projection for visualizing the anterior calcaneal process *avulsion* fracture (Figure 14-5). This view is taken with the inner border of the foot placed on the film and the sole inclined 45 degrees. *Compression* fractures of the anterior process can be seen on the lateral view of the foot. *Avulsion* fractures of the anterior process are usually small and nondisplaced and do not involve the calcaneocuboid joint (Figure 14-6). Anterior *compression* fractures are usually larger and involve the cuboid articulation. Some patients have a small accessory

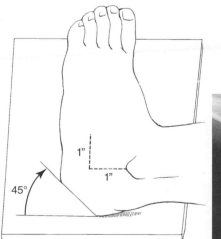

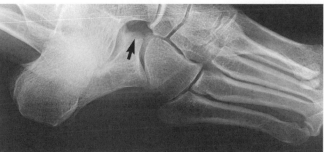

FIGURE 14-5 *Left,* Lateral oblique view of the calcaneus. The x-ray beam is centered 1 inch below and 1 inch anterior to the lateral malleolus. *Right,* The anterior process is well visualized on this view (*arrow*).

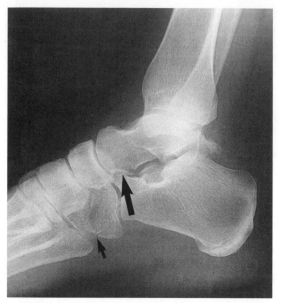

FIGURE 14-6 Lateral view of the calcaneus, demonstrating a small nondisplaced avulsion fracture of the anterior process (*large arrow*). A nondisplaced fracture of the cuboid is also present (*small arrow*).

bone just adjacent to the anterior process. The accessory ossicle can be distinguished from an avulsion fracture by its smooth, rounded contour, which differs from an irregular fracture surface.

Indications for Orthopedic Referral

Patients with large or displaced fractures of the anterior process should be referred for proper reduction and fixation. Persistent pain and nonunion are potential late complications, so some of these patients may benefit from surgical excision of the fracture fragment.

Initial Treatment

Table 14-1 summarizes management guidelines for extraarticular fractures of the calcaneus.

The initial treatment of all extraarticular fractures consists of rest, elevation, icing, and a bulky compression dressing for the first 48 to 72 hours to minimize swelling. Patients should remain non–weight bearing until definitive casting has taken place. To prevent joint stiffness, active range of motion (ROM) exercises for the foot and ankle should be started as soon as tolerated.

Table 14-1	*Management Guidelines for Extraarticular Calcaneus Fractures*
INITIAL TREATMENT	
Splint type and position	Body compression dressing
Initial follow-up visit	Within 7 days for definitive casting
Patient instruction	Non–weight bearing for 48 to 72 hours
	Icing and elevation are important to reduce swelling
	Active ROM of the foot and ankle as soon as pain permits
FOLLOW-UP CARE	
Cast or splint type and position	Anterior or medial or lateral process: SLWC
	Tuberosity: SLNWBC, 5 to 10 degrees equinus
	Sustentaculum tali: SLNWBC
	Body: no immobilization, active exercise
Length of immobilization	Anterior or medial or lateral process: 4 weeks
	Tuberosity: 6 weeks
	Sustentaculum tali: 6 to 8 weeks
Healing time	6 to 12 weeks for complete return of function
	Possible pain and stiffness for months
Follow-up visit interval	Every 2 to 4 weeks
Repeat radiography interval	For all fractures, after immobilization discontinued
	1 week after casting of tuberosity fracture to check for alignment
	Considered for delayed clinical healing
Patient instruction	ROM and strengthening exercises of the foot and ankle after immobilization
	Achilles tendon stretching is important to regain function
	Physical therapy should be considered if more aggressive rehabilitation is needed
	Heel padding as required for discomfort
Indications for orthopedic consult	Displaced fractures
	Persistent pain
	Nonunion

ROM, range of motion; SLNWBC, short-leg non–weight-bearing cast; SLWC, short-leg walking cast.

Follow-up Care

Patients should be seen within the first week after the injury for casting. Nondisplaced fractures of the anterior process heal well with immobilization in a short-leg walking cast for 4 weeks. Patients may have pain or stiffness for several months after treatment. Ankle and foot flexibility exercises should be emphasized after discontinuation of cast immobilization. Physical therapy should be considered for patients who are unable to comply with home therapy or who need assistance with rehabilitation.

Return to Work or Sports

The period of immobilization is relatively short compared with the total time required to return to a full preinjury activity level. Diligent effort during the rehabilitation period should help patients resume more physically demanding activities sooner. Those in more sedentary jobs should be able to work throughout the period of immobilization and rehabilitation. Return to activities that put the patient at risk of reinjury should be avoided for 3 to 4 weeks after immobilization is discontinued.

Extraarticular Fracture: Medial or Lateral Process

Mechanism of Injury

Medial or lateral calcaneal process fractures rarely occur. When they do, the usual cause of injury is a fall on the heel, typically from some height, while the ankle is in eversion (medial) or inversion (lateral).

Clinical Presentation

After this injury, patients complain of pain, swelling, and tenderness localized over the posteromedial or posterolateral heel. Pain may occur with forced dorsiflexion of the ankle; otherwise, joint ROM is normal.

Imaging

The axial calcaneal view is best for delineating fractures of the medial or lateral process. These fractures are rarely displaced but may on occasion be comminuted.

Indications for Orthopedic Referral

Displaced fractures can usually be reduced adequately with closed manipulation. Medial or lateral compression of the heel with the palms of the hand should produce the desired alignment. If closed reduction fails, the patient should be referred for consideration of open reduction and internal fixation (ORIF).

Follow-up Care

Use of a well-molded short-leg walking cast for 4 weeks provides protection until the fracture fragments unite. A radiograph should be obtained after this period of immobilization to document fracture union. The heel may remain tender for several weeks, and this symptom is best managed with partial weight bearing as tolerated and heel padding. Infrequently, a patient with this fracture has persistent tenderness over the fracture site. This late complication is best treated conservatively. Malunion and nonunion are uncommon.

Return to Work or Sports

Patients may have difficulty getting back to full weight-bearing or weight-loading activity for several weeks after cast immobilization because of residual heel soreness. A gradual return to activity is advisable. Modification of shoe wear with padding or orthotics may allow an earlier return to more physically demanding activity. Those in more sedentary jobs should be able to work throughout the period of immobilization and rehabilitation. Return to activities that put the patient at risk of reinjury should be avoided for 3 to 4 weeks after immobilization is discontinued.

Extraarticular Fracture: Tuberosity

Mechanism of Injury

Fractures of the tuberosity result mainly from a fall from height or striking the heel on a ledge. Most of these fractures occur from an avulsion force caused by contraction of the calf muscles while landing on the forefoot (Achilles avulsion), but shear-compression forces may also play a role. The avulsion fracture pattern is more common in elderly women, in whom osteoporosis plays a role.

Clinical Presentation

Pain, swelling, bruising, and an inability to bear weight are common symptoms of this injury. The patient may report pain and difficulty with stair climbing or walking on tiptoe as a result of weak plantarflexion. If the fracture fragment is significantly displaced, tenting of the skin posteriorly may be apparent.

Imaging

A standard lateral view of the foot demonstrates this fracture and the amount of displacement (Figure 14-7). The most important factor in the definitive management of calcaneal tuberosity fractures is the amount of displacement of the avulsed fragment.

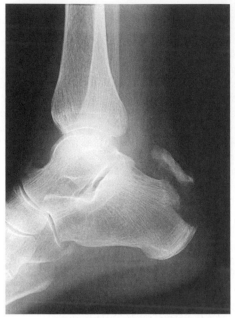

FIGURE 14-7 Avulsion fracture of the superior portion of the calcaneal tuberosity with significant displacement.

Indications for Orthopedic Referral

To restore the Achilles tendon to its original length, displaced fractures should be referred to an orthopedic surgeon within the first 7 to 10 days for ORIF.

Follow-up Care

Nondisplaced or minimally displaced fractures of the calcaneal tuberosity heal well with closed treatment. After acute treatment, the patient should be placed in a short-leg non–weight-bearing cast with the foot in 5 to 10 degrees of equinus for 6 weeks. Follow-up radiographs should be obtained 1 week after casting to ensure that the fracture fragments are still well aligned. Rehabilitation after immobilization should emphasize Achilles stretching and ankle and foot ROM and strengthening exercises.

Return to Work or Sports

The period of immobilization is relatively short compared with the total time required to return to a full preinjury activity level. Because of the length of immobilization in the equinus position, the patient requires a longer rehabilitation period to restore normal ankle motion (usually 3 to 6 months). Diligent effort during the rehabilitation period should help patients return to more physically demanding activities sooner. Those in more sedentary jobs should be able to work throughout the period of immobilization and rehabilitation. Return to activities that put the patient at risk of

reinjury should be avoided for 3 to 4 weeks after immobilization is discontinued.

Extraarticular Fracture: Sustentaculum Tali

Mechanism of Injury

Fractures of the sustentaculum tali are among the least common of all calcaneus fractures. They more often occur in combination with other fractures than as isolated fractures. The usual cause is a fall onto the heel with significant inversion of the ankle.

Clinical Presentation

This fracture usually causes pain and swelling over the medial aspect of the heel. Inversion of the ankle causes increased pain resulting from compression of the fracture against the medial malleolus. An indication of diagnosis is pain below the medial malleolus that is made worse with passive hyperextension of the great toe. This maneuver stretches the flexor hallucis longus tendon, which courses beneath the fractured sustentaculum.

Imaging

A standard calcaneal series should demonstrate this fracture, with particular attention paid to the axial view. Oblique axial views may also be helpful. If presence of this fracture is in doubt, comparison views of the uninjured foot may be necessary for confirmation.

Indications for Orthopedic Referral

If the fracture is significantly displaced (usually inferiorly), closed reduction should be attempted. Infrequently, patients with a persistently painful nonunion require late referral for consideration of surgical excision of the fracture fragment.

Follow-up Care

Isolated nondisplaced fractures of the sustentaculum tali have a good prognosis. Immobilization in a non–weight-bearing short-leg cast for 6 to 8 weeks should achieve satisfactory results. Radiographs taken at the conclusion of immobilization should demonstrate evidence of callus formation. Rehabilitation after casting includes ankle and foot ROM and strengthening exercises.

Return to Work or Sports

The total time required to return to a full preinjury activity level varies, but diligent effort during the rehabilitation should help patients return to more physically demanding activities sooner. Those in more sedentary jobs should be able to work throughout the period of immobilization and rehabilitation. Return to activities that put the patient at risk of reinjury should be avoided for 3 to 4 weeks after immobilization is discontinued.

Extraarticular Fracture: Body Not Involving the Subtalar Joint

Mechanism of Injury

Fractures of the body of the calcaneus that do not involve the subtalar joint are less common than intraarticular fractures but have a similar cause of injury. Most often, the patient reports falling from a height and landing directly on the heel.

Clinical Presentation

Patients with this fracture complain of severe pain and swelling and an inability to bear weight. Swelling and bruising may be so severe that blisters form over the heel within the first 24 hours. Ankle ROM is limited and painful. Symptoms related to this fracture are much more severe than with other extraarticular fractures.

Imaging

These fractures are usually seen on the lateral and axial views. Oblique radiographs and computed tomography (CT) should be strongly considered to rule out extension into the subtalar joint. A number of fracture configurations are possible, and the only consistent feature is lack of extension into the subtalar joint (Figure 14-8). Single oblique fracture lines behind the posterior facet and significant comminution ("cracked eggshell") are common. It is important to measure Bohler's angle because it may be decreased even though the fracture line does not involve the subtalar joint.

Indications for Orthopedic Referral

Patients with displaced extraarticular fractures of the calcaneal body should be referred for consideration of reduction. Reduction may be necessary for certain types of displacement to minimize future disability, especially in younger patients. Fracture displacement that results in abnormal widening of the heel can lead to difficulty with shoe fitting or impingement of the peroneal tendons. Flattening of Bohler's angle has the potential to shorten the Achilles tendon. Widening of the heel can usually be corrected with closed manipulation by using the palms to compress the heel medially and laterally. Restoration of Bohler's angle is usually an open reduction procedure.

Follow-up Care

Use of ice and a bulky dressing early are important to minimize blister formation and skin loss or infection. Generally, if no subtalar involvement is evident, nondisplaced fractures of the body of the calcaneus heal well regardless of treatment. Cast

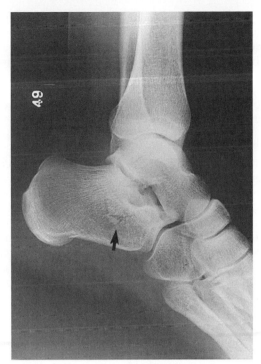

FIGURE 14-8 A slightly comminuted fracture of the body of the calcaneus posterior to the subtalar joint (*arrow*). Note that the subtalar joint is intact.

immobilization is not necessary, and an early vigorous rehabilitation program including ROM exercises of the foot and ankle is actually advantageous. Nearly all patients with this fracture have a good outcome, and nonunion is rare. Patients should use toe-touch ambulation for 4 to 6 weeks followed by gradual progression to full weight bearing. Repeat radiographs should be obtained after clinical healing has occurred or in the event of delayed clinical healing.

Return to Work or Sports

Because early motion is allowed and encouraged in the rehabilitation of this fracture, most individuals can return to a full preinjury activity level within 2 to 3 months from the date of injury. Diligent effort during the rehabilitation should help patients return to more physically demanding activities sooner. Those in more sedentary jobs should be able to work throughout the healing period. Return to activities that put the patient at risk of reinjury should be avoided for 3 to 4 weeks after clinical healing has been achieved.

Intraarticular Fractures

Mechanism of Injury

Intraarticular fractures are the most common calcaneus fractures that primary care providers encounter. This fracture nearly always occurs after the patient falls from a height and lands on the heels, which absorb the full weight of the body. The injury depends more on the vector of force directed at the calcaneus than on the distance of the fall. As a result of vertical shearing or compression forces during the fall, the calcaneus is driven into the wedge-shaped LPT (Figure 14-9).

Clinical Presentation

Patients with intraarticular fractures of the calcaneus report an inability to bear weight, moderate to severe pain, and swelling and bruising around the calcaneus. The normal contour of the heel is often distorted, with loss of the usual depression on either side of the Achilles tendon. Blistering of the skin resulting from severe soft tissue swelling may develop in the first 24 to 36 hours. Bruising that extends onto the arch of the foot within 1 or 2 days is considered a classic diagnostic sign.

Because of the high likelihood of associated injuries, patients who have fallen from a height and sustained a calcaneal fracture should be carefully evaluated for lower extremity and lumbar spine injuries. Lumbar compression fractures occur in 10% of patients, and up to 70% have other lower extremity injuries. Similarly, any patient who has spinal or lower extremity injuries after a fall should be examined for a calcaneus fracture even if the patient does not initially complain of heel pain.

Imaging

Intraarticular fractures of the calcaneus are easily diagnosed with a standard series. Bohler's angle should be measured on the lateral view and compared with the opposite side. A depressed fracture is diagnosed when the angle is less than 20 degrees (Figure 14-10). The axial view shows the amount

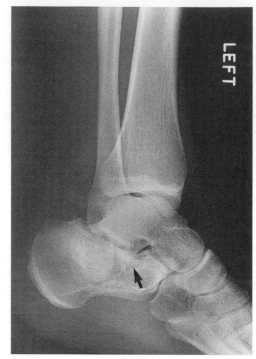

FIGURE 14-10 Depressed intraarticular calcaneus fracture with flattening of Bohler's angle (*arrow*).

of heel widening and degree of comminution and displacement of the fracture fragments. Oblique views may also be helpful. CT has become an essential tool in the assessment of the extent and severity of subtalar joint involvement. It is especially useful for preoperative planning.

Indications for Orthopedic Referral

Because of the complexity of possible fracture configurations and the usual need for open surgical repair, patients with fractures of the calcaneus involving the subtalar joint should be referred to an orthopedic surgeon for definitive care. The goal of operative repair is to achieve anatomic joint reduction and restore the normal dimensions of the calcaneus.

Initial Treatment

The acute management of intraarticular fractures of the calcaneus includes bed rest, elevation, icing, and a bulky compressive dressing. Control of soft tissue edema is paramount in the first few days, and consideration should be given to hospitalization of patients for controlled elevation and bed rest if they are unable to comply with this regimen at home.

Follow-up Care

Many different treatment methods have been used in the management of intraarticular calcaneal fractures, including no reduction and early

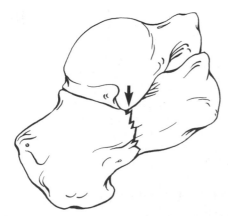

FIGURE 14-9 The lateral process of the talus acts as a driving wedge against the calcaneus with compression loading.

mobilization, cast immobilization, and ORIF. The benefit of operative compared with nonoperative treatment remains unclear.[3] However, correlation between anatomic restoration and functional outcomes has not been proven definitively, and calcaneal fractures are notorious for postoperative complications.[4] In those treated nonoperatively, it appears that if subtalar joint arthrosis does not occur, the functional outcome is likely to be satisfactory.[5]

Calcaneus Stress Fractures

Stress fractures of the calcaneus occur most often in distance runners and military recruits because of repetitive overload. Often, a rapid increase in activity level from a prior sedentary lifestyle is present. Patients may complain of an insidious onset of heel pain, which can be confused with plantar fasciitis or Achilles tendonitis; eventually, the pain persists throughout the course of the day. Tenderness usually is present along the medial and lateral walls of the calcaneus and along the plantar aspect of the tuberosity. Pain elicited by squeezing the calcaneus from both sides simultaneously can usually differentiate this condition from plantar fasciitis, retrocalcaneal bursitis, and Achilles tendinitis. Soft tissue swelling over the medial and lateral surfaces of the calcaneus may be present.

The most common stress fracture site is the upper posterior margin. Plain radiographs are often unremarkable but may show sclerotic changes perpendicular to the trabecular pattern and parallel to the posterior margin of the calcaneus (Figure 14-11, A). Advanced imaging studies such as bone scan or magnetic resonance imaging (MRI) are generally required to diagnose a calcaneal stress fracture (Figure 14-11, B).

Calcaneal stress fractures are considered "low risk" because of their propensity to heal and the relatively low likelihood of complications during that process. These injuries generally heal with activity restrictions, heel-pad inserts, and protected weight bearing. An initial period of non–weight bearing on crutches may be needed if pain with walking is more severe. When the patient is pain free and there is no local tenderness (usually within 1 to 2 weeks), activity can be gradually increased over the next 4 to 6 weeks back to preinjury levels.

CALCANEUS FRACTURES (PEDIATRIC)

Pediatric calcaneal fractures are extremely uncommon, and fractures involving displacement of the articular surface are even less common. Calcaneal fractures in children are more often the result of lower energy mechanisms than in adults. Children and adolescents exposed to higher degrees of trauma have a fracture pattern similar to that of adults.[6] Physeal injuries of the calcaneus are extremely rare. The majority of fractures have excellent outcomes.[7]

Anatomic Considerations

The differences in fracture patterns between adults and children can be explained partially by the

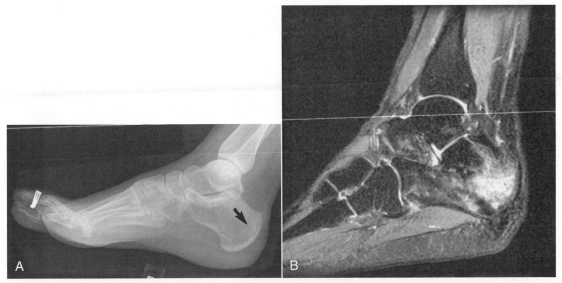

FIGURE 14-11 **A,** Lateral view of the foot showing subtle and easily missed sclerotic changes perpendicular to the trabecular pattern and parallel to the posterior margin of the calcaneus (*arrow*). **B,** Magnetic resonance image of the same foot showing changes consistent with a calcaneal stress fracture.

anatomic differences between the immature and mature talus and calcaneus. The lateral process is tiny in the immature talus, reducing the possibility of impaction injuries in the calcaneus.

The calcaneal apophysis, the site of insertion of the Achilles tendon, covers the entire calcaneal physis and demonstrates many irregularities in ossification, including fragmentation and sclerosis (Figure 14-12). The clinical condition of heel pain combined with the radiographic findings of variable ossification carries the diagnosis of Sever's disease. This condition, presumably resulting from a traction apophysitis from overuse, is analogous to Osgood-Schlatter disease at the tibial tuberosity apophysis.

Mechanism of Injury

Fractures of the calcaneus may occur in toddlers and very young children after minor falls. In older children, calcaneal fractures nearly always result from landing on the heels after a fall from a significant height. Calcaneal injuries may also be caused by vehicular or lawn mower accidents.

Clinical Presentation

Pain, swelling, an inability to bear weight, localized tenderness, and a history of a fall are clear indications of calcaneal fracture in children. Careful palpation of the heel in a child who refuses to walk is essential to exclude this diagnosis. Other associated skeletal injuries (e.g., thoracolumbar spine compression fracture, tibial plateau fracture) are present in up to half of children.[8]

Imaging

Calcaneal fractures in children can be missed if only standard foot views are taken. Axial and lateral oblique views of the calcaneus should be added. Bohler's angle is normally smaller in young children than the 20 to 40 degrees that is normal in adults, and the irregular shape of the immature calcaneus makes this angle difficult to assess. Comparison views of the uninjured foot can help exclude significant compression of the calcaneus. CT more reliably demonstrates the presence and extent of a calcaneal fracture and is the preferred definitive study because up to 50% of these fractures are missed initially in children.[9] In a young child who refuses to walk and has foot tenderness and negative plain radiograph findings, applying a short-leg walking cast for 2 weeks before obtaining a more definitive diagnostic study is a reasonable approach. If the child remains symptomatic after 2 weeks, further imaging with a CT scan is warranted. A lateral view of the spine should be obtained when patients have obvious fractures because compression fractures of the thoracolumbar spine can occur in children just as in adults.

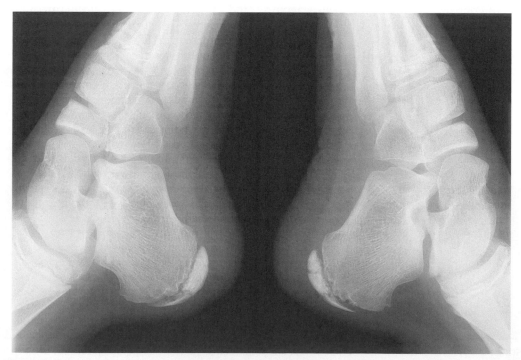

FIGURE 14-12 Fragmented and sclerotic changes in the calcaneal apophysis. These are normal changes. (*From Thornton A, Gyll C. Children's Fractures: A Radiological Guide to Safe Practice. Philadelphia, WB Saunders, 1999.*)

Indications for Orthopedic Referral

Patients with intraarticular and displaced extraarticular fractures of the calcaneus should be referred to an orthopedic surgeon for consideration of operative treatment. Patients with avulsion fractures of the tuberosity of the calcaneus should also be referred because ORIF yields the best results.

Treatment

Use of a short-leg walking cast for 3 to 4 weeks is sufficient for immobilization of most nondisplaced calcaneal fractures. The younger the children, the more likely he or she is to heal uneventfully. If nonoperative treatment is chosen for an older child, a non–weight-bearing cast should be used for immobilization. Complications such as long-term joint pain or stiffness are uncommon except in patients with displaced intraarticular fractures.

TALUS FRACTURES (ADULT)

The relative infrequency of talar fractures has complicated the management because of the lack of adequate evidence-based literature on which to base treatment decisions. Fractures of the talar neck are the most common, accounting for approximately 50% of all talar injuries.[10]

Anatomic Considerations

Minor anterior or posterior avulsion fractures of the talus are common after ankle injuries. Major fractures of the talus most frequently occur in the talar neck. Other talus fractures occur in the body, which articulates with the tibia, and the distal head, which articulates with the navicular. The lateral process, a portion of the posterior talar facet, is a large wedge-shaped prominence that

makes up almost the entire lateral wall of the talus (Figure 14-13). Fractures of the lateral process involve the posterior portion of the subtalar joint, an injury that could cause long-term complications. The vascular supply to the body of the talus enters from the distal aspect, which leads to an increased risk of avascular necrosis (AVN) after proximal body and neck fractures. The talus contains no muscle insertions and is connected to other tarsal bones by ligamentous attachments.

Mechanism of Injury

Talar avulsion fractures follow twisting injuries of the ankle, often with extreme plantarflexion or dorsiflexion. Talar neck fractures are usually the result of severe dorsiflexion of the ankle such as occurs when the foot is jammed against the floorboard during a motor vehicle accident (MVA). The force of the impact drives the neck of the talus against the anterior tibia. If the dorsiflexion force continues, the proximal fragment may dislocate posteriorly. Talar body fractures result from axial compression during a fall from height and are often comminuted and displaced. Fractures of the head are rare and usually result from compressive forces. Fractures of the LPT are increasingly being attributed to snowboarding injuries and are discussed separately. Stress fractures of the neck and body of the talus have been reported in military recruits and athletes.

Clinical Presentation

Patients with talus fractures report swelling, tenderness, and pain that may be poorly localized. The pain is exacerbated by ankle motion, with fractures of the neck and body usually the most painful. Joint locking may occur in the presence of a displaced avulsion fracture. Fractures of the neck and

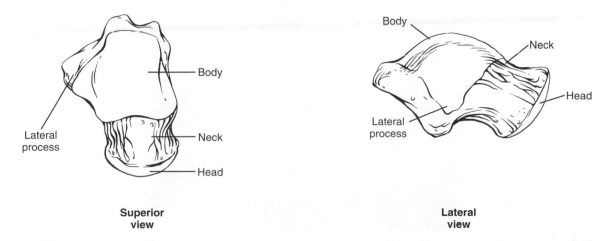

FIGURE 14-13 Superior and lateral views of the talus.

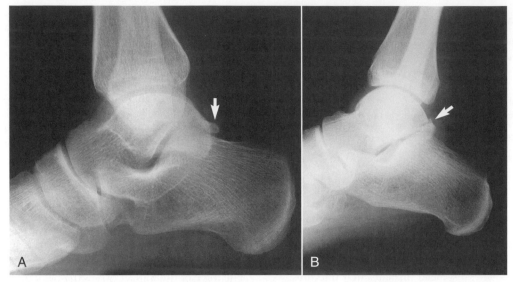

FIGURE 14-14 A, Accessory ossicle os trigonum (*arrow*). Note the smooth, rounded surface. **B,** Avulsion fracture of the posterior process of the talus (*arrow*). Note the irregular border.

body are usually the most painful. A patient with a posterior fracture dislocation of the neck of the talus has the ankle locked in dorsiflexion. Sensation and pulses in the foot should be documented because nerve or vascular injury is possible if the talus becomes dislocated.

Imaging

Avulsion fractures may be subtle and difficult to identify on a standard ankle radiograph series. Oblique views may be helpful. The accessory ossicle, os trigonum, may be confused with a posterior avulsion fracture (Figure 14-14). Fractures of the neck and body are best seen on the lateral view (Figure 14-15). Anteroposterior (AP) and oblique

views are necessary to assess the amount of displacement and the alignment of the talus in the ankle mortise. Malleolar fractures (usually medial) frequently accompany talar neck fractures. Clinicians should review radiographs carefully for both of these fractures in any patient with a hyperdorsiflexion ankle injury. Oblique views or CT may be necessary to diagnose fractures of the talar head. CT is the best diagnostic tool for detecting stress fractures of the talus.

Indications for Orthopedic Referral

Patients with displaced fractures of the neck, body, or head of the talus, especially those injuries associated with subluxation or dislocation, should be

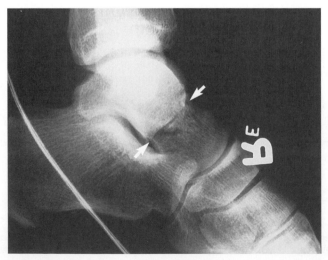

FIGURE 14-15 Lateral view reveals a nondisplaced talar neck fracture extending into the subtalar joint (*arrows*). (*From Mettler FA. Essentials of Radiology. Philadelphia, WB Saunders, 1996.*)

referred for reduction on an emergency basis to prevent soft tissue ischemia or neurovascular compromise. Comminuted fractures of the body also require anatomic reduction. Patients with fractures of the talar head that involve more than 50% of the talonavicular surface should also be referred. Displaced or large (>0.5 cm) avulsion fractures may require fixation to prevent subsequent joint locking or arthritis, so orthopedic consultation is recommended for these fractures. If the complications of AVN or delayed union develops, patients should receive orthopedic consultation.

Initial Treatment

Table 14-2 summarizes management guidelines for nondisplaced talus fractures.

Acute treatment of patients with nondisplaced fractures includes icing, elevation, analgesics, and immobilization of the ankle. The ankle should be splinted at 90 degrees (i.e., neutral position) and placed in a lower extremity splint. The first follow-up visit should be scheduled within 5 to 7 days when the swelling will have subsided to some degree. The patient should remain non–weight bearing until definitive casting is done.

Follow-up Care

Avulsion Fractures

Small, nondisplaced avulsion fractures heal well when the patient's foot is placed in a short-leg walking cast for 4 weeks. A neutral position should be used when casting anterior fractures, and 15 degrees of equinus used in casting posterior fractures.

Neck Fractures

Nondisplaced fractures of the neck should be treated with a non–weight-bearing short-leg cast for 4 to 6 weeks followed by a short-leg walking cast for an additional 4 weeks. Weight bearing is restricted until there is radiographic evidence of healing (typically 6 weeks). Repeat radiographs should be obtained every 2 to 3 weeks to assess fracture healing and ensure continued

Table 14-2	*Management Guidelines for Talus Fractures*
INITIAL TREATMENT	
Splint type and position	Lower extremity splint with ankle at 90 degrees
Initial follow-up visit	Within 7 days for definitive casting
Patient instruction	Remain non–weight bearing
	Icing and elevation are important
FOLLOW-UP CARE	
Cast or splint type and position	Avulsion: SLWC, anterior—neutral; posterior—15 degrees equinus
	Neck: SLNWBC followed by SLWC
	Body: SLNWBC
	Head: SLWC
	Talar dome (types I and II): activity restriction or SLWC
Length of immobilization	Avulsion: 4 weeks
	Neck: SLNWBC for 4 to 6 weeks; then SLWC for 4 weeks
	Body: 6 to 8 weeks
	Head: 6 to 8 weeks followed by longitudinal arch support for 3 to 6 months
Healing time	8 to 12 weeks for complete clinical healing (avulsion fractures, 6 to 8 weeks)
	Possible pain and stiffness for months
Follow-up visit interval	Every 2 to 4 weeks
Repeat radiography interval	Neck: every 2 to 3 weeks to assess healing (look for signs of AVN)
	At 4 to 6 weeks after injury (some radiographic healing should be apparent)
Patient instruction	Ankle and foot ROM exercises and calf stretching and strengthening after immobilization
	Good arch support important during rehabilitation
Indications for orthopedic consult	Displaced or comminuted fractures
	Intraarticular fractures of the talar head
	Large avulsion fractures
	Stage III or IV talar dome fractures
	Stage I or II talar dome fractures with persistent symptoms after 4 to 6 months of conservative treatment

AVN, avascular necrosis; ROM, range of motion; SLNWBC, Short-leg non–weight bearing cast; SLWC, short-leg walking cast.

nondisplacement. If no radiographic evidence of fracture union is apparent at 8 weeks, the patient should be referred to an orthopedic surgeon. CT may be necessary to demonstrate fracture union.

An accepted radiographic indicator of vascular integrity of the talus is Hawkins' sign.[11] If present, it indicates the normal process of bony absorption after cast immobilization and an intact blood supply and manifests as a subchondral radiolucency of the talar dome in the AP view at 6 to 8 weeks after the injury. MRI can also be used to assess healing and determine weight-bearing limits if radiographs are inconclusive. Increased radiodensity (sclerosis) in the talar dome just below the ankle joint suggests AVN. Malunion, delayed union, post traumatic arthritis, and infection are other long-term complications of talar neck fractures.

Body Fractures

Nondisplaced fractures of the body of the talus should be immobilized in a short-leg non–weight-bearing cast for 6 to 8 weeks with gradual return to weight bearing upon radiographic evidence of healing. AVN, malunion, and post traumatic arthritis may be late complications, especially after displaced fractures.

Head Fractures

Use of a short-leg walking cast for 6 to 8 weeks followed by longitudinal arch support for several more weeks is the recommended treatment for fractures of the talar head. These fractures may be complicated by persistent pain resulting from post-traumatic arthritis in the talonavicular joint.

Rehabilitation

After cast immobilization of talus fractures, patients should receive instruction in ankle and foot ROM exercises and calf and peroneal muscle stretching and strengthening. Good arch support is important during rehabilitation. Physical therapy should be considered for most patients because the rehabilitation period may be longer because of loss of function from prolonged immobilization. A follow-up visit 2 to 3 weeks into the rehabilitation should be scheduled to confirm adequate progress in restoring normal motion and function of the foot and ankle. Follow-up should continue until patients have near-normal return of function.

Return to Work or Sports

The total time required to return to a full preinjury activity level varies, but diligent effort during rehabilitation should help patients return to more physically demanding activities sooner. Fractures requiring immobilization in the equinus position and those requiring immobilization for 8 weeks or more will have a longer rehabilitation of up to 4 months. Those in more sedentary jobs should be able to work throughout the period of immobilization and rehabilitation. Return to activities that put the patient at risk of reinjury should be avoided for 3 to 4 weeks after immobilization is discontinued. Decisions concerning return to sports should be based on recovery of ankle function and the presence of persistent symptoms with sport activity.

Osteochondral Dome Fractures

Mechanism of Injury

The articular surface of the talar dome can be damaged from impaction against either malleolus during an inversion or eversion ankle injury. These fractures are often overlooked initially. Inversion injuries cause most of these osteochondral fractures, and they usually occur on the anterolateral or posteromedial aspect of the talus. Anterolateral fractures result from an inversion dorsiflexion force, and posteromedial fractures occur after inversion of the plantarflexed ankle.

Clinical Presentation

Prolonged pain after an inversion injury of the ankle should raise suspicion of an osteochondral talar dome fracture. The symptoms can be nonspecific and may have persisted from several weeks to months before the time of diagnosis. Patients typically report stiffness, limitation of ankle joint motion, and pain with activity with or without joint effusion. Displaced fractures may cause locking. Findings consistent with the diagnosis include point tenderness in the area of the fracture, decreased ROM, crepitus, and effusion.

Imaging

A classification system developed by Berndt and Harty is widely used to stage talar dome lesions from plain films but does not allow for definitive determination of articular cartilage integrity.[12] In general, the higher the stage, the worse the prognosis. The stages are I—compression; stage II—attached, nondisplaced fragment; stage III—detached, nondisplaced fragment; and stage IV—displaced fragment (Figures 14-16 and 14-17). If plain radiographs show no abnormality or are equivocal, an MRI can confirm the diagnosis and assist in determining the exact location and more definitively define talar dome pathology.

Indications for Orthopedic Referral

Those with stage III and IV osteochondral fractures should be referred for likely arthroscopic repair. Fractures greater than 10 mm, even if nondisplaced, should be referred.

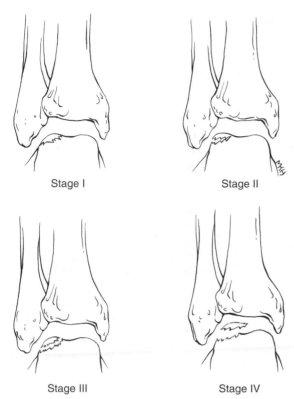

Stage I

Stage II

Stage III

Stage IV

FIGURE 14-16 Osteochondral dome fracture classified according to severity: Stage I—compression. Stage II—attached, nondisplaced. Stage III—detached, nondisplaced. Stage IV—displaced.

Treatment

The radiographic stage of the osteochondral fracture determines treatment and prognosis. The vast majority of symptomatic stage I and II fractures respond well to the conservative treatment of immobilization in a non–weight-bearing cast for 6 to 8 weeks. If symptoms persist or progress after 4 to 6 months of conservative therapy, surgical options such as arthroscopic curettage, drilling of the subchondral bone or excising a displaced fragment should be considered.

Fracture of the Lateral Process of the Talus (Snowboarder's Fracture)

Before the advent of snowboarding, fractures of the LPT were relatively uncommon. The incidence of this fracture has risen dramatically with the steady increase in the popularity of the sport. Detecting these fractures is challenging because they are notoriously difficult to recognize on plain radiographs, and clinically, they resemble an ankle sprain.

Mechanism of Injury

Before snowboarding became popular, fractures of the lateral talus were usually the result of

dorsiflexion-inversion injuries, falls from height, or high-velocity injuries such as MVAs. The exact cause of this injury during snowboarding is still uncertain, but most experts agree that impact loading and ankle dorsiflexion are highly associated.[13,14] The higher incidence of soft boot wear among snowboarders together with nonreleasable strap bindings allowing increased flexibility may explain the increased incidence of this injury.[15] As the sport of snowboarding continues to evolve to include an increasing number of aerial maneuvers and jumps, the incidence of this fracture may rise because of the increased risk of axial loading.

Clinical Presentation

The typical findings of a fracture of the lateral process can mimic those found in an inversion sprain of the ankle, making it difficult to diagnose. The clinician must be extremely suspicious of this injury in snowboarders. The patient will complain of lateral and weight-bearing pain and will usually have some swelling and bruising in this area. Point tenderness localized to the lateral talus approximately 1 cm from the tip of the lateral malleolus is an indication of the diagnosis.

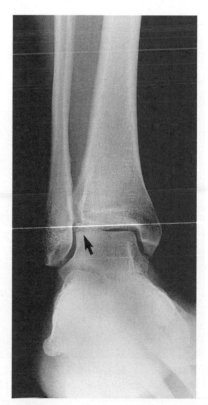

FIGURE 14-17 Stage II osteochondral dome fracture (*arrow*).

Imaging

A standard three-view ankle series should be obtained in the initial evaluation of a patient with a suspected snowboarder's fracture. This fracture is best seen on the mortise view just distal to the tip of the lateral malleolus; however, some fractures can be seen on the lateral view through the overlapping malleoli (Figure 14-18, A and B). The fracture fragment may be a single small or large avulsed piece or be quite comminuted. CT is the preferred imaging technique if this fracture is suspected but plain radiography findings are negative or equivocal. A CT scan is also useful in delineating the extent of the fracture and alignment (Figure 14-18, C).

Indications for Orthopedic Referral

Because of the need to maintain congruity of the articular surfaces to achieve good clinical healing,

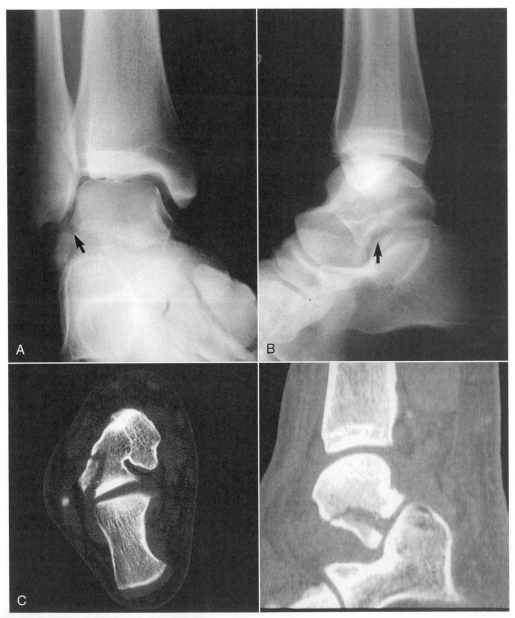

FIGURE 14-18 Snowboarder's fracture. **A,** Mortise view of the ankle showing a fracture of the lateral process of the talus. The fracture line is apparent just inferior to the lateral malleolus (*arrow*). **B,** The fracture is barely visible on the lateral view of the ankle (*arrow*). **C,** Computed tomography scan views of the same ankle show the extent of the fracture and amount of displacement. Note that the fracture did not appear significantly displaced on the mortise and lateral views. (*Photos courtesy of Keith A. Stuessi, MD.*)

patients with large, displaced, and comminuted fractures of the lateral process should be referred to an orthopedic surgeon for surgical management. The patient's foot should be placed in a posterior splint and kept non–weight bearing until evaluated by a surgeon.

Treatment

The optimal approach for treating these fractures is not known because no prospective trials have been performed. A nondisplaced small (<2 mm) fracture is probably best managed with immobilization in a short-leg non–weight-bearing cast for 4 weeks followed by 2 weeks of progressive weight bearing in a walking cast or cast boot. Most other fractures require ORIF to restore anatomic alignment. If small displaced fracture fragments or significant comminution is present, excision of the fragments is a reasonable alternative to internal fixation. Close follow-up of this fracture is important both clinically and radiographically to look for signs of fracture displacement.

Complications

An unrecognized fracture may result in malunion or nonunion with persistent pain and disability. Osseous overgrowth and malalignment are common and result in persistent pain and possibly limitation of ankle motion. Surgical management of complications may be warranted but usually only after conservative strategies such as physical therapy or orthotic correction has been tried.

TALUS FRACTURES (PEDIATRIC)

Fractures of the talus are rare in children, and most are nondisplaced fractures through the neck. Osteochondral fractures of the talar dome, although most common in young adults, can occur in teenagers. Forced dorsiflexion appears to be the usual cause of injury for neck fractures. Children with nondisplaced fractures may have minimal symptoms, but all of these fractures are accompanied by localized tenderness just distal to the ankle joint and pain with dorsiflexion.

AP, lateral, and oblique views of the foot centered on the hindfoot reveal talar neck fractures in most cases. If plain radiography findings are negative but the suspicion remains high, CT can confirm the presence of a talar fracture and provide more definitive information if operative repair is needed. Nondisplaced talar neck fractures are treated with immobilization in a short-leg non–weight-bearing cast for 4 to 6 weeks. Radiographs should be monitored for signs of AVN during the healing process.

Displaced talar fractures require ORIF, and patients with these injuries should be referred to an orthopedic surgeon for definitive management. The most significant complication of talar fractures in children is AVN. The body of the talus is vulnerable to ischemia in displaced neck fractures.

NAVICULAR FRACTURES (ADULT)

Anatomic Considerations

The midfoot, which includes the navicular, cuboid, and cuneiforms, is the least mobile of the three portions of the foot. Fractures of the navicular bone are uncommon, but four basic types can occur (listed in order of decreasing frequency): dorsal avulsion, tuberosity, body, and stress fractures. The deltoid ligament inserts into the dorsal lip and into the tuberosity of the navicular bone. Several ligaments unite the navicular bone with the adjacent talus and other midfoot bones. The posterior tibialis tendon inserts on the navicular tuberosity. The midtarsal joint involves the articulation between the distal and lateral navicular surface and the cuboid and cuneiform bones. The lateral and medial thirds of the navicular have increased vascularity compared with the middle third, thus defining a watershed area that predisposes this region to stress fractures.

Mechanism of Injury

Dorsal avulsion fractures are the result of a twisting force (usually eversion) with the foot in plantarflexion. Acute eversion of the foot places increased tension on the anterior deltoid ligament fibers or the posterior tibialis tendon, which can result in a navicular tuberosity fracture. Tuberosity fractures are often seen in conjunction with compression fractures of the cuboid. Fractures of the body of the navicular bone result from various causes, including hyperextension of the foot, direct trauma, and extreme flexion with rotation. Most of these fractures are associated with other injuries of the midtarsal joint.

Clinical Presentation

Common symptoms after a navicular fracture include localized pain and swelling over the fracture site and pain with weight bearing. Pain with eversion of the foot is most prominent in tuberosity fractures.

Imaging

Dorsal avulsion fractures are usually apparent on the lateral view (Figure 14-19). Tuberosity fractures are best seen on the AP and medial oblique views of the foot. Accessory bones commonly occur in the region of dorsal avulsion fractures (os supranaviculare) or tuberosity fractures (os tibiale externum). Accessory navicular bones are

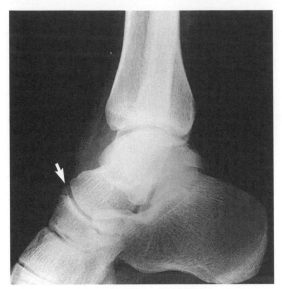

FIGURE 14-19 Dorsal avulsion fracture of the navicular bone with minimal displacement (*arrow*).

frequently bilateral and are distinguished from fractures by their smooth, rounded edges, which differ from the irregular surfaces of acute fractures. Fractures of the body of the navicular bone occasionally are seen in only one view, so careful study of AP, oblique, and lateral views is necessary for diagnosis.

Indications for Orthopedic Referral

Patients with the following fractures should be referred to an orthopedic surgeon for possible surgical repair: large, displaced dorsal avulsion fractures involving more than 20% to 25% of the talonavicular articular surface; tuberosity fractures with more than 1 cm of proximal displacement; and displaced body fractures. Patients with persistently painful avulsion or tuberosity fractures should be referred for consideration of surgical excision of the offending fragment.

Initial Treatment

Table 14-3 summarizes management guidelines for navicular fractures.

Table 14-3	*Management Guidelines for Navicular Fractures*
Initial Treatment	
Splint type and position	Lower extremity splint or bulky dressing
	Stress fractures placed in cast at initial visit
Initial follow-up visit	Within 7 days for definitive casting
Patient instruction	Icing, compression, and elevation
	Crutches as needed
Follow-up Care	
Cast or splint type and position	Dorsal avulsion: SLWC or compressive dressing
	Tuberosity: SLWC
	Body: below-knee walking cast
	Stress: SLNWBC
Length of immobilization	Dorsal avulsion: 4 to 6 weeks
	Tuberosity: 4 to 6 weeks; additional 2 to 4 weeks if symptomatic nonunion at 6 weeks
	Body: 6 to 8 weeks
	Stress: 6 to 8 weeks
Healing time	6 to 10 weeks for complete clinical healing
	Up to 6 months for complete return to activity after stress fracture
Follow-up visit interval	Every 2 to 4 weeks
Repeat radiography interval	At 6 weeks to document healing in tuberosity and body fracture
	Every 2 to 4 weeks if nonunion is apparent at 6 weeks
Patient instruction	Ankle and foot ROM exercises
	Calf muscle stretching and strengthening
Indications for orthopedic consult	Large displaced dorsal avulsion fractures
	Tuberosity fractures with >1 cm proximal displacement
	Displaced body fractures
	Nonunion or delayed union stress fracture
	Persistent symptoms after treatment of avulsion or tuberosity fractures

ROM, range of motion; SLNWBC, short-leg non–weight bearing cast; SLWC, short-leg walking cast.

Initial management of an acute navicular fracture should be symptomatic and include elevation, icing, and compression with a posterior splint or bulky dressing. Casts may be applied to stress fractures during the initial visit unless moderate to severe swelling is evident.

Follow-up Care

Dorsal Avulsion Fracture

Immobilization in a commercially available walking fracture boot or short-leg walking cast for 4 to 6 weeks should be adequate therapy for these fractures. Repeat radiographs are not necessary unless clinical healing is delayed beyond 6 weeks.

Tuberosity Fractures

Nondisplaced tuberosity fractures should be immobilized in a short-leg walking cast, well molded under the longitudinal arch, for 4 to 6 weeks. Because nonunion occasionally occurs, repeat radiographs after immobilization should be obtained to confirm fracture union. Patients with symptomatic nonunion at 6 weeks should be immobilized for an additional 2 to 4 weeks in an attempt to achieve union and be referred to an orthopedist if this treatment fails.

Body Fractures

A below-the-knee walking cast should be used to treat nondisplaced body fractures for 6 to 8 weeks or until radiographic healing is complete. Follow-up radiographs should be obtained at 6 weeks and every 2 to 4 weeks thereafter until union is ensured. After cast immobilization, patients should use a longitudinal arch support in their shoes for extra protection during weight bearing.

Rehabilitation

After cast immobilization of navicular fractures, patients should receive instruction in ankle and foot ROM exercises and calf and peroneal muscle stretching and strengthening. A follow-up visit 2 to 3 weeks into the rehabilitation should be scheduled to confirm adequate progress in restoring normal motion and function of the foot and ankle.

Return to Work or Sports

The total length of time required to return to a full preinjury activity level varies, but diligent effort during the rehabilitation should help patients return to more physically demanding activities sooner. Patients with dorsal avulsion or tuberosity fractures will usually be back to full activity within 2 to 3 months. Those with fractures of the body of the navicular will have a lengthier rehabilitation of up to 4 months because of the longer period of immobilization. Those in more sedentary jobs should be able to work throughout the period of immobilization and rehabilitation. Return to activities that put the patient at risk of reinjury should be avoided for 3 to 4 weeks after immobilization is discontinued. Decisions concerning return to sports should be based on recovery of ankle function and the presence of persistent symptoms with sport activity.

Navicular Stress Fracture

Mechanism of Injury

Stress fractures of the navicular bone are being identified with increasing frequency in those engaged in vigorous weight-bearing activities, particularly young, active runners. Overuse conditions and training errors, improper equipment, improper technique, and anatomic variants may all increase the risk of injury.

Clinical Presentation

Athletes with navicular stress fractures often seek treatment 3 to 6 months after the onset of symptoms when conservative measures have failed. They may complain of vague pain on the dorsomedial or medial aspect of the midfoot that is aggravated by activity and relieved with rest. Dorsal tenderness over the navicular bone ("the N-spot") is the most consistent finding.[16] ROM is typically normal.

Imaging

Stress fractures are difficult to identify on plain radiographs. Increased uptake on bone scan is not specific to navicular stress fractures but can at least localize the cause of the pain to the navicular (Figure 14-20). A negative bone scan essentially excludes the diagnosis of navicular stress fracture because of its high negative predictive value. Further imaging with thin-cut CT scan or MRI can distinguish a stress fracture from a stress reaction. MRI gives information similar to that of a bone scan plus CT scan.

Indications for Orthopedic Referral

Surgery should be considered for those with the rare displaced fracture, those who have difficulty complying with non–weight-bearing treatment, and failure of conservative treatment resulting in delayed union or nonunion. Typically, surgical management involves screw fixation with possible bone grafting.

Treatment

Insufficient evidence exists comparing operative and nonoperative management of acute stress fractures, so treatment of athletes should be individualized. The key to management of a navicular

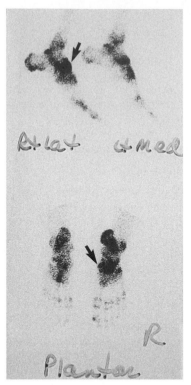

FIGURE 14-20 Bone scan of the foot demonstrating increased uptake in the right navicular bone indicative of a stress fracture (*arrows*).

stress fracture is early diagnosis. After the fracture is diagnosed, the patient should be placed in a short-leg non–weight-bearing cast for 6 to 8 weeks or until clinical healing occurs. Fracture healing can be assessed by examining for persistent tenderness over the dorsum of the foot at the "N-spot" starting at 6 weeks after treatment.[17] If tenderness persists, immobilization and non–weight bearing should be continued with follow-up every 2 weeks to reassess healing. Follow-up diagnostic imaging is not generally useful in monitoring healing because radiographic findings lag far behind clinical healing and may remain abnormal for years. Biomechanical problems and training errors leading to overuse conditions should be corrected. The average time until return to full sports participation is approximately 4 to 6 months. Long-term complications include delayed union, nonunion, and fracture recurrence.

NAVICULAR FRACTURES (PEDIATRIC)

The most common navicular fracture in children is a dorsal avulsion fracture. This fracture is best visualized on the lateral view, and significant displacement is rare. The treatment is generally uncomplicated, and most patients heal well with 3 to 4 weeks of immobilization in a short-leg walking cast or boot. Displaced fractures of the navicular in children are usually associated with severe trauma and require operative fixation.

Kohler's Disease

The ossification of the tarsal navicular bone has been shown to be quite variable and irregular. The findings associated with this process—sclerotic, thin, fragmented bone—have been termed Kohler's disease (Figure 14-21). This condition may represent an overuse syndrome from repetitive microtrauma, but some consider these findings a normal variant because they have no correlation to symptoms and radiographs of the foot taken for other reasons often show irregularity of ossification. The length of time the patient remains symptomatic can be shortened with immobilization in a short-leg walking cast for 6 to 8 weeks, but this may be unnecessary for the bone to return to its normal structure. Consultation with a pediatric orthopedic surgeon is suggested for patients with this condition.

CUBOID AND CUNEIFORM FRACTURES

Mechanism of Injury

Isolated fractures of the cuboid and cuneiform bones are uncommon. When they do occur, they are usually the result of direct trauma to the foot. Fractures of these bones may accompany fractures, subluxations, or dislocation of the midtarsal or tarsometatarsal joints. Cuboid fractures may occur in combination with some calcaneus fractures. A compression ("nutcracker") fracture of the cuboid results from a lateral stress on the midfoot, causing a crushing of the cuboid between the calcaneus and the fourth and fifth metatarsals.

Clinical Presentation

Patients with fractures of the cuboid or cuneiform bones usually complain of severe pain over the involved area typically after a direct blow to the foot. Localized tenderness, swelling, and increased pain with movement of the midfoot are apparent during physical examination. The clinician should look for any deformity of the midfoot indicating a possible dislocation.

Imaging

A standard foot series, including AP, lateral, and oblique views, is usually adequate to detect cuboid and cuneiform fractures (see Figure 14-6). Comparison views may help confirm or exclude a subluxation or dislocation of the midtarsal or tarsometatarsal joints.

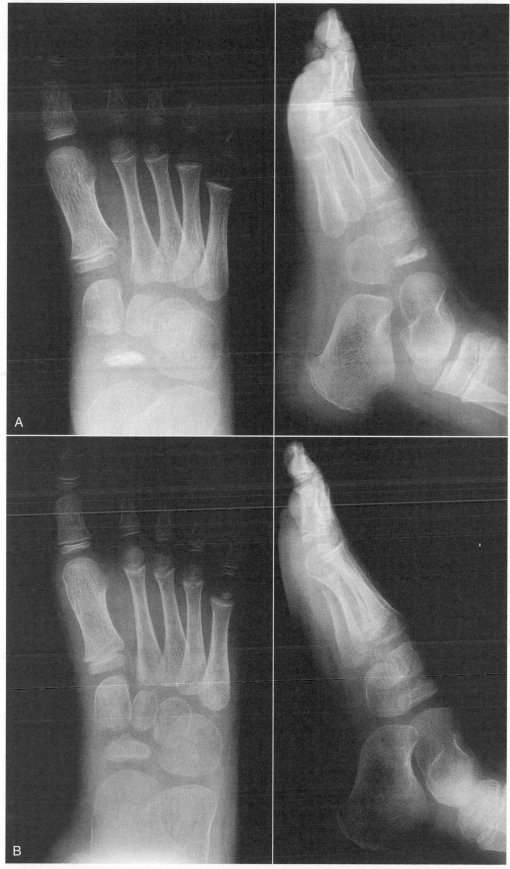

FIGURE 14-21 Kohler's disease. **A,** Anteroposterior and lateral views of the foot showing irregularity and sclerosis of the navicular in a young child. **B,** Radiographs of the same child 9 months later showing complete resolution of these changes.

Indications for Orthopedic Referral

Severe comminution, significant displacement, or concomitant dislocations are indications for orthopedic referral to restore alignment and minimize late complications.

Initial Treatment

The initial management of cuboid and cuneiform fractures is similar to the acute management of other tarsal bones and should include symptomatic treatment with elevation, icing, and compression with a posterior splint or bulky dressing. Correct identification of displacement should lead to early referral for reduction.

Follow-up Care

Nondisplaced fractures of the cuboid or cuneiform bones should be immobilized in a short-leg walking cast for approximately 6 weeks. After casting, the patient should use a longitudinal arch support for several months. Rehabilitation and return to work or sports guidelines are the same as outlined earlier for navicular fractures. Impaired function of the peroneus longus tendon is a potential late complication of cuboid fractures and results from scar formation during fracture healing.

REFERENCES

1. Schepers T, Ginai AZ, Van Lieshout EMM, Patka P. Demographics of extra-articular calcaneal fractures: including review of the literature on treatment and outcome. *Arch Orthop Trauma Surg.* 2008;128:1099-1106.
2. Judd DB, Kim DH. Foot fractures frequently misdiagnosed as ankle sprains. *Am Fam Physician.* 2002;66(5):785-794.
3. Gougoulias N, Khanna A, McBride DJ, Maffulli N. Management of calcaneal fractures: systematic review of randomized trials. *Br Med Bull.* 2009;92:153-167.
4. Bridgman SA, Dunn KM, McBride DJ, Richards PJ. Interventions for treating calcaneal fractures (Cochrane review). *The Foot.* 2002;47-61.
5. Allmacher DH, Galles KS, March JL. Intra-articular calcaneal fractures treated nonoperatively and followed sequentially for 2 decades. *J Orthop Trauma.* 2006;20:464-469.
6. Petit CJ, Lee BM, Kasser JR, Kocher MS. Operative treatment of intraarticular calcaneal fractures in the pediatric population. *J Pediatr Orthop.* 2007;27:856-862.
7. Mora S, Thordarson DB, Zionts LE, Reynolds RAK. Pediatric calcaneal fractures. *Foot Ankle Int.* 2001;22(6):471-477.
8. Ribbans WJ, Natarajan R, Alavala S. Pediatric foot fractures. *Clin Orthop Relat Res.* 2005;(432):107-115.
9. Inokuchi S, Usami N, Hiraishi E, Hashimoto T. Calcaneal fractures in children. *J Pediatr Orthop.* 1998;18:469.
10. Ahmad J, Raikin SM. Current concept review: talar fractures. *Foot Ankle Int.* 2006;27(6):475-482.
11. Hawkins LG. Fractures of the neck of the talus. *J Bone Joint Surg [Am].* 1970;52:991-1002.
12. Berndt AL, Harty M. Transchondral fractures (osteochondritis dissecans) of the talus. *J Bone Joint Surg [Am].* 1959;41:988-1020.
13. Boon AJ, Smith J, Zobitz ME, Amrami KM. Snowboarder's talus fracture: mechanism of injury. *Am J Sports Med.* 2001;29:333-338.
14. Valderrabano V, Perren T, Ryf C, et al. Snowboarder's talus fracture: treatment outcome of 20 cases after 3.5 years. *Am J Sports Med.* 2005;33(6):871-880.
15. Kirkpatrick DP, Hunter RE, Janes PC, et al. The snowboarder's foot and ankle. *Am J Sports Med.* 1998;26:271-277.
16. Gehrmann RM, Renard RL. Current concepts review: stress fractures of the foot. *Foot Ankle Int.* 2006;27(9):750-757.
17. Kahn KM, Brukner PD, Kearney C, et al. Tarsal navicular stress fractures in athletes. *Sports Med.* 1994;17:65-76.

METATARSAL FRACTURES

Co-Author: Michael Seth Smith

See Appendix for stepwise instructions for weight-bearing and non–weight-bearing short-leg casts and a lower extremity splint used in the treatment of metatarsal fractures.

See Expert Consult for the electronic version of a patient instruction sheet named "Broken Foot or Ankle," which covers the steps of care from pain relief to rehabilitation exercises. This can be copied to hand out to patients to assist them during the treatment period.

Metatarsal fractures are relatively common, making up 5% to 6% of all fractures. To the primary care provider, they offer opportunities and pitfalls. Most are best managed conservatively, producing very good outcomes and lending themselves to primary care management. Pitfalls arise from the fact that it is easy to underestimate the severity of certain metatarsal fractures. Significant angulation may go undetected, as may considerable soft tissue injury. Relatively subtle injuries such as Lisfranc fracture dislocations and stress fractures of the proximal fifth metatarsal may be missed initially, leading to prolonged recovery or long-term disability. Avulsions of the tuberosity of the fifth metatarsal may be overlooked if the primary care provider does not recognize the mechanism of injury that produces this injury. Knowledge of metatarsal fracture patterns and their associated complications helps clinicians avoid the pitfalls and select the more easily managed fractures to treat.

FRACTURES OF THE METATARSAL SHAFTS

Anatomic Considerations

The first metatarsal is an important component of the arch of the foot, and it plays a key role in weight bearing.[1] Malalignment of the first metatarsal is therefore tolerated more poorly than malalignment of other metatarsals. The dorsalis pedis artery and one of its major branches, the deep plantar artery, pass near the base of the first metatarsal (Figure 15-1). Injuries to these arteries or the arcuate artery may complicate metatarsal fractures. The splinting action of adjacent metatarsals generally prevents much displacement unless fractures are multiple or near the metatarsal head. When displacement does occur, the pull of intrinsic muscles of the foot and the flexor tendons of the toes usually causes the head of the metatarsal to displace in a plantar direction (i.e., apex dorsal angulation at the fracture site). The soft tissues of the dorsum of the foot are relatively thin. When crushed against the underlying metatarsals, these tissues may necrose and subsequently slough, converting a closed fracture into an open one.

Mechanism of Injury

Many shaft fractures result from a direct blow such as when a heavy object is dropped on the foot.[2] Twisting forces may also produce these fractures. Because of the first metatarsal's relative size and strength, considerable force is required to fracture it. Ballet dancers may fracture the distal fifth metatarsal shaft by rolling onto it while raised up on their toes or by landing on it after a jump ("dancer's fracture").

Clinical Presentation

Considerable pain and tenderness accompany most acute metatarsal fractures, and weight bearing is difficult or impossible. Direct pressure under the metatarsal head produces pain at the fracture site, as will axial loading (i.e., compressing the proximal phalanx or metatarsal head toward the calcaneus). Axial loading is useful in distinguishing soft tissue injury from a fracture. Both may have significant point tenderness on direct palpation, but axial loading should not produce significant pain unless a fracture is present. Diagnostic maneuvers should be performed gently to avoid displacing the fracture and to minimize patient discomfort. Because of the foot's dependent position, swelling and ecchymosis occur quickly and may be significant, leading to early diffuse tenderness that may obscure point tenderness at the fracture site. The swelling

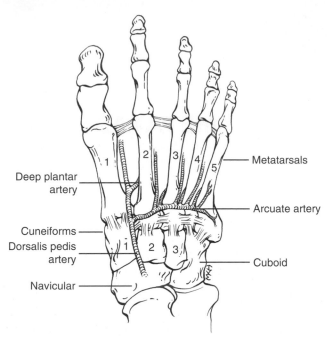

FIGURE 15-1 Anatomy of the foot, including the dorsalis pedis artery and its branches and the ligamentous attachments of the metatarsals.

may be severe enough to produce a compartment syndrome. The swelling associated with a fracture of the first metatarsal is especially pronounced, and the risk of a compartment syndrome is greater in these cases.

Imaging

Most metatarsal shaft fractures are either oblique or transverse, and they generally have at least a small amount of displacement (Figure 15-2). In many cases, overlapping shadows on the lateral view conceal significant angulation or displacement. The oblique view may best reveal fragment positions. It is important to examine the radiographs carefully to look for apex dorsal displacement because the displaced metatarsal head can cause significant disability if its position is not corrected. When fragment position is difficult to determine with anteroposterior (AP), oblique, and lateral views, it may be beneficial to obtain a modified lateral view with the metatarsals rotated slightly to avoid some shadow overlap. With crush injuries and very high forces, multiple fractures, comminution, or both are often seen (Figure 15-3).

Indications for Orthopedic Referral

Emergent Referral (Within 30 to 60 Minutes)

Patients with any open metatarsal fracture or with associated vascular compromise should be referred immediately for operative treatment.

Early Referral or Consultation (Within a Few Hours)

In some high-force injuries, the skin remains intact initially, but necroses and sloughs in the ensuing days. This may convert the injury into an open fracture and have a dismal impact on healing and outcome. Sloughing may occur even when the skin appears to have only minor damage. The provider should remain alert for this possibility and strongly consider an early consultation whenever a significant crush injury has occurred or the skin appears to be in jeopardy.

Nonemergent Referral (Within a Few Days of Injury)

Most patients with displaced fractures of the first metatarsal should be referred to an orthopedic surgeon even if the displacement appears fairly mild. Anatomic position of this bone is desirable because of its important role in weight bearing. Patients with displaced fractures of multiple metatarsals, displaced fractures that occur very close to the head, and intraarticular fractures are also best referred because these injuries usually require pin fixation. With all metatarsal fractures, the provider should be extremely suspicious of concurrent dislocation of the tarsometatarsal joint and refer the patient if this injury is suspected (see later discussion of Lisfranc dislocations).

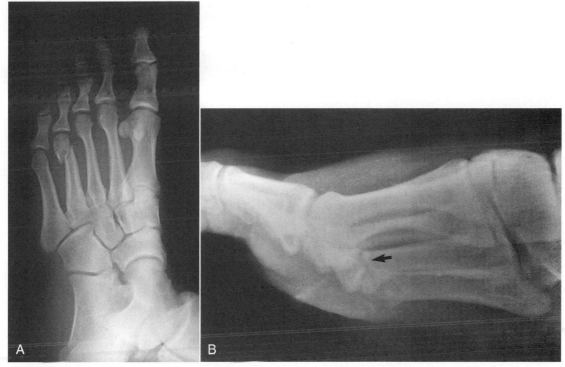

FIGURE 15-2 A, Fracture of the fourth metatarsal, oblique view. Note slight shortening and 3 to 4 mm of displacement. **B,** Lateral view. Note the double-density line at the fracture site (*arrow*) and near-normal position of the fourth metatarsal head.

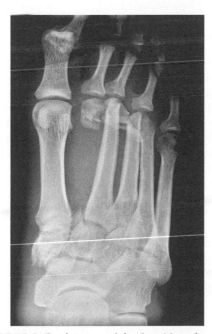

FIGURE 15-3 Crush injury of the foot. Note the marked widening of the space between the first and second metatarsals and displaced fractures of the second and third metatarsals, first toe, and first cuneiform. Although widening of the space between the first and second metatarsals is usually caused by Lisfranc fracture dislocations, it is attributable to the displaced first cuneiform fracture in this case.

Initial Treatment

Table 15-1 summarizes the management guidelines for metatarsal shaft fractures.

Before initiating treatment, the provider must assess neurovascular status and the viability of the overlying skin. Swelling is likely to be significant with these fractures, and strict elevation and icing are paramount. The patient and provider must be especially vigilant for signs and symptoms of a compartment syndrome, which may develop secondary to swelling. Immediate evaluation should be sought if indicative symptoms such as disproportionate pain, pallor, or paresthesias develop. Overnight admission to monitor vascular status should be strongly considered for first metatarsal fractures and significant crush injuries.

Nondisplaced Fractures

Initial immobilization can be achieved with a lower extremity splint, and the patient should avoid weight bearing until the next visit. Follow-up should ideally occur the next day if the skin may be in jeopardy, a cast was applied, the patient's symptoms worsen, or compliance with icing and elevation is doubtful. Otherwise, the patient may return in 3 to 5 days when decreased swelling should allow casting.

Table 15-1	*Management Guidelines for Metatarsal Shaft Fractures*
INITIAL TREATMENT	
Splint type and position	Nondisplaced: lower extremity splint with ankle at 90 degrees
	Displaced after reduction: bivalved well-molded SLNWBC
Initial follow-up visit	3 to 5 days
	If a cast is applied initially, cast check in 24 hours
Patient instruction	Elevation and icing crucial in first 2 to 3 days
	No weight bearing until follow-up
	Explain signs of compartment syndrome
FOLLOW-UP CARE	
Cast or splint type and position	Nondisplaced: firm-soled shoe, cast boot or SLWC if the patient is in severe pain
	Reduced: SLNWBC
Length of immobilization	Nondisplaced: SLWC or boot for 3 to 4 weeks if used; firm-soled shoe for 4 to 6 weeks
	Reduced: SLNWBC for 3 to 4 weeks, followed by SLWC for 3 to 4 weeks
Healing time	Nondisplaced: 6 weeks
	Reduced: 6 to 8 weeks
Follow-up visit interval	Every 1 to 2 weeks initially to assess the need for a cast change as it loosens
	Every 2 to 4 weeks after cast is removed or if a firm-soled shoe is used
Repeat radiography interval	Reduced or unstable: within 7 days to check fracture position
	4 to 6 weeks after injury to document healing
Patient instruction	Nondisplaced: advance weight bearing as tolerated
	Reduced: no weight bearing for first 3 to 4 weeks
	Ankle ROM and calf stretching and strengthening after the cast has been removed
Indications for orthopedic consult	High risk for skin necrosis
	Open fractures
	Vascular injury
	Compartment syndrome
	Fracture dislocation
	Intraarticular fractures
	Displaced, unable to reduce
	Multiple metatarsal fractures

ROM, range of motion; SLNWBC, short-leg non–weight bearing cast; SLWC, short-leg walking cast.

Displaced Fractures

Fractures with dorsal or plantar angulation greater than 10 degrees should be reduced or referred, as should fractures with fragments displaced more than 3 to 4 mm in this plane.[1,3] Care should be taken to detect and correct rotational deformity, because rotation remodels much more poorly than other types of displacement. Uncorrected displacement or angulation in the lateral or medial plane is generally well tolerated as long as displacement is not excessive (Figure 15-4). Excellent results have been obtained without reduction in a small sample of ballet dancers with displaced distal fifth metatarsal fractures.[4] Referral or consultation with an orthopedist or podiatrist is recommended if the primary care physician is uncertain about the necessity for reduction.

The practitioner can reduce most displaced metatarsal shaft fractures with the patient under local anesthesia by placing the toes in Chinese finger traps and allowing gravity to slowly reduce the fracture. In some cases, it may be necessary to apply a light weight (2 to 5 lb) around the distal tibia, perform concurrent manual manipulation, or

both to achieve the reduction. Alternatively, traction can be maintained on the appropriate toe(s) by an assistant while the operator presses the distal fragment back into position with a thumb. A highly molded, bivalved, non–weight-bearing short-leg cast should maintain most reductions, provided the fracture is neither multiple nor very near the metatarsal head. Postreduction radiographs should be obtained after casting to confirm adequate reduction. If reduction is difficult (perhaps owing to soft tissue interposition) or adequate position is not maintained after release of traction, referral for possible operative reduction is required.

Follow-up Care

Nondisplaced Fractures

Nondisplaced metatarsal shaft fractures usually heal well without cast immobilization. The patient should wear a firm-soled shoe and begin partial weight bearing as tolerated. A postoperative shoe with a wooden sole can be used if the patient does not have suitable shoes or cannot wear shoes comfortably as a result of swelling (Figure 15-5). If the patient does not tolerate this type of treatment

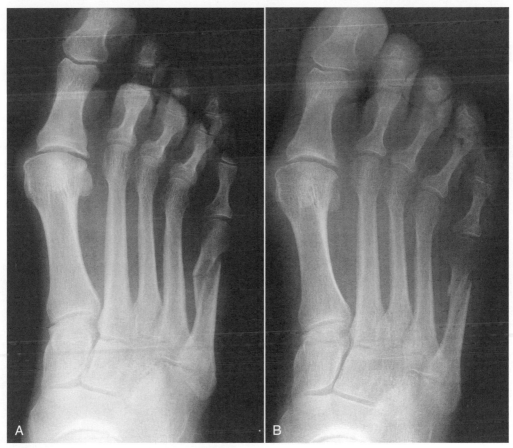

FIGURE 15-4 A, Anteroposterior view of an oblique fracture of the fifth metatarsal shaft with apex medial angulation. The patient was treated without fracture reduction and placed in a hard-soled shoe. **B,** Six weeks later, the fracture is healing with good alignment.

because of pain, a short-leg walking cast can be applied (well molded under the arch). Casts for metatarsal fractures often become unacceptably loose as swelling subsides. A cast check in 3 to 5 days is advisable. The cast may be discontinued 2 to 3 weeks after the injury, depending on the

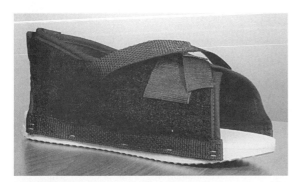

FIGURE 15-5 Postoperative wooden shoe used in the treatment of metatarsal shaft fractures.

patient's symptoms. After removal of the cast, the patient should be switched to a firm shoe that provides good arch support and begin progressive ankle range of motion (ROM) and calf stretching and strengthening exercises. Clinical healing is usually achieved within 6 weeks. Radiographs should be repeated within 1 week to confirm that the fracture remains nondisplaced and within 4 to 6 weeks after injury to document healing.[5]

Displaced Fractures after Reduction

Because casting of displaced fractures is usually done at the initial visit when further swelling is likely, the cast should be bivalved and a cast check performed the next day. The patient should not bear weight on the cast for 5 to 7 days and then should be reevaluated. Cast loosening should be checked and repeat radiographs in the cast taken to assess fracture position, followed by immobilization in a non–weight-bearing cast. If the cast has not loosened, the bivalved cast can be wrapped with additional cast material to convert the bivalved cast into a solid cast. After 2 to 3 additional weeks, the cast should be removed, radiographs obtained, and an examination performed out of the cast. The patient should be converted to a short-leg walking cast for 3 to 4 more weeks with progressive weight bearing prescribed. After discontinuing the cast, the patient can be treated as described earlier for nondisplaced fractures. If fracture position is lost during follow-up, orthopedic consultation is recommended.

Return to Work or Sports

Patients with sedentary jobs may return to work within 1 week of the fracture date, provided pain and swelling are reasonably well controlled and the patient is able to elevate the extremity much of the time. Patients may return to more active duties when weight bearing produces little or no pain as long as the duties do not expose the patient to possible foot trauma. If certain duties significantly increase the pain or swelling, these duties should be temporarily stopped. After healing has occurred (callus is present and little or no point tenderness at the fracture site exists), patients may gradually resume full regular duties. Casual athletes may cautiously start rehabilitation at this point by walking for progressively longer distances. When they can comfortably walk 1 to 2 miles without experiencing significant aching afterward, they may intersperse walking with short periods of straight running on even surfaces. The running distances may be progressively increased as tolerated. Speed work and cutting should be delayed for several weeks until stamina is regained and running modest distances is well tolerated. After speed and cutting drills are well tolerated, the patient may return to game situations. Dedicated or highly competitive athletes may wish to work with a trainer or physical therapist to begin safe resistance or cross-training activities while weight bearing is impossible and to devise a plan to return to competition as rapidly and safely as possible.

Complications

Arterial injury and compartment syndromes may occur and have dire consequences such as loss of the foot or ischemic contractures (claw foot). Osteomyelitis may complicate open fractures. Unrecognized injuries of the tarsometatarsal (Lisfranc) joint may be debilitating, producing chronic pain with weight bearing and subluxation of the metatarsals toward the sole (Lisfranc injuries are discussed in more detail later in this chapter). If the fracture heals in a position with significant plantar displacement of the distal fragment, the foot may become chronically painful and develop an intractable plantar keratosis. Malunion of the first metatarsal is also tolerated poorly. Finally, complex regional pain syndrome (CRPS) may

develop after metatarsal fractures. This should be suspected when significant pain and swelling persist 2 to 3 months after injury. This condition responds best if it is recognized early and treated aggressively with physical therapy.

Pediatric Considerations

The physis of the first metatarsal is sometimes confused with a fracture because it is located proximally rather than distally like the physes of the other metatarsals (Figure 15-6). If significant tenderness exists over the physis, it is wise to treat the condition as though a fracture is present and repeat radiographs in 2 weeks to definitively confirm or rule out a fracture. Torus fractures of the metatarsal

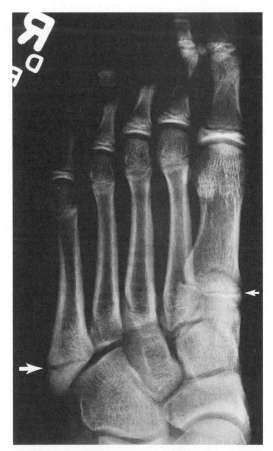

FIGURE 15-6 Oblique view of an adolescent's foot demonstrating a fracture. At first glance, the practitioner may confuse the physis of the first metatarsal (*small arrow*) with a fracture because this physis is located proximally but the physes of the other metatarsals are located distally. The physis in this example is normal. However, a styloid fracture of the proximal fifth metatarsal is present (*large arrow*). Note the contrast between the physis and the fracture line. The lucency of the physis takes a meandering course with smooth, rounded undulations. A rim of denser white bone also lines the lucency. The lucency of the fracture is more linear, and no increased density is seen at the margin.

are relatively common and often have little or no swelling. These may be quite subtle and may be missed unless the physician is highly suspicious whenever point tenderness is present. If a fracture is apparent, follow-up radiographs taken 2 to 3 weeks later should reveal unmistakable callus. An example of such a fracture with comparison views and follow-up radiographs is shown in Figure 15-7.

Children are susceptible to avascular necrosis of the distal second metatarsal, a condition known as Freiberg's disease. It is characterized by localized pain made worse by walking or running. Radiographs demonstrate sclerosis and partial collapse of the metatarsal head. Although conservative treatment is usually tried first for patients with Freiberg's disease, referral is recommended.

In children, substantial remodeling occurs after healing of metatarsal fractures. The younger the child, the greater the correction that can be expected. Children are therefore able to tolerate greater amounts of displacement than adults. Fractures having more than 20 degrees of dorsal or plantar angulation should be reduced or referred, especially if the child is older and less remodeling can be expected. Care should be taken to detect and correct rotational deformity, because rotation remodels much more poorly than other types of displacement.

Although adults with metatarsal shaft fractures may not need casting, short-leg walking casts are generally preferred in children. They offer greater protection and better initial control of symptoms than other treatment approaches. Care should be taken to maintain the foot in 90 degrees of flexion while the cast is being applied. If the cast is placed while the foot is plantarflexed and the foot lifted to 90 degrees as the cast hardens, kinking of the cast will occur. This creates pressure over the anterior ankle that can impair circulation to the foot, which can create a situation analogous to a compartment syndrome, particularly in children.

Healing is more rapid than in adults, occurring in as little as 3 weeks in young children and 5 to 6 weeks in older children. Complications are similar to those described previously for adults with two notable exceptions: malunion is less common because of remodeling, and future growth abnormalities may arise if the physis is injured. Children with any displaced physis fracture should be referred, as should children with Salter-Harris types III, IV, and V and those with conditions already indicated for referral. Primary care physicians with additional expertise often manage selected nondisplaced type I and II fractures. Care of these fractures should include confirmation of fragment position after cast application, discussion

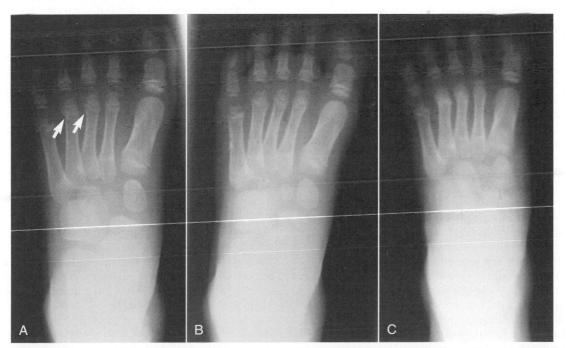

FIGURE 15-7 A, Anteroposterior (AP) view of a child's painful foot. Subtle irregularity of cortex is seen in third and fourth distal metatarsal shafts (*arrows*), but the radiograph was read as "no fracture" by the radiologist. **B,** AP view of the opposite foot showing smooth cortex in the area of interest. This suggests that the irregularities seen on the injured foot do indeed represent torus fractures. **C,** Follow-up radiograph of the injured foot 3 weeks after injury. Increased bone density, representing callus, has developed at the sites of irregularity, confirming that a fracture was indeed present.

of the possibility of future growth abnormalities with the patient and parents, and follow-up radiographs at approximately 6-month intervals for 1 to 2 years to detect growth problems early and refer the child for treatment if they should develop.

STRESS FRACTURES OF THE METATARSAL SHAFTS

The metatarsal shafts are common sites of stress fractures. Any metatarsal may be involved, with the second metatarsal most often affected. Stress fractures of the proximal fifth metatarsal, which are discussed later in this chapter, have distinct considerations and a much worse prognosis.[6] Stress fractures usually occur several weeks after an abrupt increase in activity. Metatarsal stress fractures are commonly called "march fractures" because they often occur in military recruits during basic training. These fractures also occur in athletes who have recently changed their exercise routine or who chronically overload the bone.

Symptoms related to a stress fracture have an insidious onset. Early on, only minor pain and tenderness may be present. If activities are not limited, symptoms worsen and eventually progress to swelling, point tenderness, and severe pain with weight bearing. Symptoms precede radiographic findings by approximately 2 to 3 weeks. The first radiographic sign may be a narrowing of the medullary canal, a faint lucency, or periosteal thickening (Figure 15-8, A). Callus usually is present by 4 to 5 weeks (Figure 15-8, B), and complete healing may take months (Figure 15-8, C). Although bone scans and magnetic resonance imaging (MRI) can detect stress fractures soon after symptoms develop, they are often not necessary. Presumptive treatment can be started based on history and examination alone.[7] If early diagnostic confirmation is desired, MRI is generally preferred over a bone scan. It offers greater specificity with similar sensitivity.[8]

In most cases, stress fractures can be managed without casting. If symptoms are very mild, simply eliminating running and jumping and restricting the amount of walking may suffice. Use of crutches with partial weight bearing may be necessary if routine walking is painful. Stress fractures that are very symptomatic may be treated acutely with a short-leg walking cast and crutches. After about 1 week of non–weight bearing, progressive weight bearing may be started. When walking is no longer painful, treatment may be advanced (i.e., cast removed or activity level increased). Inadequate limitation, premature resumption, or too rapid an advancement of activities may lead to a recurrence of the fracture. Nonunion may occur, so radiographic follow-up should be performed to document healing.

Pediatric Considerations

Metatarsal stress fractures in children occur most often in adolescents. Although these injuries in children are less common than in adults, diagnosis and treatment are the same. Because it may be difficult to get adolescents to adequately restrict their activities, a short-leg walking cast may be necessary if symptoms persist, even if only with more vigorous activity. Nonunion of a shaft stress fracture in a child is very unusual.

PROXIMAL FRACTURES OF THE FIRST THROUGH FOURTH METATARSALS

Anatomic Considerations

The joint between the tarsal bones and the metatarsal bases, the Lisfranc joint, is crucial to proper foot function. With each step, high forces are transmitted through this joint. The metatarsals must be firmly held in anatomic position to comfortably bear these forces. Disruption of one or more of the ligaments that attach to the proximal metatarsals can lead to disabling injuries with long-term sequelae. The attachments of the first and second metatarsals are particularly important. The first metatarsal, unlike the others, is not attached to the adjacent metatarsal proximally (see Figure 15-1). As a result, it tends to displace away from the other metatarsals when the tarsometatarsal ligaments are injured. The importance of the second metatarsal lies in its role as the "keystone" of the midfoot–forefoot junction. If the second metatarsal loses its proper alignment with the middle cuneiform, the third through fifth metatarsals generally become displaced as well.

Several arteries pass over or near the proximal metatarsals, and these may be injured at the time of fracture. Collateral arteries generally prevent vascular compromise. However, arterial injury may cause dramatic swelling, which may lead to a compartment syndrome.

Mechanism of Injury

As with other metatarsal fractures, direct blows and crush injuries cause most proximal fractures. Falling forward over a plantarflexed foot, such as occurs when missing a step on a staircase, may also result in a proximal metatarsal fracture (Figure 15-9) and is the most common cause of a Lisfranc injury. Lisfranc fracture dislocations were originally described in soldiers whose horse fell on their feet (i.e., direct blow to the top or side of a plantarflexed foot). However, the foot need not be in this position to sustain this injury, particularly when high-energy or crushing blows are involved.

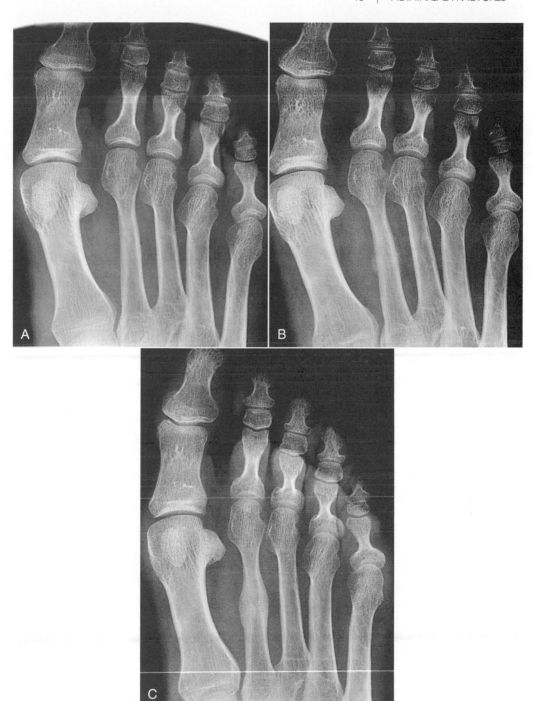

FIGURE 15-8 A, Very early stress fracture of the second metatarsal. The only hint that a stress fracture may be present is the mild medullary narrowing seen in the midshaft. A bone scan performed at this time would have shown positive findings. **B,** Follow-up radiograph obtained 24 days later. Subtle, fluffy callus and blurring of the cortex are apparent. **C,** Three months later, abundant, well-organized callus is seen, indicating a healed fracture.

Clinical Presentation

Swelling and pain are likely to be severe, causing an inability to bear weight. Because multiple bones, ligaments, or both are often involved, tenderness is likely to be diffuse. Fractures of the bases of the first four metatarsals share many signs and symptoms with tarsal fractures, Lisfranc fracture dislocations, and isolated ligament injuries. Pain at the joint produced by gentle pronation and abduction of the foot suggests a fracture dislocation or sprain. If significant tenderness and swelling are

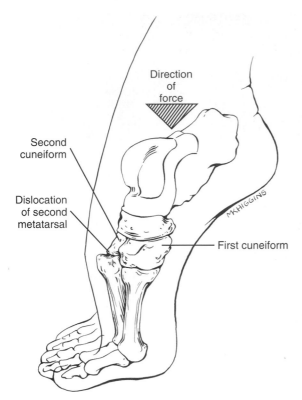

FIGURE 15-9 Typical cause of injury for a Lisfranc injury—falling forward on a plantarflexed foot.

cuboid and the medial edge of the third metatarsal with the medial edge of the third cuneiform.

A Lisfranc joint dislocation should be strongly suspected when a patient has an avulsion ("fleck") fracture of the lateral base of the first metatarsal or the medial base of the second or when the space between the first and second metatarsals is widened (Figure 15-12). The physician should also be highly suspicious of this injury in patients without an apparent fracture who have tenderness over the tarsometatarsal joint and are unable to bear weight while standing on their tiptoes. Comparison views of the other foot, with special attention paid to the oblique view, may help the physician recognize the slight displacement usually seen with Lisfranc fracture dislocations. In subtle Lisfranc injuries, an AP weight-bearing view may reveal widening not seen in standard views (Figure 15-13), and lateral weight-bearing views may reveal subluxation, seen as a stepoff between a proximal metatarsal and the adjacent tarsal. If a Lisfranc injury is strongly

present but radiographs reveal neither fracture nor abnormal spacing between metatarsal bases, an isolated sprain may be present.

Imaging

A standard foot series (AP, lateral, and oblique views) should be obtained. Proximal metatarsal fractures are often multiple (Figure 15-10) and may be accompanied by tarsal fractures. Although the fragments may appear to have little or no displacement, proximal metatarsal fractures are notorious for being associated with concurrent injuries of the tarsometatarsal ligaments (Lisfranc fracture dislocation). This injury is frequently overlooked on radiographs because the bones may spontaneously return to near-normal position after injury.

Lisfranc Joint Dislocation

The AP and oblique views should be carefully examined for proper alignment between the metatarsal bases and the tarsal bones. On both of these views, the medial edge of the second metatarsal base should be in line with the medial edge of the middle cuneiform (Figure 15-11). Displacement of a metatarsal is best seen on the oblique view where the medial edge of the fourth metatarsal base normally should be in line with the medial edge of the

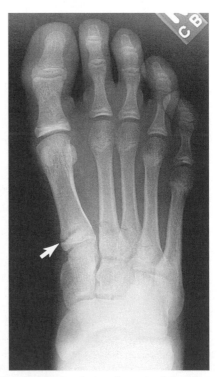

FIGURE 15-10 Nondisplaced proximal fractures of the second, third, and fourth metatarsals. The alignment between the metatarsals and tarsals is normal. The lucency in the proximal first metatarsal (*arrow*) represents a physis. From this radiograph alone, it is impossible to tell whether the physis is also fractured. Clinical examination is needed (tenderness over the physis would suggest a nondisplaced Salter I fracture). Comparison views of the opposite foot could also be obtained to help detect subtle abnormalities of the physis.

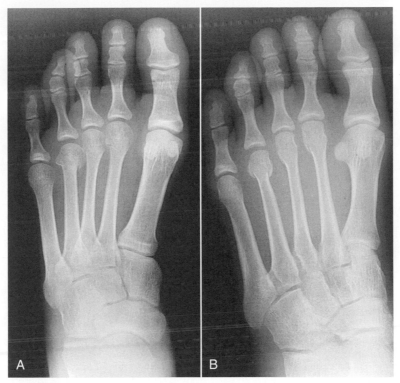

FIGURE 15-11 Anteroposterior (**A**) and oblique (**B**) views of the foot demonstrating the normal parallel alignment of the medial edge of the base of the second metatarsal with the medial edge of the middle cuneiform. A minimally displaced fracture of the fourth metatarsal neck is present.

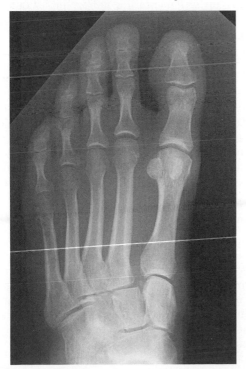

FIGURE 15-12 Anteroposterior view demonstrating a fleck fracture of the base of the second metatarsal with a Lisfranc joint dislocation. Note the widened space between the first and second metatarsals and the incongruity of the base of the second metatarsal with the middle cuneiform.

suspected but findings of weight-bearing views are normal, MRI is very good at detecting injury to the Lisfranc ligament.[9] It is superior to computed tomography (CT) for this purpose because it allows visualization of the ligaments; CT is only able to detect fractures and abnormal spacing between the bones.[9]

Indications for Orthopedic Referral

Emergent Referral (Within 30 to 60 Minutes)

Patients with any open metatarsal fracture or with associated vascular compromise should be referred immediately for operative treatment.

Early Referral or Consultation (Within a Few Hours)

In some high-force injuries, the skin remains intact initially but necroses and sloughs in the ensuing days. This may convert the injury into an open fracture and have a dismal impact on healing and outcome. Sloughing may occur even when the skin appears to have only minor damage. The primary care provider should remain alert for this possibility and strongly consider an early consultation whenever a significant crush injury has occurred or the skin appears to be in jeopardy.

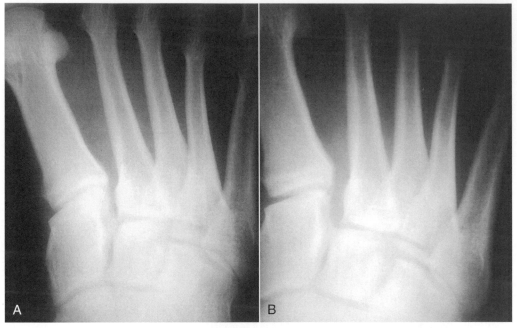

FIGURE 15-13 A, Anteroposterior (AP) non–weight-bearing view demonstrating normal alignment between the first and second metatarsals. **B,** AP weight-bearing view of the same patient reveals widening between the first and second metatarsals. This patient had a typical mechanism of injury for a Lisfranc injury that was missed initially on the standard views.

Nonemergent Referral (Within a Few Days of Injury)

Most patients with proximal fractures of the first four metatarsals should be referred. This is especially important for multiple or displaced fractures because they are frequently associated with dislocations of the Lisfranc joint. Patients with Lisfranc fracture dislocations should be referred because anatomic reduction is essential, and internal fixation is nearly always necessary. The disability that results from inadequate treatment of this injury is so severe that, during the Napoleonic Wars, Lisfranc recommended amputation as the preferred treatment. Patients with isolated sprains of this region should also be referred because even fairly subtle injuries can produce long-term consequences if not meticulously managed. Patients should be immobilized in a lower extremity splint and remain non–weight bearing until seen by an orthopedic consultant.

Treatment

If a proximal metatarsal fracture is truly nondisplaced without evidence of ligament disruption, it can be managed similar to a displaced metatarsal shaft fracture that requires reduction as described earlier. Weight bearing should be delayed until 4 to 6 weeks after injury to optimize the stability of the affected area followed by 2 to 4 weeks of weight bearing in a well-molded short-leg walking cast.

Follow-up weight-bearing radiographs should be obtained if symptoms persist for 2 weeks after discontinuation of the cast.

Return to Work or Sports

With one exception, considerations are similar to those described previously for metatarsal shaft fractures. Because treatment involves prolonged non–weight bearing, patients with nonsedentary jobs should not work for 5 to 7 weeks unless they can be temporarily reassigned to job tasks that do not require walking, standing, or using their feet. These tasks may be gradually resumed after weight bearing has begun and is well tolerated.

Complications

Complications of proximal metatarsal fractures are similar to those associated with shaft fractures. An unrecognized fracture dislocation is the most common complication and almost always results in significant long-term disability if not promptly identified and carefully treated. Skin necrosis and sloughing, vascular injury, and compartment syndromes are also possible, especially if significant fracture displacement or a crush injury exists.

Pediatric Considerations

Awareness of the usual location of the first metatarsal physis (proximal) is necessary to avoid misreading a normal physis as a fracture (see Figures 15-6 and 15-10). Point tenderness over the physis, even when findings on radiographs are apparently normal, should lead to presumptive treatment for a Salter-Harris type I fracture. The physis of the first metatarsal is more susceptible to premature closure and other growth disturbances than the other metatarsal physes, so referral is recommended for all patients with physeal injuries, including nondisplaced type I fractures. Because of its proximal location, an injury to this physis should be considered in any child with a proximal fracture of other metatarsals. Lisfranc fracture dislocations are unusual in children, but they do occur. As with adults, the bones may spontaneously return to near-anatomic position, making recognition of the injury difficult. It is said that children tolerate this injury better than adults, but referral is still highly recommended because internal fixation is often necessary, and severe future disability may occur.[10]

Fractures of the Proximal Fifth Metatarsal

Fractures of the proximal fifth metatarsal have little in common with proximal fractures of the other metatarsals and are therefore discussed separately. They are divided into three types that have distinct etiologies, prognoses, and treatments.

Table 15-2 summarizes the management guidelines for fractures of the proximal fifth metatarsal.

Anatomic Considerations

It is helpful to divide the proximal fifth metatarsal into three regions (Figure 15-14). The most proximal region, the metatarsal styloid, is susceptible to avulsion fractures from a forceful pull of the lateral band of the long plantar ligament and peroneus brevis tendon. These common fractures almost always do well with minimal treatment. The middle region, the metaphyseal–diaphyseal junction, includes the joint between the base of the fourth and fifth metatarsals. This region receives less blood supply. Consequently, fractures in this region heal more slowly and can be more problematic than styloid fractures. The third region, the proximal diaphysis, is susceptible to a specific stress fracture that is notoriously slow to heal.

Table 15-2	*Management Guidelines for Proximal Fifth Metatarsal Fractures*		
	STYLOID AVULSION	METAPHYSEAL–DIAPHYSEAL JUNCTION	DIAPHYSEAL STRESS
		INITIAL TREATMENT	
Splint type and position	Firm-soled shoe	Lower extremity splint or cast Ankle at 90 degrees	Lower extremity splint or cast Ankle at 90 degrees
Initial follow-up visit	4 to 7 days	3 to 5 days	3 to 5 days
Patient instruction	Weight bearing as tolerated	Non–weight bearing	Strict non–weight bearing
		FOLLOW-UP CARE	
Cast type and position	SLWC if significant symptoms Ankle at 90 degrees	SLNWBC Ankle at 90 degrees	SLNWBC Ankle at 90 degrees
Length of immobilization	2 weeks maximum	6 to 10 weeks	Up to 20 weeks
Healing time	4 to 8 weeks	6 to 12 weeks	Up to 20 weeks
Follow-up visit interval	Every 2 to 4 weeks	At 6 to 8 weeks to document any healing	Every 4 to 6 weeks
Repeat radiography interval	May be done at 6 to 8 weeks to document healing	At 6 to 8 weeks to document healing 4 weeks later if necessary If symptoms worsen after healing (rule out recurrence)	Every 4 to 6 weeks If symptoms worsen after healing (rule out recurrence)
Patient instruction	Advance activity as tolerated	Gradually advance activity after cast removed	Strict non–weight bearing Cautiously advance activity after cast removed
Indications for orthopedic referral	Displaced >3 mm	Displaced Nonunion at 3 months Patient reluctant to undergo up to 3 months of casting	Consider in all cases, especially types II and III Not healed at 3 to 4 months Recurrence

SLNWBC, short-leg non–weight bearing cast; SLWC, short-leg walking cast.

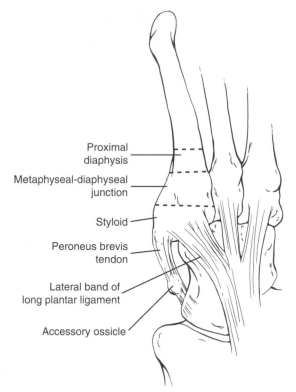

FIGURE 15-14 The three regions of the proximal fifth metatarsal. Fractures of the styloid heal well with minimal treatment. Fractures of the metaphyseal–diaphyseal junction are slow to heal. Fractures of the proximal diaphysis are at risk of delayed healing, nonunion, and recurrence.

Avulsion Fractures of the Styloid

Mechanism of Injury

Avulsion fractures of the styloid are probably the most common fractures of the lower extremity and are often missed because the cause of injury is identical to that of a lateral ankle sprain (i.e., inversion of the ankle, often with plantarflexion). In fact, patients with this fracture commonly complain mainly of having a "twisted ankle." The area of tenderness overlaps the areas of tenderness present with lateral ankle sprains, and the fracture is often inadequately detected on ankle radiographs. To avoid missing these fractures, the physician must palpate the proximal fifth metatarsal of any patient with an inversion ankle injury and order a radiographic series of the foot if tenderness is present at this site.

For many years, the avulsion fracture of the styloid was thought to result from a sudden, forceful pull of the peroneus brevis tendon. Recent studies suggest that the avulsion likely results from the pull of both this tendon and the plantar aponeurosis.[11]

Clinical Presentation

Pain, swelling, ecchymosis, and an ability to bear weight are similar to those seen with moderate ankle sprains. Compared with sprains, the swelling associated with an avulsion fracture is often localized to a smaller, more inferior area. The patient has point tenderness over the base of the fifth metatarsal.

Imaging

Avulsion fractures of the proximal fifth metatarsal occur in the styloid region and are almost always transverse (see Figures 15-6 and 15-15). Rarely are they displaced more than 1 to 2 mm. Accessory ossicles are commonly seen proximal to the base of the fifth metatarsal. In general, these are easily distinguished from fracture fragments by their smooth, rounded contour (see Figure 15-15). Fracture fragments, on the other hand, generally have one straight or irregular edge that lacks cortication. The apophysis of the fifth metatarsal, seen during childhood, also may be mistaken for a fracture. This is discussed later under Pediatric Considerations.

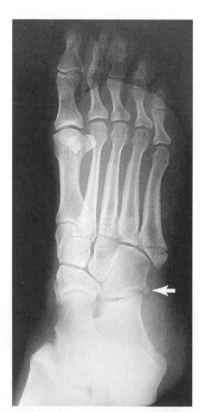

FIGURE 15-15 Minimally displaced avulsion fracture of the fifth metatarsal styloid. Note the incidental finding of an accessory ossicle adjacent to the proximal aspect of the cuboid (*arrow*). Such ossicles are common in this area and may be mistaken for fracture fragments.

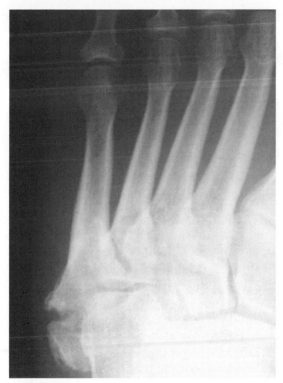

FIGURE 15-16 Nonunion of a proximal fifth metatarsal avulsion fracture 9 months after injury. Note the widened fracture line with sclerotic edges. The patient was asymptomatic except for minimal discomfort with prolonged walking.

Indications for Orthopedic Referral

Patients with avulsion fractures of the styloid rarely need referral. If the fragment is detached and displaced more than 3 mm, more aggressive treatment may be required, and referral should be considered.

Initial Treatment

If nondisplaced, these fractures nearly always do well even with minimal treatment.[6,12] In a small randomized study, treatment with a soft dressing was compared with a short-leg cast. Treatment with a soft dressing led to faster return to function with no adverse impact on healing.[13] In most cases, initial icing and elevation, followed by use of a firm-soled shoe for 4 to 8 weeks is the only treatment required. Crutches (or a walker for elderly patients) are often needed initially and may be replaced with a cane as symptoms subside. Initial follow-up can be done in 4 to 7 days to assess symptoms and mobility. At this point, some patients continue to experience significant discomfort. In such cases, a short-leg walking cast may improve symptoms substantially. Casting should be limited to 2 weeks because its drawbacks probably

outweigh its benefits if continued for a longer period of time.

Subsequent follow-up should occur at 2- to 4-week intervals until the patient has resumed most normal activities. In most cases, symptoms are minimal by 3 to 4 weeks after injury. Radiographic healing is usually apparent by 6 to 9 weeks.[13] Repeat radiographs are rarely necessary earlier unless symptoms worsen.

Return to Work or Sports

With styloid fractures, the physician need not limit the patient's weight bearing or other activities beyond what is necessary for symptom control. The patient can use comfort as a guide and progressively increase activities as tolerated. If additional activity produces greater pain or tenderness, activities should be scaled back. After symptoms subside, activity can again be gradually increased. Full recovery is likely to take several months. In a small prospective study, all patients returned to preinjury functional status by 1 year, but only 20% had done so by 3 months and 85% by 6 months.[12] As with all fractures, the more the clinician and patient focus on rehabilitation, the faster the return to full function.

Complications

The ankle's ROM may decrease during treatment, especially if casting was necessary. This condition should respond readily to appropriate ROM and stretching exercises. Occasionally, radiographic healing is delayed or does not occur. Fibrous union usually produces excellent results. Hence, patients having fractures with apparent nonunion (i.e., no apparent radiographic healing) (Figure 15-16) rarely need referral unless significant symptoms persist.

Pediatric Considerations

During late childhood and adolescence, an apophysis (growth center for a tendon insertion) is usually seen at the base of the fifth metatarsal (Figure 15-17). The apophysis is important for two reasons. First, if physicians are not aware that an apophysis is located in this area, they often misinterpret a normal apophysis as a fracture. Second, the apophysis may be fractured (avulsed) during twisting injuries. In fact, avulsions of the apophysis are the second most common fracture of the fifth metatarsal in children.[14] A normal apophysis can be differentiated from a fracture by its lack of tenderness and its orientation: the apophysis lies parallel to the long axis of the metatarsal, but styloid fractures are almost always transverse (see Figures 15-6, 15-15, and 15-16). Tenderness over the apophysis after acute injury would suggest avulsion of the apophysis. If displacement is minimal,

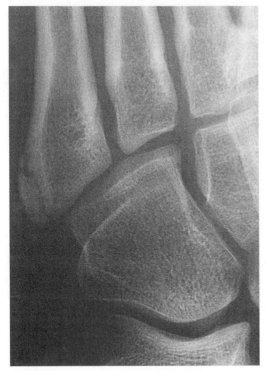

FIGURE 15-17 Apophysis of the proximal fifth metatarsal. Note that whereas the lucency is oriented parallel to the long axis of the fifth metatarsal, nearly all fractures of this area are oriented transverse to the long axis. A thickened rim, analogous to a cortex, is apparent along the length of the apophysis.

comparison views of the other foot may be helpful in evaluating the injury. Nondisplaced and minimally displaced avulsions of the apophysis are treated with a short-leg walking cast for 3 to 6 weeks.[14] Apophysitis should be considered if tenderness is present but radiographic findings are normal and no history of acute trauma exists. This condition typically responds to nonsteroidal anti-inflammatory agents and rest.

Although the apophysis is commonly fractured, it is not the most common site. As with adults, avulsion of the styloid is the most common fracture of the proximal fifth metatarsal in children (see Figure 15-6).[14] Treatment of styloid avulsions in children is similar to that in adults. However, because casts offer more protection and symptom control, they are used more commonly with children.

Fractures of the Metaphyseal–Diaphyseal Junction

Acute fracture of the metaphyseal–diaphyseal junction bears the name of Sir Robert Jones, who described it in 1902.[15] In the ensuing years, the eponym "Jones' fracture" has been applied to other fractures of the proximal fifth metatarsal. In fact,

the term is probably applied more often to stress fractures of the diaphysis than to true Jones' fractures. This, plus the fact that stress fractures may also occur at the metaphyseal–diaphyseal junction, has caused much confusion. This confusion can be avoided by describing proximal fifth metatarsal fractures by their location (styloid, metaphyseal–diaphyseal junction, or proximal diaphysis) and type (acute versus stress).

Mechanism of Injury

Acute fractures of the metaphyseal–diaphyseal junction generally result from a sudden force under the lateral aspect of the distal fifth metatarsal. This injury may occur when a person lands on the side of the foot after stumbling. Direct blows can also fracture this area, and chronic overloading may lead to stress fractures of the area.

Clinical Presentation

Pain is generally localized to the midportion of the lateral border of the foot. Swelling is initially limited to this area but may later spread, particularly if the foot is not kept elevated. Weight bearing is difficult, if not impossible, and distinct point tenderness is present at the fracture site. Most patients with stress fractures of the metaphyseal–diaphyseal junction have a prodrome of gradually increasing pain.

Imaging

A typical example is shown in Figure 15-18, A. The fracture is transverse and extends into the joint between the bases of the fourth and fifth metatarsals. Initially, the medial cortex may appear intact, but it later shows the fracture as well. In some cases, the medial border is obviously disrupted from the start, often with comminution. Significant displacement is very unusual. Stress fractures may occur in this region, although they are usually seen more distally. Radiographic findings that would suggest a stress fracture include a widened fracture line and medullary sclerosis (Figure 15-19, B). Stress fractures are discussed more fully later under Stress Fractures of the Fifth Metatarsal Diaphysis.

Indications for Orthopedic Referral

Indications for emergent referral are the same as discussed above for metatarsal shaft fractures. Displaced fractures of the junction, which are quite unusual, require internal fixation. If characteristics of a stress fracture are present (a widened fracture line or medullary sclerosis), early operative repair should be considered to avoid the possibility of prolonged immobilization and to decrease the chance of nonunion. If, however, the fracture has acute rather than stress characteristics, it will

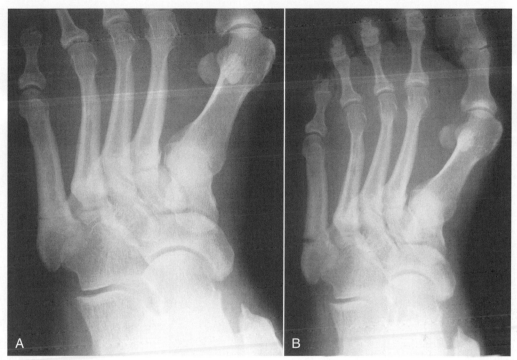

FIGURE 15-18 A, Nondisplaced fracture of the fifth metatarsal metaphyseal–diaphyseal junction. As expected with fractures in this area, the fracture line extends medially toward the joint between the bases of the fourth and fifth metatarsals. **B,** Follow-up radiograph after 6 weeks in a non–weight-bearing cast. The fracture line is now more prominent, indicating no radiographic healing. The patient was referred for internal fixation.

usually heal well. Healing may take 2 to 3 months, repeat fractures may occur, and there may be a prolonged delay in return to sports (≤6 months).[16] For these reasons, initial screw fixation may be indicated for certain individuals with acute fractures of the metaphyseal–diaphyseal junction, including patients who are unwilling to accept the prospect of prolonged immobilization or recovery (especially athletes). Conservative management includes non–weight bearing and close follow-up of healing. Unless the primary provider is comfortable providing this, patients with these fractures should be referred to an orthopedist.

Initial Treatment

Initially, a lower extremity splint can be applied. As with all lower extremity fractures, icing and elevation are particularly important to help control swelling and thereby allow timely casting on follow-up. The patient should be given crutches, bear no weight on the foot, and be reevaluated in 3 to 5 days.

Follow-Up Care

If swelling allows, a short-leg cast or boot may be applied at the first follow-up visit. Although some authorities recommend a walking cast, others recommend a non–weight-bearing cast. The

difference of opinion seems to be related to whether these fractures are discussed as distinct entities or lumped together with styloid fractures. Most experts who consider this fracture as a distinct entity recommend non–weight-bearing casts.[16-19] Recent clinicians allow use of a non–weight-bearing cast boot.[16] After 6 to 8 weeks of non-weight-bearing immobilization, the patient should be evaluated out of the cast. If neither clinical nor radiographic healing is apparent (Figure 15-18, B), a non–weight-bearing cast should be reapplied for 4 more weeks or the patient referred for consideration of internal fixation. If only clinical healing has occurred (i.e., pain and tenderness are absent or minimal but radiographs show no healing), internal fixation remains an option. Alternatively, protection could be continued with a brace or cast boot, which could be removed intermittently to allow the patient to start ROM and strengthening exercises. If radiographic healing has not occurred by 3 months, the patient should be referred to an orthopedist.

After both radiographic and clinical healing has occurred, protection may be discontinued and the patient may gradually resume activities. If activities are increased too rapidly, the fracture may recur. Referral for physical therapy may be necessary, especially if immobilization was prolonged.

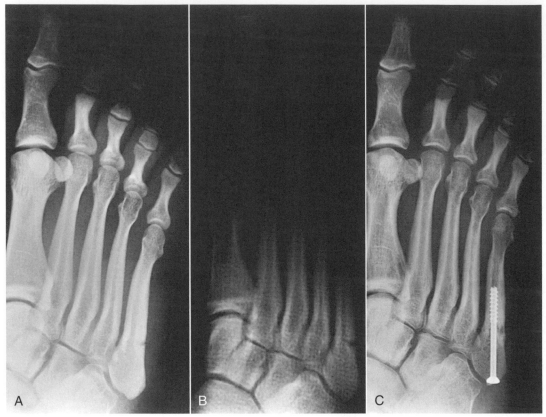

FIGURE 15-19 A, Type I stress fracture of the fifth metatarsal diaphysis. The patient sustained the fracture after minimal impact while playing basketball, suggesting that the bone had been weakened by repetitive stress. **B,** Six weeks later, a radiograph taken in the cast shows that the fracture line has widened to a type II lesion. **C,** The patient underwent screw fixation, and recovery was rapid thereafter.

Return to Work or Sports

Considerations are similar to those described previously under Metatarsal Shaft Fractures, with two exceptions. Because treatment involves prolonged non–weight bearing, patients with nonsedentary jobs should not work unless they can be temporarily reassigned to job tasks that do not require walking, standing, or use of their feet. Metaphyseal–diaphyseal fractures tend to recur, so athletes with these fractures should resume running and other sports activities much more cautiously than described for shaft fractures. A progressive increase in discomfort or tenderness at the fracture site suggests weakening of the fracture and should prompt an immediate, sharp reduction in activity. After these symptoms subside, a more gradual increase in activity can be attempted.

Complications

Delayed union and nonunion are the primary complications. Occasionally, painful disuse osteoporosis or CRPS occurs. Osteoporosis generally improves as weight bearing and activities resume.

Pediatric Considerations

Acute fractures of the metaphyseal–diaphyseal junction may occur in adolescents. If the physician can confidently differentiate these injuries from stress fractures, they may be managed as described previously for adults.

STRESS FRACTURE OF THE FIFTH METATARSAL DIAPHYSIS

Although commonly referred to as a "Jones' fracture," a stress fracture of the fifth metatarsal diaphysis is actually distinct from the fracture first described by Jones. Unlike other metatarsal stress fractures, which tend to heal well, stress fractures of the fifth metatarsal diaphysis have a pronounced tendency toward delayed healing, nonunion, and recurrence. Fortunately, these fractures are relatively uncommon.

Mechanism of Injury

Stress fractures of the fifth metatarsal diaphysis generally occur in young male athletes. They are associated with repetitive stresses on the lateral foot. Repetitive pivoting is a common cause, and basketball players are probably most susceptible to this fracture. The fracture may result from chronic overload on the bone or from a change in routine that suddenly subjects the bone to greater stress. "Acute on chronic" injuries may also occur, in which a relatively mild force fractures a bone weakened by chronic stress.

Clinical Presentation

As with other stress fractures, patients usually experience a prodrome of gradually increasing pain. Pain typically increases during activities that stress the bone. If the forces applied continually exceed the bone's ability to repair itself, symptoms gradually increase, and the cortex progressively becomes fatigued. The weakened cortex may suddenly fracture, usually as the result of relatively low forces. In most cases, the patient seeks medical treatment before a frank fracture occurs. The amount of tenderness and swelling vary, and the diagnosis is often suggested more by history than by examination. Stress fractures are often misdiagnosed as soft tissue injuries. This is especially true early in their course when symptoms are relatively mild and radiographs may appear normal.

Imaging

The fracture line is characteristically located just distal to the joint between the bases of the fourth and fifth metatarsals (see Figure 15-14). Plain radiographs have traditionally been used to stage stress fractures, and treatment recommendations are typically based on plain radiograph findings. For prognostic purposes and treatment planning, stress fractures of the proximal fifth metatarsal can be divided into three types. Type I includes early fractures, with radiographic findings ranging from normal to the appearance of a clear fracture line (Figure 15-19, A). Type II fractures have a widened fracture line and medullary sclerosis, indicating a fracture more resistant to treatment (Figure 15-19, B). If nonunion develops (type III), the intramedullary canal is obliterated.

If a stress fracture of the proximal fifth metatarsal is suspected but radiography findings are negative, confirmation of the diagnosis is desirable. Note that this contrasts with the management of stress fractures of the metatarsal shaft, in which presumptive therapy is entirely reasonable (discussed earlier in chapter). Greater certainly of the diagnosis is desirable with proximal fifth metatarsal stress fractures because they are more difficult to treat and more likely to lead to complications. Bone scans are able to detect stress fractures earlier than plain radiographs, but they are nonspecific and require several steps. MRI has largely replaced bone scans for the early detection of stress fractures because of its greater sensitivity and specificity.[8,20,21] However, the specificity of MRI is not perfect for early fractures, and clinical correlation is very important.

Indications for Orthopedic Referral

Because of the tendency toward poor healing, orthopedic consultation should be obtained for all stress fractures of the fifth metatarsal diaphysis. Many practitioners advocate early screw fixation, especially for athletes, because this allows much earlier return to sports. Type I fractures are likely to do well with conservative treatment provided the patient complies with directives, avoids weight bearing as instructed, and does not return to full activity too quickly. Even under optimal conditions, the fracture may require up to 20 weeks of immobilization, and nonunion may still occur. After a widened fracture line or nonunion is present (i.e., types II and III fractures), referral for internal fixation is recommended.

Initial Treatment

If referral is planned or swelling prevents casting at the first visit, crutches should be provided, icing and elevation initiated, and the patient instructed to strictly avoid any weight bearing on the affected foot. Although not essential, a lower extremity splint may provide some comfort and remind the patient not to bear weight. Adhering to these measures should allow any significant swelling to subside in 3 to 5 days, so follow-up and casting can take place at that time. Alternatively, a cast boot can be used. However, it is much easier to bear weight in a cast boot, and the patient must be committed to no weight bearing.

Follow-up Care

Conservative treatment with cast immobilization is an option for many type I fractures. It is also occasionally an alternative for patients with type II fractures, especially if they are less active and are not bothered by the prospect of prolonged immobilization. If conservative treatment is elected by the patient and physician, a short-leg non–weight-bearing cast or cast boot is applied and use of crutches continued. Follow-up can occur at 4 to 6 week intervals and should include radiographs and examination out of the cast at each visit. When radiographs and examinations indicate that healing is well under way, protected weight bearing may begin with use of a short-leg walking cast or boot for 2 to 4 weeks. If radiographs, symptoms, and examination findings continue to improve, protection may be discontinued, and former activities can be very gradually resumed. It is important to stress that increasing the activity level too quickly may cause a recurrence of the fracture. Orthopedic consultation should be considered if healing has not occurred by 3 to 4 months or if radiographs reveal the development of a type II or III fracture.

Return to Work or Sports

With intramedullary screw fixation, weight bearing may begin as early as 2 weeks, and running may begin as early as 7 weeks. Recovery is much more prolonged with conservative therapy, and it may take 6 to 8 months before running is possible. Patients with nonsedentary jobs should pursue temporary reassignment to alternative job tasks that do not require walking, standing, or the use of their feet. After weight bearing is begun, increases in job activities should be very gradual to avoid a recurrence of the fracture. After the cast is discontinued, physical therapy is highly recommended, especially if prolonged casting was necessary. Restricting increases in walking to 10% to 20% per week are prudent. Any recurrence of symptoms or tenderness should prompt a sharp reduction in activity and reevaluation for recurrence of the fracture. If walking is well tolerated for 1 to 2 months and does not cause a recurrence of symptoms, short periods of running on a soft, even surface may be started and progressively increased at 10% to 20% per week. Pivoting, jumping, kicking, and other activities that place high stress on the metatarsals should be postponed until late in the rehabilitation process.

Complications

Nonunion, prolonged healing times, and recurrence of the fracture are the primary difficulties encountered with stress fracture of the fifth metatarsal diaphysis. CRPS and disuse osteoporosis occasionally develop.

Pediatric Considerations

Stress fractures of the fifth metatarsal diaphysis may occur in adolescents. Nonunion of this fracture is said to be much less common than in adults, making conservative therapy a more attractive option.[12] However, essentially all adolescents with this fracture are athletes who would prefer early return to activity, and one study documented a high fracture recurrence rate in adolescent athletes who were treated conservatively.[14] Hence, referral of these patients for consideration of early internal fixation is desirable in all cases.

REFERENCES

1. Armagan OE, Shereff MJ. Injuries to the toe and metatarsals. *Orthop Clin North Am.* 2001;32:1-10.
2. Saraiya MJ. First metatarsal fractures. *Clin Podiatr Med Surg.* 1995;12:749-758.
3. Heckman JD. Fractures and dislocations of the foot. In: Rockwood CA, Green DP, Buckholz RW, Heckman JD, eds. Fractures in Adults. 4th ed. vol II. Philadelphia: Lippincott-Raven; 1996:2362-2382.
4. O'Malley MJ, Hamilton WG, Munyak J. Fractures of the distal shaft of the fifth metatarsal: "dancer's fracture." *Am J Sports Med.* 1996;24(2):240-243.
5. Greene WB, ed. Essentials of Musculoskeletal Care. 2nd ed. Rosemont, IL: American Academy of Orthopedic Surgeons; 2001:453.
6. Quill Jr GE. Fractures of the proximal fifth metatarsal. *Orthop Clin North Am.* 1995;26:353-361.
7. Simons SM. Foot injuries in the runner. In: O'Connor FG, Wilder RP, eds. Textbook of Running Medicine. New York: McGraw-Hill; 2001:213.
8. Fredericson M, Jennings F, Beaulieu C, Matheson GO. Stress fractures in athletes. *Top Magn Reson Imaging.* 2006;17:309-325.
9. Hatem SF. Imaging of Lisfranc injury and midfoot sprain. *Radiol Clin North Am.* 2008;46:1045-1060.
10. Ribbons WJ, Natarajan R, Alavala S. Pediatric foot fractures. *Clin Orthop Relat Res.* 2005;432:107-115.
11. Theodorou DJ, Thoedorou SJ, Kakitsubata Y, et al. Fractures of proximal portion of fifth metatarsal bone: anatomic and imaging evidence of a pathogenesis of avulsion of the plantar aponeurosis and the short peroneal muscle tendon. *Radiology.* 2003;226:857-865.
12. Egol K, Walsh EK, Rosenblatt K, Capla E, Koval KJ. Avulsion fractures of the fifth metatarsal base: a prospective outcome study. *Foot Ankle Int.* 2007;28:581-583.
13. Weiner BD, Linder JF, Giattini JFG. Treatment of fractures of the fifth metatarsal: a prospective study. *Foot Ankle Int.* 1997;18:267-269.
14. Herrera-Soto JA, Scherb MN, Duffy MF, Albright JC. Fractures of the fifth metatarsal in children and adolescents. *J Pediatr Orthop.* 2007;27:427-431.
15. Jones R. Fracture of the base of the fifth metatarsal by indirect violence. *Ann Surg.* 1902;35:697-700.
16. Chuckpaiwong B, Queen RM, Easley ME, Nunley JA. Distinguishing Jones and proximal diaphyseal fractures of the fifth metatarsal. *Clin Orthop Relat Res.* 2008;466:1966-1970.
17. Nunley JA. Fracture of the base of fifth metatarsal: the Jones fracture. *Orthop Clin North Am.* 2001;32:171-180.
18. Lawrence SJ, Botte MJ. Jones' fractures and related fractures of the proximal fifth metatarsal. *Foot Ankle.* 1993;14:358-365.
19. Landorf KB. Clarifying proximal diaphyseal fifth metatarsal fractures. The acute fracture versus the stress fracture. *J Am Podiatr Med Assoc.* 1999;89:398-404.
20. Umans HR. Imaging sports medicine Injuries of the foot and toes. *Clin Sports Med.* 2006;25:763-780.
21. Wall J, Feller JF. Imaging of stress fractures in runners. *Clin Sports Med.* 2006;25:781-802.

16

TOE FRACTURES

Toe fractures account for approximately 8% to 9% of fractures.[1,2] Toe fractures are relatively straightforward to treat, and the outcome is generally excellent. Hence, they are frequently managed by primary care providers. Clinicians who understand basic principles of fracture care and can recognize the occasional toe fracture that requires referral should be able to confidently manage the vast majority of closed toe fractures. In isolated settings, primary care physicians with additional experience in fracture management sometimes treat selected open toe fractures.

TOE FRACTURES

Anatomic Considerations

The second through fifth digits generally have three phalanges, and the first toe (and occasionally the fifth) has two. Extensor and flexor tendons insert on the proximal aspects of the middle and distal phalanges. These are occasionally injured in toe fractures. The interosseous, abductor, adductor, and flexor muscles insert at the bases of the proximal phalanges. The action of these muscles occasionally contributes to displacement of proximal fragments. Sesamoid bones may be present in the flexor tendons beneath the distal head of the metatarsals and are most frequently seen adjacent to the first metatarsal head.

Mechanism of Injury

Nearly all toe fractures result from either a stubbing injury or a heavy object being dropped on the toe. Infrequently, hyperextension of the toe results in avulsion or spiral fractures. Open toe fractures are often caused by lawnmower injuries or other sharp trauma.

Clinical Presentation

The severe pain experienced at the time of fracture often subsides, leading many patients to doubt the presence of a fracture. A dull throbbing usually follows, however, and most patients who do not seek care initially do so after 24 to 48 hours. When examined, the fractured toe usually appears swollen, and point tenderness is present at the fracture site. Ecchymosis, a subungual hematoma, or both may be present. Injuries to the nail and nail plate are commonly associated with toe fractures, and a laceration of the nail plate often indicates an open fracture. In the case of the great toe, tense swelling may be apparent, particularly if a crushing injury has occurred. Significant crushing of overlying soft tissue and subsequent necrosis and sloughing may convert a closed fracture to an open one. The neurovascular status of the toes should be documented, although nerve or arterial injury associated with toe fractures is rare except with severe displacement and lawnmower-type injuries.

Because the bones are small and tenderness is generally diffuse, it is often difficult to pinpoint or confirm a nondisplaced toe fracture on clinical grounds alone. Displaced toe fractures, on the other hand, are generally quite evident. Not enough soft tissue exists to disguise the rotation, angulation, or shortening that accompanies most displaced toe fractures.

Imaging

In most cases, anteroposterior (AP), lateral, and oblique views are necessary to diagnose toe fractures. The oblique view is often more helpful than the lateral because overlying shadows may make the lateral view difficult to interpret. Most toe fractures are nondisplaced or minimally displaced. Spiral fractures may show shortening and rotation, and transverse fractures occasionally have significant angulation. Toe fractures are frequently comminuted, particularly if the distal phalanx is involved. Two phalanges are often fractured simultaneously, and intraarticular fractures are fairly common (Figure 16-1).

Indications for Orthopedic Referral

Open toe fractures involving the proximal phalanx should be referred promptly, as should severe crush injuries and those with vascular compromise. Open

319

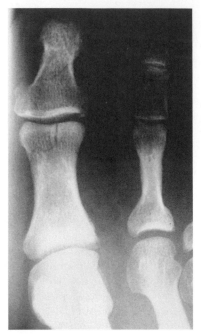

FIGURE 16-1 Fracture of the great toe with involvement of proximal and distal phalanges. Note that the distal phalanx fracture is comminuted with two separate fracture lines extending into the interphalangeal joint. The proximal phalanx fracture also extends into the joint.

fractures of the distal phalanx should either be referred right away or treated promptly as described below. Referral is preferable if the patient is diabetic or immunocompromised, the wound is grossly contaminated, or presentation is delayed.

The great toe plays an important weight-bearing role. Because deformity, decreased range of motion, and degenerative changes may interfere with patients' activities, great toe fractures are much more likely than other toe fractures to require referral.[3] Displaced intraarticular fractures of the great toe generally require internal fixation, as do great toe fractures that spontaneously become displaced when traction is released after reduction. Compared with the great toe, the lesser toes are extremely forgiving. Referral is rarely necessary unless the fracture is open or difficult to reduce. Other indications for referral (greater and lesser toes) include fracture dislocations and nondisplaced intraarticular fractures with fragments that involve more than 25% of the joint surface.

Initial Treatment

Table 16-1 summarizes management guidelines for toe fractures.

Nondisplaced Fractures

Most nondisplaced toe fractures can be treated by buddy taping to the adjacent toe (Figure 16-2).

Table 16-1	*Management Guidelines for Toe Fractures*
	INITIAL TREATMENT
Splint type and position	Buddy taping to adjacent toe
	Consider SLWC with toe platform for great toe fracture
Initial follow-up visit	Within 1 to 2 weeks
	Within 3 to 5 days for open fracture to assess wound
Patient instruction	Elevation and icing essential to reduce swelling
	Hard-soled or postoperative shoe
	FOLLOW-UP CARE
Cast or splint type and position	Buddy taping with hard-soled shoe
Length of immobilization	Buddy taping: 3 to 6 weeks
	SLWC with toe platform: 2 to 3 weeks followed by buddy taping and hard-soled shoe
Healing time	4 to 6 weeks
Follow-up visit interval	Every 2 to 4 weeks
Repeat radiography interval	7 to 10 days for intraarticular fractures or fractures requiring reduction only
Patient instruction	Persistent pain possible for several weeks or months
	Hard-soled shoe worn as much as possible during healing
Indications for orthopedic consult	Displaced intraarticular fractures
	Fracture dislocations
	Intraarticular fractures involving >25% of the joint
	Unstable displaced fracture of the first toe
	Open fractures of the proximal phalanges
	Open fracture of the distal phalanx with gross contamination or delayed treatment

SLWC, short-leg walking cast.

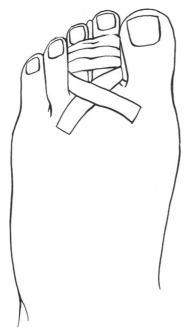

FIGURE 16-2 Buddy taping of the second and third toes. Gauze padding is inserted between the toes to prevent maceration, and the nail beds are exposed to avoid concealing rotational deformity.

Gauze padding should be placed between the two toes. The tape should not cover the nail beds to avoid obscuring rotational deformity until it is too late to correct the problem. After buddy taping, pain can be minimized by using ice, elevation, and appropriate medication (over-the-counter analgesics or mild narcotics for the first few days). Overzealous application of ice could potentially injure a digit, so direct contact of ice with skin should be avoided, and icing should be limited to 20 minutes per hour. Elevation should be strongly encouraged to help reduce pain and swelling.

Pain control and early mobility can be greatly enhanced by having the patient wear firm-soled shoes that have had part of the top cut out to uncover the injured toe. Patients can be instructed to do this at home with a pair of shoes they do not mind sacrificing. A wooden postoperative shoe is a good alternative. Some patients require crutches initially. A subungual hematoma or nail bed injury should be managed as described in Chapter 3.

Many fractures of the great toe require a short-leg walking cast with a toe platform (Figure 16-3). Some authorities recommend this type of immobilization for better pain control in great toe fractures.[4] Other experts favor buddy taping.[3,5,6] Overall, a cast with a platform provides better immobilization. It is usually the preferred initial treatment for nondisplaced intraarticular fractures of the great toe and for great toe fractures that require reduction and are stable. Cast immobilization also should be considered for lesser toe fractures if buddy taping does not provide adequate pain relief.

Displaced Fractures: Closed Reduction Technique

Displaced fractures can almost always be reduced by use of longitudinal traction, either manual or with finger traps. An object such as a pencil may be placed in the webspace to stabilize the proximal fragment, act as a fulcrum, and assist with the reduction.[7] In most cases, applying an ice pack for 10 to 20 minutes beforehand provides adequate anesthesia. A digital nerve block may be required for a more difficult reduction. A satisfactory position is nearly always maintained with buddy taping alone in the lesser toes. The great toe may require casting (Figure 16-3). For great toe fractures, if displacement recurs when traction is released (i.e., the reduction is not stable), the patient should be referred for open reduction or percutaneous pinning.

Treatment of Open Distal Phalanx Toe Fractures

Open toe fractures are fairly common and are easier to treat than other open fractures. They demand prompt definitive treatment and fairly close follow-up, which pose a dilemma for patients who live in isolated areas. Consequently, some primary care physicians manage these fractures.

Open toe fractures usually result from crushing or slicing injuries to the distal phalanx. Often, either the overlying skin is gone or its viability is questionable. After a digital block is performed, the first priority is to aggressively clean the wound followed by profuse irrigation with sterile saline. Any nonviable tissue should be debrided, with the exception of thicker flaps of skin that may be used later to close the defect. Next, the wound should

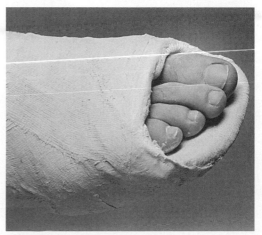

FIGURE 16-3 Toe platform extension of cast used in the treatment of great toe fractures.

be closed so that no bone is exposed to air. In many cases, this can be done by suturing the remaining skin and soft tissue into positions that close the defect and cover the exposed bone. A flap of skin may be hanging by only a small anchor or may even be completely detached when the patient arrives for treatment. Even if long-term viability is in doubt, reattaching the skin is often worthwhile. The reattached skin will at least provide a temporary physiologic covering that will later slough or be debrided. Surprisingly often, it will reestablish itself and heal nicely. When the skin is missing, the physician can only approximate the underlying soft tissue and allow the wound to heal by secondary intention.

If the bony edge of the fractured phalanx protrudes up to or beyond the margins of the soft tissue, simple closure is impossible. In these cases, it is necessary to debride the bone back to a point that allows complete closure. This can be done rather easily under digital block anesthesia. A rongeur (Figure 16-4) is used to progressively

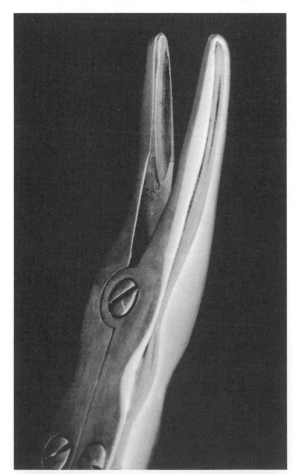

FIGURE 16-4 A rongeur used to debride the edge of exposed fractures. Note the scooped-out recess within the jaws and the sharp jaw edges.

remove small chunks of bone until the tissues beside the bone can be pulled together and closed over the bone without creating too much tension on the skin or soft tissue.

Although the effectiveness of prophylactic antibiotics for such wounds is not clear, prescribing an antibiotic effective against common skin flora is standard practice. Oral cephalexin has been a common choice, sometimes in conjunction with an initial one-time dose of intravenous cefazolin. However, with the rising prevalence of community acquired methicillin-resistant *Staphylococcus aureus* (MRSA), coverage for this would be prudent. Patient instructions should emphasize elevation of the injured toe as much as possible until follow-up. The patient should be told to return promptly if signs of infection develop. Unless swelling becomes very problematic, ice should probably not be used if the skin or soft tissue overlying the fracture appears at high risk of necrosis. Follow-up should take place in 3 to 5 days and then weekly thereafter, with suture removal in 10 to 14 days. Follow-up radiographs should be performed approximately every 2 weeks until healing occurs to monitor for evidence of osteomyelitis. Purulent drainage or other signs of infection would necessitate referral or change of antibiotics. If symptoms persist more than a few days after treatment or if radiographic changes suggest osteomyelitis, referral or appropriate osteomyelitis treatment should be instituted. Referral is recommended for most diabetic patients, patients with advanced peripheral vascular disease, and immunocompromised patients.

Follow-up Care

Buddy taping, maintained for at least 3 to 4 weeks, constitutes definitive care for most toe fractures. If healing is slow or pain is persistent, taping may be needed for up to 6 weeks. If a walking cast with toe plate is used, immobilization should be continued for 2 to 3 weeks and then replaced with buddy taping and a hard-soled shoe. Patients should ideally be seen within 1 to 2 weeks after injury. However, many patients with toe fractures fail to return for scheduled appointments unless they are wearing a cast or experience bothersome symptoms. Follow-up radiographs are generally not needed unless the fracture is intraarticular or involves the great toe or the patient is failing to improve with treatment. Only great toe fractures that require reduction or involve a substantial area of the joint surface are likely to require radiographs 7 to 10 days after injury to ensure good alignment before healing.

Return to Work or Sports

Patients with lesser toe fractures may set their own pace for returning to activities using their symptoms as a guide. Speed of recovery varies widely. For patients who are returning to running or kicking sports, some authorities recommend an additional 3 weeks of immobilization. Activities should be resumed more gradually with first toe fractures, especially unstable ones. Significant stresses on the first toe should be avoided until healing is complete.

Complications

In general, toe fractures heal well. Fractures involving joint surfaces may lead to severe degenerative changes, and malunions with significant angulation may interfere with normal function of the foot. The second through fifth toes withstand degenerative changes and decreased motion extremely well unless the metatarsophalangeal (MTP) joint is involved. The lesser toes also tolerate angulation well unless it leads to excessive contact and friction with the ground or top of the shoe. Unacceptable angulation of a lesser toe is rare if the fracture is reduced and buddy taped. Angulation and degenerative changes of the great toe more often cause persistent symptoms. Thus, near-anatomic reduction of great toe fractures is preferable, particularly if joint surfaces are involved. Uncommon complications include osteomyelitis after an open fracture and vascular injury associated with crush or severe lacerating injuries.

Pediatric Considerations

Treatment of pediatric toe fractures, which is similar to that described previously for adults, requires a few special considerations. The epiphysis of the proximal phalanx of the first toe is often bipartite, simulating a Salter-Harris type III fracture. If the toe is nontender, no treatment is indicated. If tenderness is present, comparison views of the other great toe, comparison with an atlas of normal radiographic variants, or referral to an orthopedic surgeon can help discern whether a fracture is indeed present. With the exception of first toe fractures in older children, few pediatric toe fractures need reduction. Remodeling will restore the vast majority to acceptable if not perfect position.

Because of the first toe's critical role in the normal gait, patients with displaced first toe fractures should usually be referred. In the management of first toe fractures, it is crucial to look for and correct any rotational deformity. This deformity, which is present with most spiral fractures, does not remodel well and can seriously impair normal function of the first toe. It can generally be detected by comparing the nails of the first and second toes. After reduction, both should lie in the same plane. The nails of the opposite foot can be used for comparison if needed. Casting with a toe platform (Figure 16-3) or leaving the nail beds exposed after buddy taping allows monitoring for loss of position after taping or reduction. A cast with toe platform is recommended for active children.[7] Pediatric toe fractures are generally healed in 3 weeks. Follow-up can cease at 3 weeks unless concern exists about possible injury to a physis. In this case, periodic follow-up over 1 to 2 years allows early detection and intervention should abnormal growth occur.

TOE DISLOCATIONS

Dislocations of the interphalangeal (IP) or MTP joints are fairly common. They usually result from hyperextension during a stubbing or kicking injury. Although the diagnosis may be obvious on inspection, it is still important to obtain radiographs before treatment to detect fracture dislocations (for which patients should usually be referred) and to avoid misdiagnosing a displaced fracture as a dislocation. Figure 16-5 shows a dislocation of the proximal IP joint, demonstrating the importance of multiple views.

Dislocated toes are generally easy to reduce. After a digital block, longitudinal manual traction is applied to the distal portion of the digit and it is manipulated back into position. It may be necessary to slightly accentuate the deformity before applying traction or manipulation.[6] Closed reduction may be prevented by interposition of soft tissue between the dislocated bones or by button-holing of the proximal bone through the plantar plate–sesamoid complex. Open reduction is generally necessary if initial closed attempts fail.

Buddy taping for 3 weeks is used to maintain the reduction. Longer periods of taping may be needed for very active people and athletes. No special considerations are necessary for pediatric toe dislocations except for being especially alert to the possibility of concurrent injury to the physis adjacent to the dislocated joint.

SESAMOID FRACTURES

Mechanism of Injury

The sesamoid bones are occasionally fractured when subjected to a direct blow during jumping. However, stress fractures are more common and result from chronic repetitive trauma during activities such as long-distance running or dancing.[8] The medial sesamoid of the great toe is subject to the most force and is most commonly fractured. However, fractures may occur of the lateral sesamoid as well as the sesamoids of the lesser toes.

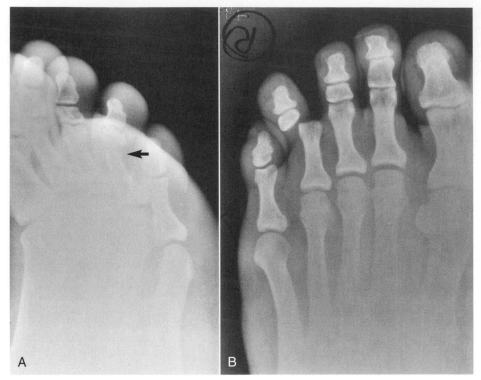

FIGURE 16-5 A, Oblique view of an injured fourth toe. Apart from narrowing or disappearance of the proximal interphalangeal (IP) joint space (*arrow*), the radiograph appears normal. **B,** Anteroposterior view of the same toe shows obvious dislocation of the proximal IP joint.

Clinical Presentation

Based on history, sesamoid fractures may be confused with toe fractures. However, the tenderness associated with sesamoid fractures is generally located more proximally, with point tenderness beneath the metatarsal head, directly below the sesamoid. Prodromal symptoms are often present, and swelling is often minimal. Because sesamoid bones are enclosed in the flexor tendons, extension of the toe at the MTP joint is painful. Rising up on the tiptoes is also painful. Inflammation of the structures adjacent to a sesamoid (sesamoiditis) may be difficult to distinguish from an early stress fracture, but initial treatment is the same for both conditions.

Imaging

Sesamoid fractures are usually transverse. The fracture may be difficult to detect on radiographs because of overlying shadows, so tangential views of the sesamoids may be helpful. When evaluating radiographs, the examiner should remember that bipartite and tripartite sesamoids are common. These have smooth, rounded, corticated surfaces and are bilateral in 85% of patients (Figure 16-6). Fractures have abrupt edges and no cortication along the inner edges of the fragments (Figure

16-7). Comparison views can help distinguish an acute fracture from a partite sesamoid if doubt remains after examination of the initial radiographs. Rarely, magnetic resonance imaging may be needed to distinguish the two. Stress fractures are unlikely to be visible on plain radiographs until symptoms have been present for several weeks. If no fracture is visible initially, radiographs may be repeated after 2 to 3 weeks of conservative treatment.

Indications for Orthopedic Referral

The rare sesamoid fracture that is either open or displaced requires referral. Nonunion after 4 to 6 months and persistent symptoms after 4 to 6 months also merit referral.

Treatment

Several treatment options exist, including immobilization with either a well-padded walking cast or a hard soled shoe (or molded orthotic) combined with a "donut" or "C" pad over the area of the sesamoid.[3,8] Rest is also important and may require partial or complete non–weight bearing if needed for symptom control. Treatment is generally required for 6 to 8 weeks. If a cast is used initially, it should be discontinued after 3 to 4 weeks

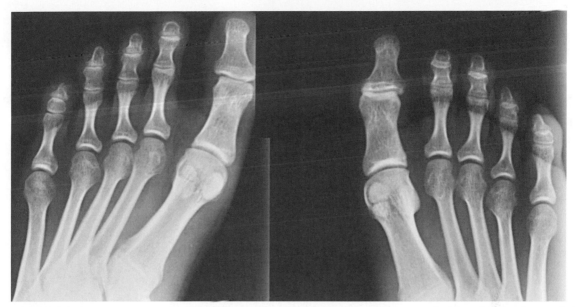

FIGURE 16-6 Anteroposterior views of both feet demonstrating bilateral bipartite sesamoids. Note the smooth, rounded edges.

and the patient switched to a firm shoe with donut pad for another 4 to 6 weeks for comfort. The clinician can generally treat early stress fractures by prescribing a firm shoe, a donut pad, and avoidance of high-impact activities. Stress fractures may take

3 to 6 months to heal. In some patients with sesamoid fractures, significant pain persists after treatment. Excision or bone grafting of the sesamoid may be indicated but only if symptoms have been present for more than 6 months.

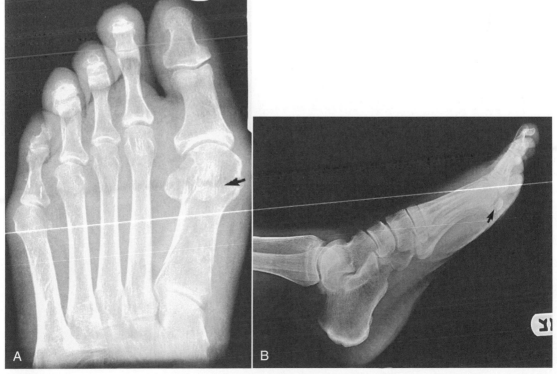

FIGURE 16-7 Anteroposterior (A) and lateral (B) views of the foot showing a transverse fracture of the medial sesamoid (*arrows*). Note the irregular, noncorticated fracture line. A nondisplaced fracture of the first metatarsal shaft is also present.

REFERENCES

1. Hatch RL, Rosembaum CI. Fracture care by family physicians. A review of 295 cases. *J Fam Pract.* 1994;38: 238-244.
2. Eiff MP, Saultz J. Fracture care by family physicians. *J Am Board Fam Pract.* 1993;6:179-181.
3. Mittlmeier T, Haar P. Sesamoid and toe fractures. *Injury.* 2004;35(suppl 2):S87-S97.
4. Elleby DH, Marcinko DE. Digital fractures and dislocations. *Clin Podiatr.* 1985;2:233-245.
5. Ly PN, Fallat L. Hallus fractures: diagnosis and treatment. *J Foot Surg.* 1992;31:332-341.
6. Armagan OE, Shereff MJ. Injuries to the toes and metatarsals. *Orthop Clin North Am.* 2001;32:1-9.
7. Schnaue-Constantouris EM, Birrer RB, Grisafi PJ, Dellacorte MP. Digital foot trauma: emergency diagnosis and treatment. *J Emerg Med.* 2002;22:163-170.
8. Hockenbury RT. Forefoot problems in athletes. *Med Sci Sports Exerc.* 1999;31(7 suppl):S448-S458.

17

FACIAL AND SKULL FRACTURES

Co-Author: John Malaty

As long as they are aware of certain pitfalls, primary care providers can manage nasal fractures, including reduction of selected displaced fractures. Fractures of other facial bones and the skull are rarely seen in primary care settings but are commonly encountered in rural, emergency department, and urgent care settings. In these instances, primary care clinicians will be called on to evaluate the patient for other serious associated injuries, stabilize the patient, provide initial care of the fracture, and arrange appropriate specialty evaluation and treatment. This chapter focuses on the management of nasal fractures and on the recognition of other facial and skull fractures and the potentially serious injuries that often accompany them.

In adults, nasal fractures are the most common fracture of the face and skull and rank third in incidence of any fracture (only clavicle and wrist fractures are more common).[1-3] The mandible and zygoma are also frequently fractured. Facial fractures are encountered fairly frequently in primary care and sports medicine settings. Sports-related facial fractures account for 10% to 42% of all facial fractures.[4] Other common etiologies include motor vehicle accidents (MVAs), altercations and assaults, and falls. Facial fractures are two to three times more common in males than in females, and the incidence of each type of fracture is related to each bone's anatomic location and strength.[5] The force required to cause fractures of the face and skull increases as follows: nasal bones, zygoma, mandible (angle), frontal bone, maxilla and mandible (midline), and supraorbital rim.

Facial and skull fractures are less common in children than in adults and follow a different pattern. In the age group 0 to 18 years, mandible fractures are most common (32.7%), followed by nasal (30.2%) and maxillary or zygoma (28.6%) fractures. The likelihood of these fractures increases with age. In adolescents, these fractures are more common, and mandible fractures predominate. In toddlers and infants, cranial and central facial injuries are more common. Unless the cause of injury is obvious (e.g., MVAs), one must always consider the possibility of child abuse when evaluating such fractures. As with adults, boys experience more facial fractures than girls (5:3 ratio).[6,7]

Many fractures in adults and children can be prevented. It is estimated that more than 250,000 people per year in the United States (many of whom are children) have sports-related facial trauma because of inadequate safety equipment such as improper seat belt or helmet use.[8]

NASAL FRACTURES

Anatomic Considerations

External Nose

The paired nasal bones lie at the top of the nose (Figures 17-1 to 17-3), encompassing approximately one-third of the nose's length. Each nasal bone attaches superiorly to the frontal bone and inferiorly to an upper lateral cartilage, a curved triangular cartilage that articulates in the midline. The paired upper lateral cartilages are critical in defining nasal appearance, and fractures involving these can lead to significant cosmetic deformity. They also articulate with the paired lower lateral cartilages at a complex fibrous joint that functions as a nasal valve, a critical region that affects nasal airflow (see Figure 17-2). Fracture involving the nasal valve can cause problems with nasal obstruction (chronic nasal congestion). The external cartilage structure of the nose (upper and lower lateral cartilages) encompasses approximately two-thirds of the length of the nose. The medial canthal ligament of the eye attaches near the base of the upper nose (see Figure 17-1). After significant trauma to this area, this ligament may rupture or be displaced, which causes the globe to move laterally. This produces an abnormally wide spacing of the eyes, referred to as telecanthus.

Nasal Septum and Surrounding Structures

The nasal septum is composed of cartilage and bone, similar to the external nose. The cartilaginous septum is the primary structure separating the

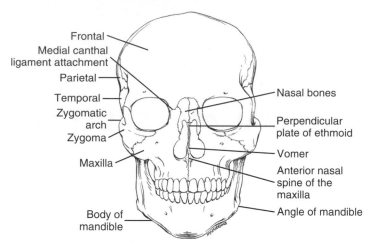

FIGURE 17-1 Anterior view of the skull and facial bones.

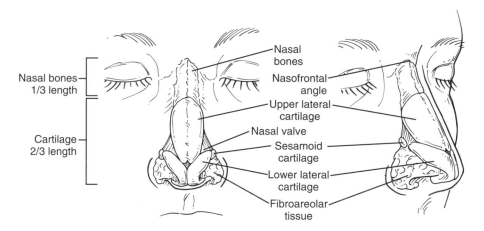

FIGURE 17-2 Anatomy of the external nose.

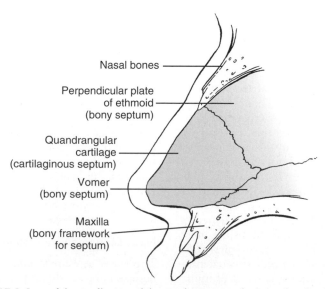

FIGURE 17-3 Lateral (sagittal) view of the nasal septum and surrounding bony framework.

right and left nasal passages and is composed of the quandrangular cartilage (which is quandrangular shaped, as the name implies). This is the structure that you first see when you look at the septum during an internal nasal examination. This is also the structure that typically causes congenital septal deviation. Thus, when fractured or dislocated, it causes nasal obstruction (chronic nasal congestion). The quadrangular cartilage is supported by the anterior nasal spine of the maxilla inferiorly and by the bony septum (perpendicular plate of the ethmoid posteriorly and the vomer inferiorly) (see Figures 17-1, 17-3, and 17-4). The cartilaginous and bony septum is lined by mucoperichondrial and mucoperiosteal soft tissue, respectively, that has a robust vascular supply. This is responsible for epistaxis at the time of injury. This can also cause a septal hematoma, which if not immediately treated can lead to necrosis of the cartilaginous septum with resulting severe cosmetic deformity and functional impairment.

Mechanism of Injury

Nasal fractures result from direct blows. The direction and force of the blow determine the injury pattern. Lateral blows of moderate force result in a depressed, inward fracture of the ipsilateral nasal bone. With greater forces, the contralateral nasal bone may outfracture or the septum may fracture. Inferior blows commonly result in isolated septal fractures as the quandrangular cartilage is torn from its inferior attachment to the anterior nasal spine of the maxilla, vomer, or both. Frontal blows, if sufficiently forceful, may produce a septal

fracture with splaying of the nasal bones. These fractures have a higher likelihood of being comminuted. If the injury was caused by very high force, it is important to consider the possibility of concomitant serious injuries to the neck, face, or skull.

Clinical Presentation

The primary goal of the initial visit is to assess the patient adequately. Clots and dried blood (both internal and external) should be removed to allow adequate visualization. Topical decongestants can be used to control epistaxis and should be used to improve visualization during internal nasal examination (anterior rhinoscopy). Examination of the cranial nerves is advisable, with particular attention paid to cranial nerves II to VIII (vision, extraocular movements, facial sensation, facial movement, and hearing and balance). Associated injuries may include septal hematoma, fractures of other facial bones, dental fractures or injuries, and cerebrospinal fluid (CSF) leakage. CSF leakage sometimes is not evident until several days after acute injury. If evident on initial presentation, the patient needs careful evaluation and management to decrease the risk of associated complications.

Typical symptoms of a nasal fracture include localized pain and edema. Visual inspection and palpation should be performed systematically to evaluate for nasal bone depression, displacement, or mobility. These findings confirm nasal bone fracture in the majority of cases. A major pitfall is not doing this portion of the examination adequately in the presence of edema, which can mask

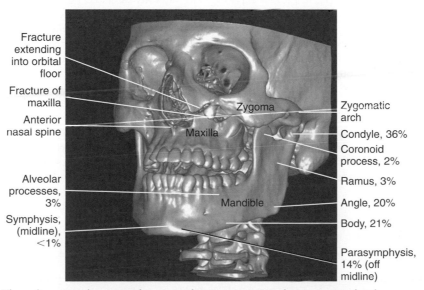

FIGURE 17-4 Three-dimensional computed tomography reconstruction demonstrating facial anatomy, including the different regions of the mandible with their incidence of fractures. Fractures of the maxilla are also visualized.

a fracture during an inadequate examination. One must also visually inspect and palpate the nasal cartilage (upper and lower lateral cartilages) and septal cartilage (quadrangular cartilage) for fracture or dislocation from their fibrous attachments. Both epistaxis and ecchymosis around the nose or eyes suggest the presence of a nasal fracture, although one can have a nasal fracture without these. Overlying abrasions or lacerations may also be noted. Patients generally report difficulty breathing through the affected side(s) of the nose. The patient (or a companion if present) commonly reports that the shape of the nose has changed. Visual changes, telecanthus (abnormally wide spacing of the eyes), paresthesias, or altered sensorium strongly suggests other potentially serious injuries.

Hematomas of the nasal septum are relatively common. They require drainage as soon as possible to prevent necrosis of the cartilaginous septum and a saddle deformity that is difficult to correct surgically. After draining the septal hematoma, packing or nasal splints should be used to compress the septum on both sides to prevent reaccumulation of the hematoma (see below for more details). An early septal hematoma may be mistaken for a deviated septum. Palpating the septum can help distinguish between the two: an acute hematoma will feel soft, fluctuant, and raised. If a hematoma cannot be excluded, otolaryngology consultation is recommended.

Imaging

Radiographs are not required in the assessment of nasal fractures. History and physical examination is more accurate for the detection of a clinically significant fracture. In fact, some clinicians report that radiographs fail to show 47% to 60% of clinically detectable fractures. Furthermore, radiographs of the nose are often misleading and difficult to interpret. After studying the time and expense of radiographs, many surgeons have concluded that radiographs are not justified in the evaluation of nasal fractures.[9] The primary role of imaging in patients with suspected nasal fractures is to evaluate for fractures of other facial bones. Computed tomography (CT) scans are superior to plain radiographs for this purpose, especially when assessing patients with more serious injuries or concerning signs or symptoms such as visual complaints or facial paresthesia.

Indications for Referral

Emergent Referral (Within 30 to 60 Minutes)

Blows to the face that fracture the nose may cause other more serious injuries. A history of loss of consciousness or neck pain necessitates

appropriate workup, referral, or both. Fractures of other facial bones and any neurologic or cranial nerve deficit also require emergency consultation. The most common cranial nerve-related signs and symptoms are visual impairment, diplopia, facial paresthesia or numbness, facial paresis, and hearing or balance problems). Telecanthus should be suspected whenever the distance between the eyes (from the medial canthus of the right eye to the medial canthus of the left) exceeds the distance from the medial canthus to the lateral canthus of each eye. This condition should also prompt emergency consultation. Patients with septal hematomas should immediately be referred to an otolaryngologist for drainage if one is uncomfortable doing this procedure. If adequate drainage has been performed (as described below), close follow-up should be scheduled as a nonemergent referral.

Nonemergent Referral (Within Several Days)

Patients with complex nasal fractures should be referred to an otolaryngologist or plastic surgeon for consideration of open reduction or repair. These include septal fractures and dislocations, the presence of a septal hematoma, and nasal bone fractures with external nasal deviation greater than half of the width of the nasal bridge (the nasal bridge is the widest part of the top third of the nose). In these cases, open reduction or repair is recommended. A fractured or dislocated septum can interlock with the nasal bones when twisted, which makes successful closed reduction improbable. Furthermore, if the septum is fractured or dislocated, open reduction is necessary to avoid further damage to the septum. If the nasal bones are laterally deviated by more than half the width of the nasal bridge, successful closed reduction is also unlikely. Open fractures (lacerations that communicate with the fracture site) generally do well with vigorous irrigation, repair of the laceration, and a course of oral antibiotics, but telephone consultation in such cases is recommended, at a minimum. Otolaryngology or plastic surgery consultation is also advisable for lacerations involving the nasal cartilage. If a septal hematoma has been drained or packed by a primary care provider, prophylactic oral antibiotics for staphylococci and streptococci is recommended with close otolaryngology follow-up, both to reevaluate the septum and consider open reduction or repair.

Initial Treatment

Epistaxis

In the majority of cases, epistaxis is well controlled with topical decongestant sprays with or without direct pressure. Short-term, liberal use of these sprays is safe in the absence of hypertensive urgency or emergency. If epistaxis is persistent, one may reapply topical decongestant and hold direct pressure for 5 to 10 minutes (the patient or a staff member can assist with direct pressure). Direct pressure should be applied by squeezing at the lower third of the nose (at the junction of the upper and lower lateral cartilages, applying firm pressure unto the septum). This area is compressible and often helps reduce bleeding while minimizing discomfort for the patient (as opposed to the upper third of the nose, which is not compressible and more likely to be painful). Both for safety and to reduce epistaxis, it is important to ensure the patient does not have uncontrolled hypertension (treat hypertension if systolic blood pressure >160 mm Hg or diastolic blood pressure >110 mm Hg).

If the patient has brisk epistaxis not responding to the above measures, nasal packing may be required. If nasal packing is used, prophylactic oral antibiotics to cover staphylococci and streptococci should be considered (while nonabsorbable packing is in place) given the potential risk of toxic shock syndrome. Although no large trials have addressed the prevalence of toxic shock syndrome with nonabsorbable nasal packing, case reports have been published in the adult and pediatric literature, and information has been extrapolated from similar cases with tampon use.[10,11] Given the potential to prevent a life-threatening complication and medicolegal concerns, prophylactic antibiotics are suggested. If packing is required, other factors must also be considered. If the patient is taking an antiplatelet agent or anticoagulant, one should assess the risks and benefits in that particular patient and consider holding the medication. Nasal packing should not performed if one suspects a LeFort fracture (dissociation of the maxilla from the skull). A LeFort fracture can be recognized clinically by forward motion of the maxilla when one stabilizes the skull and gently pulls the upper teeth forward. This fracture (discussed below under Fractures of Other Facial Bones: Clinical Presentation) must be stabilized before nasal packing.

Septal Hematoma

These need to be drained immediately. The technique for this drainage is similar to an incision and drainage of an abscess, a skill possessed by most primary care providers. One important difference is that the mucoperichondrial lining overlying the quadrangular cartilage is very thin. Thus, after local anesthesia is given (described below under Indications and Technique for Closed Reduction), the incision is made superficially through this thin mucoperichondrium to avoid scoring the underlying cartilage. Injection of adequate local anesthetic between the mucoperichondrium and underlying cartilage helps separate the two anatomic layers. After the hematoma is drained, Silastic splints or packing must be placed bilaterally to firmly support both sides of the cartilaginous septum to prevent reaccumulation of the hematoma (described below under Indications and Technique for Closed Reduction). If drainage of a septal hematoma is performed, referral to an otolaryngologist for close follow-up and consideration of open reduction or repair of the fracture is needed. At the time of drainage, a minimum of telephone consultation is recommended. Oral antibiotics are recommended for staphylococci and streptococci coverage while the nonabsorbable packing is in place.

Isolated, Simple Nasal Bone Fractures

Nasal fractures are considered simple if external nasal deviation is less than half the width of the nasal bridge, the nasal septum is not fractured or dislocated, septal hematoma is not present, the fracture is closed, and no other facial fractures are present. Simple fractures may be either unilateral or bilateral. Nondisplaced simple fractures require no specific treatment other than control of epistaxis (if present) and ice or analgesia because these patients do not have nasal obstruction or cosmetic deformity. Closed reduction is recommended for displaced simple fractures. The best time for successful reduction is within 3 hours of injury before the onset of significant edema. If this is not possible, reduction should be delayed 3 to 7 days to allow edema to improve and facilitate improved reduction.[12] If reduction is delayed, closed reduction within 2 weeks of injury yields the best results. After associated injuries have been excluded and epistaxis is controlled, the patient may be discharged with instructions. Go to Expert Consult for the electronic version of a patient instruction sheet for nasal fractures.

Informed Consent Before Closed Reduction

Patients should be counseled that they may have persistent cosmetic deformity or nasal obstruction (chronic nasal congestion) after closed reduction but that it is being offered to give them a chance at improved cosmesis or function without requiring an open procedure. These are the main points of patient dissatisfaction and must not be underemphasized. If the patient is dissatisfied after closed reduction, he or she still has the option to have an open septorhinoplasty procedure in the future by an otolaryngologist or plastic surgeon. Patients should also be counseled on other risks, including unsuccessful closed reduction necessitating open reduction, increased epistaxis, infection, and allergic reaction to medication.

Indications and Technique for Closed Reduction of Isolated, Simple Nasal Fractures

Closed reduction is indicated if significant cosmetic deformity or significant functional impairment (obstruction of the nasal passage) is present. Closed reduction provides good results in approximately three-fourths of these patients, provided the reduction is timed as described above. Injuries that are more complex or older may require open reduction under general anesthesia. Open reduction may also be necessary if closed reduction does not produce acceptable results.

Although the operating room with short-term anesthesia may seem like the optimal setting for closed reduction of simple nasal fractures, this is rarely done unless other surgeries are needed simultaneously. Data do not demonstrate better outcomes for closed reduction performed in the operating room under sedation compared with other settings with local anesthesia. If feasible, premedication should be done with an oral or intravenous benzodiazepine 30 minutes before reduction. Topical lidocaine, cocaine, benzocaine, or tetracaine should be obtained to obtain intranasal anesthesia. Using bayonet forceps, the practitioner should layer thin gauze packing soaked with the anesthetic in the nose and remove the packing after 5 minutes. The anesthetic must extend far enough into the nose to reach the mucosa underlying the nasal bones because this area must be anesthetized. Some also advocate supplementing topical anesthesia with injection of 1% lidocaine with 1:100,000 epinephrine along the dorsum of the nose (externally) lateral to the midline bilaterally and at the base of the anterior septum (internally). This optional, additional anesthesia can further block the infratrochlear, infraorbital, greater palatine, and superior alveolar nerves. If these injections are performed, the practitioner should wait 10 to 20 minutes before reduction. After removing the anesthetic-soaked gauze, the practitioner should measure the distance from the external nostril rim to the top of the nasal bone, where the nasal bone articulates with the frontal bone (may be measured externally using the instrument). A blunt instrument such as an elevator (if available) or the rigid steel handle of a scalpel is inserted into the nasal cavity to a point that is 1 cm less than the previously measured distance (nasal fracture rarely involves the strong nasofrontal suture and manipulation of this area produces unnecessary mucosal damage or bleeding). The depressed nasal bone fragment is elevated by applying a moderate amount of force in the direction opposite the fracturing force (almost always anterolaterally). At the same time the instrument is being moved laterally, if the contralateral nasal bone is displaced laterally, it should also be pushed medially into proper alignment by the contralateral hand with the fingers placed gently over the fracture site to feel when the bone is adequately reduced. If not adequately reduced, a repeat attempt should be made (through whichever nostril will best facilitate reduction, which is often the nostril ipsilateral to the worst fracture).

The cosmetic result should be assessed by the physician and patient. The nose should be examined internally to be sure the nasal passages are adequately patent and the septum is not significantly deviated. If the septum is found to be deviated after reduction, it should be relocated in the maxillary groove. Bleeding is likely to occur after reduction, but this can generally be controlled with a topical decongestant spray (see Epistaxis above).

After reduction, an external nasal splint should be applied. If prefabricated nasal splints are not available, a splint may be made as follows: The practitioner cuts several layers of plaster cast material into a triangular shape 2 inches in length. He or she covers the surface of the nose with tape (applying it in left-to-right direction), wets the splint material, gently molds the splint over the nose (paying particular attention to the upper third of the nose where the nasal bones have been reduced), and holds it in place with tape (applied in a left-to-right direction). The splint should be removed in 1 to 2 weeks. If there is concern that the reduction of the nasal bones is unstable or that the septum may be unstable, one may place Silastic septal splints covered in antibiotic ointment for 3 to 7 days or pack the nose with antibiotic ointment-soaked gauze strip packing for 2 to 3 days to support the reduction. This may be challenging because the packing must be inserted high into the nose to support the nasal bones. Referral may be preferable if instability is anticipated.

Follow-up Care

Patients will need follow-up to have the external nasal splint or nasal packing removed at the time intervals noted above. At that time, one can start gentle normal saline nasal irrigations twice daily, as tolerated, to decrease nasal obstruction from blood clots or debris. The final cosmetic and functional result should be assessed approximately 1 month after reduction, at which time a repeat external and internal nasal examination should be performed. If the patient is not satisfied with the cosmetic result or a nasal passage is significantly obstructed, the patient should be referred for consideration of operative repair. As already discussed, patients accept this referral much better if the possibility was explicitly discussed before the initial reduction.

Return to Work or Sports

Most individuals with an isolated, simple nasal fracture can return to work in 1 to 2 weeks after the acute healing period and to noncontact sports in 2 weeks. It takes approximately 3 weeks for initial healing of a nasal fracture in a healthy adult. Nasal fractures are relatively common in contact sports. Athletes who are anxious to return to contact sports before a nasal fracture is fully healed should ensure they have adequate head and face protection. They may benefit from use of a facial brace that covers the nose. Ready-made braces are available and work well if a good fit can be found. If an athlete is unable to find a commercial brace that fits well, an orthotist can make custom facial protection. After a patient has a nasal fracture, he or she is more prone to having a recurrent fracture in the setting of nasal trauma. The risk for recurrent fractures increases if open surgery was required.

Complications

The most common complication is a lingering unsatisfactory result (cosmetic or functional), which may necessitate open reduction. Another typical complication is persistent epistaxis (managed as discussed above). Necrosis of the septum after septal hematoma and complications resulting from unrecognized associated injuries may also occur. If the patient has evidence of new, clear rhinorrhea after a nasal fracture, one must consider a CSF leak. This often results from a fracture of the cribriform plate of the ethmoid or anterior cranial fossa (see Figure 17-5). If not recognized and managed properly, this injury can lead to potentially fatal meningitis or pneumocephalus. A salty taste or new anosmia may also be found in patients with CSF leaks, but these are often not present.

Pediatric Considerations

Nasal fractures are less common in children than in adults. This is not surprising because children's noses do not protrude as far, and they have an increased cartilage-to-bone ratio (more flexible). This also explains why children have more cartilaginous septal fractures and fewer nasal bone fractures.

Pediatric nasal fractures are more challenging to manage than those of adults. The nasal fracture may be subtle and may injure a growth center. In addition, an adequate examination can be difficult to perform without placing the patient under sedation or general anesthesia. Septal hematomas are also more common in children. Referral for evaluation and treatment is preferable. If this is not possible, pediatric nasal fractures may be managed as described previously for adults. Open reduction of a nasal fracture in a child is rarely indicated because of the risk of growth center injury during surgery.

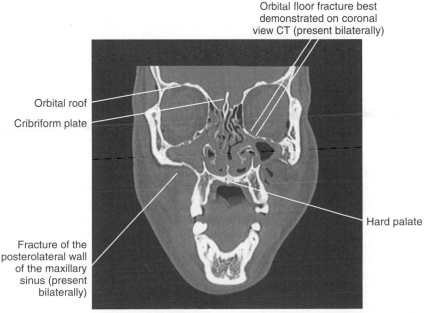

FIGURE 17-5 Coronal computed tomography scan demonstrating the anatomy of the cribriform plate and fractures of the orbital floor and maxillary sinus (posterolateral wall). This image highlights the importance of coronal imaging to evaluate horizontally oriented fractures and structures.

Fractures of Other Facial Bones

The other bones of the face are less exposed than the nasal bones and, with the exception of bones lining the orbit, are substantially stronger. Hence, these bones fracture less often. When they fracture, the injury is usually caused by high-force trauma and may be accompanied by other serious injuries that can be life threatening. A detailed discussion of the management of these fractures is beyond the scope of this book. Virtually all of them require the expertise of an otolaryngologist, maxillofacial surgeon, or plastic surgeon. Therefore, this section focuses on the recognition of these injuries and their potential complications. General management considerations are also discussed.

Anatomic Considerations

The facial bones are illustrated in Figures 17-1 and 17-4. Although not as exposed as the nasal bones, the zygoma and the angle of the mandible are considerably more exposed than the other facial bones. They protrude away from the face to form its distinct contour (see Figure 17-4). The zygoma and portions of the mandible also have decreased strength compared with some of the other facial bones. These bones, therefore, fracture more often than other facial bones. The U-shaped mandible is composed of two hemimandibles fused at the midline. The mandible articulates with the skull, forming a ringlike structure. As such, it usually fractures in two places, much like the ringlike structure of the pelvis. Figure 17-4 illustrates the different portions of the mandible and the frequency at which they fracture in adults.[13] The fracture rate correlates to the strength of that portion of the mandible and its exposure to injury. The midline symphysis of the mandible, where a strong fusion of the two hemimandibles occurs developmentally, is more resistant to fracture than the other parts of the mandible. The condyle requires the least amount of force to fracture and is the most commonly fractured part of the mandible. It articulates with the skull at the temporomandibular joint (TMJ), which can be palpated immediately anteriorly to the tragus during deglutition (chewing). The TMJ is composed of the mandibular condyle articulating with the temporal bone, an articular cartilage disc between the two, a joint capsule, three ligaments, and the lateral pterygoid muscle. Each of these has an important role in deglutition. A fracture, disruption, or malfunction of any of these portions of the TMJ can lead to future pain and dysfunction of the TMJ (TMD). Dental injury and malocclusion may also lead to TMD.

The bones that form the floor and walls of the orbit are exceptionally thin. They can be fractured by forces as small as a finger jabbed into the eye.

A branch of the second division of cranial nerve V exits the skull through the infraorbital foramen. Fractures of this region of the face may affect this nerve, leading to paresthesia of the cheek.

Mechanism of Injury

Facial fractures result from forceful, direct blows to the face. Common causes include automobile accidents, falls, sports injuries, and direct blows from weapons or fists. Fractures to the floor and medial wall of the orbit usually result from milder trauma such as a modest blow to the globe or eye socket. The force of the blow is transmitted to these very thin bones, causing them to collapse downward or outward. In edentulous patients, the mandible becomes substantially weaker, predisposing it to fracture with comparatively small forces.

Clinical Presentation

In addition to inspection and palpation, assessment of patients with suspected facial fracture should include a careful oral and cranial nerve examination. Cranial nerves II to XII should be assessed, including sensation in all three divisions of the trigeminal nerve (V1–V3). Facial fractures may be accompanied or suggested by abnormalities found on these examinations. The clinician should also be alert for the presence of altered mental status, shock, paralysis, respiratory distress, and other symptoms of serious injury that may accompany facial fractures.

With most facial fractures, swelling and ecchymosis develop rapidly. If oral examination reveals ecchymosis of the gums of the upper teeth, a maxillary fracture is likely. Ecchymosis of the floor of the mouth is virtually pathognomonic for mandible fracture. However, this sign is often absent, and its absence does not exclude a mandible fracture. Oral examination should also evaluate for oral mucosal lacerations requiring suturing, lip lacerations, and dental injury (especially to prevent risk of tooth aspiration). Loss of sensation in the distribution of the third division of the trigeminal nerve (lower lip and chin region) suggests mandibular fracture, with disruption of the inferior alveolar nerve as it runs through the mandibular canal. Trismus (difficulty opening the mouth normally) is highly suggestive of a mandible or lover maxillary fracture, as is a sensation of malocclusion (i.e., the bite is abnormal and the teeth do not meet properly). With greater displacement, an open bite deformity may be present. This occurs when the teeth on one side come together normally but the teeth on the fractured, depressed side do not (Figure 17-6).

Midface

The midface includes the zygoma, maxilla, and naso-orbital area. When these are fractured,

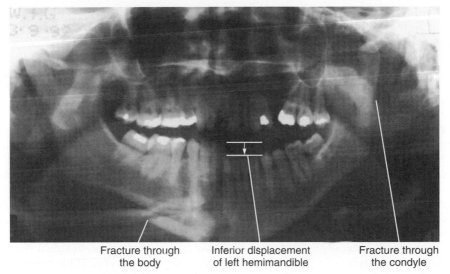

Fracture through   Inferior displacement   Fracture through
the body   of left hemimandible   the condyle

FIGURE 17-6 Fractures through both the right body of the mandible and the left condyle. This condyle is also displaced. These fractures cause inferior displacement of the left hemimandible, producing a left-sided open bite deformity. (*From Raby N, Berman L, DeLong G*. Accident and Emergency Radiology: A Survival Guide. *Philadelphia, WB Saunders, 1995.*)

obvious asymmetry of the face may exist. This is especially true if the zygomatic arch is fractured because it significantly contributes to facial contour. Palpation of the face often reveals a stepoff or focal pain or crepitus at the fracture site. With severe injuries to the midface, the face may be abnormally elongated or flattened. Fractures of the maxilla can affect the second division of cranial nerve V, causing numbness or paresthesias of the upper cheek.

Fractures of the midface may also dissociate the maxilla from the rest of the head (LeFort fractures, discussed below under Classifications). When this has occurred, it can be diagnosed clinically. In these fractures, the maxilla can be pulled forward by stabilizing the head with one hand, grasping the upper teeth with the other, and gently pulling forward. Maxillary fractures may also produce periorbital ecchymosis ("raccoon eyes"), as well as a cracked pot sound when the upper teeth are tapped with a metal instrument. Swelling, bleeding, and secretions may compromise the airway. In the presence of a LeFort fracture, epistaxis should not be controlled with nasal packing. The fracture must be stabilized before nasal packing because even in a LeFort I fracture, the maxilla is mobile. Intubation should be performed to protect the airway and emergent specialty consultation obtained. While waiting for specialty management, gauze bandage rolls may be placed in the mouth to push the soft palate upward, which may help reduce the epistaxis and stabilize a portion of the LeFort fracture. A large gauze bandage roll is preferable to 4 × 4 gauze to decrease the risk of aspirating individual pieces of gauze.

Telecanthus, an abnormally wide spacing between the eyes, may also occur with midface fractures. It should be suspected whenever the distance between the eyes (from the medial canthus of the right eye to the medial canthus of the left) exceeds the distance from the medial canthus to the lateral canthus of each eye. When present after acute trauma, this likely indicates naso-orbital fracture and possible disruption of the medial canthal ligament (see Figure 17-1).

CSF rhinorrhea or middle ear effusion or otorrhea may also occur if the fracture extends into the cranial vault. Thus, anterior rhinoscopy should be performed to look for clear rhinorrhea (CSF leak) or epistaxis (nasal fracture). Similarly, clear middle ear effusion or otorrhea can also indicate CSF leakage, with CSF entering the middle ear space via the eustachian tube (which connects the nose to the middle ear space). This violation of the cranial vault puts patients at increased risk for intracranial complications.

Orbital Floor (Blowout) Fractures

These fractures may be subtle initially. Although periorbital edema and ecchymosis are usually noted, the orbital rim may remain intact without stepoff or point tenderness. Recognition of orbital floor fractures can be improved by suspecting these injuries in all patients who have sustained a blow to the eye and by remaining alert to three important indicators of injury. First, the infraorbital nerve is commonly damaged by blowout fractures. Hence, paresthesia of the cheek should prompt consideration of an orbital blowout fracture. Second, the globe on the fractured side usually sits lower or farther inside (enophthalmos) compared with the normal eye. Third, orbital floor fractures may produce entrapment of the inferior rectus muscle with resulting diplopia, which may only be noted when the patient gazes upward. Similar entrapments of the other extraocular muscles can occur with fractures of the medial wall, lateral wall (Figure 17-7), or roof of the orbit. Thus, when assessing potential facial fractures, it is important to carefully assess and document globe position, extraocular movements, and visual acuity.

Imaging

Interpreting radiographs of the facial bones is challenging. Multiple overlying shadows are apparent, and fractures may be subtle. If a facial fracture is suspected, CT imaging is generally needed to characterize the injury adequately.

Mandible

The mandible is difficult to evaluate fully on the standard Waters, Caldwell, and lateral views of the face. A panoramic radiograph (see Figure 17-6). provides the best plain radiographic visualization of the mandible.[14] Figure 17-6 highlights the ring-like structure of the mandible resulting in two fractures. The combination of these fractures causes inferior displacement of the left hemimandible, which would produce a visible open bite deformity on examination (right-sided teeth would come together, but left-sided teeth would not). This image also demonstrates how overlying shadows can make it challenging to evaluate facial fractures on plan radiographs. Despite its limitations, the panoramic radiograph is the one plain radiograph that provides adequate visualization of all the portions of the mandible, including the ramus, condyle, and TMJ. Panoramic radiographs can be used to further characterize suspected fractures and to rule out occult fractures in patients with suggestive symptoms. Because single fractures of the ring-like mandible are unusual, the physician should always look for a second fracture (as seen in Figure 17-6). With simple mandible fractures, panoramic radiography can fully visualize the fracture. With more complex mandible fractures, CT is a very useful modality (Figure 17-8). If panoramic radiography equipment is unavailable and a mandible fracture is suspected clinically, CT can be used for evaluation. Because CT is frequently used before definitive management by specialists, one should not be hesitant to obtain this if there is a reasonable suspicion of a mandible fracture.

Other Facial Bones

CT has long been recognized as the modality of choice in evaluating patients with craniofacial trauma and is the current standard of care.[15] In emergent situations, initial imaging with 5-mm axial slices may be performed to quickly evaluate for intracranial pathology and facial fractures. However, for complete evaluation of facial fractures in a stable patient, smaller maxillofacial axial slices (i.e., 2-3 mm) should be requested in addition to 5-mm axial slices of the head. When evaluating facial fractures, both coronal and axial views should be obtained. Coronal views (Figure 17-5) better demonstrate fractures of horizontal structures (e.g., the cribriform plate, orbital floor, orbital roof, hard palate, and mandibular rami).

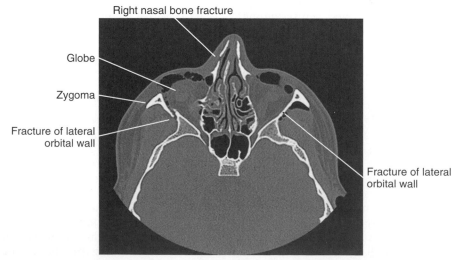

FIGURE 17-7 Axial computed tomography scan demonstrating lateral orbital fractures bilaterally and right nasal fracture.

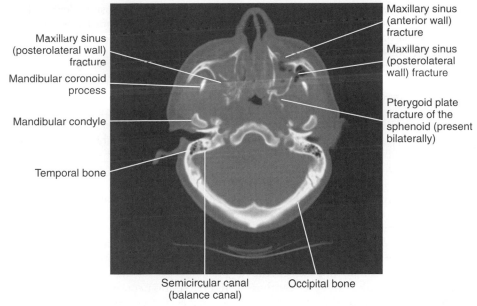

Maxillary sinus (posterolateral wall) fracture
Mandibular coronoid process
Mandibular condyle
Temporal bone

Maxillary sinus (anterior wall) fracture
Maxillary sinus (posterolateral wall) fracture
Pterygoid plate fracture of the sphenoid (present bilaterally)

Semicircular canal (balance canal)
Occipital bone

FIGURE 17-8 Axial computed tomography (CT) scan demonstrating fractures of the maxillary sinuses and pterygoid plates (sphenoid). It also demonstrates the value of CT in visualization of the mandible and skull (temporal bone and occipital bone).

Classification

In midface fractures, the maxilla may become dissociated from the rest of the face and even from the skull. It may, on rare occasion, become impacted. Midface fractures are classified according to the LeFort classification system.

1. A LeFort I fracture is a low maxillary fracture that separates the maxilla at the level of the nasal floor (separation of the lower third of the face from the midface).
2. A LeFort II fracture results in a separation of the central third of the face from the base of the skull.
3. A LeFort III fracture causes a complete separation of the zygomaticomaxillary complex from the base of the skull (separation of the face from the skull).

An injury may produce fractures at different levels on each side of the face, such as a LeFort II on the right and LeFort III on the left.

Indications for Referral

Emergent Referral (30 to 60 Minutes Depending on the Stability of the Patient)

Except with selected nasal fractures, referral is recommended for essentially all patients with fractures of a facial bone. Many need acute or even emergency evaluation by an otolaryngologist, maxillofacial surgeon, or plastic surgeon. At a minimum, virtually all of these fractures should be discussed with a specialist at the time of diagnosis. Some facial fractures can be observed and managed expectantly, but intervention will be necessary if the fracture causes a functional or cosmetic problem.

Initial Treatment

When evaluating a patient with a suspected facial fracture, the primary care provider's initial responsibility is to consider and rule out other more serious injuries. Because the facial injury may be striking, the physician must guard against being distracted from more serious, but less obvious, associated injuries. The principles of advanced trauma support should be applied, first focusing on airway, breathing, and circulation and then performing a brief neurologic assessment and surveying the body for other injuries. Careful attention should be paid to assessing for cervical spine and cerebral injuries. The mouth should be examined. If necessary, gentle suction should be used, and any loose teeth or objects removed to decrease the risk of aspiration. An oral airway can be used provided no fracture of the midface or upper face exists. These injuries are commonly associated with a free-floating maxilla, which can be detected by grasping the upper teeth and pulling forward on the maxilla while steadying the patient's head with the other hand (if mobile, a LeFort fracture is suspected). If not contraindicated by other injuries, rolling the patient over into a semiprone position (head looking downward and to the side) can help maintain the airway. This position allows blood and secretions to flow out with gravity. Intubation should be performed if the airway is compromised or in jeopardy. The nasotracheal route should be avoided because it may result in intracranial placement of the endotracheal tube if the fracture extends into the cranial vault. Cricothyroidotomy may be necessary if oral intubation is impossible.

After other potentially serious injuries have been ruled out or addressed, attention is paid to assessing the fracture and checking for other facial injuries. The cranial nerves, vision, and pupil reactivity should be assessed in all patients. If the eye has been traumatized, a hyphema, lens dislocation, and retinal detachment should be suspected. In patients with more severe facial trauma, the intercanthal distance should be measured. The distance from the inner canthus of the left eye to the inner canthus of the right eye should not exceed the distance from the inner canthus to outer canthus of either eye.

Clear nasal discharge associated with a facial fracture should be assumed to be CSF rhinorrhea until proven otherwise. CSF rhinorrhea, which is commonly associated with LeFort fractures, should also be suspected if bloody secretions produce a halo when dropped onto a piece of tissue or filter paper ("halo" or "ring" sign). The presence of glucose in nonbloody nasal secretions strongly suggests CSF rhinorrhea because nasal mucus normally contains little, if any, glucose. A sample can be sent for evaluation of beta-transferrin for definitive confirmation. Some clinicians recommend antibiotic prophylaxis for patients with a CSF leak, but prospective studies have shown no benefit. Epistaxis may be treated as outlined earlier in this chapter, but it is important to reiterate that nasal packing should be avoided if a LeFort fracture is suspected or present until the patient is stabilized.

Until definitive care can be achieved, treatment should focus on control of pain and swelling. Ice packs and elevation of the patient's head can help alleviate some symptoms.

Follow-up Care

Definitive treatment may be deferred for 3 to 10 days to allow swelling to subside, but many fractures can be treated acutely. Lower maxillary and mandible fractures are usually treated acutely. The most common approach is to use arch bars. One is attached to the upper teeth (maxilla) and one to the lower teeth (mandible). Reduction is accomplished by positioning the fractured bony fragments in such a way that the patient's normal bite is reestablished. The bars are then wired together to maintain this position (maxillomandibular fixation [MMF]). While MMF is being used, it is important to emphasize dental hygiene with routine use of oral antibacterial rinses, such as chlorhexidine, to reduce dental caries.

Return to Work or Sports

Decisions regarding return to work or sport activity are carried out by the specialist caring for the patient and depend largely on the fracture pattern and presence of associated injuries. For athletes, face shields are available to protect the fractured bone and allow earlier return to play.

Complications

The primary complications of facial fractures are those resulting from acute associated injuries. Infections of facial wounds or of the sinuses may also occur. If the fracture extends into the cranial vault, a CSF leak with associated meningitis or pneumocephalus may occur. CSF leaks usually resolve spontaneously after 3 to 10 days if fractures are stable. Patients with CSF leaks must be monitored closely because intervention, including possible repair of the leak, may be required if the leak does not stop spontaneously. Malunion of the mandible or maxilla may cause problems with mastication. TMD and degenerative joint disease may result from fractures involving the TMJ. Patients with orbital floor fractures may continue to have diplopia even after surgical repair of the floor defect. Cosmetic deformity can occur with all facial fractures, even after repair.

Pediatric Considerations

Specialists should be involved in the care of all children with facial fractures. Their management is more complicated, partly because injury to growth centers may lead to future problems.

Skull Fractures

Anatomic Considerations

The skull consists of several large, platelike bones joined together to form an intact enclosure (see Figure 17-1). In early childhood, the joints between these bones, the cranial sutures, are somewhat flexible. However, the skull bones soon become rigidly attached and then behave like a single continuous bone. Vascular structures that lie close to the skull, such as the middle meningeal artery and the dural venous sinuses, may be injured by a skull fracture, leading to life-threatening intracranial bleeding. A distinction is often made between basilar skull fractures, which involve the floor of the skull, and other fractures that involve either the sides or top of the skull. The cranial nerves exit the skull via foramina in the base of the skull and may be injured during fractures to this area.

Mechanism of Injury

The skull, especially in an adult, is a strong structure. Significant force is required to fracture it. Common causes include falls, MVAs, and forceful blows.

Clinical Presentation

The initial force of the blow usually, but not always, causes loss of consciousness. It is estimated that one quarter of patients with depressed skull fractures do not lose consciousness.[16,17] Loss of consciousness ranges from brief to prolonged, depending on the extent of cerebral injury. Short periods of retrograde amnesia are common. Anterograde amnesia can also occur. The patient's mental status initially may range from fully alert and oriented to unresponsive. Local swelling and tenderness is usually noted, and overlying lacerations are common. The following signs and symptoms strongly suggest the presence of a basilar skull or temporal bone fracture: raccoon eyes (periorbital ecchymosis), Battle's sign (ecchymosis over the mastoid or postauricular region), CSF leaks (clear rhinorrhea or otorrhea), hemotympanum, bloody otorrhea, tympanic membrane perforation or ossicle disruption, facial nerve paresis or paralysis, hearing loss, vertigo, and nystagmus. Other cranial nerve injuries can also occasionally accompany basilar skull fractures. Thus, it is important to perform a thorough neurologic assessment (including mental status and cranial nerve examination), otoscopy, and anterior rhinoscopy.

Imaging

Plain radiographs are suboptimal in evaluating skull fractures and not indicated in either low- or high-risk patients.[18] CT is the preferred modality to evaluate skull fractures and associated intracranial pathology. Temporal bone fractures are encountered in 75% of basilar skull fractures. As with facial fractures, if a temporal bone fracture is suspected, both coronal and axial images should be obtained. Furthermore, dedicated temporal bone CT should be requested if there is a concern for temporal bone fracture clinically or if the temporal bone needs further evaluation based on suspicious findings on head CT.

Skull fractures may be linear, stellate, or comminuted. In adults, the fracture typically does not follow a suture line. It is important to distinguish between depressed fractures and nondepressed fractures because depressed skull fractures usually require more aggressive treatment. A fracture should be considered depressed if part of any fragment lies lower than the surrounding bone.

Indications for Referral

Neurologic deficits, intracranial bleeding, pneumocephalus, open fractures, CSF leaks and fractures with depressed fragments require immediate consultation or referral to a neurosurgeon. If the patient is stable and lacks these concerns and complications, a neurosurgeon should be consulted in a routine fashion.

Initial Treatment

The first priority in treating patients with skull fractures is to evaluate and address other potentially more serious injuries. Indications for head CT include current altered mental status, neurologic symptoms or signs, loss of consciousness of longer than 5 minutes, or a suspected depressed fragment. Fractures that require immediate attention include depressed or open fractures and those with a CSF or air leak. Depressed fragments generally need operative repair to restore their normal position. Open fractures need thorough irrigation before closure of the scalp wound. Open fractures that are comminuted, contaminated, or both may require operative debridement and closure. CSF leaks and pneumocephalus both indicate open fractures (i.e., connection of the cranial vault with the outside). They put the patient at risk for meningitis and generally require inpatient observation. Air is usually rapidly reabsorbed, so persistent pneumocephalus indicates an ongoing connection that may need intervention. CSF leakage is initially managed by keeping the patient's upper body semierect. Prophylactic antibiotics have not been shown to be helpful. If the leak persists beyond a few days, reduction of CSF pressure by drainage may be necessary, and repair of the leak may ultimately be required.

After it has been determined that the fracture is uncomplicated, the first concern is to observe the patient for changes in neurologic status. Subarachnoid, subdural, or epidural bleeding can lead to neurologic decline that necessitates emergency intervention. Patients with epidural hemorrhage can have a lucid interval between the initial trauma and subsequent neurologic deterioration, so close observation is important. These bleeding complications are much more common if the fracture line crosses the vascular channels of the skull or brain. After observation confirms that the patient is neurologically stable, uncomplicated fractures generally require only analgesics for pain and outpatient follow-up. The patient should be seen in 1 to 2 weeks, with follow-up imaging obtained in 2 to 3 months to document healing. Failure to heal may indicate the development of a leptomeningeal cyst. In this condition, the fracture line gradually expands because of herniation of intracranial contents through the fracture line.

Complications

In addition to traumatic brain injury, patients with skull fractures are at risk for other potentially serious injuries caused by the initial trauma. They are also prone to vascular injuries leading to subarachnoid, subdural, or epidural bleeding. Cranial nerves are occasionally injured, especially with basilar skull fractures. The facial nerve is most susceptible to this type of injury. Fortunately, the deficit often resolves spontaneously over time. Surgical intervention may be necessary, however. Other potential complications include CSF leaks, meningitis, pneumocephalus, hydrocephalus, and leptomeningeal cyst development.

Return to Work or Sports

Patients who sustain uncomplicated skull fractures may gradually resume their usual activities as soon as symptoms allow. Activities that pose a high risk of significant blows to the head should be avoided until healing is well under way.

Pediatric Considerations

In the pediatric age group, falls, including those involving a short distance (<3 feet) are the most common causes of isolated skull fractures.[19] Child abuse is an important cause of skull fractures, especially in young children. Therefore, any skull fracture in a child should prompt suspicion of child abuse. Unless the injury is clearly the result of an accident, a skeletal survey should be strongly considered, especially in young children. As in adults, CT is the preferred modality to diagnose skull fractures and other intracranial injuries.

With two exceptions, the fracture patterns in children are similar to those in adults. When children's sutures have not yet fused, fractures may separate the bones along the suture lines (diastatic fractures). The very soft skulls of infants are susceptible to a depressed plastic deformity. This creates a hollowed-out defect with a pondlike appearance or an appearance similar to the depression produced by pressing firmly on a ping pong ball.

Indications for referral to a neurosurgeon include depressed, basilar, widely diastatic, or open skull fractures. Children with an isolated nondepressed skull fracture with less than 3 mm of separation without an associated intracranial injury are at low risk for complication and do not require admission to the hospital, provided child abuse is not suspected.[20] After the mental status has returned to normal and the child is tolerating liquids, he or she may be discharged home with instructions to the parent to look for

any worrisome signs such as lethargy, vomiting, confusion, or seizures. A follow-up visit should occur 1 to 2 months after the injury to check for healing (i.e., no palpable defect).

REFERENCES

1. Alvi A, Doherty T, Lewen G. Facial fractures and concomitant injuries in trauma patients. *Laryngoscope.* 2003;113:102-106.
2. Daw JL, Lewis VL. Lateral force compared with frontal impact nasal fractures: need for reoperation. *J Craniomaxillofac Trauma.* 1995;1:50-55.
3. Bailey BJ, Calhoun KH, Johnson JT, et al. Head & Neck Surgery-Otolaryngology. 3rd ed. Philadelphia: Lippincott Williams & Wilkins; 2001:793.
4. Romeo SJ, Hawley CJ, Romeo MW, Romeo JP. Facial injuries in sports: a team physician's guide to diagnosis and treatment. *Phys Sportsmed.* 2005;33(4):45-53.
5. Iida S, Kogo M, Sugiura T, Mima T, Matsuya T. Retrospective analysis of 1502 patients with facial fractures. *Int J Oral Maxillofac Surg.* 2001;30(4):286-290.
6. Imahara SD, Hopper RA, Wang J, Rivara FP, Klein MB. Patterns and outcomes of pediatric facial fractures in the United States: a survey of the National Trauma Data Bank. *J Am Coll Surg.* 2008;207(5):710-716.
7. Gassner R, Tuli T, Hachl O, Moreira R, Ulmer H. Craniomaxillofacial trauma in children: a review of 3,385 cases with 6,060 injuries in 10 years. *Oral Maxillofac Surg.* 2004;62(4):399-407.
8. Laskin DM. Protecting the faces of America. *J Oral Maxillofac Surg.* 2000;58(4):363.
9. Sharp JF, Denholm S. Routine x-rays in nasal trauma: the influence of audit on clinical practice. *J R Soc Med.* 1994;87:153-154.
10. Barbour SD, Shlaes DM, Guertin SR. Toxic-shock syndrome associated with nasal packing: analogy to tampon-associated illness. *Pediatrics.* 1984;73(2):163-165.
11. Hull HF, Mann JM, Sands CJ, Gregg SH, Kaufman PW. Toxic shock syndrome related to nasal packing. *Arch Otolaryngol.* 1983;109(9):624-626.
12. Colton JJ, Beekhuis GJ. Management of nasal fractures. *Otolaryngol Clin North Am.* 1986;19:73-85.
13. Stacey DH, Doyle JF, Mount DL, et al. Management of mandible fractures. *Plast Reconstruc Surg.* 2006;117:48e-60e.
14. Raby N, Berman L, de Long G. Accident and Emergency Radiology. Philadelphia: WB Saunders; 1999:37-49.
15. Laine FJ, Conway WF, Laskin DM. Radiology of maxillofacial trauma. *Curr Probl Diagn Radiol.* 1993;22(4):145-188.
16. Brown L, Moynihan JA, Denmark TK. Blunt pediatric head trauma requiring neurosurgical intervention: how subtle can it be? *Am J Emerg Med.* 2003;21(6):467-472.
17. Moran SG, McCarthy MC, Uddin DE, Poelstra RJ. Predictors of positive CT scans in the trauma patient with minor head injury. *Am Surg.* 1994;60(7):533-535.
18. Masters SJ, McClean PM, Arcarese JS, et al. Skull x-ray examinations after head trauma. Recommendations by a multidisciplinary panel and validation study. *N Eng J Med.* 1987;316(2):84-91.
19. Greenes DS, Schutzman SA. Infants with isolated skull fracture: what are their clinical characteristics, and do they require hospitalization? *Ann Emerg Med.* 1997;30:253-259.
20. Vogelbaum MA, Kaufman BA, Park TS, Winthrop AL. Management of uncomplicated skull fractures in children: is hospital admission necessary? *Pediatr Neurosurg.* 1998;29:96-101.

RIB FRACTURES

Rib fractures are some of the most common thoracic injuries, but diagnosing them can be difficult because reliable clinical examination findings are lacking and radiographs are specific but not very sensitive. Certain types of rib fractures are associated with an increased risk of organ injury, and up to 50% are related to significant pulmonary trauma. Primary care providers must remain alert to the possibility of associated serious injuries such as pneumothorax, hemothorax, and vascular or abdominal organ laceration in the management of rib fractures. The principal goal in evaluating rib fractures is to detect complications. In the absence of complications, the goal is pain relief. Rib fractures in children after reportedly minor trauma should raise suspicion of child abuse.

Anatomic Considerations

The rib cage consists of true ribs and false ribs. The true ribs (1 to 7) have cartilage at the end of the ribs that attach directly to the sternum. The false ribs (8 to 12) attach to the costochondral cartilage of the superior rib. Fractures may occur anywhere along the rib cage but are somewhat more common in the posterior and middle third of the fourth through the ninth ribs. Fractures in the lateral aspect of the ribs are more common because they have less protection from the overlying chest musculature. Fractures in the upper ribs suggest that the patient has experienced a significant degree of trauma because the ribs are well protected by surrounding musculoskeletal structures, and the ribs are short and broad. Fractures in this location may be associated with arterial and bronchial trauma. Fractures of the lower ribs are associated with upper abdominal organ injury such as liver and spleen lacerations.

Mechanism of Injury

Rib fractures are the most common anatomic deformity resulting from blunt trauma but are rarely life threatening. Whereas blunt trauma to the chest is the most common cause of injury in rib fractures, less common causes include stress from severe or prolonged coughing and overuse stress in certain sports such as rowing, baseball

(pitching), and golf. Rib stress fractures are discussed at end of the chapter in greater detail. Rib fractures can result from pathologic processes such as cancers that metastasize to bone such as breast, prostate, and renal cancer.

RIB FRACTURES AFTER TRAUMA

Clinical Presentation

Because the severe pain that accompanies a rib contusion is indistinguishable from that caused by a fracture, clinical impression is unreliable in identifying a rib fracture. Point tenderness, splinting, and referred pain on chest compression are common physical findings, but they are not specific enough to indicate a fracture. Decreased breath sounds may reflect splinting but could also be a sign of more significant injury (e.g., pneumothorax) and warrant further evaluation with radiographs.

Imaging

The main reason to obtain a routine posteroanterior (PA) and lateral chest radiograph is to look for signs of intrathoracic complications of rib fractures such as pneumothorax or hemothorax. Although its role has been called into question, chest radiography is still standard practice in the emergency department evaluation of victims of major trauma.[1] Trauma patients suspected of having a significant intrathoracic injury should undergo a computed tomography (CT) scan of the chest. A follow-up, two-view chest radiograph is recommended 6 hours after the initial evaluation to rule out a delayed hemothorax or pneumothorax.[2] After high-energy injuries, multiple fractures in adjacent ribs usually occur. A flail chest results when three or more adjacent ribs fracture in two separate places on the same rib, creating a free-floating segment. Rib fractures are often detected coincidentally during the course of CT evaluation of the traumatized chest.

It is usually unnecessary to obtain dedicated rib films in addition to a standard chest series when evaluating a patient with a suspected rib fracture. Whereas routine chest radiographs demonstrate major intrathoracic complications of rib fractures, they are insufficient to detect all rib fractures. The routine chest radiograph allows for an excellent view of the posterior portion of the ribs above the diaphragm, but it does not adequately portray the lateral portion of the ribs. Lateral rib fractures must be significantly displaced before they can be detected on a routine chest radiograph. The anterior and posterior portions of the ribs can be seen in profile (the best way to see rib fractures) on the standard PA view. An oblique view of the ribs must be obtained to view the lateral portion of the ribs. A rib series is only indicated if suspicion is high for multiple fractures or pathologic fractures not apparent on plain radiographs.

A nondisplaced rib fracture is typically seen as a vertical or oblique fracture line with a slight offset that is more easily identified at the superior margin (Figure 18-1). Nondisplaced or minimally displaced rib fractures may be detected more easily by looking for the surrounding soft tissue density of the hematoma that is usually associated with the fracture (Figure 18-2). Rib fractures are often more obvious on follow-up radiographs because of displacement at the fracture margins caused by respiratory motion (Figure 18-3). Nondisplaced fractures may only appear as callus at the fracture site 10 to 14 days after injury.

Ultrasonography has been used to evaluate rib fractures, but further study is needed to determine its clinical utility compared to plain radiographs.[3,4]

Indications for Orthopedic Referral

The need for referral or consultation with a specialist depends on the presence of associated chest injuries such as airway obstruction, pneumothorax, hemothorax, cardiac tamponade, or abdominal organ laceration. Emergency consultation is required for any patient who is hemodynamically unstable. Orthopedic consultation is rarely needed

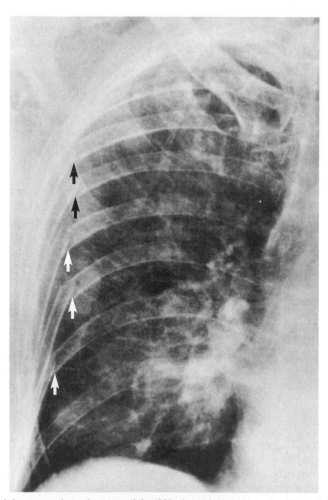

FIGURE 18-1 Fractures of the posterolateral aspect of the fifth through the ninth ribs (*arrows*). Note that the fractures lie in an approximately vertical line. (*From Rogers LE [ed]. Radiology of Skeletal Trauma, 3rd ed, vol 1. New York, Churchill Livingstone, 2001.*)

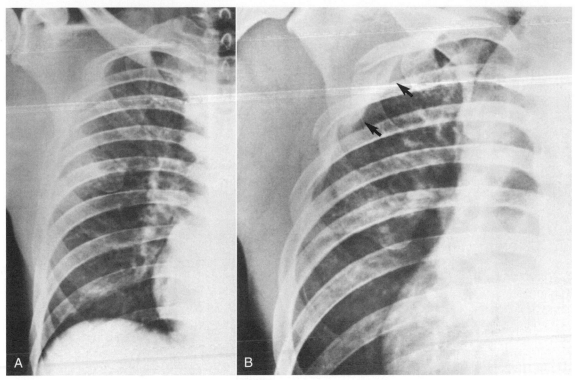

FIGURE 18-2 A, Anteroposterior view shows only minimal extrapleural density. The fractures are not demonstrated. **B,** Right posterior oblique view shows fractures of the second through fifth right ribs with a surrounding hematoma manifested by extrapleural density (*arrows*). *(From Rogers LE [ed].* Radiology of Skeletal Trauma, *3rd ed, vol 1. New York, Churchill Livingstone, 2001.)*

because the majority of rib fracture complications are pulmonary, vascular, or abdominal.

Initial Treatment.

Emergent Treatment

The acute management of the patient with a rib fracture depends in large part on whether any complications have developed. An aggressive search must be made for the source of life-threatening injury in a patient who is hemodynamically unstable after chest trauma. Patients with two or more rib fractures at the same level are at increased risk of pneumothorax, hemothorax, and abdominal organ injury and thus higher morbidity and mortality.[5] The morbidity and mortality risk is even greater in elderly patients who sustain blunt trauma with rib fractures.[6] All patients with three or more rib fractures should be hospitalized for observation and treatment because of the higher risk of complications in this group.

Nonemergent Treatment

The mainstay of treatment for uncomplicated rib fractures is pain control. Patients with rib fractures often require narcotic medication for adequate analgesia in the acute treatment period to avoid splinting and subsequent atelectasis. A rib belt may provide additional pain relief by limiting chest movement, although use of the belt may be uncomfortable for some patients and compromise breathing, and use of these devices has not been shown to have superior outcomes.[7,8]

Invasive forms of pain control that are often used in the management of patients with multiple rib fractures include intercostal nerve block using local anesthetic agents and epidural analgesia These methods of analgesia can minimize the use of narcotics during the acute treatment phase and allow the patient to perform breathing exercises that help avoid atelectasis and pneumonia. Consultation with an anesthesiologist is recommended if invasive pain control measures are being considered.

Although delayed intrathoracic complications are unusual, they can occur during the first few days after an acute rib fracture. A follow-up clinical evaluation is warranted in the first 72 hours or at any time the patient experiences increased difficulty breathing or other worrisome symptoms to reassess the patient's symptoms and condition and determine the need for further imaging.

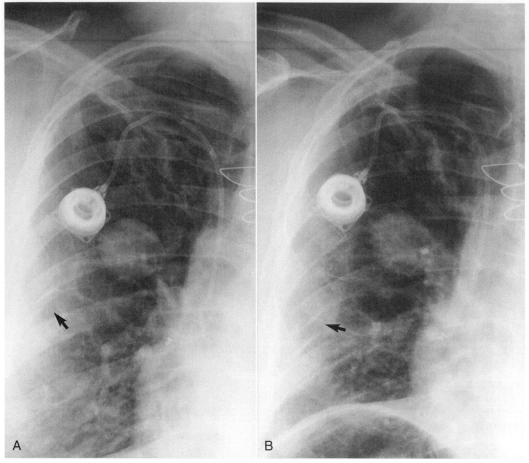

FIGURE 18-3 A, Posteroanterior (PA) view of the chest shows a nondisplaced fracture of the posterior aspect of the right seventh rib (*arrow*). Multiple pulmonary metastases are also present, raising the possibility of a pathologic fracture. **B,** PA radiograph taken 5 days later shows displacement of the fracture fragments caused by respiratory movement (*arrow*). (*From Rogers LE [ed].* Radiology of Skeletal Trauma, *3rd ed, vol 1. New York, Churchill Livingstone, 2001.*)

Definitive Treatment

No specific treatment has been shown to be superior in the management of uncomplicated rib fractures. The vast majority of these injuries heal without difficulty despite constant respiratory movement. The intercostal muscles provide natural protection and relative immobilization during the healing phase. The primary goal of treatment is adequate pain relief that allows satisfactory pulmonary function to prevent basilar atelectasis and pneumonia. Liberal use of ice, analgesic medication, and activity restriction are the cornerstones of treatment. The duration of symptoms varies, but most rib fractures heal within 6 weeks. Follow-up radiographs are unnecessary unless indicated by physical findings (e.g., decreased breath sounds, severe persistent pain).[9]

Return to Work or Sports

Return to work or sports after a rib fracture depends largely on the patient's level of pain and the demands of the activity. When pain free at rest, the patient can begin to increase activity. Restricted contact activity is advised for at least 3 weeks after the injury. Use of a rib protector or flak jacket during contact sports can allow the athlete to return to competition sooner and should be worn for 6 to 8 weeks after the injury.

Complications

The more ribs that are fractured, the greater the likelihood of complications.[10] The most common initial complications are pneumothorax, pleural effusion, and hemothorax. Delayed complications include pneumonia, pulmonary contusion, and pulmonary embolus. Malunion or nonunion are uncommon and rarely cause symptoms if they do occur. Resection of the rib or bone grafting should be considered only for patients with a *symptomatic* nonunion.

Pediatric Considerations

Accidental rib fractures are rare in infancy and result from severe trauma. The detection of a rib fracture after a fall or minor trauma should raise the suspicion of child abuse.[11] The ribs are a common site for skeletal injury in abused children, and the majority of abuse-related rib fractures are in children younger than 2 years of age. Children younger than 14 years of age have more compliant rib cages than adults. Thus, rib fractures in a younger child indicate that the child's chest has sustained significant trauma.

Squeezing the chest, compressing the front of the chest, hitting the child from behind, or stepping on the chest causes injury in abuse-related rib fractures. Anterior rib fractures are more common in abuse, and lateral fractures are more common in nonabuse.[12] Inflicted rib fractures usually are nondisplaced and involve multiple sequential ribs.

When child abuse is suspected, the addition of oblique views or a bone scan is warranted because rib fractures are highly associated with abuse, and identifying such fractures with routine chest radiographs is difficult.

Stress Fractures of the Ribs

Cough-Induced Stress Fracture

A cough-induced rib fracture should be considered in the patient with severe localized chest pain that occurs suddenly after prolonged or severe coughing.[13] Because the symptoms of a cough-induced fracture occur simultaneously with symptoms of an underlying disorder (e.g., pneumonia), initial diagnosis of a rib fracture is difficult and often delayed. Most cough-induced stress fractures are subtle and nondisplaced. Callus may be the only fracture indication revealed on follow-up radiographs. Using bone scintigraphy to confirm the diagnosis of fracture may be clinically important to avoid an unnecessary search for a pulmonary or cardiac condition. Helical CT can also exclude other rib lesions such as metastatic tumor. Management of cough-induced fractures of the ribs consists of adequate analgesia, cough suppression, and treatment of the underlying cause of the cough.

Sports-Related Fracture

Sports-related stress fractures have been reported in throwing sports, golf, rowing, and swimming. Various theories have been proposed to explain the cause of stress fractures of the ribs during these sports. In a significant majority of cases, a rapid increase in activity is the precipitating factor. In rowers, actions of the serratus anterior and external oblique muscles on the ribs during repetitive bending forces may cause stress fractures.[14] Stress fractures in rowers occur most commonly in the anterolateral and posterolateral aspects of ribs 5 through 9. The cause of injury in golf may be force exerted by contraction of the serratus, latissimus dorsi, and abdominal muscles

and bending of the upper body during the swing phase. Most rib stress fractures in golfers occur on the leading side of the trunk (i.e., the same side as the golfer's dominant hand).[15]

Gradual onset of pain associated with activity, especially twisting motions, typically is a symptom of rib stress fracture. The diagnosis is often confused with an intercostal muscle strain. Because stress fractures of the ribs are often missed on plain radiographs, a bone scan should be obtained if a stress fracture of the rib is suspected.

Healing usually occurs without complication if the athlete can refrain from the causative activity for 4 to 6 weeks. When the fracture site is nontender and no pain occurs with the motion that originally caused the fracture, gradual rehabilitation can begin. Strengthening of the serratus anterior muscle is especially important. No cases of malunion or nonunion of lower rib stress fractures have been reported.

REFERENCES

1. Sears BW, Luchette FA, Esposito TJ, et al. Old fashion clinical judgment in the era of protocols: is mandatory chest X-ray necessary in injured patients? *J Trauma.* 2005;59:324-330.
2. Misthos P, Kakaris S, Sepsas E, et al. A prospective analysis of occult pneumothorax, delayed pneumothorax and delayed hemothorax after minor blunt thoracic trauma. *Eur J Cardiothorac Surg.* 2004;25:859-864.
3. Hurley ME, Keye GD, Hamilton S. Is ultrasound really helpful in the detection of rib fractures? *Injury.* 2004;35:562-566.
4. Griffith JF, Rainer TH, Ching AS, et al. Sonography compared with radiography in revealing acute rib fracture. *AJR Am J Roentgenol.* 1999;173:1603-1609.
5. Sirmali M, Turut H, Topcu S, et al. A comprehensive analysis of traumatic rib fractures: morbidity, mortality and management. *Eur J Cardiothorac Surg.* 2003;24:133-138.
6. Stawicki SP, Grossman MD, Hoey BA, et al. Rib fractures in the elderly: a marker of injury severity. *J Am Geriatr Soc.* 2004;52:805-808.
7. Lazcano A, Dougherty JM, Kruger M. Use of rib belts in acute rib fractures. *Am J Emerg Med.* 1989;7:97-100.
8. Quick G. A randomized clinical trial of rib belts for simple fractures. *Am J Emerg Med.* 1990;8:277-281.
9. Bansidhar BJ, Lagares-Garcia JA, Miller SL. Clinical rib fractures: are follow-up chest X-rays a waste of resources? *Am Surg.* 2002;68:449-453.
10. Flagel BT, Luchette FA, Reed RL, et al. Half-a-dozen ribs: the breakpoint for mortality. *Surgery.* 2005;138:717-723.
11. Cadzow SP, Armstrong KL. Rib fractures in infants: red alert! The clinical features, investigations and child protection outcomes. *J Paediatr Child Health.* 2000;36:322-326.
12. Barsness KA, Cha ES, Bensard DD, et al. The positive predictive value of rib fractures as an indicator of nonaccidental trauma in children. *J Trauma.* 2003;54:1107-1110.
13. Hanak V, Hartman TE, Ryu JH. Cough-induced rib fractures. *Mayo Clin Proc.* 2005;80:879-882.
14. Karlson KA. Rib stress fractures in elite rowers: a case series and proposed mechanism. *Am J Sports Med.* 1998;26:516-519.
15. Lord MJ, Ha KI, Song KS. Stress fractures of the ribs in golfers. *Am J Sports Med.* 1996;24:118-122.

APPENDIX (CASTING AND SPLINTING)

Co-Author: Michael J. Petrizzi

This appendix provides a step-by-step, how-to guide for the application of the following casts and splints:

Short-arm cast
Short-arm cast with thumb spica
Long-arm cast
Long-arm thumb spica cast
Short-leg cast, weight bearing and non–weight bearing
Long-leg cast
Ulnar gutter splint
Upper extremity sugar tong splint
Thumb spica sugar tong splint
Lower extremity splint

Go to Expert Consult for an electronic version of a patient education handout titled "Cast Care Instructions."

GENERAL PRINCIPLES ABOUT SPLINTING AND CASTING

Fiberglass Splint Rolls

Some basic important principles to be used include using the right-sized material, which can often be done by using an elastic wrap to measure the area to be splinted. Fiberglass can start to set with just ambient humidity. Therefore, it is important to have all of the necessary supplies on hand before starting to apply the splint. Depending on the particular manufacturer's specifications, the appropriate use of clips or closures to keep the remaining splint material fresh for its next use is also important. Most materials now come with at least one side with padding, and this obviously should be applied to the patient. The extremity should always be in the neutral or functional position. When splint rolls are used, there is no need to dip the entire length into a bucket of water as with a manufactured fiberglass casting tape roll. Never use water hotter than room temperature because the setting of fiberglass is an exothermic reaction and can cause burns on the patient. When rolling the elastic wrap to keep the splint in place, one should use enough pressure that provides a comfortable application but does not cause any potential harm to the neurovascular status of the extremity. Roll away from the patient. The elastic wrap should overlap approximately half the width, as it is wrapped from distal to proximal to aid with the edema being pushed up and out of the extremity. One can always rewrap the elastic roll if the patient feels it is on too tightly. The patient should demonstrate how he or she would remove and replace the wrap. Keep in mind that the use of any pinpoint pressure from fingertips can leave deep impressions in the fiberglass, causing friction points and either discomfort or ulceration and should be avoided. Patients should receive education about the device that they have, including warning signs of neurovascular compromise or other issues that would require immediate attention. If the splint is being used for definitive immobilization of a fracture, advise that it not be removed and therefore should be protected from getting excessively wet.

Although fiberglass splint roll products are readily available, we include the technique to fashion your own splint with padding material and rolls of fiberglass casting tape if you do not have access to a splint roll.

Creating Your Own Splint

1. Roll out four to eight layers of padding and set aside an extra layer of padding. When the padding is ready, using gloves, roll out four to eight layers of fiberglass alongside (not onto) the padding. Take care not to stretch the material while rolling it out.

2. When ready to apply the splint, dip the fiberglass or plaster layers into lukewarm water, squeeze out the excess water, place the material onto the padding, and then place the extra layer of padding on top. Ideally, the padding should completely cover the splinting material.

    NOTE: Dipping fiberglass splinting material in water allows it to set more quickly. Fiberglass splinting material may be applied without soaking in water; this allows for more time to apply the material, which may be especially useful for less experienced operators.

    The warmer the water temperature, the faster the casting material will set. However, never use water hotter than lukewarm because the heat emitted from the hardening splint may burn the patient.

3. Apply the splint to the patient using an elastic wrap to keep it in place.

Casts

Casts in general provide superior strength, durability, and immobilization than splints but can also cause more complications. Benefits provided by casts include preventing loss of position and additional soft tissue, vascular, or nerve damage and can provide considerable pain relief while the fracture is healing. Because the cast cannot allow for further edema, if further swelling is expected, a cast should not be applied for 24 to 48 hours. A cast should also not be applied if there is significant soft tissue damage or if there is concern that the patient will be unable to comply with the recommendation of elevation. A cast check should be performed at 24 hours, and the need for a replacement cast is specific to the particular area of the body and type of fracture.

Additional materials needed when applying casts include stockinettes and cast padding as well as a bucket for the water and the fiberglass role of cast tape. It is often helpful to think of the stockinette as the first layer of protection for the skin and the cast padding as a way to further protect the skin as well as provide protection over bony prominences and to prevent burns when the cast saw is used to remove the cast. The first one to two layers of cast should be considered as the treatment of the fracture, and the second or third layers, depending on the area of the body, should be viewed as protecting that first layer of cast from trauma from the environment. Although fiberglass does breathe easier and even with the new synthetic stockinette materials, water that gets inside the cast can frequently lead to skin breakdown.

When the extremity is in a proper position, the length of the stockinette should be measured to extend 1 to 2 inches past the ends of the area to be casted. Padding should be rolled on from distal to proximal overlapping by half the width. Care should be taken to avoid wrapping the padding on too tightly. A small amount of extra padding over bony prominences such as the elbow, heel, or tibial tuberosity can reduce complications. Padding should only be applied to the area where the casting tape will be rolled. After the padding has been applied, do not allow the patient to move out of position because this will lead to creases and a very uncomfortable interface with the skin.

Applying the first wrap without dipping it in water will give you more time. As with all rolls, casting material should be applied from the distal end of the extremity and overlapping half the width on the way up. The cast tape can be applied in two ways. The first method involves unrolling the tape as one does with an elastic wrap. Sometimes this can cause the tape to be applied too tightly. Another method uses unrolling some of the tape and more gently applying the tape onto the extremity. It is also very important to avoid leaving impressions in the cast from fingertip pressure because this can lead to skin irritation. However, one must mold the cast after just the first roll is on. This is a critical component to making the cast comfortable and protecting the skin from rubbing against casting material. Again, never use fingertip pressure; rather, the base of the hand to provide the molding, which can be done at the wrist, around the forearm, into the arch of the foot, around both sides of the Achilles tendon, and around the malleoli. Then roll back the ends of the stockinette at both the proximal and distal ends of the cast and incorporate the stockinette into the next roll. As with splints, education is key for the patient's comfort and safety, and written cast care instructions are helpful. Because the fiberglass material does not have any give and it completely encompasses the injured extremity, a repeat neurovascular examination must be performed and documented before the patient leaves.

Cast Removal

Cast removal is accomplished with a cast saw. Patients mistakenly believe the blade rotates. The teeth penetrate the cast by vibrating and significant amounts of heat are generated, so it behooves one to avoid contact with the patient's skin.

To remove or bivalve a cast, the patient should position the affected extremity on a level surface. Have the patient "push down" into the surface while applying even pressure to the cast on the side opposite the surface. Remove the saw immediately when there is no longer any resistance. Move down the cast in small increments. Repeat these steps on the other side. Sometimes a tongue depressor can be gingerly inserted between the skin and cast along the cut line to help gain the trust of the patient. Use a cast spreader to separate the halves. Carefully place a blunt-edged bandage scissors underneath the stockinette and padding and carefully cut with upward pressure. The extremity can then be examined.

SHORT-ARM CAST CPT 29075

Indications. Fractures of the distal radius, ulna, or both; fractures of the carpals, excluding scaphoid fractures; may be used with an outrigger for distal fourth and fifth metacarpal fractures or stable fractures to the base of the proximal phalanx of the fourth and fifth fingers

Advantages. Allows extensive ROM of the elbow and fingers

Disadvantages. Allows some supination/pronation of the forearm

Materials. 2- or 3-inch-wide fiberglass casting material; 2- or 3-inch-wide cast padding; 2- or 3-inch stockinette; 1-inch tube gauze to make a collar over the thumb

Instructions

1. Measure from just past the MCP joint (Fig. SAC-1) to 3 finger breadths below the antecubital fossa (Fig. SAC-2). Position the patient's affected forearm in the neutral or functional position. The elbow should be at 90 degrees. The radial surface should be up. The hand should be slightly dorsiflexed as in a "handshake" position.
2. Use 1-inch tube gauze to make a collar over the thumb (Fig. SAC-3). Cut a length of stockinette sufficient to extend from just above the antecubital fossa to just past the MCP joints (Fig. SAC-4). Pinch the stockinette over the thumb (Fig. SAC-5). Cut a small hole for the thumb (Fig. SAC-6).
3. Wrap on the cast padding, starting at the hand and overlapping 50 percent up the arm. The padding should extend from the last palmar crease to three fingers below the antecubital space (Fig. SAC-7).
4. Dip the cast material in water and roll the material on over the same area covered by the cast padding. Anchor the cast tape at the wrist as you proceed around the ulnar side of the hand and approach the web space (Figs. SAC-8 to SAC-10). While wrapping, maintain a moderate tension and avoid creases or divots, overlapping by 50% each rotation.

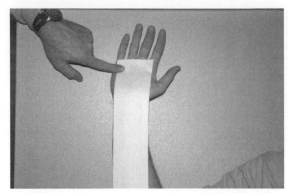

FIGURE SAC-1 Measure from right past the MCP joints.

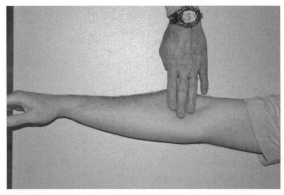

FIGURE SAC-2 Measure to a point 3 finger breadths from the antecubital fossa.

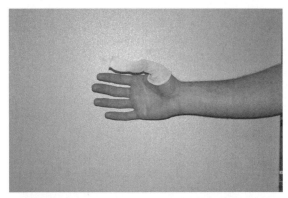

FIGURE SAC-3 Tube gauze as collar for the thumb.

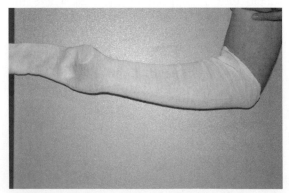

FIGURE SAC-4 Extend the stockinette from the MCP joints to just above the antecubital fossa and place over the thumb.

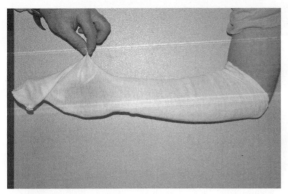

FIGURE SAC-5 Pinch the stockinette over the thumb.

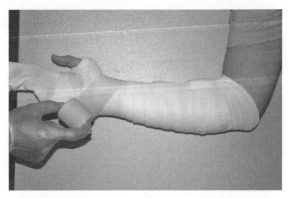

FIGURE SAC-9 Wrap to the ulnar side of the hand.

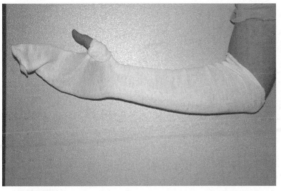

FIGURE SAC-6 Cut a small whole and push the thumb through.

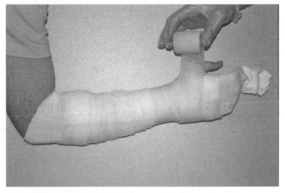

FIGURE SAC-10 Approach the web space.

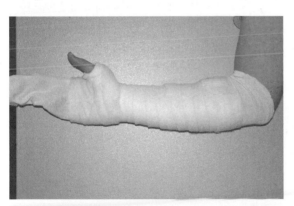

FIGURE SAC-7 Place cast padding from three palmar crease to three fingers below the antecubital space.

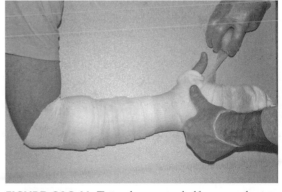

FIGURE SAC-11 Twist the tape a half turn each time through the web space.

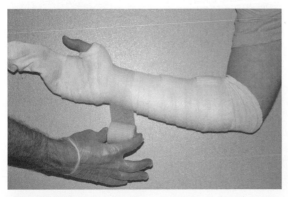

FIGURE SAC-8 Anchor the casting material at the wrist.

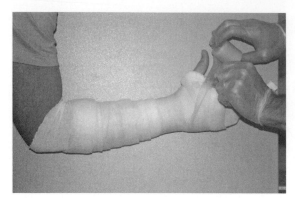

FIGURE SAC-12 Pinch the cast tape.

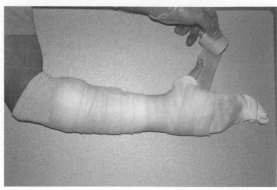

FIGURE SAC-13 Cut half the width of the tape for the length of the thumb.

5. Be careful to avoid impinging on the web space of the thumb or the dorsal base of the thumb. Move the wrap distally, passing the casting material over the web space between the thumb and forefinger at least twice. Any of three different techniques may be used to get the casting material through the web space without impingement: (1) twist the roll as the casting material is being unrolled through the web space (Fig. SAC-11), (2) pinch the casting material together as it is being unrolled through the web space (Fig. SAC-12), or (3) trim the material on the side that passes by the thumb by cutting a notch extending half the width of the roll up to the top of the thumb each time you go through the web space (Fig. SAC-13).
6. The cast should go up to the second palmar crease on the volar side and right to the MCP joints on the dorsal side. Be sure to apply an even thickness of casting material over the length of the area casted because areas where thicknesses vary are potential points of cast fracture.
7. After the first layer of casting material has been applied, mold the cast by gripping the patient's hand with your hand while placing your other palm in the dorsal aspect of the patient's wrist to provide for moderate dorsiflexion (Fig. SAC-14). Mold the forearm area of the cast into an oval around the radius and ulna (Fig. SAC-15).
8. Fold back the ends of the stockinette and roll on the final layer of cast material, tacking down the stockinette at the ends (Fig. SAC-16 and SAC-17). As you approach the web space, use the pinch technique because it will be on the surface of the cast (Figs. SAC-18 and SAC-19). Finish off the remaining cast material (Figs. SAC-20 and SAC-21).

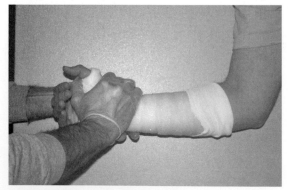

FIGURE SAC-14 Mold around the hand by gripping the patient's hand around the thumb.

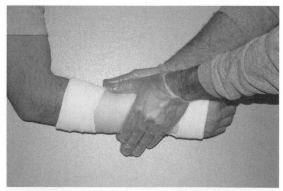

FIGURE SAC-15 Mold the cast around the forearm into an oval.

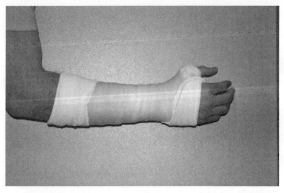

FIGURE SAC-16 Fold back the ends of the stockinette.

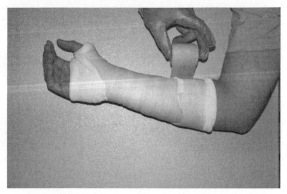

FIGURE SAC-17 Second roll captures the stockinette at the proximal portion of the cast.

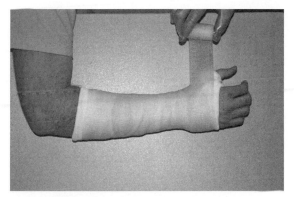

FIGURE SAC-18 Approach the web space.

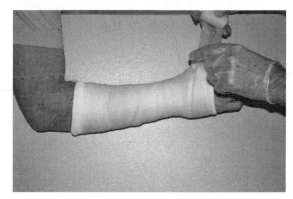

FIGURE SAC-19 Pinch the casting tape as you go through the web space.

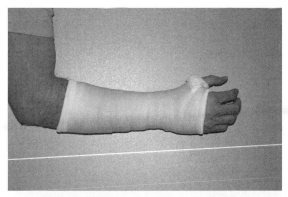

FIGURE SAC-20 Dorsal view, finished cast.

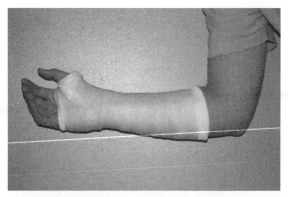

FIGURE SAC-21 Volar view, finished cast.

SHORT-ARM THUMB SPICA CAST
CPT 29075

Indications. Scaphoid or to rule out scaphoid fractures, thumb fractures

Advantages. Allows extensive ROM of the elbow and fingers

Disadvantages. Allows some supination/pronation of the forearm

Materials. 2- or 3-inch-wide fiberglass casting material; 2- or 3-inch-wide cast padding; 2- or 3-inch stockinette; 1-inch tube gauze to make a collar over the thumb

Instructions

1. Place 1-inch tube gauze over the thumb. Cut a length of stockinette sufficient to extend from just above the antecubital fossa to just past the MCP joints (Fig. TSC-1). Cut a hole for the thumb and put the thumb through the hole (Fig. TSC-2).
2. Position the patient's forearm and thumb in the neutral position. The thumb should *not* be pointed upward.
3. Wrap on the cast padding, starting at the hand and overlapping 50% up the arm. The padding should cover from the last palmar crease to two fingers below the antecubital space (Figs. TSC-3 and TSC-4). Be careful to avoid impinging on the web space of the thumb or the dorsal base of the thumb.

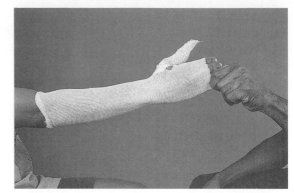

FIGURE TSC-2 Place the stockinette from just past the MCP joints to just above antecubital fossa. Cut a hole for the thumb.

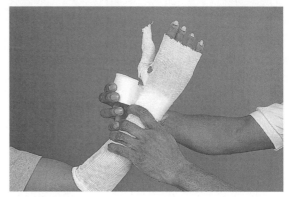

FIGURE TSC-3 Begin application of padding by anchoring at the wrist.

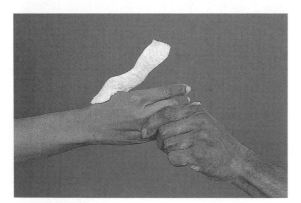

FIGURE TSC-1 Place tube gauze over the thumb.

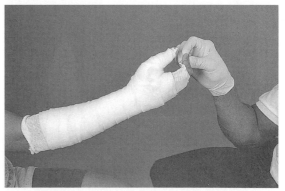

FIGURE TSC-4 Apply cast padding around the wrist up to the tip of the thumb.

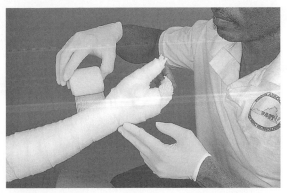

FIGURE TSC-5 Anchor casting material at the wrist.

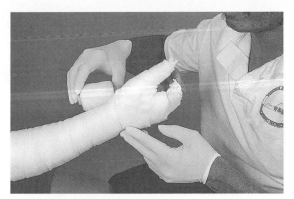

FIGURE TSC-6 Proceed around the wrist.

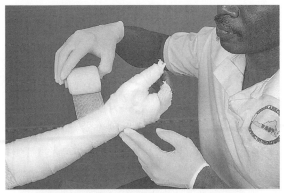

FIGURE TSC-7 Continue around the wrist.

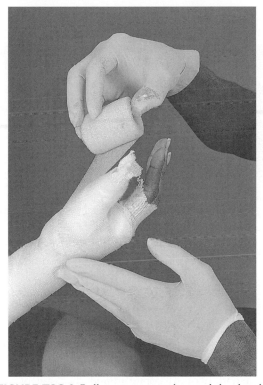

FIGURE TSC-9 Roll casting material around the thumb.

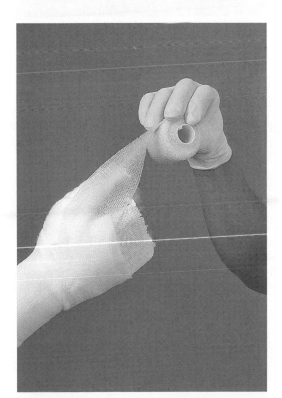

FIGURE TSC-8 Advance casting material over the thumb by using a half twist.

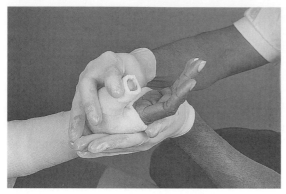

FIGURE TSC-10 Fold the stockinette down and mold around the thumb.

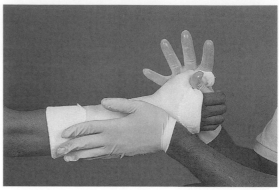

FIGURE TSC-11 Mold the cast so the wrist is in moderate dorsiflexion in the hand grip position.

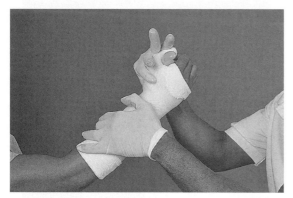

FIGURE TSC-12 Mold the cast around the forearm.

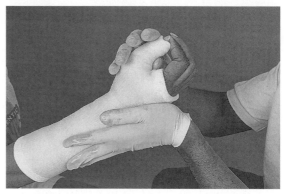

FIGURE TSC-13 Mold the cast on the top of the hand.

4. Dip the cast material in water and roll the material on over the same area covered by the cast padding. Anchor at the wrist (Fig. TSC-5). While wrapping, maintain a moderate tension and avoid creases or divots, overlapping by 50% each rotation (Figs. TSC-6 and TSC-7). Make a half twist to come around the base of the thumb (Fig. TSC-8). Continue around the thumb up to the tip (Fig. TSC-9).
5. After the first layer of casting material has been applied, fold the stockinette down over the cast tape and mold the cast by gripping the patient's hand with your hand while placing your other palm in the dorsal aspect of the patient's wrist to provide for moderate dorsiflexion into a hand grip position (Fig. TSC-10). Mold the forearm area of the cast into an oval around the radius and ulna (Figs. TSC-11 to TSC. 13).
6. Place your final layer of cast material, tacking down the stockinette at the ends usually starting at the thumb (Fig. TSC-14).

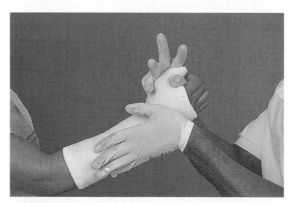

FIGURE TSC-14 Finish molding with hand grip and the hand over dorsum of forearm after the second layer of cast is over the stockinette at both ends.

LONG ARM CAST CPT 29065

Indications. Fractures of the radius, ulna, or both; elbow fractures

Advantages. Prevents flexion/extension at the elbow and supination/pronation of the forearm

Disadvantages. Can cause decreased ROM of affected arm shoulder, elbow, or both

Note. Usually worn in a sling for at least the first 1 to 2 weeks

Materials. 2- or 3-inch-wide fiberglass casting material; 2- or 3-inch-wide cast padding; 2- or 3-inch stockinette

Instructions

1. Stockinette should extend from just distal of the MCP joints to the shoulder. Cut the slit at the antecubital space (Figs. LAC-1 and LAC-2).
2. Position the patient in the neutral position (Fig. LAC-3).
3. Padding should extend from the last palmar crease to midway up the deltoid. Be sure to provide extra padding at the elbow (Fig. LAC-3).
4. Dip the cast material in water and roll on the material over the same area covered by the cast padding. While wrapping, maintain a moderate tension and avoid creases or divots, overlapping by 50% each rotation. When putting on the first layer of a long-arm cast, it is often helpful to complete a short-arm cast first (Fig. LAC-4), mold it, and then continue up the arm with the next roll (Fig. LAC-5).

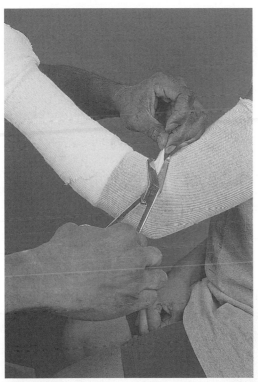

FIGURE LAC-1 Cut slit in the stockinette at the antecubital space.

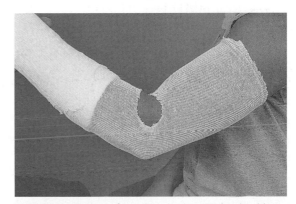

FIGURE LAC-2 Stockinette extending to the shoulder.

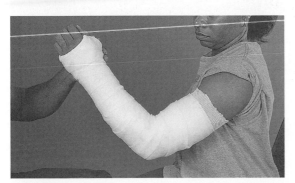

FIGURE LAC-3 Position the patient in neutral position and extend padding above the elbow.

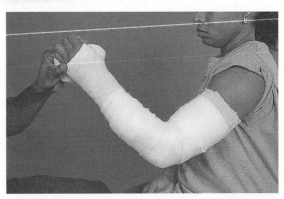

FIGURE LAC-4 Begin application of casting material at the wrist.

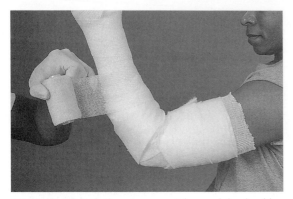

FIGURE LAC-5 Roll casting material toward the shoulder.

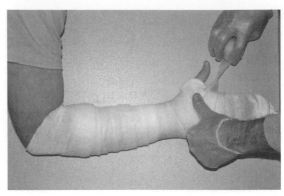

FIGURE LAC-6 Twist tape a half turn each time through the web space.

5. Be careful to avoid impinging on the web space of the thumb and the dorsal base of the thumb. Move the wrap distally, passing the casting material over the web space between the thumb and forefinger at least twice. Any of three different techniques may be used to get the casting material through the web space without impingement: (1) twist the roll as the casting material is being unrolled through the web space (Fig. LAC-6), (2) pinch the casting material together as it is being unrolled through the web space (Fig. LAC-7), or (3) trim the material on the side that passes by the thumb by cutting a notch extending half the width of the roll up to the top of the thumb each time you go through the web space (Fig. LAC-8).

6. After the first layer of casting material has been applied, mold the cast by gripping the patient's hand with your hand while placing your other palm in the dorsal aspect of the patient's wrist to provide for moderate dorsiflexion Mold the forearm area of the cast into an oval around the radius and ulna (Fig. LAC-9). After the second roll has been applied, the cast should be molded around the distal humerus epicondyles and the elbow (Fig. LAC-10).

7. Next fold back the ends of the stockinette and place your final layer of cast material, tacking down the stockinette at the ends. (For adults, a long-arm cast may require three cast rolls.)

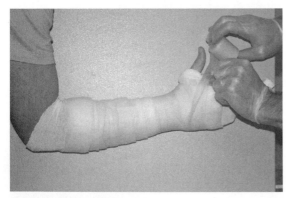

FIGURE LAC-7 Pinch the cast tape.

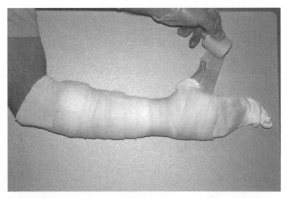

FIGURE LAC-8 Cut half the width of the tape for the length of the thumb.

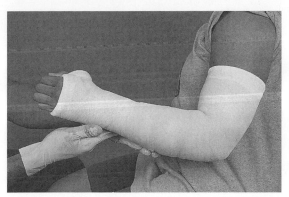

FIGURE LAC-9 Mold the cast around the forearm into an oval.

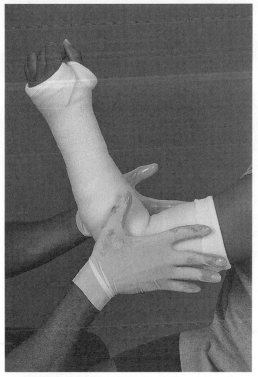

FIGURE LAC-10 Mold the cast around the elbow.

Long-Arm Thumb Spica Cast
CPT 29065

Indications. Fractures of scaphoid, some first metacarpal fractures

Advantages. Prevents flexion/extension at the elbow and supination/pronation of the forearm

Disadvantages. Can cause decreased ROM of affected arm shoulder, elbow, or both

Note. Usually worn in a sling for at least the first 1 to 2 weeks

Materials. 2- or 3-inch-wide fiberglass casting material; 2- or 3-inch-wide cast padding; 2- or 3-inch stockinette; 1-inch tube gauze

Instructions

1. Place 1-inch tube gauze over the thumb (Fig. LATS-1). Cut a hole for the thumb and put the thumb through the small hole (Fig. LATS-2). The stockinette should extend from just distal of the MCP joints to the shoulder. Cut the slit at the antecubital space (Figs. LATS-3 and LATS-4).
2. Position the patient in neutral position, including the forearm and thumb. The thumb should *not* be pointed upward (Fig. LATS-2).
3. Cast padding should be anchored at the wrist, go around the thumb, progress through the web space, and extend to midway up the deltoid. Be sure to provide extra padding at the elbow (Figs. LATS-5 and LATS-6).

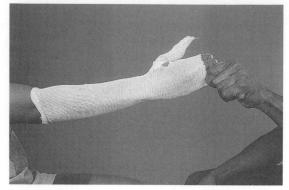

FIGURE LATS-2 Put the thumb through the hole in the stockinette.

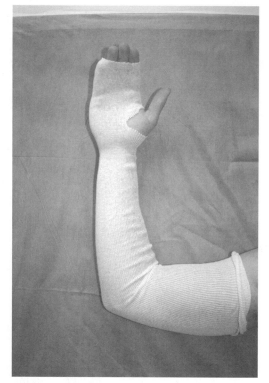

FIGURE LATS-3 Place the stockinette from just past the MCP joints to the shoulder.

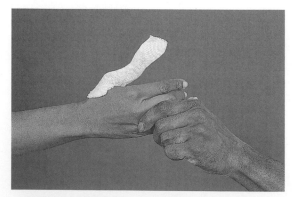

FIGURE LATS-1 Place tube gauze over the thumb.

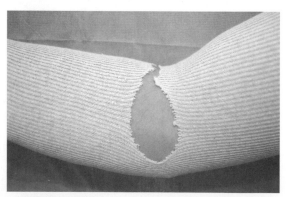

FIGURE LATS-4 Cut a slit at the antecubital fossa.

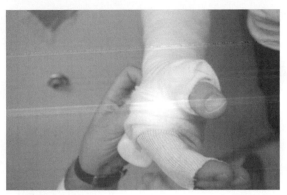

FIGURE LATS-5 Apply padding at the thumb and wrist.

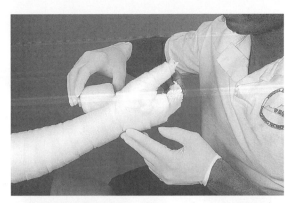

FIGURE LATS-7 Begin application of casting material at the wrist.

4. Dip the cast material in water and roll on the material over the same area covered by the cast padding. Anchor the cast at the wrist. While wrapping, maintain a moderate tension and avoid creases or divots, overlapping by 50% each rotation (Figs. LATS-7 and LATS-8). Make a half twist to come around the base of the thumb (Fig. LATS-9). Continue around the thumb up to the tip (Fig. LATS-10). Pinch the cast to go back through the web space and progress back up forearm. When putting on the first layer of a long-arm spica cast, it is advisable to complete a short arm spica cast first, mold it, and then continue up the arm with the next roll.

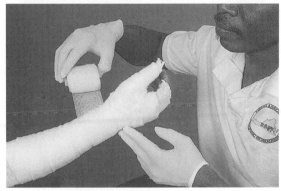

FIGURE LATS-8 Roll casting material around the wrist and thumb.

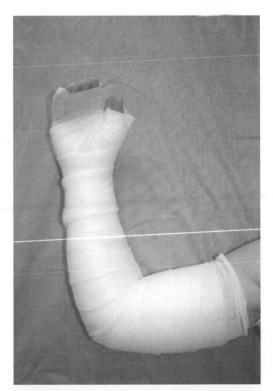

FIGURE LATS-6 Roll padding up to the middle of the biceps.

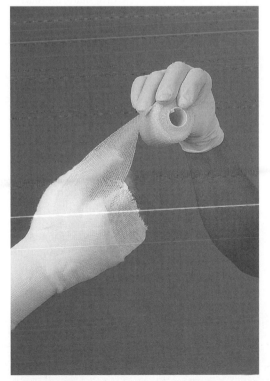

FIGURE LATS-9 Advance casting material over the thumb by using a half twist.

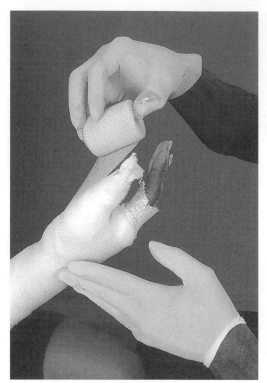

FIGURE LATS-10 Roll casting material around the thumb.

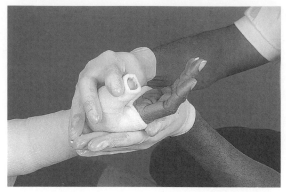

FIGURE LATS-11 Mold the cast so the wrist is in moderate dorsiflexion in hand grip position.

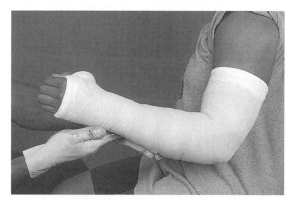

FIGURE LATS-12 Mold the cast around the forearm.

5. After the first layer of casting material has been applied, mold the cast by gripping the patient's hand with your hand while placing your other palm in the dorsal aspect of the patient's wrist to provide for moderate dorsiflexion into a hand grip position (Fig. LATS-11). Mold around the thumb. Mold the forearm area of the cast into an oval around the radius and ulna (Fig. LATS-12). After the second roll has been applied, the cast should be molded around the distal humerus epicondyles and the elbow (Fig. LATS-13).
6. Fold back the ends of the stockinette and place your final layer of cast material, tacking down the stockinette at the ends. For adults, a long-arm cast may require three cast rolls.
7. After finishing the application, check for areas of impingement and make sure the forearm is at 90 degrees and there is no pronation or supination at the wrist.

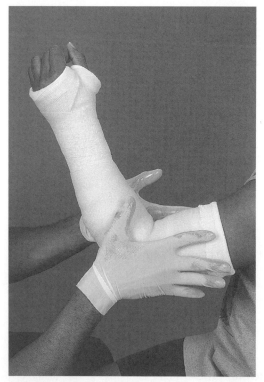

FIGURE LATS-13 Mold the cast around the elbow.

Short-Leg Cast: Non–Weight Bearing (CPT 29405) and Weight Bearing (CPT 29425)

Indications. Malleolar fractures, nondisplaced distal fibula fractures with no involvement of the tibia, and midfoot fractures

Advantages. Allows flexion/extension of the knee

Disadvantages. Allows some rotation of the lower leg below the knee

Materials. 3- or 4-inch cast tape (may need three rolls in an adult), 3- or 4-inch cast padding, 3-inch stockinette

Instructions

Non–Weight Bearing

1. Cut a length of stockinette so it extends from just past the toes up to the knee. Place the foot and ankle in the neutral position with the knee flexed at 90 degrees. Cut a slit across the front of the ankle to eliminate any folds or creases (Fig. SLC-1).
2. Wrap the cast padding on starting at the distal end of the foot and overlapping 50 percent from the metatarsal heads up to two fingers below the fibular head (Fig. SLC-2). Be sure to provide extra padding around the heel and malleoli, the distal metatarsal heads, and the proximal anterior tibia (Fig. SLC-3).

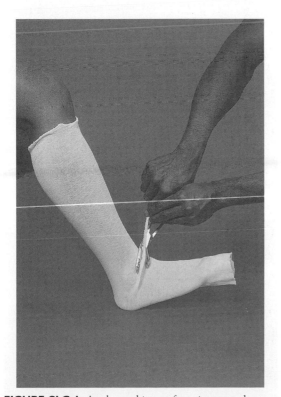

FIGURE SLC-1 Apply stockinette from just past the toes to the knee and cut a slit in front of the ankle.

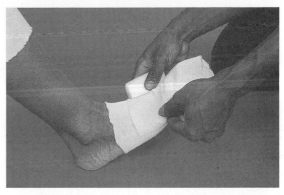

FIGURE SLC-2 Begin application of padding at the distal foot.

3. Dip the cast material in water and roll the material on over the same area covered by the cast padding. Start at the toes, leaving enough room so they are not cramped but coming forward on the plantar surface enough to prevent breakdown of the edge of the cast (Fig. SLC-4). While wrapping, maintain a moderate tension and avoid creases or divots, overlapping by 50% each rotation (Fig. SLC-5).
4. After the first layer is on, roll down the stockinette at the top and over the toes (Fig. SLC-6). The cast should end two finger widths below the tibial tuberosity. Ensure that the foot and ankle remain in proper neutral position and mold an arch under the medial aspect of the foot (Fig. SLC-7), mold around the Achilles tendon and the heel, and mold around the malleoli. Incorporate stockinette at the top of the cast with the next roll. It may take a third roll to create a cast of equal thickness throughout the length of the cast.

Add this Step for a Weight-Bearing Cast

5. If this is to be a walking cast, add four to six additional reinforcing strips of casting material to the bottom of the foot and heel (Fig. SLC-8) and incorporate them with your final roll and mold it to the bottom of the cast (Figs. SLC-9 and SLC-10). Be sure to have the patient wear a cast shoe.

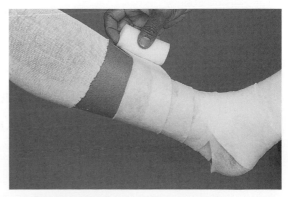

FIGURE SLC-3 Roll padding toward the knee.

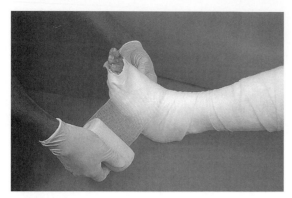

FIGURE SLC-4 Begin application of casting material at the distal foot.

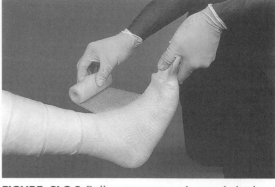

FIGURE SLC-5 Roll casting material toward the knee while maintaining a moderate tension and avoid creases or divots, overlapping by 50% each rotation.

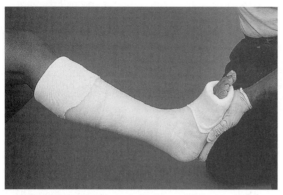

FIGURE SLC-6 Ensure that the ankle is at 90 degrees. Fold down the stockinette at the knee and toes.

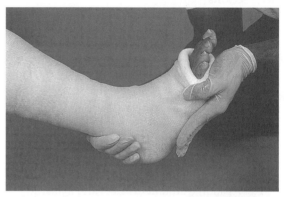

FIGURE SLC-7 Mold an arch on the bottom of the foot.

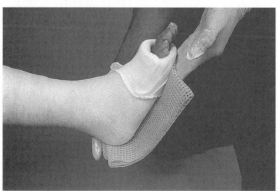

FIGURE SLC-8 Add four to six additional reinforcing strips of casting material to the bottom of the foot and heel.

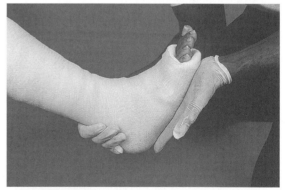

FIGURE SLC-9 Incorporate additional reinforcing strips into the final roll of casting material.

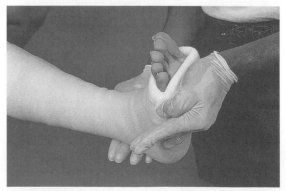

FIGURE SLC-10 Mold the reinforcing strips onto the bottom of the cast.

LONG-LEG CAST CPT 29345,355 OR 365

Indications. Stable fractures of the tibia and fibula, fractures of the patella, stable fractures of the distal shaft of the femur

Advantages. Controls motion at the knee, foot, and ankle

Disadvantages. Bulky and difficult to get around and attend to daily activities and hygiene

Materials. 4-inch stockinette, padding material, cast tape

Instructions

1. Stockinette should reach from just past the toes to the groin. Place the foot and ankle in a neutral position with the knee flexed at 25 to 45 degrees (full extension for patellar fractures). Cut a slit across the front of the ankle to eliminate any folds or creases.
2. Cast padding extends from distal metatarsal heads to four fingers below the groin. Extra padding is needed around the heel and malleoli and over the distal femoral condyles (Fig. LLC-1).
3. Dip the cast material in water and roll on the material over the same area covered by the cast padding. While wrapping, maintain a moderate tension and avoid creases or divots, overlapping by 50% on each rotation (Fig. LLC-2). Mold the layer of the short-leg portion and then complete the upper leg.
4. For the short-leg portion, after the first layer is on, ensure proper neutral position and mold an arch under the medial aspect of the foot, mold around the Achilles tendon and the heel, and mold around the malleoli (Figs. LLC-3 and LLC-4). For the upper leg, mold above the femoral condyles and around the knee (Fig. LLC-5).
5. Fold back the ends of the stockinette and apply one to two more layers. Note: If this to be a walking cast, add four to six additional reinforcing strips to the bottom of the foot and heel and incorporate them with your final roll (Fig. LLC-6). Be sure to have the patient wear a cast shoe.

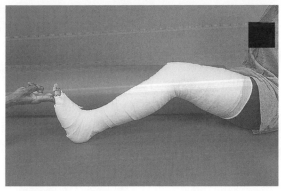

FIGURE LLC-1 Stockinette and padding from just past the toes to the groin.

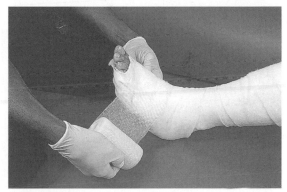

FIGURE LLC-2 Begin application of casting at the foot.

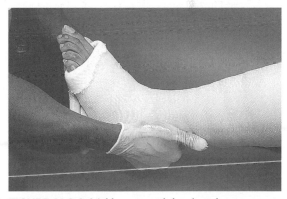

FIGURE LLC-3 Mold casting of the short-leg portion in neutral position before completing the upper leg.

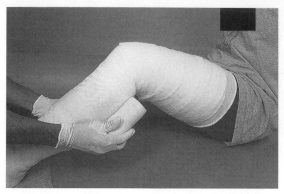

FIGURE LLC-4 Roll casting material toward the groin.

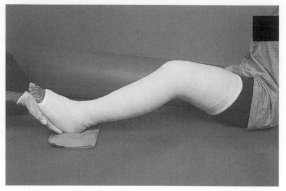

FIGURE LLC-5 Ensure neutral position of the foot after casting is complete.

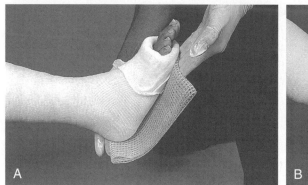

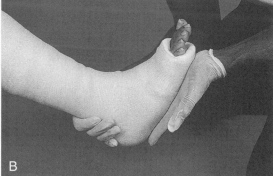

FIGURE LLC-6A, B Add four to six additional reinforcing strips to the bottom of the foot and heel and incorporate them with your final roll.

ULNAR GUTTER SPLINT
CPT 29125

Indications. Fractures of the fourth or fifth metacarpal

Advantages. Can be used in the acute setting and also serves as the definitive immobilization; for metacarpal fractures, quickly applied ulnar gutter splints dipped in cold water allow for fracture reduction in the splint

Materials. 3- or 4-inch fiberglass splint roll, 3-inch elastic wrap, 1-inch cast padding

Instructions

1. Position the hand with the fourth and fifth MCP flexed to 90 degrees (Fig. UG-1) and the wrist at 10 to 15 degrees dorsiflexion (Fig. UG-2).
2. Place a small amount of padding between fourth and fifth finger (Fig. UG-3).
3. Measure from the tip of the fourth finger to within 2 finger breadths of the antecubital fossa (Fig. UG-4).
4. Apply a thin line of water to the fiberglass on the side that will be away from the patient and then pat it dry.
5. Apply the splint with the thickest padded side toward the patient (Fig. UG-5).
6. Wrap with elastic bandage, starting at the fingertips. It is easiest if an assistant can keep the MCP as close to a 90-degree angle as possible, with the wrist at 10 to 15 degrees of dorsiflexion and the PIP at 20 to 30 degrees of flexion and hold the splint in this position until it hardens (Fig. UG-6).
7. Finally, after the splint has hardened, check to see if the initial wrap is too tight and needs to be unwrapped and reapplied before the patient leaves the office.

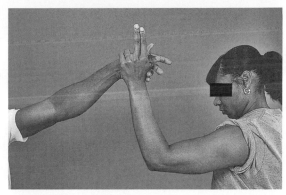
FIGURE UG-1 Position the hand with the fourth and fifth MCPs flexed to 90 degrees.

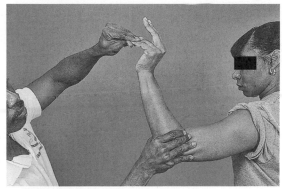
FIGURE UG-2 Position the hand with the MCP flexed and the wrist at 10 to 15 degrees of dorsiflexion.

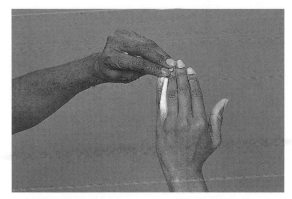
FIGURE UG-3 Place a small amount of padding between fourth and fifth fingers.

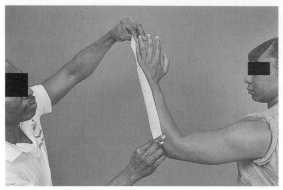

FIGURE UG-4 Measure from the tip of the fourth finger to within 2 finger breadths of the antecubital fossa.

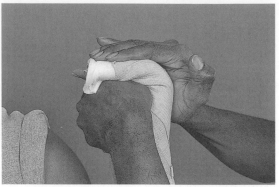

FIGURE UG-6 Wrap with elastic bandage, starting at the fingertips. Keep the MCP as close to a 90-degree angle as possible, with the wrist at 10 to 15 degrees of dorsiflexion and the PIP at 20 to 30 degrees of flexion. Hold the splint in this position until it hardens.

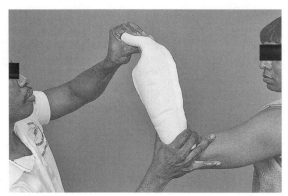

FIGURE UG-5 Place the fiberglass roll padded side to patient along the ulnar side of the hand and forearm.

UPPER EXTREMITY SUGAR TONG SPLINT CPT CODE 29125

Indications. Distal radius or ulna fractures, fractures of the wrist and elbow

Advantages. Limits flexion/extension at the elbow and supination/pronation of the forearm while allowing for edema and providing excellent strength

Disadvantages. Allows some flexion/extension of the elbow and minimal supination/pronation (depending on the quality of application)

Note. Generally used with arm sling

Materials. 3- or 4-inch fiberglass splint roll; 3- or 4-inch elastic wrap

Instructions

1. Unless contraindicated, position the arm at 90 degrees with no supination or pronation of the forearm. The wrist should be slightly dorsiflexed (10-15 degrees) to attain the position of function.
2. Measure splint length using cast padding. For the forearm, the splint should extend from just proximal to the MCP joints on the dorsal surface around the elbow and back down to the distal palmar crease on the volar surface.
3. Put a stream of water on the side of the splint that will not go against the patient and pat out the excess moisture with a paper towel.
4. Place the splint roll from just below the MCP joints on the dorsal surface (Fig. ST-1).
5. Go around the elbow and back down to the distal palmar crease. Fold enough of the splint away from the thumb to allow the thumb to be in a functional position (Fig. ST-2).
6. Apply the elastic wrap starting at the hand and wrap from distal to proximal; use a figure 8 technique to go around the elbow. It is easiest if an assistant holds the splint in place while you wrap on the elastic wrap (Figs. ST-3 and ST-4).

7. After the splint is securely wrapped on, ensure correct positioning of the arm and mold the splint around the elbow, hand, and wrist.
8. After the splint has hardened, check to see if the initial wrap is too tight and needs to be unwrapped and reapplied before the patient leaves the office.

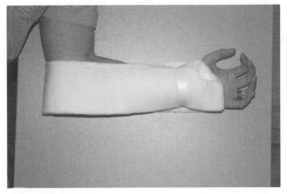

FIGURE ST-2 Go around the elbow and back down to the distal palmar crease. Fold enough of the splint away from the thumb to allow the thumb to be in a functional position.

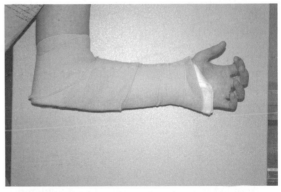

FIGURE ST-3 Dorsal view. Apply the elastic wrap starting at the hand and wrap from distal to proximal and use a figure 8 technique to go around the elbow.

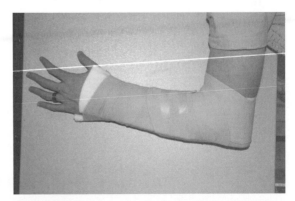

FIGURE ST-4 Volar view. Apply the elastic wrap starting at the hand and wrap from distal to proximal and use a figure 8 technique to go around the elbow. It is easiest if an assistant holds the splint in place while you wrap on the elastic wrap.

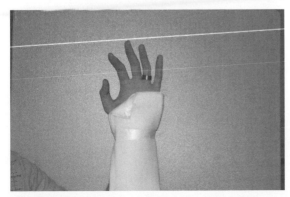

FIGURE ST-1 Place the splint roll from just below the MCP joints on the dorsal surface.

THUMB SPICA SUGAR TONG SPLINT CPT CODE 29105

Indications. "Gamekeeper's thumb" (injury of the ulnar collateral ligament of the thumb), fracture at the base of the first metacarpal, suspected scaphoid fractures

Advantages. Almost complete immobilization of thumb and prevention of supination and pronation

Disadvantages. Can be taken off by the patient

Materials. 2- or 3-inch-wide fiberglass splint roll, 2- or 3-inch elastic wrap

Instructions

1. Unless contraindicated, position the arm at 90 degrees with no supination or pronation of the forearm. The wrist should be slightly dorsiflexed (10-15 degrees) to attain the position of function. Position the forearm with the radial surface up. The thumb should be in a position of function (as if grabbing a pen).
2. Use an elastic wrap to determine the appropriate width for the splint. Place it under the forearm and select the roll that is as wide as the forearm.
3. Measure the splint length to be slightly longer than from the thumb down over the thenar eminence along the volar surface of the forearm and around the elbow to just proximal to the MCP joints on the dorsal surface.
4. When ready to apply the splint, apply a thin stream of water to the side of the material that will be facing away from the patient and pat out the excess moisture with a paper towel.
5. Apply the splint material over the thumb, molded to completely cover its circumference (Fig. TSST-1).
6. Mold the splint down over the thenar eminence of the hand (Fig. TSST-2).
7. Continue down the forearm on the volar surface and go around the elbow and place the splint roll just below the MCP joints on the dorsal surface (Fig. TSST-3).

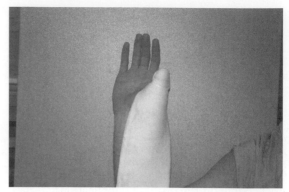

FIGURE TSST-1 Apply the splinting material over the thumb, molded to completely cover its circumference.

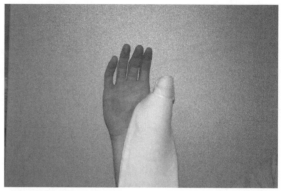

FIGURE TSST-2 Mold the splint down over the thenar eminence of the hand.

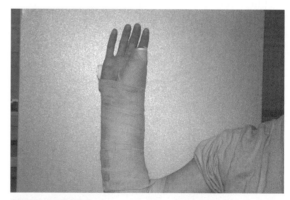

FIGURE TSST-3 Continue down the forearm on the volar surface and go around the elbow and place the splint roll just below the MCP joints on the dorsal surface.

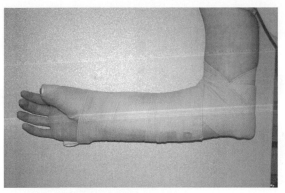

FIGURE TSST-4 Volar view.

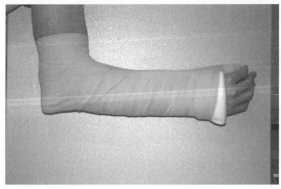

FIGURE TSST-5 Dorsal view. Apply the elastic wrap starting at the thumb and wrap from distal to proximal. Use a figure 8 technique to go around the elbow.

8. Apply the elastic wrap starting at the thumb and wrap from distal to proximal and use a figure 8 technique to go around the elbow. It is easiest if an assistant holds the splint in place while you wrap on the elastic wrap (Figs. TSST-4 and TSST-5).
9. After the splint is securely wrapped on, ensure correct positioning of the arm and mold the splint around the elbow, wrist, and thumb. This is especially important at the thumb, but it should be in a "pen grasp" position. Also avoid leaving impressions or "divots" in the splint from fingertip pressure.
10. After the splint has hardened, check to see if the initial wrap is too tight and needs to be unwrapped and reapplied before the patient leaves the office.

LOWER EXTREMITY SPLINT (THREE-SIDED IMMOBILIZATION) CPT 29505

Indications. Distal fibula fractures and tibial avulsion fractures, ankle fractures awaiting surgery, significant trauma to the ankle without immediate access to radiographs

Advantages. Allows for swelling; durable

Materials. 3- and 4-inch fiberglass splint roll (that can be opened on one side); one or two 6-inch elastic wraps; 3-inch stockinette and 3-inch cast padding

Instructions

1. The posterior component of the lower extremity splint should be measured from a point 3 finger breadths below the fibular head to 2 finger breadths beyond the great toe (Fig. LE-1).The sugar tong portion of the device, which provides support on the medial and lateral sides of the leg, should be measured from 3 finger breadths below the fibular head to down around the foot and back up to a position exactly across from the lateral aspect (Fig. LE-2).
2. Stockinette can be used and measured from the back of the knee to below the toes and pulled on (Fig. LE-3).
3. Apply cast padding at least from the mid arch and use either a figure 8 technique or successive strips of cast padding (Fig. LE-4). Provide a gentle but consistent amount of pressure to minimize edema formation. Pay careful attention to providing material underneath one or both malleoli, depending on the extent of the injury.

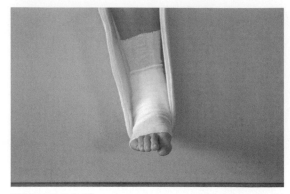

FIGURE LE-2 The sugar tong portion of the device should be measured from 3 finger breadths below the fibular head to down around the foot and back up to a position exactly across from the lateral aspect.

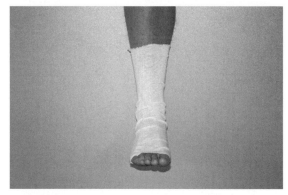

FIGURE LE-3 Apply stockinette from the back of the knee to below the toes.

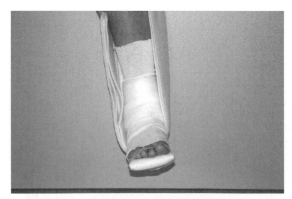

FIGURE LE-1 Measure the splint material for the posterior component from below the fibular head to beyond the great toe.

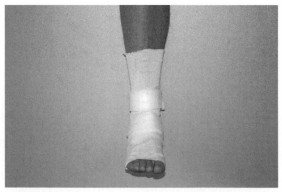

FIGURE LE-4 Apply cast padding around the malleoli and over the dorsum of the foot.

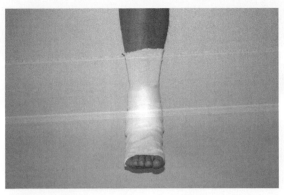

FIGURE LE-5 Apply additional padding up the lateral third of the leg in front of the fibula and in the spaces around the Achilles tendon.

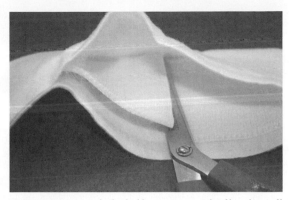

FIGURE LE-6 Mark the halfway point on the fiberglass roll of sugar tong component; open the fiberglass roll and only cut the fiberglass at the halfway point.

4. Always extend the padding over the dorsolateral portion of the foot. If appropriate, additional padding can be applied up the lateral third of the leg in front of the fibula and in the spaces around the Achilles tendon (Fig. LE-5).
5. Take the fiberglass roll that will be used as the sugar tong component and mark a point on the fiberglass exactly halfway. Open up the tape side of the roll of fiberglass and place a clean cut with scissors through the fiberglass, being careful not to affect the padding (Fig. LE-6).
6. Reclose the roll with its two-sided tape. Grab each end of the roll and pull the ends apart briskly, which allows a space wide enough for the foot and posterior splint to fit underneath (Fig. LE-7).
7. Place a stream of water on the side opposite from the application to the patent. Never use water warmer than room temperature to avoid burning the patient. Blot with a towel or other appropriate material.
8. Position sugar tong component from at least 3 finger breadths below fibular head down around the foot and back up to the same height on the medial side. The foot should fit into the gap created by pulling the ends apart. Have the patient or an assistant hold it in place (Fig. LE-8). Grasp the posterior component of the splint. Apply from the area 3 finger breadths below the fibular head and construct a toe plate at the distal end. Again with the use of the assistant, keep this in place (Fig. LE-9).
9. Take the 6-inch elastic wrap and apply from distal to proximal with a gentle amount of pressure. Start from the medial side of the foot. Overlap the wrap each successive time around the leg by 50% (Figs. LE-10 and LE-11). Be

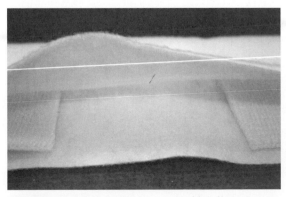

FIGURE LE-7 Pull the ends apart briskly, allowing space for foot and posterior splint.

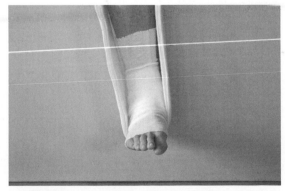

FIGURE LE-8 Position the sugar tong component of the three-way splint with the foot in the gap created by pulling the ends apart.

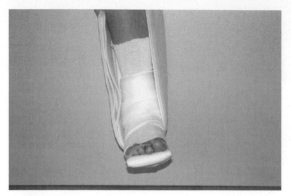

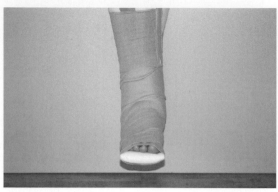

FIGURE LE-9 Position posterior component of three-way splint from the same point on the calf as the sugar tong starts from to the tip of the toes folding an end piece down as a toe plate.

FIGURE LE-10 Frontal view: elastic wrap from distal to proximal applied from the medial aspect of the foot and around the ankle.

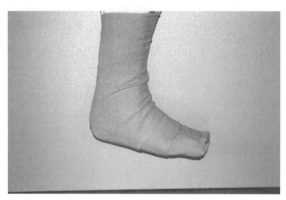

FIGURE LE-11 Lateral view: elastic wrap from distal to proximal applied from the medial aspect of the foot and around the ankle.

careful when applying the elastic wrap around the ankle so that the three sides of the splint are rounded into shape around the tibia and fibula. If necessary, use a second elastic wrap and overlap by one full length below the last roll of the first application.

10. Be certain to maintain the patient's ankle at 90 degrees without any pronation or supination of the foot.

11. Using the palm of the hand, mold an arch into the posterior component. Mold around the malleoli and over the cast padding. Use the palms of the hands to mold around the Achilles tendon.

index

Page numbers followed by "f" indicate figures, "t" indicate tables, and "b" indicate boxes.